Tumors of the Soft Tissues

Atlas
of
Tumor Pathology

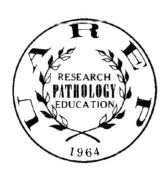

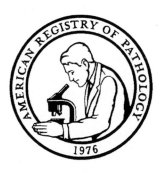

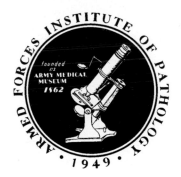

ATLAS OF TUMOR PATHOLOGY

Third Series
Fascicle 30

TUMORS OF THE SOFT TISSUES

by

Richard L. Kempson, M.D.
Professor of Pathology; Co-Director, Surgical Pathology
Stanford University Medical Center
Stanford, California

Christopher D. M. Fletcher, M.D., FRCPath
Professor of Pathology, Harvard Medical School
Director of Surgical Pathology, Brigham and Women's Hospital
Boston, Massachusetts

Harry L. Evans, M.D.
Professor of Pathology
The University of Texas MD Anderson Cancer Center
Houston, Texas

Michael R. Hendrickson, M.D.
Professor of Pathology, Co-Director, Surgical Pathology
Stanford University Medical Center
Stanford, California

Richard K. Sibley, M.D.
Professor of Pathology; Co-Director, Surgical Pathology
Stanford University Medical Center
Stanford, California

Published by the
ARMED FORCES INSTITUTE OF PATHOLOGY
Washington, D.C.

Under the Auspices of
UNIVERSITIES ASSOCIATED FOR RESEARCH AND EDUCATION IN PATHOLOGY, INC.
Bethesda, Maryland
2001

Accepted for Publication
1998

Available from the American Registry of Pathology
Armed Forces Institute of Pathology
Washington, D.C. 20306-6000
www.afip.org
ISSN 0160-6344
ISBN 1-881041-60-3

ATLAS OF TUMOR PATHOLOGY

EDITOR
JUAN ROSAI, M.D.

Department of Pathology
Memorial Sloan-Kettering Cancer Center
New York, New York 10021-6007

ASSOCIATE EDITOR
LESLIE H. SOBIN, M.D.

Armed Forces Institute of Pathology
Washington, D.C. 20306-6000

EDITORIAL ADVISORY BOARD

EDITORS' NOTE

The Atlas of Tumor Pathology has a long and distinguished history. It was first conceived at a Cancer Research Meeting held in St. Louis in September 1947 as an attempt to standardize the nomenclature of neoplastic diseases. The first series was sponsored by the National Academy of Sciences-National Research Council. The organization of this Sisyphean effort was entrusted to the Subcommittee on Oncology of the Committee on Pathology, and Dr. Arthur Purdy Stout was the first editor-in-chief. Many of the illustrations were provided by the Medical Illustration Service of the Armed Forces Institute of Pathology, the type was set by the Government Printing Office, and the final printing was done at the Armed Forces Institute of Pathology (hence the colloquial appellation "AFIP Fascicles"). The American Registry of Pathology purchased the Fascicles from the Government Printing Office and sold them virtually at cost. Over a period of 20 years, approximately 15,000 copies each of nearly 40 Fascicles were produced. The worldwide impact that these publications have had over the years has largely surpassed the original goal. They quickly became among the most influential publications on tumor pathology ever written, primarily because of their overall high quality but also because their low cost made them easily accessible to pathologists and other students of oncology the world over.

Upon completion of the first series, the National Academy of Sciences-National Research Council handed further pursuit of the project over to the newly created Universities Associated for Research and Education in Pathology (UAREP). A second series was started, generously supported by grants from the AFIP, the National Cancer Institute, and the American Cancer Society. Dr. Harlan I. Firminger became the editor-in-chief and was succeeded by Dr. William H. Hartmann. The second series Fascicles were produced as bound volumes instead of loose leaflets. They featured a more comprehensive coverage of the subjects, to the extent that the Fascicles could no longer be regarded as "atlases" but rather as monographs describing and illustrating in detail the tumors and tumor-like conditions of the various organs and systems.

Once the second series was completed, with a success that matched that of the first, UAREP and AFIP decided to embark on a third series. A new editor-in-chief and an associate editor were selected, and a distinguished editorial board was appointed. The mandate for the third series remains the same as for the previous ones, i.e., to oversee the production of an eminently practical publication with surgical pathologists as its primary audience, but also aimed at other workers in oncology. The main purposes of this series are to promote a consistent, unified, and biologically sound nomenclature; to guide the surgical pathologist in the diagnosis of the various tumors and tumor-like lesions; and to provide relevant histogenetic, pathogenetic, and clinicopathologic information on these entities. Just as the second series included data obtained from ultrastructural (and, in the more recent Fascicles, immunohistochemical) examination, the third series will, in addition, incorporate pertinent information obtained with the newer molecular biology techniques. As in the past, a continuous attempt will be made to correlate, whenever possible, the nomenclature used in the Fascicles with that proposed by the World Health Organization's International Histological Classification of Tumors. The format of the third series has been changed in order to incorporate additional items and to ensure a consistency of style throughout. Close cooperation between the various authors and their respective liaisons from the editorial board will be emphasized to minimize unnecessary repetition and discrepancies in the text and illustrations.

To its everlasting credit, the participation and commitment of the AFIP to this venture is even more substantial and encompassing than in previous series. It now extends to virtually all scientific, technical, and financial aspects of the production.

The task confronting the organizations and individuals involved in the third series is even more daunting than in the preceding efforts because of the ever-increasing complexity of the matter at hand. It is hoped that this combined effort—of which, needless to say, that represented by the authors is first and foremost—will result in a series worthy of its two illustrious predecessors and will be a suitable introduction to the tumor pathology of the twenty-first century.

Juan Rosai, M.D.
Leslie H. Sobin, M.D.

ACKNOWLEDGMENTS

The authors wish to express their appreciation to the residents and fellows who have trained in our departments through the years. It is their insistence on precise definitions and practical differential diagnoses that has been a prime motive for us to write a book that focuses on these issues. Our debt to the many pathologists who have shared their cases with us is enormous. Consultation cases are not only the source of many of the illustrations in most surgical pathology books, they allow investigators to study the clinical biology of rare and unusual lesions. Without consultation cases, progress in surgical pathology would be significantly impeded.

We would like to acknowledge Siloo B. Kapadia, M.D., for allowing us to review her collection of fetal rhabdomyomas.

It fell to Kristen Jensen to do much of the typing of the seemingly endless revisions. This she did with consummate skill and good grace while providing useful editorial suggestions. We are most grateful. Following the completion of the text, Ms. Jensen entered medical school, whether because of, or in spite of, this Fascicle is not clear.

Finally, but certainly not least, we wish to thank our colleagues and chairpersons for providing an environment conducive to clinical research and scholarship. The production of a book such as this can only be accomplished in this setting.

Richard L. Kempson, M.D.
Christopher D. M. Fletcher, M.D., FRCPath
Harry L. Evans, M.D.
Michael R. Hendrickson, M.D.
Richard K. Sibley, M.D.

Table of Contents

TUMORS OF THE SOFT TISSUES

1
INTRODUCTION

CLASSIFICATION

The large number of soft tissue tumor types, the relative rarity of most of these, and the often subtle histologic differences between them may produce anxious moments for the pathologist faced with an unfamiliar soft tissue tumor. However, a knowledge of the primary conventions of the classification system, an understanding of which histopathologic diagnostic decisions are important and which are not, and an organized approach to the interpretation of the myriad histologic patterns found in soft tissue tumors will go a long way toward reducing this anxiety and increasing diagnostic accuracy.

In this chapter, we first distinguish between two complementary purposes of oncologic classification: scientific (or explanatory) and clinical managerial. With this background we then focus on the scientific classification of soft tissue tumors, point out some of the important definitions and conventions that are used to place tumors in the major categories of this classification, and suggest that, when possible, locating a soft tissue tumor in the scientific classification is a useful first step in its evaluation. We then emphasize the importance of formulating a clinical managerial classification that in a therapeutically useful way elaborates the definitions of the terms "benign," "intermediate" (or "borderline"), and "malignant" as they apply to soft tissue tumors. Because grading is thought by many to provide further insight into the aggressive potential of adult sarcomas, we outline some of the higher profile grading schemes. Next, we explore the morphologic features that we think are helpful in distinguishing clinically benign lesions (including both benign neoplastic and reactive lesions) from those with aggressive potential. This is followed by a discussion of more mundane but extremely important practical matters including the clinical information that is essential in arriving at a clinicopathologic diagnosis, the utility of the various biopsy procedures currently available, and the handling of resection specimens and reporting the results of their examination. Last, we describe a step-by-step systematic approach to the microscopic evaluation of neoplasms encountered in the soft tissues which we find useful, particularly when faced with difficult cases.

The Purposes of Classification

Human neoplasms are classified for two very different purposes: one scientific, the other managerial (21). Briefly, purely scientific classification schemes, at the most primitive level, group tumors on the basis of perceived shared morphologic features when viewed with conventional light microscopy. In recent years, this characterization has been supplemented by ultrastructural, immunophenotypic, and cytogenetic features. This initial separation is typically supplemented by a further stratification within each differentiated group into morphologically benign and morphologically malignant. As discussed below, this may or may not correlate with clinical behavior. Scientific classifications tend to be relatively elaborate and provide a suitable taxonomic scaffolding to support investigations into the etiology, pathogenesis, and epidemiology of the neoplasms being classified. They also provide an "in-house" vocabulary for pathologists to discuss differential diagnostic problems. As discussed below, the current scientific classification of soft tissue neoplasms is based upon presumed histogenesis (in reality, it is based upon cellular differentiation).

Purely managerial classifications, in contrast, capture only those aspects of neoplasms that bear on the clinical course of patients who harbor them. Their primary focus is on prognosis and treatment and the number of categories in the classification tends to be much more limited than those of scientific classifications. This simplification reflects the lamentable fact that the medical community is better at coming up with scientific distinctions than developing treatments. The traditional managerial distinction has been into "(clinically) benign" and "(clinically) malignant." In recent years this dichotomous classification has been expanded into a number of other clinically relevant categories.

The existing classification schemes for soft tissue proliferations such as that of the World Health Organization (WHO) are chimeric in that their primary scientific stratification is in terms of differentiated features, but engrafted on this is a secondary classification within most differentiated types which places the tumors into benign, intermediate, and malignant groups (40,41). Thus, classifications such as the WHO attempt to serve both masters—scientific investigators and clinicians—but in doing so meet with limited success. These chimeric classifications are faulted on occasion by the scientists for not including enough scientific detail and at the same time by the clinicians for being unwieldy and overly complicated for clinical management purposes. Moreover, these mixed classifications have difficulty with neoplasms that *look* malignant morphologically such as leiomyosarcoma of the skin and infantile fibrosarcoma but *behave* in a clinically benign fashion under current therapies. In some scientific sense it may be useful to regard these as malignant; in a managerial sense, they should be treated as benign neoplasms despite their alarming microscopic appearance. Also difficult to place in such chimeric classifications are tumors that are histologically bland but that can recur aggressively such as the bland smooth muscle tumors of the retroperitoneum, and those that are bland and recur but do not metastasize unless recurrences are morphologically malignant such as atypical lipomatous tumors (well-differentiated liposarcoma).

Scientific Classification

Since the 19th century, scientific tumor classification has been shaped by the now-familiar approach of trying to establish the histogenesis ("cell of origin") of a tumor and fashioning a classification scheme (and associated set of labels) that reflect the various possible pedigrees. Operationally, of course, this really amounts to characterizing as completely as possible (using available technology) the phenotype of the constituent cells of the neoplasm and with this information in hand, turning to a stock of normal cell phenotypes and searching for a good match. If a successful match is identified, two things occur: first, the histogenetic inference is that the normal cell gave rise to the class of neoplasms under study, and second, a label is concocted that reflects these beliefs about differentiation and histogenesis. It is important to emphasize that this talk of "histogenesis" is largely talk about phenotypes; the "it looks like therefore it came from" part is an inference. In reality, the scientific classification of soft tissue neoplasms is based whenever possible on the phenotype of the tumor cells (1).

Many subsets of soft tissue proliferations exhibit specific cytoplasmic differentiation (e.g., cytoplasm containing filaments arranged as cross striations or cytoplasmic lipid vacuoles) or distinctive extracellular matrix material from which the phenotype of the associated cells can be inferred (e.g., bone, cartilage). Thus, the assignment of a tumor to the fatty, muscular, cartilaginous, or osseous group requires, with some exceptions, evidence of cellular differentiation along each of these lines by at least some of the neoplastic cells. Unfortunately, the current taxonomies seldom specify the minimum number of differentiated cells required. When tumors are composed of cells that do not possess features that provide either direct or indirect evidence of some normal mesenchymal phenotype, their classification may be based upon the presence of a distinctive architectural arrangement of the constituent cells that resembles normal tissues (e.g., vessel formation by the cells composing vascular tumors, some neural tumors). When neither the appearance of the tumor cells nor their arrangement provide clues to their direction of differentiation, tumors may be named on the basis of a distinctive microscopic appearance for which there is no normal counterpart (e.g., alveolar soft part sarcoma, small cell desmoplastic tumor, epithelioid sarcoma). A few neoplasms whose direction of differentiation was not apparent when the tumor was first described are labeled with a physician's name (e.g., Bednar's tumor, Ewing's sarcoma). The major phenotypic categories that comprise the scientific soft tissue classification are presented in Table 1-1, which also contains a miscellaneous category for those tumors composed of cells whose direction of differentiation is

Table 1-1
MAJOR CATEGORIES IN THE SCIENTIFIC CLASSIFICATION OF SOFT TISSUE TUMORS*

I	Fibrous and myofibroblastic tumors
II	Tumors included in the fibrohistiocytic category
III	Lipomatous tumors
IV	Smooth muscle tumors
V	Skeletal muscle tumors
VI	Vascular tumors
VII	Perivascular tumors
VIII	Synovial tumors
IX	Neural tumors (see the Fascicle, Tumors of the Peripheral Nervous System)
X	Extraskeletal osseous and cartilaginous tumors
XI	Miscellaneous tumors**
XII	Unclassified†

*The individual lesions that compose each of these major categories are specified in a table in the chapter that pertains to the category.
**Included in this category are tumors whose direction of differentiation is uncertain but whose pattern is distinctive as well as those whose differentiation is nonmesenchymal such as epithelioid sarcoma and clear cell sarcoma.
†See discussion of undifferentiated (unclassified) soft tissue neoplasms in the text.

uncertain or nonmesenchymal, i.e., epithelial or melanocytic. Histochemistry, electron microscopy, immunohistochemistry, and cytogenetic or molecular techniques may be utilized to detect differentiation not apparent by conventional light microscopy (16).

The customary first step when confronted with a soft tissue proliferation is to search for distinctive phenotypic features that allow placement within one of the major phenotypic groups in the scientific classification listed in Table 1-1. A default group, unclassified tumor, should be used infrequently; strategies for further characterizing this group are detailed in the Managerial Classification section below. When placing soft tissue neoplasms in one or another named group it is, of course, important that pathologists use the same definitions for the different categories of cellular differentiation, and that they be aware of the conventions that modify these def-

initions. While some of these definitions and conventions are well known, others are underspecified in the literature. Brief definitions of the main types of soft tissue tumors are presented here and in more detail in the chapters concerning each of the tumor types.

Fibrous, Myofibroblastic, and Fibrohistiocytic Tumors. The phenotypic differences exploited by soft tissue tumor taxonomists in their classificatory efforts must appear relatively subtle to their colleagues who labor in other parts of the oncologic vineyard because in their more bland forms many soft tissue proliferations are composed of otherwise undistinguished spindled cells arranged in nonspecific bundles within varying amounts of fibrous-appearing connective tissue or myxoid matrix, while many sarcomas strike the newcomer to the field as undifferentiated collections of pleomorphic anaplastic spindled and rounded cells again embedded in varying amounts of collagen or myxoid matrix. Soft tissue pathologists have handled this problem by relegating tumors with these relatively nondescript mesenchymal features to the fibrous, myofibroblastic, and fibrohistiocytic tumor groups. The taxonomic boundaries that subdivide this collection have shifted over the years so it is important to be aware of the current rules and conventions that apply to these groups. These are presented in the Introduction to the chapter on fibrous and myofibroblastic tumors as well as in the chapter on the fibrohistiocytic tumors.

Lipomatous Tumors. Fatty differentiation is relatively straightforward. It requires that at least some of the constituent tumor cells contain single or multiple clear cytoplasmic vacuoles that distort or deform the nucleus, which then may be pushed to one side of the cell by the vacuole(s); i.e., at least some tumor cells must be differentiated as lipocytes or lipoblasts. The cytoplasmic vacuoles must not contain stainable material other than lipid. Brown fat, characterized by round cells with granular eosinophilic cytoplasm between multiple clear fat vacuoles and a central nucleus, can also be seen in some lipidic tumors such as hibernoma. Lipoblasts differ from lipocytes by a larger and often more coarsely grainy nucleus and the frequent presence of multiple cytoplasmic vacuoles. Exceptions to this rule that tumors in the lipidic category must be composed at least in part of cells differentiated as fat cells should be rare and mainly involve tumors that are otherwise typical myxoid liposarcomas (e.g., possess arborizing vasculature and extensive myxoid lakes that produce a pulmonary edema pattern, etc.) but lack demonstrable lipoblasts after a reasonable number of sections have been examined. Tumors that are composed at least in part of lipidic cells are then subclassified within the fatty tumor category based on the type of lipidic cells, the type of nonlipidic cells, and the architectural arrangements and cytologic features of these cells, e.g., lipoma, myxoid liposarcoma, atypical lipomatous tumor, etc.

Muscle Tumors. The definition of tumor muscle differentiation is variable. For an adult sarcoma to be placed in the skeletal muscle category, there must be cross-striations identified in at least some tumor cells by light microscopy (a rare to nonexistent occurrence), ultrastructural evidence of skeletal muscle differentiation (e.g., thick and thin myofilaments), or immunologic support for muscle differentiation coupled with an appropriate histologic pattern for a skeletal muscle tumor. Desmin expression by tumor cells is supportive of skeletal muscle differentiation but is not usually considered to be diagnostic; however, desmin staining plus staining with myoglobin, fast myosin, or myoD1 is considered by many observers as solid evidence of muscle differentiation. Childhood rhabdomyosarcomas are identified by location, histologic pattern, and immunohistochemical staining; cells with cross-striations are not required for the diagnosis although some tumors contain them (hence their classification as rhabdomyosarcomas). Essentially all childhood rhabdomyosarcomas contain desmin-positive cells, a feature that should be used in their identification. Serious consideration should be given to other diagnostic possibilities if the cells in a putative childhood rhabdomyosarcoma are desmin negative.

What counts as evidence of smooth muscle differentiation is somewhat imprecise but essentially requires cells that "look like" smooth muscle cells arranged, at least focally, in bundles. Because neoplastic smooth muscle cells can lose some of their normal smooth muscle features and come to resemble myofibroblasts, the dividing line between a myofibroblastic tumor and a smooth muscle one is not always crisp. Consequently, one pathologist's smooth muscle tumor may be

another's myofibroblastic proliferation. Fortunately, there is usually very little at stake managerially when the question is smooth muscle versus a myofibroblastic or fibroblastic tumor. The important parameter is the malignant potential which is usually a matter of assessing the tumor's cytologic features, size, and anatomic location (skin versus superficial soft tissue versus deep soft tissue). The latter is important because bland smooth muscle and myofibroblastic tumors in some parts of the soft tissues can recur while those with an alarming appearance that are superficially situated are often clinically benign after excision. The role of desmin in the definition of smooth muscle differentiation has not been resolved to everyone's satisfaction, but most pathologists consider desmin expression to be supportive of smooth muscle differentiation if the cells and their arrangement are otherwise characteristic. Almost all smooth muscle cells also express an antigen recognized by smooth muscle actin antibodies, but this is less specific than desmin because fibroblasts and myofibroblasts are commonly smooth muscle actin positive and much less frequently desmin positive.

Vascular Tumors. Vascular differentiation basically requires vessel formation by tumor cells but slit-like spaces and intracellular "lumens" also count. Reactivity with immunohistochemical endothelial markers currently is considered supportive of vascular differentiation and diagnostic as long as the histologic features are those of a defined vascular tumor. CD31 is the most sensitive endothelial marker and for this reason we think it is the antibody of choice to identify vascular differentiation (10). Factor VIII is as specific as CD31, but less sensitive and CD34 is less specific than either.

Neural Tumors (see also Fascicle, Tumors of the Peripheral Nervous System [35a]). Benign nerve sheath tumors are recognized on the basis of their nuclear features, their stroma, and the arrangement of the tumor cells. Tumor cell reactivity for S-100 protein is, for all practical purposes, definitional for neurofibroma, schwannoma, and other benign neural tumors except for perineurioma which is S-100 protein negative and epithelial membrane antigen positive. Therefore, benign neoplasms which meet the histologic and cytologic definitions of neurofibroma or schwannoma are placed in the neural category and S-100 protein stains can be used when there is diagnostic uncertainty. Malignant peripheral nerve sheath tumors (MPNSTs) can have a variety of different histologic patterns varying from nerve sheath-like to those that resemble pleomorphic malignant fibrous histiocytoma (MFH) or fibrosarcoma, but definitionally they also must meet one or more of the following requirements: 1) arise from a nerve, 2) arise from a neurofibroma, 3) develop in a patient with neurofibromatosis, or 4) have ultrastructural features of neural differentiation. S-100 protein expression is supportive and present in about 50 percent of otherwise typical MPNSTs.

Extraskeletal Osseous and Cartilaginous Tumors. As is well known, a necessary condition for the assignment of a soft tissue neoplasm to the osseous or cartilaginous category is that at least some tumor cells produce bone or cartilage ("tumor bone/cartilage"). Confusingly, tumor bone and/or cartilage formation is not a sufficient condition; several lesions classified as other than bony, such as giant cell sarcoma and ossifying fasciitis, are allowed to contain cells that produce bone or cartilage. These exceptions to the classificatory rule for bony and cartilaginous tumors have no obvious rational explanation and simply represent taxonomic conventions promoted by investigators who, when classifying tumors possessing small amounts of tumor bone, chose to focus on the non-bone forming cells. In contrast to tumor bone, metaplastic bone is allowed in tumors in all categories. Distinguishing between tumor bone and metaplastic bone is not always possible but the latter is usually focal, located at the periphery of the tumor, and elaborated by bland cells.

Synovial and Perivascular Tumors. Some soft tissue tumors do not sit comfortably in the current WHO classification. Presumably for historical reasons, the WHO classification places synovial sarcoma in a synovial tumor category, although there is no evidence that the tumor cells in synovial sarcoma are differentiating as synovial cells. In fact, the current evidence indicates the epithelioid cells are indeed epithelial (2,29). Consequently, we have moved synovial sarcoma to the miscellaneous category. Hemangiopericytomas are in a similarly uncomfortable position in the perivascular category. There is

little evidence that the constituent cells are differentiating as pericytes; rather they appear to be primitive mesenchymal cells which often express CD34 (38). Because the direction of differentiation of the constituent cells in hemangiopericytoma is not clear we have left it in the pericytic category.

Mesenchymoma. This term has been used by some for both benign and malignant tumors whose constituent cells demonstrate more than one line of differentiation. Unfortunately, there are enough such tumors that the terms benign and malignant mesenchymoma have lost specificity. Consequently we do not use them, and tumors will not be described with this label in this Fascicle. For some such tumors the multiple lines of differentiation are expressed in the label, e.g., angiomyolipoma, or the label, while not expressing the lines of differentiation, applies to only one neoplasm, e.g., Triton tumor. For the remainder, either of two equally acceptable courses can be taken: 1) classify the tumor on the basis of the predominant pattern of differentiation and mention the other, e.g., leiomyosarcoma with cartilaginous metaplasia (or with chondrosarcoma), or 2) label the tumor as a mixed mesenchymal neoplasm and specify the lines of differentiation that are present, e.g., mixed leiomyosarcoma and chondrosarcoma. Whatever labels are used, these are rare neoplasms and their expected behavior should be described in the comment section of the pathology report.

Immunocytochemistry and Ultrastructure in Establishing Phenotype. When the direction of differentiation of the cells in a soft tissue tumor is not apparent on the basis of hematoxylin and eosin (H&E)-stained sections and the pattern is not recognizable, immunohistochemistry may be helpful. Commonly available antibodies useful in the diagnosis of soft tissue tumors are presented in Table 1-2 (5). However, there is considerable overlap in the expression of antigens by the cells of different types of soft tissue tumors and this fact emphasizes the primary importance of morphologic features in diagnosis. Actin and desmin are both expressed by normal muscle cells, and actin is often expressed by fibroblasts and myofibroblasts. Much less frequently, desmin can be expressed by fibroblasts and myofibroblasts. Consequently, antibodies against these antigens are

Table 1-2

USEFUL ANTIBODIES IN THE DIAGNOSIS OF SOFT TISSUE SARCOMAS*[†]

Tumor	Main Markers	Other Markers
Leiomyosarcoma	90% SMA+; 90% muscle actin+; 75% desmin+	30% cytokeratin+ Occasional cases S-100 and CD34+
Biphasic synovial sarcoma	>95% EMA+; 95-100% cytokeratin+	Rare cases S-100+; 60-70% CD99+
Monophasic synovial sarcoma	50% cytokeratin or EMA+	Same
Malignant peripheral nerve sheath tumor	50% S-100+	Leu-7; very rare cases cytokeratin and muscle actin+
Childhood rhabdomyosarcoma	95% desmin+; 90% muscle actin+; 30-40% myoglobin+	Rare cases can be cytokeratin, neurofilament, NSE, or S-100+
Ewing's sarcoma/PPNET[‡]	>95% CD99+	Synaptophysin, S-100, neurofilament Occasional cases cytokeratin+
Angiosarcoma	90% CD31+; 80% CD34+	Epithelioid angiosarcomas often cytokeratin and EMA+
Epithelioid sarcoma	>90% EMA and cytokeratin+	50% CD34+
Clear cell sarcoma	80% S-100 and HMB45+	

*Modified from reference 5.
[†]Vimentin is positive in most of these lesions and has no discriminant value. See also Table 1-3 for CD34-positive tumors.
[‡]PPNET = Peripheral primitive neuroectodermal tumor.

Table 1-3

SOFT TISSUE TUMORS AND CD34 EXPRESSION*

Tumor	Approximate % of Tumors that Stain
Dermatofibrosarcoma protuberans (DFSP)	95
Solitary fibrous tumor	90
Spindle cell lipoma	95
Nerve sheath tumor	Common
Hemangiopericytoma	50
Epithelioid sarcoma	50
GI stromal tumor	85
Smooth muscle tumor	30
Angiosarcoma	60
Epithelioid angiosarcoma	80
Other soft tissue tumors	Rare
Carcinoma	Very rare
Melanoma	Very rare
Lymphoma	Lymphoblastic only

*Table data from reference 38.

often useful in the diagnosis of spindled soft tissue tumors. S-100 protein is expressed by the cells of many neural tumors and in fact its expression is definitional for neurofibroma and schwannoma. Of course, S-100 protein is also expressed by the cells of other soft tissue tumors. CD34 is expressed by a number of soft tissue tumors but it practically never stains melanoma, carcinoma, or the fibrous histiocytomas (see Table 1-3) (38). Because of what it does and does not stain and because CD34 is the only positive marker for some soft tissue tumors, it has rapidly become a widely used antibody in soft tissue tumor diagnosis. CD31 is an endothelial cell marker that has largely replaced factor VIII and ULEX (*Ulex europeaus*) (10). The ubiquity of vimentin expression, particularly in soft tissue neoplasms, greatly limits its usefulness except to determine whether lesional cells are immunoreactive; we seldom employ it.

An equally or even more important use of immunohistochemistry is to assist in excluding metastasis and lymphoma. We think a panel composed of antibodies against keratin, S-100 protein, and common leukocyte antigen should be applied whenever metastasis or lymphoma is a possibility in the differential diagnosis. Keratin can be expressed by primary soft tissue tumors, S-100 protein is expressed by several types of mesenchymal tumor cells including cartilaginous and fat cells, and not all lymphoma cells express common leukocyte antigen. As a result, this basic panel should be expanded to include multiple keratin stains, epithelial membrane antigen, and B- and T-cell markers whenever indicated and the results must always be interpreted in conjunction with the H&E morphology.

With the advent of immunohistochemistry, a subset of soft tissue tumors has emerged whose members are not only composed of cells with epithelioid cytomorphology but also express cytokeratin, i.e., they have an epithelial phenotype. Such tumors and their epithelioid counterparts that do not contain keratin-positive cells raise the important differential diagnostic considerations of metastatic carcinoma or sweat gland carcinoma (see Table 1-6) (11).

Today electron microscopy is used infrequently to detect differentiation in a hard-to-classify soft tissue tumor, but it can be helpful at times, particularly to search for evidence of muscle differentiation in a small round cell tumor or neural differentiation in a spindle cell neoplasm.

Placing Tumors Within the Major Phenotypic Categories of the Scientific Classification. Within each of the major phenotypic categories of soft tissue tumors listed in Table 1-1 are variable numbers of different neoplasms and tumor-like lesions whose constituent cells display the differentiated features indicated by the major category. For example, the different tumor types in the fatty tumor category have different histologic patterns and sometimes different clinical behaviors but they have in common cells that demonstrate lipocytic differentiation. After identifying the major phenotypic category of a soft tissue tumor, the next step is to match the histologic pattern with one of the tumors within the category. In this Fascicle each major phenotypic type of soft tissue tumor is assigned a chapter and at the beginning of that chapter there is a table listing the tumors within the category and assigning them to one of the managerial classes outlined in Table 1-10. The remainder of the chapter describes the clinical and pathologic features of each of these tumors in detail. Whenever possible we have followed the WHO classification but where

we think that classification does not stratify or name tumors according to current concepts and practice we have taken the liberty to change it.

The Unclassified (Undifferentiated) Soft Tissue Neoplasm. Unfortunately, for some soft tissue tumors no distinctive cellular differentiation, matrix, or architectural arrangement of the cells can be discerned either by conventional light microscopy, electron microscopy, or immunohistochemical techniques. Strategies for further characterizing these for clinical management purposes are set out in the Managerial Classification section below. Typically, the neoplasms that resist characterization are obvious high-grade sarcomas occurring in adults and nothing of managerial importance is discovered in this process. Thus, from the perspective of patient care, however scientifically unsatisfying the designation "unclassified soft tissue tumor" or "undifferentiated sarcoma" might be, it is a good enough diagnosis to proceed with therapy and render a prognosis as long as the tumor can be placed in an appropriate managerial category (34). It is useful to describe in the comment section of the pathology report the procedures performed in an attempt to classify such neoplasms and a description of the tumor cells is often useful, e.g., "unclassified small round blue cell tumor" or "unclassified spindle cell tumor."

An Approach to the Scientific Classification of Soft Tissue Tumors when Proper Placement in the Scientific Classification Is Not Apparent. The constituent cells of a soft tissue tumor usually can be broadly characterized as monomorphous spindled, epithelioid, pleomorphic mixed spindled, and round cell or "small round cell," and these cells may be arranged in fascicular, alveolar, palisading, storiform, cording, acinar, plexiform, or pericytoma patterns. The stroma may be myxoid, granulation tissue-like, collagenous, or osseous or cartilaginous. Tables 1-4 to 1-9 present some of the tumors characterized by these features (13,39). These tables can be used both to aid in the formulation of a differential diagnosis and as a memory jogger when evaluating morphologic features of a difficult-to-classify soft tissue tumor.

Cytogenetic Abnormalities. Clonal, nonrandom chromosomal abnormalities are common in both benign and malignant soft tissue tumors, including tumors that occur predominantly in

Table 1-4

**PATTERN RECOGNITION:
SOFT TISSUE TUMORS COMPOSED
OF MONOMORPHIC SPINDLED CELLS**

Nodular fasciitis
Cellular fibroma of tendon sheath
Benign nerve sheath tumors
Palmar and plantar fibromatosis
Leiomyomas
Dermatofibrosarcoma protuberans (DFSP)
Desmoid fibromatosis
Fibrosarcoma
Leiomyosarcoma*
Synovial sarcoma
Malignant peripheral nerve sheath tumor*
Spindle cell (embryonal) rhabdomyosarcoma

*These tumors also may be pleomorphic (see Table 1-7).

Table 1-5

**PATTERN RECOGNITION:
ROUND CELL NEOPLASM**

Round Cell Neoplasms of the Soft Tissues

Small round cell tumors: childhood rhabdomyosarcoma, PPNET/Ewing's, desmoplastic small cell
tumor
Cellular myxoid liposarcoma (round cell liposarcoma)
Mesenchymal chondrosarcoma

Nonmesenchymal Round Cell Neoplasms

Lymphoma
Neuroblastoma
Metastatic carcinoma
Melanoma

Table 1-6

**PATTERN RECOGNITION: SOFT TISSUE
EPITHELIOID NEOPLASMS**

**Epithelioid Neoplasms that
Do Not Contain Keratin- or EMA-Positive Cells**

Alveolar soft part sarcoma
Epithelioid malignant peripheral nerve sheath
tumor (11)

**Epithelioid Neoplasms that Often Contain
Keratin- or EMA-Positive Cells**

Epithelioid sarcoma
Synovial sarcoma*
Epithelioid vascular tumors
Glandular malignant peripheral nerve sheath tumor*
Malignant tumor with rhabdoid features (many
examples in adults are metastases)
Epithelioid leiomyosarcoma
Carcinoma either extending into the region from an
organ in the area or metastatic to the site from
a remote primary site

*These tumors almost always also have a spindle cell
component.

Table 1-7

**PATTERN RECOGNITION: TUMOR
COMPOSED OF PLEOMORPHIC
SPINDLED AND/OR ROUND CELLS**

Pleomorphic malignant fibrous histiocytoma
Pleomorphic leiomyosarcoma
Pleomorphic liposarcoma
Pleomorphic rhabdomyosarcoma
Pleomorphic malignant peripheral nerve sheath tumor
Be careful about metastasis

adults as well as those that have a predilection for children. Because many of these chromosomal abnormalities are less complex than those found in carcinoma, they have been extensively studied and as a result we know a great deal about the chromosomal deletions, rearrangements, and amplifications that occur in soft tissue tumors. Information about clonal abnormalities is provided in the Special Studies section for each tumor type. Many clonal chromosomal ab-

normalities are specific for a tumor type and some appear to have prognostic significance, so potentially this information could be used to classify a difficult to diagnose tumor or to estimate prognosis. However, currently this technology is expensive, is available in only a few laboratories, has a false positive-false negative rate that is largely unknown, and in most instances does not provide information that cannot be obtained by standard histologic examination. Consequently, it is now largely a research tool used

Table 1-8

PATTERN RECOGNITION: TUMORS THAT MAY HAVE A MYXOID STROMA

Benign
(Managerial Groups Ia, Ib, and Ic, see Table 1-10)

Nodular fasciitis

Intramuscular myxoma

Neurofibroma

Superficial angiomyxoma

Myxoid spindle cell lipoma

Lipoblastoma

Myxoid smooth muscle tumors

Neurothekeoma (nerve sheath myxoma)

Intermediate
(Managerial Groups IIa, IIb, and IIc, see Table 1-10)

Aggressive angiomyxoma

Myxoid dermatofibrosarcoma protuberans

Ossifying fibromyxoid tumor

Juxta-articular myxoma

Inflammatory myxohyaline tumor

Malignant
(Managerial Group III, see Table 1-10)

Myxoid liposarcoma*

Myxoid chondrosarcoma*

Myxoid malignant fibrous histiocytoma (myxofibrosarcoma)*

Embryonal rhabdomyosarcoma

Myxoid smooth muscle tumors

Myxoid metastatic neoplasms, especially carcinoma and melanoma*

Myxoid malignant peripheral nerve sheath tumor

Low-grade fibromyxoid sarcoma*

---

*Whenever a myxoid neoplasm is encountered in the deep soft tissues these should always be in the differential diagnosis.

to better understand neoplastic transformation and to more accurately classify tumors in a research setting. Nonetheless, this will change when technical advances lower the cost if it is shown that chromosomal specific break points provide information concerning response to therapy or prognosis not provided by histologic and immunohistochemical examination. Fletcher (17) has recently published an excellent review of the chromosomal aberrations found in soft tissue tumors.

Table 1-9

PATTERN RECOGNITION: ARRANGEMENT OF CELLS

Alveolar	Alveolar soft part sarcoma Alveolar rhabdomyosarcoma
Glands	Synovial sarcoma (rule out metastatic carcinoma or sweat gland carcinoma) Glandular malignant peripheral nerve sheath tumor
Fascicular or bundles	Desmoid Smooth muscle tumor Cellular benign nerve sheath tumor Synovial sarcoma Malignant peripheral nerve sheath tumor Fibrosarcoma
Lobular	Myxoid chondrosarcoma Clear cell sarcoma Epithelioid sarcoma
Palisading	Nerve sheath tumors Smooth muscle tumors Spindle cell lipoma Synovial sarcoma (rarely)
Plexiform	Nerve sheath tumors Plexiform fibrous histiocytoma
Arborizing or plexiform vascular	Myxoid liposarcoma Nodular fasciitis Myxoid malignant fibrous histiocytoma (MFH) (myxofibrosarcoma)
Storiform	Some fibrous histiocytomas: dermatofibrosarcoma protuberans (repetitive), dermal fibrous histiocytomas, pleomorphic MFH (focal) Perineurioma Low-grade fibromyxoid sarcoma Dedifferentiated liposarcoma

Managerial Classification

In contrast to the considerable effort that has gone into constructing elaborate scientific classifications of soft tissue tumors and the time and financial resources that are often expended detecting differentiation that allows placement of a hard-to-classify soft tissue tumor in one of these categories, substantially less attention has been given to the equally important task of constructing a clinically relevant managerial classification of soft tissue neoplasms (33). Some managerial information is provided by the existing classification of soft tissue tumors, since tumors within each major differentiated group are further stratified into benign or malignant. However, in recent years it has become apparent that there are degrees of clinical malignancy and the simplistic

Table 1-10

MANAGERIAL DISEASE CATEGORIES

Group	Outcome	Usual Therapy	Examples
Clinically Benign			
Ia	Local excision is almost always curative Metastasis never occurs	Local excision	Nodular fasciitis; dermal fibrous histiocytoma, dermatofibroma type
Ib	Recurrences do occur but are not destructive Never metastasizes	Local excision; treat recurrences if they occur	Aneurysmal fibrous histiocytoma; superficial angiomyxoma
Clinically Intermediate			
IIa	Local recurrence very common and may be destructive Never metastasizes	Local excision with attention to margins	Desmoid fibromatosis
IIb	Local recurrence very common Metastasis vanishingly rare unless tumor "dedifferentiates" to a process in group III	Local excision with attention to margins Adjuvant therapy usually not warranted	Atypical lipomatous tumor ("well-differentiated liposarcoma"); dermatofibrosarcoma protuberans (DFSP)
IIc	Local recurrence common Metastasis can rarely occur without dedifferentiation	Local excision with attention to margins Adjuvant therapy not warranted	Ossifying fibromyxoid tumor; plexiform fibrous histiocytoma
Clinically Sarcoma			
III	Local recurrence common Metastasis occurs	Local excision with compulsive attention to margins Consideration given to adjuvant therapy	Pleomorphic malignant fibrous histiocytoma; malignant peripheral nerve sheath tumor; myxoid liposarcoma
IV	Systemic disease assumed to be present at the outset	Adjuvant therapy usual	Embryonal rhabdomyosarcoma; primitive neuroectodermal tumor

and clinically unhelpful view that neoplasms can be sorted into "benign" and "malignant" is increasingly giving way to a more nuanced treatment of this issue. In response to problems of this sort, a borderline or intermediate category has been delineated for most tumor types. What is required from a patient care perspective is a classification that further elaborates this approach and explicitly defines the several clinical behaviors that are encompassed by the terms benign, intermediate, and malignant. This can be accomplished by collapsing the long list of soft tissue tumors that the scientific classification recognizes into seven categories that capture most of the clinically relevant features that guide clinical care. These categories can be thought of as comprising a clinical management classification that is distinct from, but complimentary to, the scientific classification discussed above; this classification along with examples is set out in Table 1-10. For convenience, each of the categories has been designated with a group number and these group numbers are used in the classification table in each chapter.

Benign tumors are cured by simple excision or they may recur but they do not recur in an uncontrolled fashion or destroy significant amounts of normal tissue. Intermediate neoplasms recur commonly and are sometimes destructive but metastasis is rare in the absence of the development of a new component in the neoplasm. This latter phenomenon has been given the not altogether happy label "dedifferentiation." Metastasis never occurs in group IIa tumors.

Sarcomas fall into either group III or IV. Some of these management groups are, of course, further subdivided for the purposes of therapy. For example, within group IV it is important to distinguish peripheral primitive neuroectodermal tumor (PPNET)/Ewing's sarcoma from rhabdomyosarcoma since the chemotherapeutic approach and associated prognosis is substantially different. It is crucial to distinguish *morphologically* malignant from *clinically* malignant because some morphologically malignant neoplasms such as atypical fibroxanthoma are not clinically malignant while some morphologically bland neoplasms such as well-differentiated smooth muscle tumors in the retroperitoneum may pursue a clinically malignant course.

Prognostically important morphologic features vary from one differentiated tumor group to another, so taking reasonable steps to determine the direction of a neoplasm's differentiation or to recognize a named histologic pattern may be required before a credible statement about the neoplasm's malignant potential can be made. If the scientific name of a well-known tumor provides all of the managerial information needed for patient care, it will also suffice as the managerial classification (e.g., lipoma). However, when rare and unusual tumors are encountered (and many soft tissue tumors fall into this category) or when a single tumor behaves in a variety of ways, then the WHO name should be supplemented with a more elaborate managerial assessment. Table 1-10 provides a guide for such an assessment. For example, atypical lipomatous tumor (also known as well-differentiated liposarcoma) may be cured by excision, it may recur nonaggressively, recur aggressively, recur in an uncontrolled fashion and cause patient death, or dedifferentiate and metastasize after dedifferentiation. Moreover, the probability of dedifferentiation and uncontrolled growth depends on its anatomic location (it is more common in the retroperitoneum than in the deep soft tissues of the extremities). The possible behaviors for atypical lipomatous tumor in any given location and the pathologist's assessment of their relative likelihood always should be carefully spelled out in the pathology report in addition to using whichever of the two scientific names, atypical lipomatous tumor or well-differentiated liposarcoma, one prefers.

GRADING SARCOMAS

Some investigators believe that further prognostic information can be extracted from grading the adult sarcomas that are group III neoplasms (Table 1-10). To grade a group III adult sarcoma is to attempt to predict the likelihood of metastasis or recurrence on the basis of morphologic features such as the degree of pleomorphism, mitotic activity, cellularity, extent of tumor cell necrosis, and degree of differentiation. Whether adult soft tissue sarcomas should be graded is controversial and hotly contested. In one camp are those who have concluded that all of the information relevant to estimating the risk of recurrence and metastasis depends solely on the histologic type of the sarcoma (14,20). In the opposing camp are those who think grading contributes significantly toward predicting the behavior of most adult soft tissue sarcomas, but even they concede that grading is useful only for adult sarcomas that fall into the group III category in Table 1-10, and that some of these sarcomas, notably alveolar soft part sarcoma, epithelioid sarcoma, myxoid chondrosarcoma, and clear cell sarcoma, should not be graded because grading has not identified significant differences within these differentiated tumor types (1,4,6,9, 12,22,24,25,30,36,37). The middle camp concedes useful information may be obtained by grading some adult sarcomas, but points out that the sarcomas to be graded have not been generally agreed upon, that no single grading scheme is universally satisfactory to the majority of soft tissue pathologists, and that grading criteria are poorly defined and not equally applicable to all tumor types.

The first grading scheme for soft tissue tumors that gained general attention was that developed by Russell et al. (35) who utilized seven morphologic grading features but did not provide detailed instructions for assessing and quantifying these features; they also did not analyze them in a multivariate fashion in order to determine the relative contribution (if any) of each feature. The American Joint Committee incorporated the grade determined by this scheme as a major parameter in determining stage (3) (Table 1-11). In 1984, Costa and associates (9) analyzed the impact of six histologic parameters on predicting time to recurrence for a variety of adult soft tissue sarcomas and found

Table 1-11

AMERICAN JOINT COMMITTEE STAGING SYSTEM OF SOFT TISSUE SARCOMAS*

Definitions of TNM

Primary Tumor (T)

TX	Primary tumor cannot be assessed
T0	No evidence of primary tumor
T1	Tumor 5 cm or less in greatest dimension
T1a	superficial tumor**
T1b	deep tumor**
T2	Tumor more than 5 cm in greatest dimension
T2a	superficial tumor**
T2b	deep tumor**

Regional Lymph Nodes (N)

NX	Regional lymph nodes cannot be assessed
N0	No regional lymph node metastasis
N1	Regional lymph node metastasis

Distant Metastasis (M)

MX	Distant metastasis cannot be assessed
M0	No distant metastasis
M1	Distant metastasis

Histopathologic Grade (G)

GX	Grade cannot be assessed
G1	Well differentiated
G2	Moderately differentiated
G3	Poorly differentiated
G4	Undifferentiated

Stage Grouping

Stage I

Stage IA Low grade, small, superficial, and deep	G1-2, T1a-1b,	N0,	M0
Stage IB Low grade, large, superficial	G1-2, T2a,	N0,	M0

Stage II

Stage IIA Low grade, large, deep	G1-2, T2b,	N0,	M0
Stage IIB High grade, small, superficial, and deep	G3-4, T1a-b,	N0,	M0
Stage IIC High grade, large, superficial	G3-4, T2a,	N0,	M0

Stage III

Stage III High grade, large, deep	G3-4, T2b,	N0,	M0

Stage IV

Any metastasis	any G, any T,	N1,	M0
	any G, any T,	N0,	M1

*Data compiled from reference 8.

**Superficial tumor is located exclusively above the superficial fascia without invasion of the fascia; deep tumor is located either exclusively beneath the superficial facia, or superficial to the fascia with invasion of or through the fascia, or superficial and beneath the fascia. Retroperitoneal, mediastinal, and pelvic sarcomas are classified as deep tumors.

that tumor cell necrosis was the single best predictor. They proposed a grading scheme (NCI) for soft tissue sarcomas based mainly on the extent of tumor cell necrosis: grade I sarcomas were a defined group of known low-grade sarcomas (myxoid liposarcoma, well-differentiated neural and smooth muscle tumors, and paucicellular myxoid chondrosarcoma) without tumor cell necrosis; grade II tumors were all other sarcomas with either no necrosis or less than 15 percent tumor cell necrosis; and grade III sarcomas were those in which more than 15 percent of the tumor was necrotic. Unfortunately, a detailed method for determining the extent of necrosis (gross, microscopic, or both) was not provided and, of course, the total extent of necrosis in a tumor is not evaluable in a biopsy specimen. Moreover, necrosis cannot be utilized as a grading parameter for patients who receive preoperative therapy and it is not clear that extent of necrosis is independent of tumor size. This scheme was later modified by Lack and colleagues (25) and more details about how the extent of necrosis was evaluated were included.

Table 1-12

GUIDELINES FOR GRADING SOFT TISSUE SARCOMAS*

Tumors which are definitionally high grade
    Ewing's sarcoma/MPNET
    Rhabdomyosarcoma (all types)
    Angiosarcoma
    Pleomorphic liposarcoma
    Soft tissue osteosarcoma
    Mesenchymal chondrosarcoma
    Desmoplastic small cell tumor
    Extra-renal rhabdoid tumor

Tumors which are definitionally low grade
    Well-differentiated liposarcoma/atypical lipo-
       matous tumor
    Dermatofibrosarcoma protuberans
    Infantile fibrosarcoma
    Angiomatoid "MFH"

Tumors which are not gradable but which often metastasize within 10–20 years of follow-up
    Alveolar soft part sarcoma
    Clear cell sarcoma
    Epithelioid sarcoma
    Synovial sarcoma
    "Low-grade" fibromyxoid sarcoma

Tumors of varying behavior for which grading may be prognostically useful
    Myxoid liposarcoma
    Leiomyosarcoma
    Malignant peripheral nerve sheath tumor
    Fibrosarcoma
    Myxofibrosarcoma (myxoid MFH)

Tumors of varying behavior for which grading parameters are not yet established
    Hemangiopericytoma
    Myxoid chondrosarcoma
    Malignant granular cell tumor
    Malignant mesenchymoma

*Table 3 from Association of Directors of Anatomic Pathology. Recommendations for reporting soft tissue tumors (2a).

Also in 1984, Trojani et al. (36) evaluated seven histologic parameters by multivariate analysis and found that three were independent predictors of metastasis for adult soft tissue sarcomas: the number of mitotic figures per 10 high-power fields, the extent of tumor cell necrosis, and the differentiation of the tumor. Their proposed grading system involves adding the scores of these three parameters to provide three grades in a manner similar to the scoring system used in the Bloom-Richardson grading scheme for breast carcinoma. The reproducibility of this scheme was tested by 15 pathologists and the interobserver agreement for each of the three parameters was reported to be 75 to 80 percent (7). Instructions on how to determine the extent of necrosis were significantly understated and the definition of tumor differentiation was vague. In a recent update, these concerns have been addressed but this scheme is still time consuming (19).

There is yet a fourth approach, a two-tier scheme that sorts adult sarcomas into "high grade" and "low grade" by placing those with tumor cell necrosis, high cellularity, numerous mitotic fig-

ures, and easily discernible pleomorphism in the high-grade category while the remainder are classified as low grade. Guidelines for using such a grading scheme have been presented by the Association of Directors of Anatomic and Surgical Pathology (Table 1-12) (2a). Whatever grading scheme is used it is generally agreed that childhood sarcomas, alveolar soft part sarcoma, clear cell sarcoma, myxoid chondrosarcoma, and epithelioid sarcoma are not graded. When these four grading schemes, and for that matter most of the other grading schemes reported in the literature, are applied to test cases, they stratify them into groups with respectable differences in metastasis and recurrence rate between grades (1,4,6,9,12,19,22,24,25,30,32,36,37).

Does this mean we should be expected to grade adult sarcomas? The answer is not clear and the question remains contentious. However, both staging systems currently in use in the United States require a tumor grade and clinicians often ask whether adult sarcomas are high grade or low grade when considering various therapy options (4,25). We think grading is useful for some

Table 1-13

FRENCH FEDERATION OF CANCER CENTERS SYSTEM GRADING SCHEME FOR ADULT SARCOMAS*

Grading Parameter

I **Tumor Differentiation** (Table 1-14 will be needed to assign a tumor differentiation score)

    Score 1 = Sarcomas closely resembling normal adult tissue (i.e., low-grade sarcomas)

    Score 2 = Sarcomas not in score 1 for which histologic typing is certain (i.e., they fit a category in the WHO classification)

    Score 3 = Undifferentiated sarcomas and sarcomas of uncertain type plus synovial sarcoma, PPNET/Ewing's sarcoma, and some types of pleomorphic differentiated adult sarcomas, e.g., pleomorphic liposarcoma

II **Mitotic Index**

    Score 1 = 0-9 mf/10 hpf**

    Score 2 = 10-19 mf/10 hpf

    Score 3 = >20 mf/10 hpf

III **Tumor Cell Necrosis[†]**

    Score 0 = No necrosis on any slide

    Score 1 = 50% of the tumor is necrotic in the slides examined

    Score 2 = 50% of the tumor is necrotic in the slides examined

Final Grade - add the three scores

    Grade 1 = When sum of scores equals 2 or 3

    Grade 2 = When sum of scores equals 4 or 5

    Grade 3 = When sum of scores equals 6, 7, or 8

---

*Data from references 7, 19, and 36.
**Mitoses per high-power field. High-power field area = 0.1744 mm^2.
[†]To estimate tumor cell necrosis a minimum of one section per 2 cm of tumor diameter is suggested.

adult soft tissue sarcomas and should be provided when oncologists use grade to plan therapy. As recently modified, the best analyzed and most reproducible scheme is that of Trojani et al. (19) now known as the French Federation of Cancer Centers System and we think if grading is performed it is a useful scheme to consider (Table 1-13). However, the two-grade system also is attractive because it is faster, commonly used by clinicians for treatment planning, and does a respectable job of stratifying sarcomas with significant differences in metastatic and recurrence rates (Table 1-12) (32). To determine tumor differentiation as Trojani et al. do it, one needs to use the table provided in their most recent publication (Table 1-14) because their assignment of differentiation scores cannot be determined otherwise. Moreover, microscopic field size must be adjusted for mitotic counting, and there must be at least one section for each 2 cm of maximum diameter of tumor to insure adequate sampling for estimating the extent of tumor cell necrosis.

BEYOND BENIGN AND MALIGNANT

The importance of encoding managerially relevant information by expanding the dichotomous classification of benign/malignant cannot be overemphasized. We pathologists tend to focus our attention and interest on scientific classifications and these have a tendency to become highly detailed and sensitive to the latest technologic developments. Although scientific classifications provide the necessary scaffolding for exploring the biology of similar tumors, managerial information that is complete, readily understood, and clinically useful is vital for patient care. We cannot always depend on clinicians to accurately translate scientific classifications into managerial classifications. As the eminent oncologist Saul Rosenberg has written about the REAL lymphoma classification presented in 1994: "A clinico-pathologic classification must have more than scientific accuracy and interest, it must be clinically useful. It must be reproducible by average well-trained pathologists

Table 1-14

TUMOR DIFFERENTIATION SCORE ACCORDING TO HISTOLOGIC TYPE IN THE UPDATED VERSION OF THE FRENCH FEDERATION OF CANCER CENTERS SARCOMA GROUP SYSTEM*

Histologic Type	Tumor Differentiation Score
Well-differentiated liposarcoma	1
Myxoid liposarcoma	2
Round cell liposarcoma	3
Pleomorphic liposarcoma	3
Dedifferentiated liposarcoma	3
Well-differentiated fibrosarcoma	1
Conventional fibrosarcoma	2
Poorly differentiated fibrosarcoma	3
Low-grade malignant peripheral nerve sheath tumor	1
Conventional malignant schwannoma	2
Poorly differentiated malignant schwannoma	3
Epithelioid malignant schwannoma	3
Malignant triton tumor	3
Well-differentiated malignant hemangiopericytoma	2
Conventional malignant hemangiopericytoma	3
Myxoid malignant fibrous histiocytoma (MFH)	2
Typical storiform/pleomorphic MFH	2
Giant cell and inflammatory MFH	3
Well-differentiated leiomyosarcoma	1
Conventional leiomyosarcoma	2
Poorly differentiated/pleomorphic/epithelioid leiomyosarcoma	3
Biphasic/monophasic synovial sarcoma	3
Embryonal/alveolar/pleomorphic rhabdomyosarcoma	3
Well-differentiated chondrosarcoma	1
Myxoid chondrosarcoma	2
Mesenchymal chondrosarcoma	3
Conventional angiosarcoma	2
Poorly differentiated/epithelioid angiosarcoma	3
Extraskeletal osteosarcoma	3
Primitive peripheral neuroectodermal tumor (PPNET)/Ewing's sarcoma	3
Alveolar soft tissue sarcoma	3
Epithelioid sarcoma	3
Malignant rhabdoid tumor	3
Clear cell sarcoma	3
Undifferentiated sarcoma	3

*Table 1 from Guillou L, Coindre JM, Bonichon F, et al. Comparative study of the National Cancer Institute and French Federation of Cancer Centers Sarcoma Group grading systems in a population of 410 adult patients with soft tissue sarcoma. J Clin Oncol 1997;15:350–62.

Table 1-15

MORPHOLOGIC FEATURES THAT SUGGEST A REACTIVE OR BENIGN LESION (GROUPS Ia AND Ib)

Nuclear uniformity (nuclei may well be enlarged)
Delicate or vesicular chromatin
If mitotic figures are present they are normal
Small size
Superficial location

Table 1-16

MORPHOLOGIC FEATURES THAT SUGGEST THE POSSIBILITY OF AN ADULT SARCOMA (GROUP III)

Pleomorphism and nuclear irregularity
Coarse, grainy, dense nuclei
Large size
Located deep to the fascia
Tumor cell necrosis

using easily available and easily learned techniques and predict clinical behavior" (33).

Even when a tumor's location in a scientific classification cannot be established with certainty, a descriptive managerial category still may be provided. In this circumstance, careful evaluation of cellular features often, but not always, allows proper managerial classification (Tables 1-15, 1-16). Most benign tumors are composed of cells with fine, delicate or vesicular chromatin. The nuclei in benign tumors may be enlarged, but they are seldom significantly pleomorphic. Mitotic figures, if present, are normal. On the other hand, malignant tumors tend to be composed of cells with coarse, grainy nuclei, and the nuclei in a significant proportion of sarcomas are pleomorphic. Abnormal mitotic figures are not uncommon in sarcomas. Although benign processes may be cellular, not many sarcomas are paucicellular. Benign tumors tend to be smaller than 3 cm and most are superficial to the fascia; in contrast, most sarcomas are larger than this and they tend to arise in the deep soft tissues. Evaluating just six features—nuclear uniformity, abnormal mitotic figures, chromatin characteristics, size, cellularity, and location—in a hard-to-classify soft tissue tumor often gives a good idea of its potential for clinical aggressiveness. For example, the constituent cells of clinically benign tumors may indeed be unexpectedly pleomorphic and have dense nuclear chromatin, but the cells in morphologically benign soft tissue tumors do not divide abnormally. Exceptions, such as atypical fibroxanthoma, are morphologic sarcomas that are clinically benign because they are limited to the dermis. Most intermediate tumors have morphologic features that suggest benignity, but their size and degree of infiltration provide clues to their behavior even if they do not have the

specific arrangements of cells that identifies the tumor. A few sarcomas are paucicellular (i.e., some examples of myxoid malignant fibrous histiocytoma) but they can be identified because of pleomorphism or abnormal mitotic figures.

Of course, this approach can be used to assign the managerial class before the scientific category is determined and, in fact, many experienced pathologists prefer to first gain an impression of whether a tumor is benign, intermediate, or a sarcoma either before, or concurrently with, the determination of its differentiated type. When the lesion in question has spindled cells without obvious differentiating features other than that the cells resemble fibroblasts, myofibroblasts, or fibrocytes, an initial managerial approach is often useful. In this situation, the most important differential diagnostic considerations are a reactive process such as nodular fasciitis and its close relations, proliferative fasciitis, proliferative myositis and cellular fibroma of tendon sheath, an intermediate tumor such as a desmoid, or a sarcoma.

CLINICAL INFORMATION NEEDED TO DIAGNOSE SOFT TISSUE TUMORS

When a soft tissue tumor is received in the laboratory, certain clinical information should be obtained. We think it unwise to render a diagnosis on a soft tissue neoplasm without knowing: 1) its site in the body, i.e., extremities, trunk, etc.; 2) whether it is dermal, subcutaneous, or in the deep soft tissues; 3) its size; 4) the age of the patient harboring the lesion; 5) the results of clinical examination and/or imaging studies that exclude the possibility that the process is arising from underlying bone or other organs in the neighborhood (e.g., kidney when a retroperitoneal tumor is evaluated); and 6) any history of prior malignancies or radiation therapy. It is of course important to know whether the patient has an inherited disorder such as neurofibromatosis or Gardner's syndrome and at times the duration of the lesion can be helpful. The reasons for needing this information are many. In general, more distal sarcomas have a better prognosis than proximal ones and the retroperitoneum and mediastinum are the worst sites in which to have a sarcoma. Many dermal mesenchymal lesions are usually clinically benign, even if they are judged on morphologic grounds to be malignant (e.g., atypical fibroxanthoma and leiomyosarcoma), although there are exceptions such as angiosarcoma. Subcutaneous soft tissue tumors also are more likely to be benign while deep soft tissue tumors, particularly if they are large, are more likely to be sarcoma. Small lesions are more likely to be benign or intermediate than sarcoma. In fact, only a rare sarcoma is small enough at the time of initial excisional biopsy to totally fit into one cassette, an observation that can be very helpful, although there are exceptions. The age of the patient is important, because adult-type sarcomas are rare in children and when they occur they often do not behave as aggressively as they do in adults. Likewise, childhood sarcomas are rare after the age of 20. Equipped with a knowledge of the patient's past medical history of prior malignancies and the findings of available imaging studies the pathologist can often avoid the serious error of interpreting a metastasis or a lymphoma as a primary soft tissue tumor.

OBTAINING SPECIMENS FOR A DIAGNOSIS OF A SOFT TISSUE TUMOR

The particular technique used to biopsy a soft tissue mass can have important prognostic implications (15,39). If done improperly it may complicate subsequent therapy or reduce its effectiveness. Small, superficial masses usually can be completely excised safely with a small rim of normal tissue. Most are benign or intermediate and if sarcoma is encountered in this location, suitable reexcision is almost always feasible. Large subcutaneous tumors and all deep-seated tumors, unless they are small, should be subjected to an incisional or core needle biopsy prior to excision. Debulking diagnostic procedures ("shelling out") of deep sarcomas typically compromise subsequent attempts at wide excision and are discouraged. Careful planning of the biopsy site is important so its excision (including the overlying skin) can be accomplished as part of the definitive resection if the tumor turns out to be malignant. If the tumor is in an extremity the alignment of the biopsy incision should be along the long axis, not a transverse cut.

In general, we do not advocate the use of fine needle aspiration (FNA) to make an initial diagnosis of a soft tissue tumor unless there is suspicion that the tumor is a metastasis or a lymphoma because the specimen received from fine needle biopsies is frequently too scanty to allow for confident classification of a primary soft tissue neoplasm. In some circumstances, FNA can be used to document recurrence and as a screening tool to aid in planning more extensive biopsy procedures. In spite of these reservations, there are special circumstances in which an FNA biopsy provides all the information about a soft tissue tumor that is needed to initiate therapy (23,26,31) and there are specialized centers which have had success using FNA for primary diagnosis. This is particularly true for childhood sarcomas.

Core needle biopsy is becoming an increasingly popular method for diagnosing soft tissue tumors, particularly at institutions where preoperative chemotherapy is given for high-grade sarcomas. Core needle biopsies, in conjunction with immunohistochemistry, often reveal whether the tumor is a sarcoma and if so whether it is low grade or high grade even if exact classification of the tumor is not possible. Many times this information is sufficient for clinicians to initiate preoperative therapy for high-grade lesions and excise low-grade ones. Childhood sarcomas often can be accurately classified using immunohistochemical techniques. Interpretation of core needle biopsies requires some experience and the technique reaches its highest potential when there is a close working relationship between pathologists and clinicians.

We do not think frozen sections should be utilized to make an initial diagnosis of a soft tissue mass if this diagnosis will lead to an immediate therapeutic procedure. There are several reasons for this conclusion. Most pathologists have limited experience with the diagnosis of soft tissue tumors and there are many benign lesions which mimic sarcomas and many malignant processes that present as soft tissue masses that are not primary soft tissue neoplasms. We think it best that patients with soft tissue tumors have a permanent section diagnosis of their tumor followed by discussion of the therapy options available to them. Frozen sections however can, and probably should, be used to determine if a biopsy specimen contains viable and representative tissue. Smears can also be used for this purpose. Frozen sections are also used by some surgeons to evaluate the distance of tumor from the margins of excision (18). This works well for many high-grade lesions, but for low-grade tumors, particularly low-grade fibrous tumors such as desmoid fibromatosis, well-differentiated angiosarcoma, or low-grade fibrous histiocytoma, it may be impossible to distinguish reactive mesenchymal tissue and scar from tumor.

HANDLING THE RESECTION SPECIMEN

With the exception of superficial, grossly classic lipomas, the surgical margins of all intact excision specimens of soft tissue tumors should be inked and the distance from the tumor to the nearest margin determined grossly and microscopically if it is malignant or has recurring potential. When tumor is close to a margin, we determine if it is less than or greater than 2 cm from that margin and measure the distance if it is less than 2 cm. Upon incising the specimen, the appearance of the tumor should be noted and its size recorded. Because the extent of necrosis is often used to grade sarcomas, this feature should be determined both grossly and microscopically. If a patient has received preoperative therapy the extent of necrosis is unreliable as a grading parameter, but it may be useful in evaluating the effectiveness of the preoperative therapy. Size is an important predictor of clinical outcome as well as a staging parameter in the TNM system. T1 tumors are less than 5 cm while T2 tumors are larger (Table 1-11). The relationship of the tumor to nearby structures should be recorded. It is particularly important to note if nerves and vessels have been invaded grossly.

Section selection for histologic evaluation of soft tissue tumors varies depending on the type and the size of tumor. Small tumors should be totally submitted and at least 1 section per cen-

timeter of diameter up to 3 to 4 sections should be taken of any soft tissue tumor. One might question why an otherwise grossly banal specimen such as a lipoma should be so sectioned, but the changes of atypical lipomatous tumor can be focal and missed by a single section. For tumors that are diagnostic problems and for those in which high-grade areas may develop only focally, we recommend 1 section per centimeter of tumor up to about 10 sections, with a minimum of 5 sections. In many instances, pilot sections may be taken to determine the final number of sections needed. For example, it is unnecessary to extensively section a high-grade sarcoma beyond that needed to determine the extent of tumor cell necrosis (one section for each 2 cm of tumor diameter) but a myxoid liposarcoma that can have focal cellular (round cell) areas needs extensive sectioning to determine the extent of such areas, if any, in order to grade the tumor and better predict outcome. Areas of necrosis noted during gross examination should be documented. Selection of sections to document margins should be guided by the gross examination. Obviously the margins nearest the tumor are the ones that need to be sampled the most thoroughly. We take margin sections at right angles to the margin of nearest grossly visible tumor.

THE CONTENT OF THE SURGICAL PATHOLOGY REPORT FOR SOFT TISSUE TUMORS

The surgical pathology report should contain all of the information needed by clinicians to plan therapy and estimate prognosis for a patient with a soft tissue tumor. Since this is also true for almost all tumors that arise in any organ, it may be difficult to remember all the important features that need to be included in the surgical pathology report for each type of tumor. Checklists are a useful solution to this problem and our checklist for soft tissue tumors is provided in Table 1-17. The Association of Directors of Anatomic and Surgical Pathology have also presented recommendations for reporting soft tissue tumors (2a).

In study after study in the literature, three variables emerge as the most important in predicting outcome for patients with sarcomas: tumor size, extent of necrosis (which can be incorporated

Table 1-17
CONTENT OF THE SURGICAL PATHOLOGY REPORT*

Histologic type

Managerial category (see Table 1-10)

Grade where appropriate (see Tables 1-12, 1-13, and text)

Extent of tumor cell necrosis (may be incorporated into the grade: see Tables 1-12 and 1-13)

Size

Depth: dermis, subcutis, below fascia, body cavity

Location, i.e., extremities, retroperitoneum, etc.

Type of resection

Margins
　Involved
　Negative (if tumor is less than 2 cm from any margin record the site and the distance of the tumor from
　　　the margin; if all margins are greater than 2 cm from the nearest tumor measure the distance to the
　　　closest margin)

Results of ancillary studies, particularly immunohistochemistry

*More detailed recommendations for reporting soft tissue sarcomas are presented in reference 2a.

into the grade [see Grading above]), and status of the margins (3,4,6,9,12,24,25,27,28,30,32,36). Consequently, we think these three items must be in every surgical pathology report that concerns the resection of a sarcoma. Obviously, tumor type is essential when it can be determined and we think providing the managerial category of the tumor is essential. Sometimes, the scientific name provides adequate managerial information but when it does not the managerial category should be fully described in the comment section of the report.

A CAPSULIZED APPROACH TO THE DIAGNOSIS OF SOFT TISSUE TUMORS

Have the necessary clinical history available. At a minimum this should include the age of the patient, the location in the body, the depth (dermal versus subcutaneous versus deep), and the size. Other clinical features as outlined above may be useful or even critical.

Determine if any tumor cells demonstrate evidence of differentiation indicative of one of the major tumor types, i.e., fatty, smooth muscle, neural, vascular, skeletal muscle, or bone or cartilage. Use histochemistry and immunohistochemistry as indicated. If the tumor does fit into one of the major differentiated categories, is the pattern

that of one of the known tumor types included within this major tumor category? If all the tumor cells appear to be fibroblasts and myofibroblasts, determine if the pattern fits any of the fibrous or fibrohistiocytic tumors. Check the miscellaneous tumors to determine if the pattern fits any tumor in that category.

If these maneuvers do not result in a classificatory match, evaluate the proliferation at low-power microscopy to determine the shape and arrangement of the cells and the character of the stroma. Soft tissue tumors can roughly be grouped according to the shape and architectural arrangement of their cells and the character of their stroma. These features then can be matched to lists of tumors with similar features. Tables 1-4 to 1-9 present the more common soft tissue tumors matched with their histologic patterns and type of stroma. Histochemical and immunohistochemical stains are used as indicated.

Determine the managerial category (see Table 1-10). Essentially, this amounts to determining whether the tumor falls into the benign, intermediate, or malignant category and then placing it in one of the six managerial categories in Table 1-10. If the tumor is one of the known tumor types in the scientific classification, selection of the proper managerial category is fairly straightforward unless the tumor is so rare that few patients have been followed for any length of time (e.g., ossifying fibromyxoid tumor) or unless the tumor has variable potential. In the latter circumstances, the possible clinical outcomes should be fully explained in the comment section of the pathology report.

Some soft tissue tumors do not have histologic features that allow them to be placed confidently into a recognizable category in the scientific classification. When such a tumor is encountered, the managerial class often can be reasonably estimated by evaluating the features presented in Tables 1-15 and 1-16. Then, a reasonable estimate of which one or more of the six managerial categories presented in Table 1-10 apply to the tumor in question can be made. We think it is better to give those soft tissue tumors that do not fit into any

of the categories in the scientific classification a descriptive managerial label rather than forcing them into a scientific category which may not reflect their clinical potential.

Before reaching a final decision about any soft tissue tumor, always ask: 1) Is this apparent sarcoma in reality a benign or intermediate tumor mimicking a sarcoma? and 2) Does this apparently benign or intermediate tumor in reality have significant metastatic capacity?

If a soft tissue tumor is malignant (or even intermediate) always ask: Is this a metastasis or a hematolymphoid process mimicking a sarcoma? Could this be an extension of a neoplasm from a nearby organ into the soft tissue?

REFERENCES

1. Angervall L, Kindblom LG. Principles for the pathologic diagnosis of soft tissue sarcomas. Acta Oncol 1989;28:9–17.
2. Arber DA, Kandalaft PL, Mehta P, Battifora H. Vimentin-negative epithelioid sarcoma. The value of an immunohistochemical panel that includes CD34. Am J Surg Pathol 1993;17:302–7.
2a. Association of Directors of Anatomic and Surgical Pathology. Recommendations for the reporting of soft tissue sarcomas. Mod Pathol 1998;11:1257–61.
3. Bell RS, O'Sullivan B, Liu FF, et al. The surgical margin in soft-tissue sarcoma. J Bone Joint Surg [Am] 1989;71:370–5.
4. Brennan MF, Shiu MH. Presentation, demographics and prognostic factors of soft tissue sarcoma. In: Shiu MH, Brennan MF, eds. Surgical management of soft tissue sarcoma. Philadelphia: Lea & Febiger, 1989:45–57.
5. Calonje E, Fletcher CD. Immunohistochemistry and DNA flow cytometry in soft-tissue sarcomas. Hematol Oncol Clin North Am 1995;9:657–5.
6. Coindre JM. Pathology and grading of soft tissue sarcomas. In: Verweij J, Pinedo H, Suit H, eds. Multidisciplinary treatment of soft tissue sarcomas. Boston: Kluwer Academic Publishers, 1993:1–22.
7. Coindre JM, Trojani M, Contesso G, et al. Reproducibility of a histopathologic grading system for adult soft tissue sarcoma. Cancer 1986;58:306–9.
8. Cooper JS, Hensen DE, Hutter RU, et al. Manual for staging of cancer, 5th ed. Philadelphia: JB Lippincott, 1997:149–53.
9. Costa J, Wesley RA, Glatstein E, Rosenberg SA. The grading of soft tissue sarcomas. Results of a clinic-ohistopathologic correlation in a series of 163 cases. Cancer 1984;53:530–41.
10. De Young BR, Wick MR, Fitzgibbon JF, et al. CD31: an immunospecific marker for endothelial differentiation in human neoplasms. Appl Immunohistochem 1993;1:97–100.
11. Di Carlo EF, Woodruff JM, Bansal M, Erlandson RA. The purely epithelioid malignant peripheral nerve sheath tumor. Am J Surg Pathol 1986;10:478–90.
12. el-Jabbour JN, Akhtar SS, Kerr GR, et al. Prognostic factors for survival in soft tissue sarcoma. Br J Cancer 1990;62:857–61.
13. Enjoji M, Hashimoto H. Diagnosis of soft tissue sarcomas. Pathol Res Pract 1984;178:215–26.
14. Evans HL. Classification and grading of soft-tissue sarcomas. A comment. Hematol Oncol Clin North Am 1995;9:653–66.
15. Fine G, Hajdu SI, Morton DL, et al. Soft tissue sarcomas. Classification and treatment (a symposium). Pathol Annu 1982;17:155–96.
16. Fisher C. The value of electron microscopy and immunohistochemistry in the diagnosis of soft tissue sarcomas: a study of 200 cases. Histopathology 1990;16:441–54.
17. Fletcher JD. Cytogenetics and molecular biology of soft tissue tumors. In: Weiss SW, Brooks JJ, eds. Soft tissue tumors. Baltimore: Williams & Wilkins, 1996:37–64.
18. Golouh R, Bracko M. Accuracy of frozen section diagnosis in soft tissue tumors. Mod Pathol 1990;3:729–33.
19. Guillou L, Coindre JM, Bonichon F, et al. Comparative study of the National Cancer Institute and French Federation of Cancer Centers Sarcoma Group grading systems in a population of 410 adult patients with soft tissue sarcoma. J Clin Oncol 1997;15:350–62.

20. Hashimoto H, Daimaru Y, Takeshita S, et al. Prognostic significance of histologic parameters of soft tissue sarcomas. Cancer 1992;70:2816–22.

21. Hendrickson MR, Longacre T. Classification of surface epithelial neoplasms of the ovary. In: Hendrickson MR, ed. Surface epithelial neoplasms of the ovary. Philadelphia: Hanley & Belfus, 1993:189–254.

22. Jensen OM, Hogh J, Ostgaard SE, et al. Histopathological grading of soft tissue tumours. Prognostic significance in a prospective study of 278 consecutive cases. J Pathol 1991;163:19–24.

23. Kissin M, Fisher C, Carter R, et al. Value of tru-cut biopsy in the diagnosis of soft tissue tumors. Br J Surg 1986;73:742–4.

24. Kulander BG, Polissar L, Yang CY, Woods JS. Grading of soft tissue sarcomas: necrosis as a determinant of survival. Mod Pathol 1989;2:205–8.

25. Lack EE, Steinberg SM, White DE, et al. Extremity soft tissue sarcomas: analysis of prognostic variables in 300 cases and evaluation of tumor necrosis as a factor in stratifying higher-grade sarcomas. J Surg Oncol 1989;41:263–73.

26. Layfield LJ, Anders KH, Glasgow BJ, Mirra JM. Fine-needle aspiration of primary soft-tissue lesions. Arch Pathol Lab Med 1986;110:420–4.

27. Lewis JJ, Brennan MF. Soft tissue sarcomas. Curr Probl Surg 1996;33:817–72.

28. Mandard AM, Petiot JF, Marnay J, et al. Prognostic factors in soft tissue sarcomas. A multivariate analysis of 109 cases. Cancer 1989;63:1437–51.

29. Manivel JC, Wick MR, Dehner LP, Sibley RK. Epithelioid sarcoma. An immunohistochemical study. Am J Clin Pathol 1987;87:319–26.

30. Markhede G, Angervall L, Stener B. A multivariate analysis of the prognosis after surgical treatment of malignant soft-tissue tumors. Cancer 1982;49:1721–33.

31. Pettinato G, Swanson PE, Insabato L, et al. Undifferentiated small round-cell tumors of childhood: the immunocytochemical demonstration of myogenic differentiation in fine-needle aspirates. Diagn Cytopathol 1989;5:194–9.

32. Pisters PW, Leung DH, Woodruff J, et al. Analysis of prognostic factors in 1,041 patients with localized soft tissue sarcomas of the extremities. J Clin Oncol 1996;14:1679–89.

33. Rosenberg SA. Classification of lymphoid neoplasms [Editorial]. Blood 1994;84:1359–60.

34. Ross JC, Hendrickson MR, Azumi N, Kempson RL. The problem of poorly differentiated sarcoma. In: Fer MF, Greco FA, Oldham RK, eds. Poorly differentiated neoplasms and tumors of unknown origin. Orlando: Grune & Stratton, 1986:217–70.

35. Russell WO, Cohen J, Enzinger F, et al. A clinical and pathological staging system for soft tissue sarcomas. Cancer 1977;40:1562–70.

35a. Scheithauer BW, Woodruff JM, Erlandson RA. Tumors of the peripheral nervous system. Atlas of Tumor Pathology. 3rd Series, Fascicle 24. Washington, D.C.: Armed Forces Institute of Pathology, 1999.

36. Trojani M, Contesso G, Coindre JM, et al. Soft-tissue sarcomas of adults: study of pathological prognostic variables and definition of a histopathological grading system. Int J Cancer 1984;33:37–42.

37. Tsujimoto M, Aozasa K, Ueda T, et al. Multivariate analysis for histologic prognostic factors in soft tissue sarcomas. Cancer 1988;62:994–8.

38. van de Rijn M, Rouse RV. CD34: a review. Appl Immunohistochem 1994;2:71–80.

39. Weiss SW, Enzinger FM. Approach to the diagnosis of soft tissue tumors. In: Weiss SW, Enzinger FM, eds. Soft tissue tumors. 3rd ed. St. Louis: Mosby, 1995:131–8.

40. Weiss SW, Enzinger FM. General considerations. In: Weiss SW, Enzinger FM, eds. Soft tissue tumors. 3rd ed. St. Louis: Mosby, 1995:1–16.

41. Weiss SW, Sobin L. WHO classification of soft tissue tumors. Berlin: Springer-Verlag, 1995.

2

FIBROUS AND MYOFIBROBLASTIC TUMORS

INTRODUCTION

Many different types of soft tissue tumors contain elongate cells that resemble fibrocytes, fibroblasts, and myofibroblasts, but most such tumors also are composed of cells that demonstrate cytologic or immunohistochemical features which allow classification as another type of tumor, such as a smooth muscle tumor, neurofibroma, or monophasic synovial sarcoma. Left within the fibrous tissue category are a group of tumors and tumor-like conditions composed entirely of fibrocytes, fibroblasts, and myofibroblasts, or mixtures of these three (Table 2-1). However, not all tumors composed of these cells are classified as fibrous; for example, investigation has revealed that the histiocyte-like cells in most fibrous histiocytomas are not bone marrow–derived histiocytes but rather primitive mesenchymal cells, fibroblasts, and myofibroblasts that take on phagocytic function. As a consequence, such tumors could just as well be classified as "fibrous" or "myofibroblastic." In spite of these revelations, we think little practical benefit would come from breaking up the fibrous histiocytoma category and reassigning most of its members to the fibrous tissue category because stability of classificatory systems is important to clinical care. These concepts are also discussed in the introduction to the fibrous histiocytoma chapter.

The term "fibroma" has been used for so many different benign soft tissue tumors and tumor-like conditions that any specificity the term may have once had has been lost. Consequently, we think that fibroma as a label for soft tissue and skin lesions should never be employed without a modifier, such as dermatofibroma, elastofibroma, or fibroma of tendon sheath (3). We part company with the World Health Organization (WHO) classification, which has a "fibroma" category, presumably to accommodate the humble skin tag or fibroepithelial polyp. This Fascicle does not include a discussion of any tumor designated solely as fibroma.

Early in the twentieth century, it was observed that fibrous proliferative disorders of the soft tissues demonstrated clinical behaviors that ranged from lesions that after excision are completely harmless and nonrecurring, to those with a variable incidence of recurrence, but not destructive recurrence, to those that display destructive and sometimes uncontrolled recurrence, to those capable of metastasis. Subsequently, the fibrous tumors were divided into three clinical management ("managerial") categories: benign, fibromatosis (intermediate), and fibrosarcoma which were intended to capture some of this varied behavior. Unfortunately, three categories inadequately described the clinical potential of fibrous tumors. As a result, tumors that don't fit well into one category sometimes get moved to another based on the latest information and the bias of the groups proposing the new classification. This trend can be seen most clearly among those fibrous proliferations that usually occur in infants and children. When these were initially described, they were placed in the fibromatosis category because many demonstrated recurring potential, even though the recurrences were seldom destructive or uncontrolled. In recent years, some soft tissue pathologists have preferred to label the fibrous proliferations of infancy and childhood that do not feature destructive recurrence as "benign." The WHO has codified this latter practice in their most recent classification by moving all the fibrous tumors that occur predominantly in infants and children (with the exception of digital fibromatosis and infantile desmoid fibromatosis) into the benign category. This taxonomous move still leaves the recurring but nondestructive plantar and palmar fibromatoses within the fibromatosis category and places lesions with fibromatosis in their label outside the fibromatosis category. We are not sure this is a significant advance and it is potentially confusing. These considerations notwithstanding, we have decided to follow the WHO classification with the exception of moving digital fibromatosis into the benign category.

Benign fibrous and myofibroblastic tumors as currently defined can be conveniently divided into two distinct clinical groups based on age at presentation. The first group is composed of tumors and

Table 2-1

FIBROUS AND MYOFIBROBLASTIC TUMORS

Benign
(Managerial Groups Ia and Ib, Table 1-10)

Nodular fasciitis, including cranial fasciitis
Proliferative myositis
Proliferative fasciitis
Ischemic fasciitis
Fibroma of tendon sheath
Elastofibroma
Desmoplastic fibroblastoma
Calcifying fibrous tumor/pseudotumor
Nuchal fibroma
Pleomorphic fibroma of skin
Solitary fibrous tumor of the soft parts*
Calcifying aponeurotic fibroma
Fibromatosis colli
Fibrous hamartoma of infancy
Inclusion body (digital) fibromatosis
Myofibroma, solitary and multicentric
Hyaline fibromatosis

Intermediate
(Managerial Groups IIa and IIc, Table 1-10)

Fibromatosis
  Superficial
    Palmar
    Plantar
  Deep
    Extra-abdominal (desmoid) fibromatosis
    Abdominal fibromatosis
    Intra-abdominal fibromatosis: pelvic, retro-
      peritoneal, and mesenteric
Inflammatory myofibroblastic tumor
Inflammatory myxohyaline tumor of distal extrem-
  ities (acral myxoinflammatory fibroblastic
  sarcoma)

Malignant
(Managerial Group III, Table 1-10)

Adult fibrosarcoma
Infantile and childhood fibrosarcoma**
Low-grade fibromyxoid sarcoma
Malignant solitary fibrous tumor (described in the
  solitary fibrous tumor sections)

---

*It is increasingly apparent that SFT with bland histology belongs in managerial group IIc, Table 1-10, i.e., among the "intermediate" tumors because rare examples can metastasize, but it is left here until the incidence is better known. The histologically malignant examples belong in the malignant category as noted in this table.
**This tumor belongs in managerial group IIc because metastases are so rare. We have left it in the group III (malignant) category because tumors with "sarcoma" in their title are definitionally "malignant." It is probably time to change the classification of this tumor.

tumor-like (reactive) conditions that occur more frequently in adults and includes nodular fasciitis, proliferative fasciitis, proliferative myositis, fibroma of tendon sheath, elastofibroma, desmoplastic fibroblastoma, solitary fibrous tumor, and keloid. Nodular fasciitis, proliferative fasciitis, and proliferative myositis share many histologic features and are undoubtedly variations of the same reparative theme. Historically, the creation of the several subdivisions of these reactive lesions was prompted by differential diagnostic considerations: for example, proliferative myositis mimicked rhabdomyosarcoma and nodular fasciitis mimicked fibrosarcoma. Accordingly, once a proliferation is recognized as reactive, little purpose is served by obsessing over its assignment to one of these groups. Again, what is important is recognizing the lesion as benign and harmless (1a). As a result of these observations Dahl and Angervall (2) suggested combining nodular fasciitis, proliferative fasciitis, and proliferative myositis under the term pseudosarcomatous proliferative lesions. While this suggestion has merit, it has not become popular. Myositis ossificans also is a part of this reactive group, but because the constituent cells form osteoid and bone, it is traditionally classified as a benign bony lesion.

The second group of fibrous proliferations currently classified as benign are those that occur predominantly in infants and children. While these are clinically benign in the sense they do not metastasize, some can recur, but the recurrences are practically never uncontrolled or destructive. The childhood fibrous proliferations currently placed in the benign category are fibrous hamartoma of infancy, calcifying fibrous tumor/ pseudotumor, myofibromatosis, fibromatosis colli, calcifying aponeurotic fibroma, hyaline fibromatosis and, by us, digital fibromatosis.

Intermediate fibrous tumors are divided into three categories: fibromatoses, inflammatory myofibroblastic tumors (inflammatory fibrosarcomas), and inflammatory myxohyaline tumor (acral myxoinflammatory fibroblastic sarcoma). The fibromatoses can recur, sometimes aggressively, but they do not metastasize. They are subdivided into the superficial growths, palmar and plantar fibromatoses, and the deep growths, which may be in the abdominal wall, intra-abdominal, or in the extra-abdominal soft tissues. The deep fibromatoses are variously labeled aggressive fibromatosis, extra-abdominal desmoid, or extra-abdominal fibromatosis when they occur outside the abdomen, abdominal fibromatosis or abdominal desmoid when they occur in the abdominal wall, and intra-abdominal and mesenteric fibromatosis when they occur within the abdominal cavity. The similar lesion that occurs in the soft tissues of infants and children is labeled infantile fibromatosis. Because of the fibromatoses' tendency to recur but their consistent failure to metastasize, it is very important that they be distinguished from benign fibrous proliferations on the one hand and from fibrosarcoma on the other. The frequency of recurrence and the potential for destructive or uncontrolled growth of any fibromatosis depends on the type of fibromatosis and its anatomic location. Consequently, fibromatosis, like fibroma, should not be used as a diagnosis without a modifier such as extra-abdominal fibromatosis or mesenteric fibromatosis; it is this modifier that carries the relevant prognostic information.

A recent addition to the intermediate category of fibrous and myofibroblastic tumors is extrapulmonary inflammatory myofibroblastic tumor, which has also been labeled "inflammatory pseudotumor" and "inflammatory fibrosarcoma." We agree with Coffin and associates (1) that the best label is inflammatory myofibroblastic tumor because while it definitely has recurring potential and, on rare occasions recurrences may be unmanageable, metastases are rare.

Until recently the only malignant member of the fibrous tumor family was fibrosarcoma. Because the metastasizing capability of this neoplasm is a strong function of the age of the patient (fibrosarcomas in individuals under the age of 5 years rarely metastasize), fibrosarcomas are subdivided into adult and congenital (or infantile) types. The other malignant fibrous tumor is the recently described low-grade fibromyxoid sarcoma.

Ultrastructurally, the constituent cells of all the fibrous lesions have the features of fibroblasts, myofibroblasts, or both, although in some lesions "primitive" mesenchymal cells have been described. Consequently, the ultrastructural features of the various lesions will not be further discussed except where they deviate from this basic pattern. Ultrastructurally, myofibroblasts differ from fibroblasts by their irregular "accordion-like" nuclei, abundant cytoplasmic fibrils, sometimes containing contractile bodies, discontinuous basal lamina, and subplasmalemmal attachment plaques. They differ from smooth muscle cells by having plentiful endoplasmic reticulin, a discontinuous basal lamina, and collagen production. Moreover, myofibroblasts may form cell surface structures known as fibronexus junctions in which intracytoplasmic filaments come in contact with plasmalemmal plaques attached to colinear extracellular fibronectin filaments. These are apparently unique to myofibroblasts.

The current WHO classification contains only one tumor classified as myofibroma(tosis), solitary and multicentric, and none as myofibroblastoma or myofibrosarcoma. However, there are reports in the literature of inflammatory myofibroblastic tumors (inflammatory fibrosarcomas) and a few tumors classified as myofibrosarcomas as well as reports of palisaded myofibroblastic tumors in lymph nodes (intranodal myofibroblastoma), myofibroblastomas of the breast, angiomyofibroblastomas of the vulva and vagina, dermatomyofibromas of the skin, and myofibroblastomas of the heart. The reader is referred to the appropriate Fascicle for a discussion of these proliferations. Given the ubiquitous nature of the myofibroblast, we anticipate that the number of tumors reported with myofibro- in their title may well reach considerable proportions in the near future (4).

BENIGN FIBROUS TUMORS (MANAGERIAL GROUPS Ia AND Ib, TABLE 1-10)

The tumors and tumor-like conditions that are included in the benign fibrous category are listed in the classification in Table 2-1.

Nodular Fasciitis

Definition. Nodular fasciitis is a non-neoplastic, reactive process composed of fibroblasts and myofibroblasts with uniform, vesicular to dense nuclei arranged in gently undulating "C-" and "S-" shaped bundles (5,6,11,14,18–20). Neither significant nuclear pleomorphism or abnormal mitotic figures are definitionally allowed in nodular fasciitis.

General Considerations. Nodular fasciitis is a common lesion and is notorious for the ease with which it can be misinterpreted by the inexperienced, and sometimes by the experienced pa-

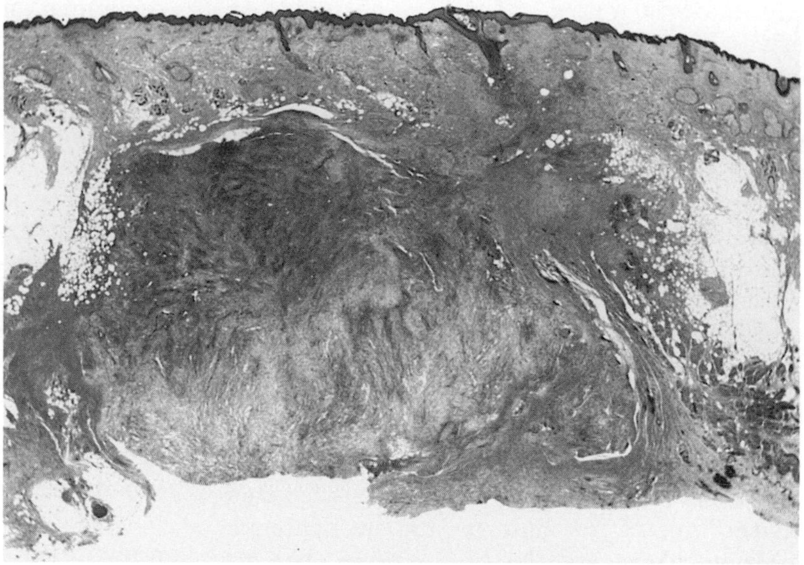

Figure 2-1
NODULAR FASCIITIS
Subcutaneous nodular fasciitis showing a partially circumscribed nodule infiltrating focally along fascial planes.

thologist, as a malignant neoplasm. However, it is also easy to make the opposite mistake: misinterpreting a malignant neoplasm or a neoplasm with recurring potential as nodular fasciitis. Traditionally, proliferations with the features of nodular fasciitis have been labeled ossifying fasciitis or fasciitis ossificans when they contain metaplastic bone, parosteal fasciitis when they are located in the periosteum and contain bone, intravascular fasciitis when they intrude into vascular lumens, intramuscular fasciitis when they involve skeletal muscle, and cranial fasciitis when they involve the skull and soft tissues of the scalp of infants and children. Moreover, further splitting has been occasioned by the variable histologic appearance of nodular fasciitis. These subspecies include the hyaline variant and the giant cell variant of nodular fasciitis; they are described in the Pathologic Findings section below.

Clinical Features. Nodular fasciitis occurs at all ages, but it most commonly develops between 20 and 40 years of age. It is uncommon in infants and children and rare past the age of 65 or 70. It can occur in so many sites that the location of the lesion is not diagnostically helpful, but the upper extremities, particularly the forearms, are the most frequently involved, followed by the trunk. For some unknown reason, nodular fasciitis is unusual in the lower extremities and it is reported to be rare on the hands

and feet. Most cases of nodular fasciitis in the head and neck occur in infants and children.

Nodular fasciitis also occurs at different anatomic depths in soft tissues. The subcutaneous tissue is the most common site of involvement but intramuscular lesions are relatively frequent and sometimes nodular fasciitis occurs along fascial planes. Intermuscular and periosteal lesions have also been described. Intradermal lesions are uncommon (9).

Nodular fasciitis grows rapidly so that most patients give a history of a lump of at most a few weeks' duration. Pain is not usually a complaint but the lesions are often tender. Multiple lesions are rare.

Gross Findings. At the time of removal, nodular fasciitis often appears infiltrative and gross inspection of the lesion almost always fails to reveal a capsule. The lesion is usually small, less than 3 cm in diameter; in fact, most examples are 2 cm or less. We think a diagnosis of nodular fasciitis should be made with great caution when the lesion is greater than 4 or 5 cm in diameter. Indeed, consultation may be considered if a diagnosis of nodular fasciitis is being entertained for a lesion larger than 4 to 5 cm. On cut section, nodular fasciitis varies from mucoid or myxoid to fibrous.

Microscopic Findings. The typical case of nodular fasciitis has several features that aid in its recognition (figs. 2-1–2-5). First, the constituent cells have uniform elongate nuclei; significant

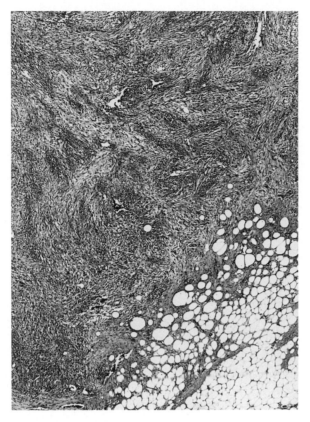

Figure 2-2
NODULAR FASCIITIS
Focal infiltration into subcutaneous fat. In this relatively mature example, granulation tissue-like vessels are distributed uniformly throughout the lesion.

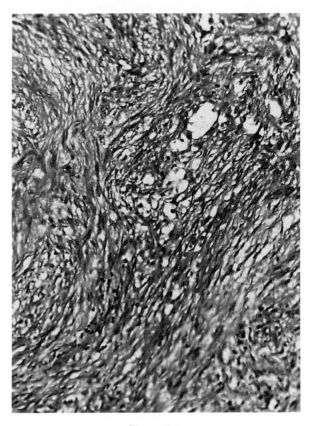

Figure 2-3
NODULAR FASCIITIS
Gently curving C- and S-shaped fascicles of myofibroblastic cells exhibit the characteristic "torn Kleenex" pattern of nodular fasciitis featuring myxoid change.

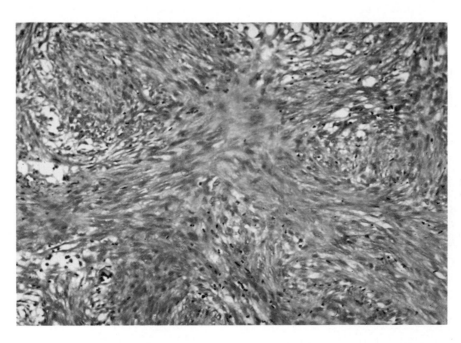

Figure 2-4
NODULAR FASCIITIS
A focal storiform pattern raises the possibility of a fibrous histiocytoma.

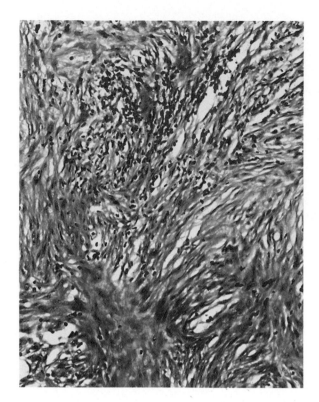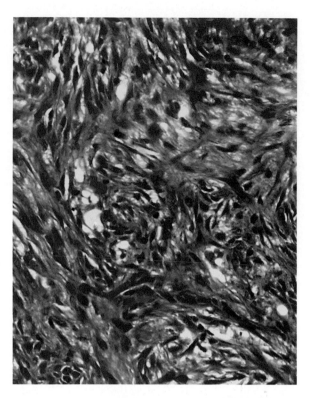

Figure 2-5
NODULAR FASCIITIS
Left: Plump spindled myofibroblastic cells and scattered extravasated red blood cells are seen.
Right: Mitotic figures may be numerous but abnormal forms are not present.

pleomorphism is not present. These nuclei are often enlarged and when they are, they are usually vesicular with an easily seen small nucleolus; smaller, more dense nuclei are less common and when cells with such nuclei are plentiful and set within a collagenous stroma, an alternative diagnosis should be considered, particularly fibromatosis or some type of fibrous histiocytoma. Cytoplasmic margins are most often indistinct, but the cells can, on occasion, possess abundant, lightly eosinophilic cytoplasm. Second, the uniform cells that compose nodular fasciitis are most often loosely arranged in C- or S-shaped bundles that intersect one another at various angles; a storiform pattern is not uncommon (fig. 2-4). Third, in many examples, stromal mucin accumulates in small irregular pools, giving rise to what appears to be "holes" or "tears" in the fabric of the tumor (fig. 2-5). This appearance has been characterized as "feathery" or "tissue culture-like." Fourth, normal and sometimes easily found mitotic figures are sufficiently

common to serve as a useful clue that one might be dealing with nodular fasciitis when other features are consistent (fig. 2-5). If abnormal mitotic figures are found in a purported nodular fasciitis, one should strongly consider the possibility of a malignant neoplasm, particularly myxoid malignant fibrous histiocytoma. Fifth, the blood vessels in nodular fasciitis are small and thin-walled and, in many examples, have an arborizing pattern. Sixth, extravasated intact red blood cells, presumably dislodged from these delicate vessels by the sectioning, are commonly scattered about the stroma, but hemosiderin and foamy macrophages are rare (fig. 2-5). Finally, inflammatory cells, usually lymphocytes, can be scattered through the tumor, but when present, are more common at the periphery.

The "buzz" words, then, for nodular fasciitis are: cells with enlarged, vesicular but uniform nuclei, arranged in gently undulating C- or S-shaped bundles; a torn or feathery background; easily found normal mitotic figures; an organized vascular

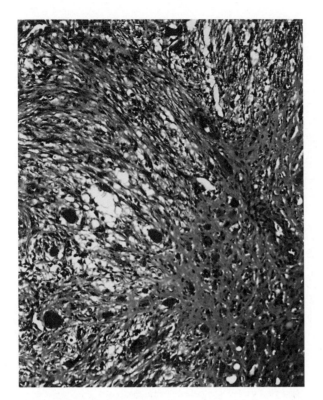 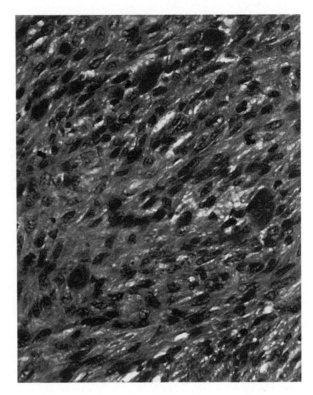

Figure 2-6
NODULAR FASCIITIS

Left: This example has a more collagenous stroma focally and involves skeletal muscle.

Right: Osteoclastic giant cells are present in the less collagenous areas. When osteoclastic giant cells are found it raises the possibility of giant cell tumor of soft parts, a subtype of malignant fibrous histiocytoma that, unlike nodular fasciitis, features nuclear pleomorphism and abnormal mitotic figures.

pattern; extravasated red blood cells; and scattered inflammatory cells. The edges of the lesion blend into or infiltrate the surrounding normal tissue. Variations are common and have given rise to the practice of naming morphologic "variants" of nodular fasciitis. Multinucleated giant cells usually resembling osteoclasts (giant cell variant), and rarely, foam cells, may be found in some cases (fig. 2-6). When nodular fasciitis is intramuscular, damaged muscle fibers with enlarged dense and sometimes multiple nuclei may be present at the edge of the lesion and can raise the possibility of sarcoma. Hyalinization in the form of smooth, amorphous, faintly pink-staining material or thick hyalinized collagen bundles is not infrequently seen and can be prominent in some examples (hyaline variant) (figs. 2-7, 2-8). Sometimes the hyaline is so extensive that the lesion resembles a keloid. Sometimes the constituent cells may surround fibrin and mucin in a pattern

reminiscent of a healing wound (repair variant). Arborizing vessels are particularly prominent in this variant. Sometimes connective tissue mucin accumulates to such an extent that large spaces are formed (cystic variant) (fig. 2-8).

Bone formation in nodular fasciitis is unusual, but occurs most commonly when the lesion is in or near the periosteum (fig. 2-9) (7,10,12). Either parosteal fasciitis or fibro-osseous pseudotumor of the digits is the term usually used when nodular fasciitis in this location contains bone; when nodular fasciitis away from the periosteum contains bone, the lesion is sometimes classified as ossifying fasciitis. Ossifying fasciitis shares many features with, and is basically the same lesion as, myositis ossificans except that the zonal arrangement of bone often found in myositis ossificans is largely absent in ossifying fasciitis, and myositis ossificans by definition occurs within skeletal muscle. We use the label myositis ossificans

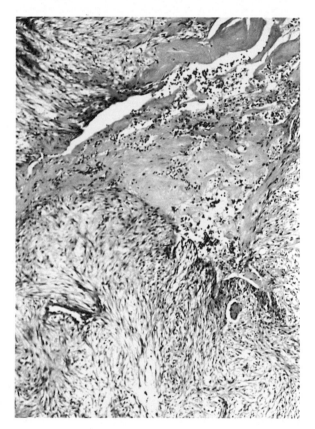

Figure 2-7
NODULAR FASCIITIS,
HYALINE VARIANT
As nodular fasciitis matures it
becomes hyalinized and may sim-
ulate keloid or fibromatosis.

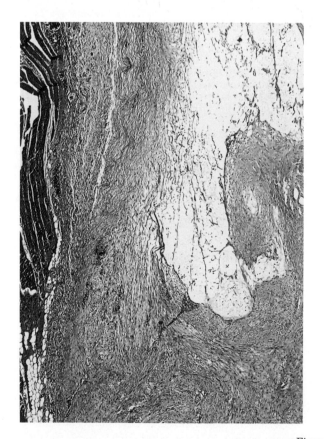

Figure 2-8
NODULAR FASCIITIS WITHIN SKELETAL MUSCLE
Cystic degeneration can be seen in the center of the lesion, a common development in nodular fasciitis.

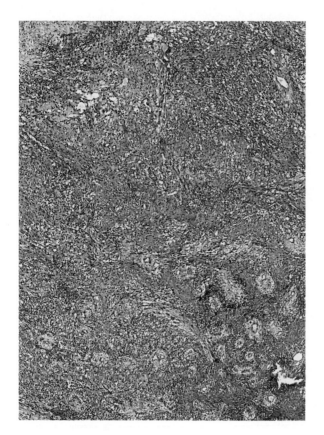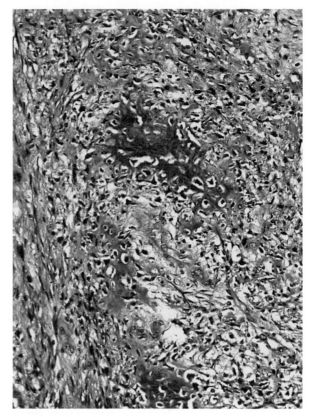

Figure 2-9
PAROSTEAL FASCIITIS
Left: A cellular proliferation features a vague zonation pattern, with nodular fasciitis regions in the upper left and new bone formation in the lower right.
Right: An island of new bone set within a sea of myofibroblastic cells.

when the X ray reveals the very characteristic veil-like pattern of ossification of this intramuscular lesion and the histologic sections reveal prominent and diffuse bone formation. Nodular or ossifying fasciitis is the term used when bone is focally present in a lesion that is otherwise nodular fasciitis either within or away from muscle.

Rarely, nodular fasciitis grows within the lumens of small veins and arteries (fig. 2-10) (16). When it does so, three different patterns may be observed. In the first, the lesion has the appearance of ordinary nodular fasciitis except that there is focal intrusion of lesional tissue into vessels, usually at the edge. In the second, there is considerable lesional tissue within vascular lumens but there are also areas of nodular fasciitis outside vessels. In the third, the lesion is predominantly or exclusively intravascular. In the latter situation, the tumor often becomes multinodular and plugs

of lesional tissue may extend along the lumens of the vessels. Histologically, the only difference the intravascular component displays is a greater tendency for multinucleated osteoclast-like giant cells to develop. Cranial fasciitis involves both the skull and the soft tissues of the scalp, usually in infants (13,17). It grows rapidly and characteristically erodes the outer and sometimes the inner table of the skull. In the latter circumstance, the dura and meninges may be involved. The histologic appearance is that of classic nodular fasciitis, although giant cells are common, necrosis may be present, and reactive bone may form, particularly at the edges of the lesion.

Special Studies. Immunohistochemistry is of limited value in diagnosing nodular fasciitis because the constituent cells are fibroblasts and myofibroblasts, the same cells that populate the many other types of soft tissue proliferations

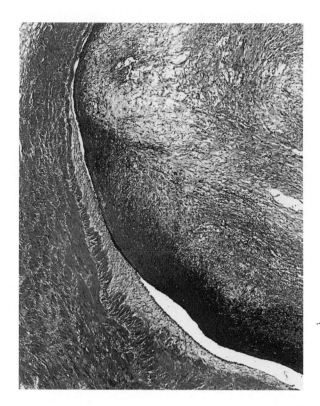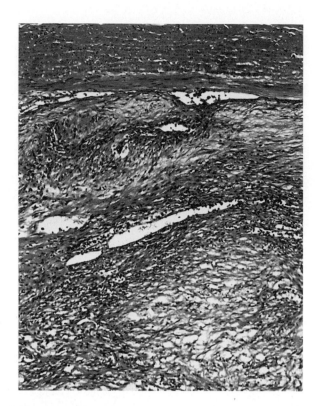

Figure 2-10
INTRAVASCULAR FASCIITIS
Left: A large focus of nodular fasciitis protrudes into a vascular space.
Right: The proliferation features the edematous background characteristic of nodular fasciitis.

with which nodular fasciitis may be confused. Immunohistochemistry can be important, however, in excluding another type of tumor that expresses antigens not expected in fibroblasts and myofibroblasts. Reports indicate that, not surprisingly, the cells in nodular fasciitis almost always (more than 95 percent) express actin (both smooth muscle actin [SMA] and muscle-specific actin [MSA]) and CD68 (KP1). They do not express S-100 protein or keratin (15). Nodular fasciitis has a flow cytometric profile compatible with a reactive process (8).

Differential Diagnosis. Nodular fasciitis can mimic lesions in all three managerial classes: 1) other benign processes, 2) lesions with recurring potential, and 3) sarcomas. Nodular fasciitis has features in common with proliferative fasciitis/ myositis and fibroma of tendon sheath. Each of these is described in this chapter; however, distinguishing among them is of little clinical importance, except to note that about a quarter of

fibromas of tendon sheath recur but not destructively. The nonosseous stroma of myositis ossificans is essentially identical to that of nodular fasciitis, but myositis ossificans is an intramuscular lesion which also features a diffuse zonal distribution of osteoid and bone that is frequently appreciated radiographically. Intramuscular myxoma and juxta-articular myxoma can resemble nodular fasciitis because of their myxoid stroma, but the former is usually far less cellular, and neither have cells arranged in bundles, a tissue culture appearance, or significant mitotic activity.

Benign neural tumors usually can be easily distinguished from nodular fasciitis on the basis of hematoxylin and eosin (H&E)-stained sections, but if there is doubt, an S-100 protein stain can be performed. This is essentially always positive in benign neural tumors and negative in nodular fasciitis. Among the lesions with recurring potential that can be confused with nodular fasciitis, the most difficult to distinguish are the subcutaneous and deep benign fibrous histiocytomas and plexiform fibrous histiocytoma. These fibrous histiocytomas have a more well-developed, solid collagenous stroma than nodular fasciitis and their constituent spindled cells usually have, at least focally, smaller and denser nuclei characteristic of mature fibrocytes. Mitotic figures are usually numerous in nodular fasciitis and often difficult to find in fibrous histiocytomas. Rounded histiocyte-like cells with abundant, easily discerned cytoplasm are prominent in many fibrous histiocytomas and rare in nodular fasciitis, although multinucleated giant cells may be found in both. Foam cells favor a fibrous histiocytoma. Not infrequently, it is impossible to distinguish between a benign fibrous histiocytoma and nodular fasciitis and in this case, we state the uncertainty and warn that recurrence is possible. This differential diagnosis is also discussed in the fibrous histiocytoma chapter and summarized in Table 3-3.

Desmoid fibromatosis is almost always over 3 cm; usually it is around 8 to 10 cm. Although focal myxoid areas are not uncommon in these tumors, the stroma also contains abundant birefringent collagen, a feature not present in nodular fasciitis, and the constituent cells are more often than not mature fibrocytes with small dense nuclei. Larger cells with open nuclei identical to those found in nodular fasciitis can be found in desmoid tumors but the cells are seldom arranged in undulating short bundles; rather they are arranged in larger, more linear fascicles and the "tearing" appearance so often seen in nodular fasciitis is usually inconspicuous or absent.

We think distinction of nodular fasciitis from sarcoma is aided by evaluating four features: size of the lesion, cellular pleomorphism, abnormal mitotic figures, and chromatin abnormalities. Sarcomas are usually over 4 cm, whereas nodular fasciitis is almost always smaller than this. Abnormal mitotic figures are common in sarcoma; for all practical purposes, they are not found in nodular fasciitis. The chromatin in the cells of many sarcomas is coarse, granular, dense, and irregularly distributed. It is fine, pale, and evenly distributed in most examples of nodular fasciitis. Pleomorphism is a common feature of sarcoma; significant pleomorphism is not present in nodular fasciitis.

Low-grade fibrosarcoma is the sarcoma most likely to be confused with nodular fasciitis. However, in fibrosarcoma the nuclear chromatin of the constituent cells is denser, the myxomatous and "torn" background of nodular fasciitis is missing, and the cells are arranged in more orderly and well-formed bundles than those that develop in nodular fasciitis. Moreover, fibrosarcoma is far less common than nodular fasciitis.

Low-grade fibromyxoid sarcoma features whirled fibrous tissue with a collagenous stroma focally, lacks the tissue culture appearance of nodular fasciitis, and it is usually larger and deeper than most cases of nodular fasciitis.

Treatment and Prognosis. Nearly 99 percent of patients with nodular fasciitis are cured by the initial excision. Recurrence is so rare that it should prompt a reevaluation of the histologic sections of the original lesion. Bernstein and Lattes (6) reported that all cases purported to be a recurrence of nodular fasciitis in their files were actually another lesion, but we have observed recurrences in rare cases that have been incompletely excised. Spontaneous regression of nodular fasciitis has been observed and it is probable that reexcision of incompletely removed lesions is not necessary.

Proliferative Myositis

Definition. Proliferative myositis is an intramuscular reactive process in which variable numbers of round cells with large nuclei, prominent nucleoli, and abundant amphophilic cytoplasm ("ganglion-like cells") are interspersed among generally elongate fibroblasts and myofibroblasts, and bundles of residual skeletal muscle fibers. The lesion is identical in appearance to proliferative fasciitis except for its location in skeletal muscle.

Clinical Features. Patients are usually seen by a physician because they have detected a mass that characteristically has been present for only a short time; pain is unusual (23,24). Most patients are middle-aged or older and the upper arm and trunk are the most commonly involved sites, although some lesions develop in the lower extremities. On rare occasions children develop this lesion (26).

Pathologic Findings. Grossly, proliferative myositis is a firm, irregularly shaped mass seated

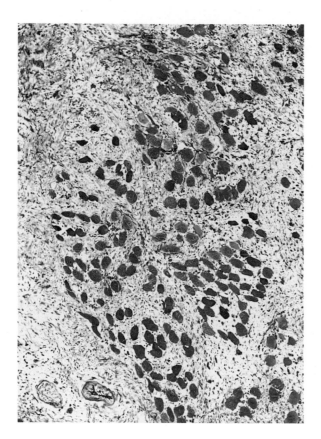 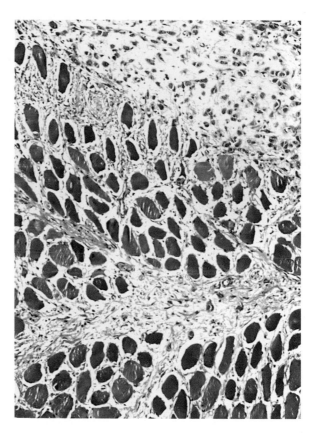

Figure 2-11
PROLIFERATIVE MYOSITIS
The characteristic checkerboard pattern is produced by the expansion of the space between muscle bundles and between individual muscle fibers by this reactive proliferation.

within skeletal muscle; most lesions are 3 to 4 cm in diameter. Histologically, plump fibroblasts and myofibroblasts accompanied by variable numbers of ganglion-like cells expand the connective tissue space separating muscle fibers, which remain relatively unchanged by this process. When fully developed, this expansion of the endomysium produces the celebrated "checkerboard" pattern in which patches of residual muscle represent the red squares of the checkerboard (figs. 2-11, 2-12). The constituent fibroblasts have nuclei whose appearance ranges from enlarged, uniform, and vesicular to small, uniform, and dense, but the striking feature is the sprinkling of large ganglion-like cells. They cause this reactive process to be pleomorphic because they are large in comparison to the smaller fibroblasts, and pleomorphism can be worrisome because it is a feature of some sarcomas. However, close inspection fails to reveal convincing nuclear features of

malignancy. The ganglion-like cells possess large, round, generally smooth nuclei with prominent nucleoli, basophilic cytoplasm, and evenly dispersed chromatin (fig. 2-12). Mitotic figures may be present, but are invariably normal. Occasionally, these cells form clusters and mimic epithelial cells by molding to one another. Reactive bone or cartilage is present in about 20 percent of the cases, providing a link to myositis ossificans (fig. 2-13). The residual muscle ordinarily does not demonstrate evidence of injury; that is, there is no sarcolemmal proliferation, no multinucleation, no nuclear enlargement, and no evidence of muscle necrosis. The overall appearance is one which suggests the proliferating reactive cells are expanding the space between intact muscle cells. The lesion in children differs from that in the adult in its better circumscription, its lobularity, its greater cellularity, and the presence of focal necrosis (26).

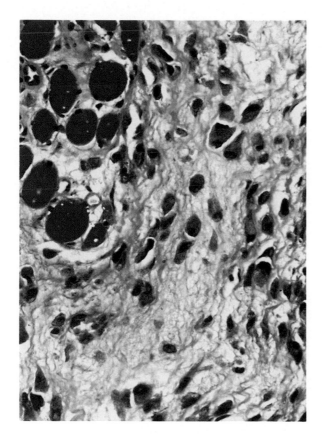
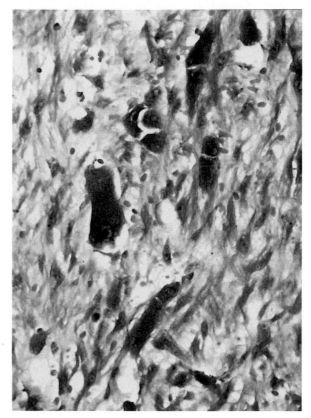

Figure 2-12
PROLIFERATIVE MYOSITIS

Large ganglion-like cells are the hallmark of this reactive proliferation. They may, as in this example, crowd and mold one another thereby simulating an epithelial malignancy (left). These myofibroblastic ganglion-like cells feature amphophilic cytoplasm and prominent nucleoli (right).

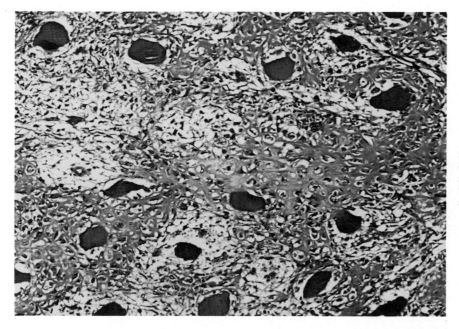

Figure 2-13
PROLIFERATIVE MYOSITIS WITH METAPLASTIC BONE

Metaplastic bone of the sort seen in myositis ossificans may be encountered. This emphasizes the substantial morphologic overlap of the reactive proliferations of the soft tissues.

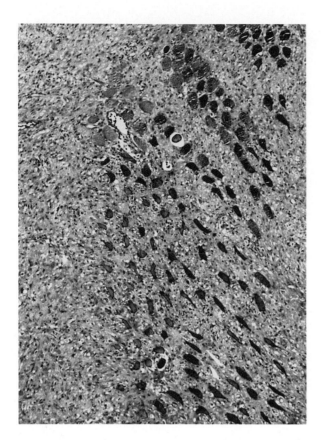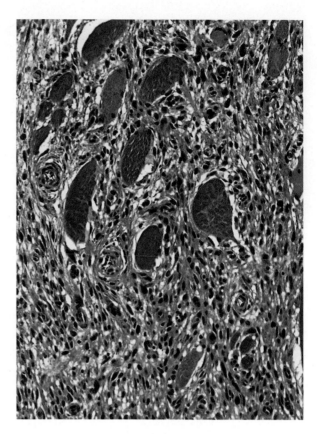

Figure 2-14
A MIMIC OF PROLIFERATIVE MYOSITIS
Left: This spindle cell sarcoma has infiltrated skeletal muscle without producing myocyte death, thereby producing a checkerboard pattern.
Right: Higher power view shows high cellularity and atypical spindle cells.

Special Studies. The spindled cells of proliferative myositis express actin but, in the few tumors which have been examined, they do not express desmin (22). The ganglion-like cells may be actin negative (25). Neuron-specific enolase and S-100 protein are also negative. Ultrastructurally, the ganglion-like cells are enlarged, rounded fibroblasts (22,27,28). Proliferative myositis has a flow cytometric profile consistent with a reactive process (21,25).

Differential Diagnosis. Proliferative myositis differs from proliferative fasciitis only by its location within skeletal muscle. It differs from intramuscular nodular fasciitis by its ganglion-like cells and characteristic pattern of involvement of muscle whereby skeletal muscle fibers are left intact within the lesion. Nodular fasciitis almost always completely obliterates muscle except at the edges of the lesion and nodular fasciitis

does not contain ganglion-like cells. Desmoid fibromatosis completely replaces muscle except at its borders, does not contain ganglion-like cells, and its stroma is mainly collagenized and only focally myxoid. Moreover, skeletal muscle fibers at the edge of fibromatosis almost always reveal evidence of injury, a feature not seen in proliferative myositis. Desmoid tumors are almost always over 3 cm in diameter.

The features discussed in the differential diagnosis section of nodular fasciitis that help distinguish sarcoma from reactive processes also apply to proliferative myositis. Although sarcomas usually destroy all skeletal muscle fibers in their path, a checkerboard pattern can occasionally be found when a malignant neoplasm infiltrates skeletal muscle (fig. 2-14). Similarly, invasive carcinoma may produce this pattern. Therefore, a checkerboard pattern is not specific for proliferative myositis and when it is encountered, there should be a careful consideration of the size of the lesion, the size and shape of the constituent cells, their nuclear chromatin patterns, and the presence and appearance of mitotic figures.

The other differential diagnoses for proliferative myositis are the same as for nodular fasciitis.

Treatment and Prognosis. Proliferative myositis is a reactive process cured by excision. If a lesion diagnosed as proliferative myositis recurs, the initial sections should be carefully reevaluated because a diagnostic error has probably occurred.

Proliferative Fasciitis

Definition. Proliferative fasciitis is a subcutaneous or fascial reactive process in which variable numbers of round cells with large nuclei, prominent nucleoli, and abundant amphophilic cytoplasm ("ganglion-like cells") are interspersed among generally elongate fibroblasts and myofibroblasts. The process is identical to proliferative myositis except for its extramuscular location.

Clinical Features. Proliferative fasciitis occurs mainly in middle-aged and older individuals and is rare in children (29,37). This is in contrast to nodular fasciitis, which is most common in adolescents and young adults and also occurs in children. Most of the lesions occur in the forearm and thigh and, like nodular fasciitis, most measure under 3 cm. It is extremely rare for a lesion of proliferative fasciitis to be over 4 cm. This lesion often has a rapid clinical evolution over 1 to 3 weeks and, by definition, it involves fascia or subcutaneous tissue. A related condition, *atypical decubital fibroplasia* or *ischemic fasciitis,* is a reactive process that occurs in regions prone to develop decubitus ulcers (34,36).

Pathologic Findings. The gross appearance is usually similar to that of nodular fasciitis, but when proliferative fasciitis involves fascia it may extend in a linear fashion. The microscopic appearance is identical to that of nodular fasciitis except that variable numbers of ganglion-like cells with abundant amphophilic to basophilic cytoplasm and large nuclei with prominent nucleoli are scattered throughout the lesion (figs. 2-15–2-17). These can vary in number from sparse to so numerous they dominate the lesion or are the exclusive cell type. Most of the ganglion-like cells are mononuclear, but some may be binucleate or even trinucleate. An arborizing vascular pattern resembling that in granulation tissue is often present and fibrin may be present centrally. Involvement of long segments of fascial planes is common, as is infiltration (fig. 2-16). The matrix is usually myxoid or edematous, but collagen is present in some lesions and hyalinization may be prominent. Grouping of cells and molding may be seen occasionally and raises the possibility of an epithelial proliferation.

Proliferative fasciitis in children tends to be more lobular than infiltrating and to be highly cellular, with a predominant population of ganglion-like fibroblasts, some of which may be elongate (33). Consequently, granulation tissue type fibroblasts, as seen in nodular fasciitis and in adult lesions of proliferative fasciitis, are sparse or absent. Acute inflammation and necrosis are also common in childhood cases.

Special Studies. Immunohistochemically, the elongate cells express smooth muscle actin (SMA), while ganglion-like cells are frequently actin negative. Desmin and S-100 protein have been reported to be negative in both types of cells (32). Ultrastructurally, the ganglion-like cells of proliferative fasciitis have the features of modified myofibroblastic cells (30,32). Proliferative fasciitis has a flow cytometric profile consistent with a reactive process (31,32,35).

Differential Diagnosis. Distinction from nodular fasciitis is based on the presence of ganglion-like cells. Proliferative fasciitis and proliferative myositis are identical histologically, only their location differs: proliferative fasciitis occurs in the subcutaneous tissue and fascia, while proliferative myositis occurs within skeletal muscle. It is possible that the ganglion-like cells in proliferative fasciitis could be confused with the ganglion cells in ganglioneuroma, but the stromal background is wrong for that tumor and the cells in proliferative fasciitis do not express ganglionic markers immunohistochemically. The ganglion-like cells sometimes cause the observer to think of rhabdomyoblasts, but they do not demonstrate cross-striations histologically or skeletal features ultrastructurally, and immunohistochemically desmin is absent. The remaining differential diagnoses of proliferative fasciitis are the same as those for nodular

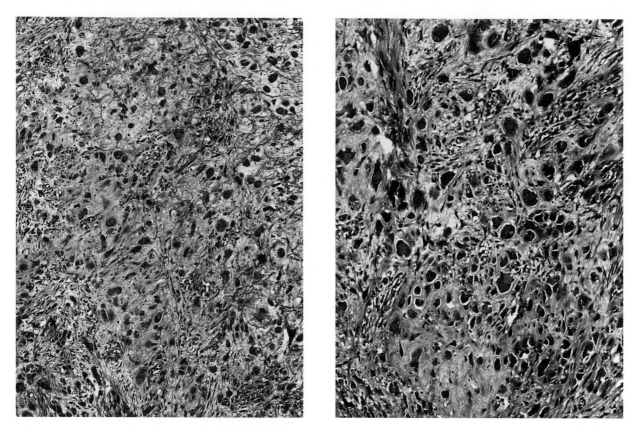

Figure 2-15
PROLIFERATIVE FASCIITIS
Left: Large ganglion-like cells are admixed with inflammatory cells and set within a vaguely hyalinized to myxoid stroma.
Right: The ganglion-like cells have amphophilic cytoplasm and prominent nucleoli.

Figure 2-16
PROLIFERATIVE FASCIITIS
A low-power view shows prominent hemorrhage and a vague centering of a cellular proliferation on the interlobular septa of the subcutaneous fat.

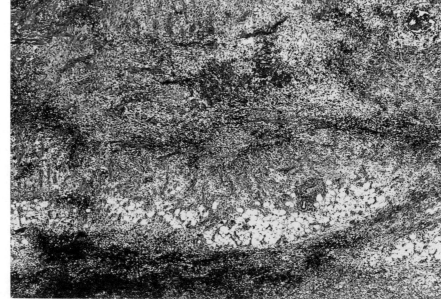

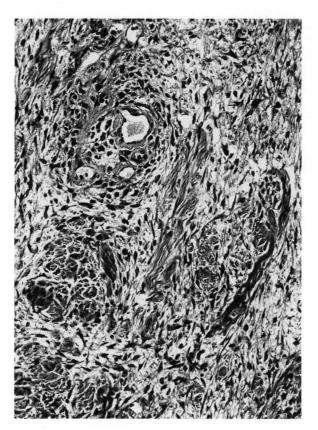 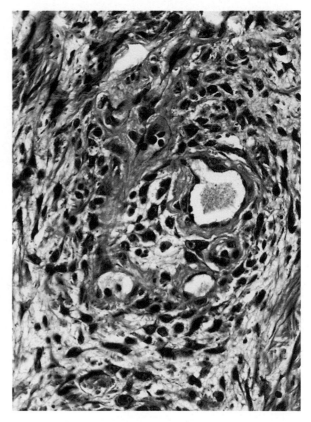

Figure 2-17
PROLIFERATIVE FASCIITIS
Left: Higher power view of figure 2-16 shows the typical admixture of ganglion-like cells, myofibroblastic cells, and inflammatory cells of proliferative fasciitis.
Right: Ganglion-like cells are condensed around a thin-walled vascular channel.

fasciitis. Sarcoma is a particularly pertinent part of the differential diagnosis because the dual population of cells might be construed as evidence of pleomorphism. Abnormal mitotic figures, nuclear chromatin abnormalities, nuclear membrane irregularities, and a large mass are features commonly present in sarcoma but not in proliferative fasciitis (see figs. 2-20, 2-21).

Treatment and Prognosis. Proliferative fasciitis is benign and does not recur after excision.

Ischemic Fasciitis
(Atypical Decubital Fibroplasia)

Definition. Ischemic fasciitis is a fibroblastic reactive mass lesion that occurs over bony prominences or in relationship to periosteum.

Clinical Features. Almost all the patients are elderly and immobilized (34,36). Most of the lesions develop over bony prominences, usually around the hips and shoulders, and present as nonulcerated masses. The chest wall may also be involved.

Pathologic Findings. Grossly, ischemic fasciitis is a mass that measures 1 to 9 cm, with a median size of about 4 cm (34,36). Histologically, the lesions are multinodular with rims of granulation tissue growing around lobules of adipose tissue that are necrotic or demonstrate myxoid change (fig. 2-18). The necrosis varies from fibrinoid to coagulative, and "ghosts" of fat cells are often visible within the necrosis. The reactive areas peripheral to the necrosis or myxoid tissue resemble granulation tissue or proliferative fasciitis and ganglion-like cells are often present (fig. 2-19). The ganglion-like cells can have quite large, irregular nuclei with dense, but often smudged chromatin and prominent nucleoli so they appear more atypical than the ganglion-like cells seen

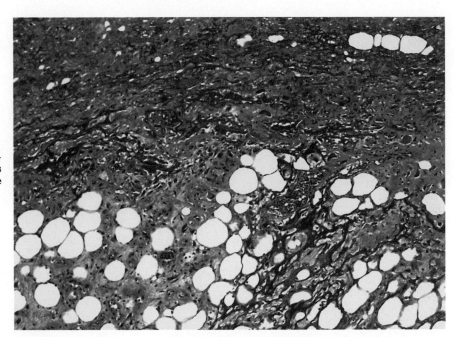

Figure 2-18
ISCHEMIC FASCIITIS
(ATYPICAL DECUBITAL
FIBROPLASIA)

A cellular, fibrin-rich proliferation is centered on a subcutaneous fibrous septum and extends into the adjacent fat.

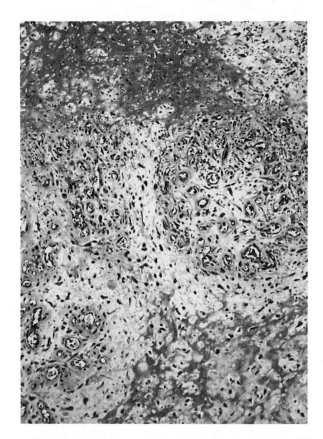

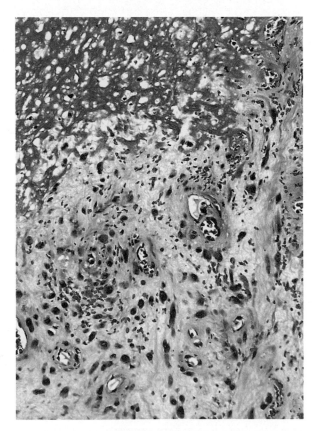

Figure 2-19
ISCHEMIC FASCIITIS (ATYPICAL DECUBITAL FIBROPLASIA)

Left: A hyalinized focus with large ganglion-like cells is reminiscent of proliferative fasciitis.
Right: Fibrin is adjacent to a collection of ganglion-like myofibroblastic cells embedded in collagenized stroma.

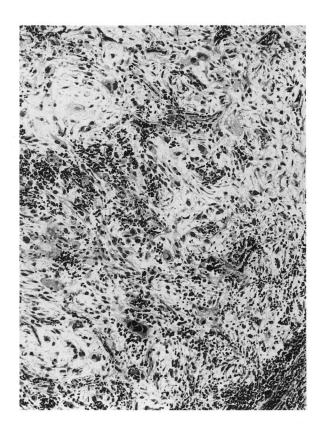 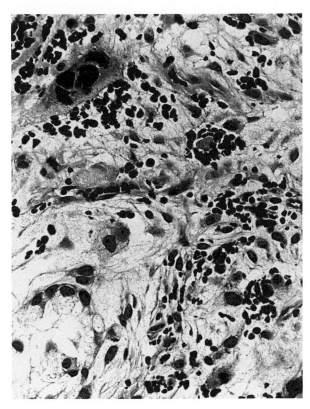

Figure 2-20
MYXOID MALIGNANT FIBROUS HISTIOCYTOMA
Left: This mimic of ischemic or proliferative fasciitis has a low density of ganglion-like cells distributed in a myxoid stroma.
Right: Bizarre cells such as this should prompt consideration of malignant myxoid lesions other than fasciitis.

in the usual proliferative fasciitis. Perivascular cuffing by ganglion-like cells is sometimes prominent and fibrin thrombi may be present. Mitotic figures are often easily found but abnormal forms are distinctly rare. Overall, the appearance of the reactive areas closely resembles proliferative fasciitis except for the more atypical appearance of the ganglion-like cells.

Immunohistochemical staining reveals that some but not all lesions contain actin and CD68-positive cells; these are usually focal.

Differential Diagnosis. The main differential diagnostic consideration is to avoid interpreting ischemic fasciitis as a sarcoma. The combination of enlarged pleomorphic ganglion-like cells, easily found mitotic figures, and an often sizable mass all contribute to the mimicry of sarcoma. However, ischemic fasciitis is usually less cellular than most sarcomas, does not feature abnormal mitotic figures, and overall closely resembles (and is probably a form of) proliferative fasciitis.

The cells in myxoid liposarcoma are not as pleomorphic as those in ischemic fasciitis and the latter lacks the arborizing vascular pattern of the former. The cells in myxoid chondrosarcoma are more uniform than those in ischemic fasciitis and the stroma is more uniformly myxoid. Myxoid MFH (myxofibrosarcoma) often contains cells whose nuclei are cytologically malignant and such cells seldom resemble ganglion cells (figs. 2-20, 2-21). Abnormal mitotic figures are common in myxoid MFH and this tumor is usually more cellular than ischemic fasciitis.

Misinterpretation of ischemic fasciitis as another type of reactive or reparative process is of little importance if infection is excluded. The most likely benign lesion to be mistaken for ischemic fasciitis is proliferative fasciitis.

Treatment and Prognosis. Ischemic fasciitis may recur but does not do so aggressively and does not metastasize (34,36). Incompletely resected lesions may not increase in size.

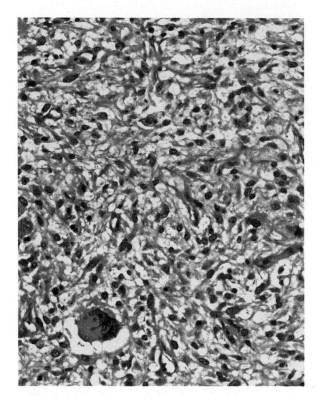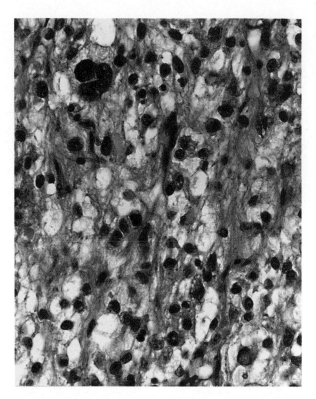

Figure 2-21
MYXOID MALIGNANT FIBROUS HISTIOCYTOMA

Left: Same case as figure 2-20 showing more typical cellular areas of myxoid malignant fibrous histiocytoma containing giant cells similar to those encountered in the myxoid areas.

Right: Higher power view.

Fibroma of Tendon Sheath

Definition. Fibroma of tendon sheath (FTS) is a circumscribed, often multinodular, fibroblastic process that almost always occurs in the extremities, most often in the hand and wrist. It typically features a prominent hyalinized stroma, at least focally.

Clinical Features. FTS occurs at all ages, but is most common in adults between 20 and 50 years of age (38–41). More than three fourths develop in the wrist, hand, and fingers; occasional examples are encountered in the forearms and toes, but essentially in no other sites. FTSs grow more slowly than the usual nodular fasciitis; it is not uncommon for patients to have been aware of the mass for over 6 months and sometimes for years. These lesions are seldom painful. It is rare for FTS to be over 2 cm in diameter and none of the reported examples have been over 6 cm.

Gross Findings. Although many FTSs are attached to a tendon sheath, not all are in that location. Outside the tendon sheath, the most common location is the superficial soft tissues. All examples are well circumscribed and most are multinodular. The cut surface is tan-white and the consistency is rubbery to firm.

Microscopic Findings. At low-power magnification the hallmark of FTS is circumscription and lobularity (fig. 2-22). The lobules of tumor are separated by thin spaces; if the lobules separate during processing, they may appear on the slide as separate. At higher magnification, the lesion ranges from paucicellular with a prominence of collagenized fibrous tissue to highly cellular with inconspicuous background collagen (fig. 2-23). The cellular areas have all or nearly all the features of nodular fasciitis. Although the paucicellular pattern usually predominates, in most tumors the two patterns blend into one another, at least focally. This results in considerable variation in cellularity from lesion to lesion and from area to area within the same lesion.

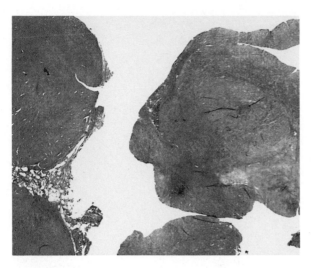 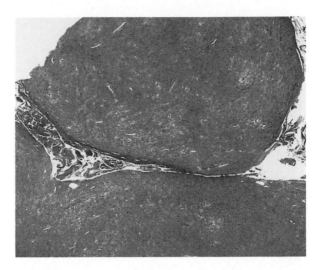

Figure 2-22
FIBROMA OF TENDON SHEATH

Left: A characteristically multinodular proliferation.

Right: The extensive collagenization of the nodules produces this typical, eosinophilic, paucicellular appearance at low power. Incomplete separation of the nodules produces cleft-like spaces.

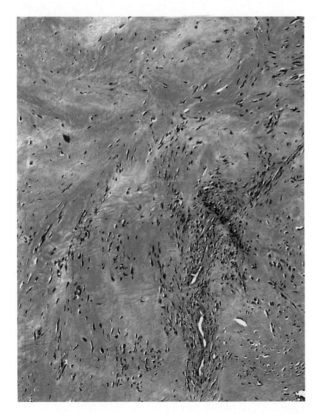 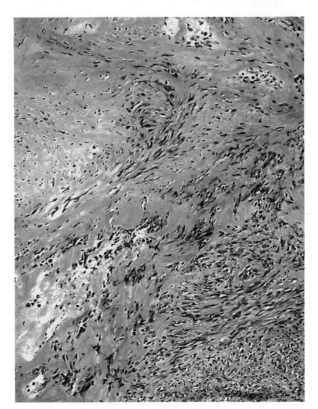

Figure 2-23
FIBROMA OF TENDON SHEATH

Left: Most examples are paucicellular with only scattered spindled fibroblasts set within a densely collagenized matrix. Scattered small calibered vessels are present.

Right: Transition from a collagenized to a more cellular area of the lesion.

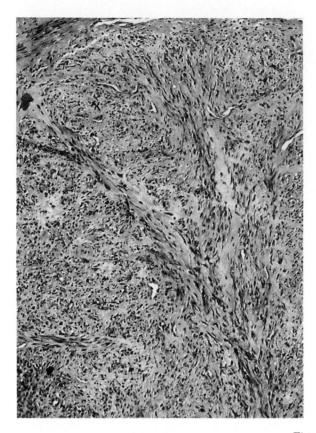 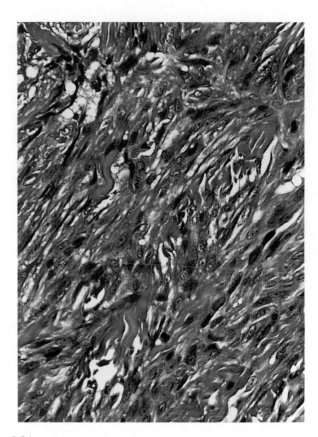

Figure 2-24
FIBROMA OF TENDON SHEATH, CELLULAR AREAS
Left: A cellular region raises the possibility of leiomyosarcoma or fibrosarcoma, neoplasms distinctly uncommon in the hands and feet.
Right: Cytologically bland fibroblasts are separated by collagen. The absence of cytologic atypia is against a diagnosis of sarcoma.

The usual FTS is mostly collagenized and paucicellular, but rare lesions are entirely cellular (fig. 2-24). The latter are sometimes designated as cellular FTS or fasciitis-like variants (38,39,41). Myxoid areas may be encountered, particularly in cellular foci.

The constituent cells of FTS have uniform, usually elongate nuclei and scant cytoplasm that sometimes is arranged as elongate polar processes. The nuclei range from large and vesicular to small and dense. Chromatin is evenly distributed and fine to smooth and dense. Mitotic figures are usually present, but are invariably normal. In the cellular areas, the uniform fibroblasts are often arranged in loops or S- and C-shaped bundles, and extravasation of red blood cells may occur, features reminiscent of nodular fasciitis. Indeed, some authors have suggested that such lesions should be considered the tenosynovial

counterpart of nodular fasciitis (41). Intralesional slit-like vascular spaces are prominent in many tumors and may be the most striking low-power microscopic finding. Rarely, a few multinucleated giant cells are found, but easily found xanthoma cells, hemosiderin and hemosiderin-laden macrophages, and large numbers of giant cells are not features of FTS and should raise consideration of localized tenosynovial giant cell tumor of tendon sheath.

Differential Diagnosis. Lesions with the classic pattern of nodular fasciitis are unusual in the hands and feet and those that do occur are usually classified as cellular FTS. It is, of course, most important not to mistake FTS for a sarcoma. This error is much more likely to occur when the pathologist is dealing with a cellular FTS and fibrosarcoma or synovial sarcoma are the most likely sarcomas to be considered. However, sarcomas of all types are rare in the hands and wrists, and, unlike FTS, are usually large and contain cells whose nuclei demonstrate chromatin abnormalities. Sarcomas also may contain abnormal mitotic figures.

Benign fibrous histiocytomas also share features with FTS; however, dermal fibrous histiocytomas are unusual in the hands and feet and FTS rarely involves the skin. Benign subcutaneous fibrous histiocytoma must be considered in the differential diagnosis of FTS, but histiocyte-like cells are not seen in FTS and giant cells, foam cells, and hemosiderin, often found in benign fibrous histiocytomas, are rare to absent in FTS. CD68 is often positive in benign fibrous histiocytomas. Localized tenosynovial giant cell tumors (giant cell tumors of tendon sheath) frequently arise in the hands and are often circumscribed and multinodular, but the constituent cells have short, plump, histiocyte-like nuclei; giant cells are almost invariably present and are usually numerous; and very often foam cells and hemosiderin deposits are identified. Slit-like vascular spaces, a prominent feature of FTS, are inconspicuous or absent in giant cell tumor of tendon sheath. However, there is overlap between cellular FTS and tenosynovial giant cell tumor and occasionally a sharp distinction between the two is not possible. Fortunately, both have about the same incidence of nonaggressive local recurrence.

Treatment and Prognosis. About a quarter of FTSs recur, presumably because of failure to remove some of the lobules of the lesion in the initial surgery; they do not recur aggressively, nor do they grow so as to interfere with function (39). They do not metastasize.

Elastofibroma

Definition. Elastofibroma is a fibrous reactive process that occurs almost exclusively in the soft tissues around the scapula and is characterized by large numbers of prominent enlarged elastic fibers.

General Considerations. One report suggests elastofibroma may be a response to repeated trauma, but this has never been confirmed (45). A familial history has been demonstrated in about a third of the large number of patients who have developed this lesion in Okinawa, supporting a theory of familial susceptibility in at least some patients (50). The large number of elastic fibers in the lesion seems to be the result of abnormal elastogenesis rather than a degenerative change in preexisting elastic fibers. Large abnormal elastic fibers resembling those seen in elastofibroma have been found in tissue removed at autopsy from the thoracic fascia of individuals who died of other causes and who did not have a mass (45).

Clinical Features. This slowly growing mass lesion occurs almost exclusively in individuals over the age of 55 and almost always is located on the trunk between the lower scapula and the chest wall. It is unilateral in over 90 percent of cases (49). The proliferation lies deep to the latissimus dorsi and rhomboid muscles, often attaching itself to the ribs. Rare examples have been reported around the hip and the upper arm. Other parts of the chest may also be involved and a few examples have been observed in the viscera. Most patients come to the attention of a physician because a painless mass is discovered. The magnetic resonance imaging (MRI) and computerized tomographic (CT) characteristics of elastofibroma are distinctive but not pathognomonic (47).

Pathologic Findings. Grossly, elastofibromas are gray-white, poorly demarcated, rubbery masses that often contain yellow streaks of elastin (fig. 2-25). Microscopically, the most striking feature is the absence of anything distinctive about the paucicellular, hyalinized, collagenous stroma that forms the mass until one notices the large, coarse, pale eosinophilic fibers scattered throughout (fig. 2-26). Sometimes the fibers are fragmented into small, often linearly arranged globules resembling beads on a string. Focally, the stroma may be myxoid and trapped residual fat cells are often within the lesion. Elastic stains are striking and reveal the large (20 to 30 μm) fibers to have a dense core and serrated or beaded margins (fig. 2-27). Ultrastructural examination confirms the presence of a central core surrounded by a fibrillary substance (42–46,48). The cell processes of the surrounding fibrocytes usually are attached to the elastin fibers, suggesting that new elastin is laid down on preexisting fibers. Ultrastructurally, the constituent cells have the features of fibroblasts and myofibroblasts, and some contain granular bodies, thought to represent elastin precursors.

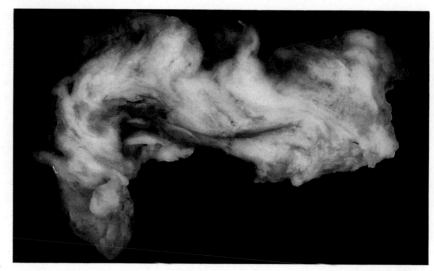

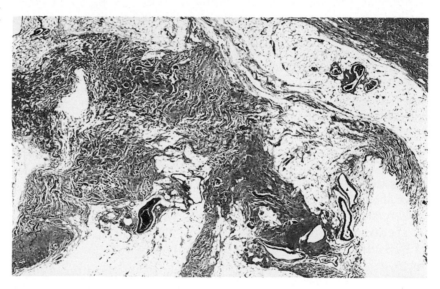

Figure 2-25
ELASTOFIBROMA
Top: The fibrocollagenous proliferation blends with fat.
Bottom: At low power the lesion looks deceptively nondescript: an admixture of paucicellular fibrous tissue admixed with mature fat.

Differential Diagnosis. Elastofibroma should always be considered whenever an asymptomatic periscapular mass is excised from the chest wall of a middle-aged or older individual. Once the possibility of elastofibroma is considered, identification of the large, coarse, elastic fibers makes the diagnosis straightforward. The lesion most likely to be confused with elastofibroma is nuchal fibroma, a rare, benign, reactive collagenized lesion that usually develops in people younger than 55 and occurs in the region between the scapula and the vertebrae. Instead of elastin fibers, the stroma contains dense collagen bundles. Since both lesions are benign the distinction is not clinically critical. Fibrolipoma enters the differential diagnosis of elastofibroma because fat is often trapped within the elastofibroma; however, the presence of altered elastic fibers as described above is definitional for elastofibroma. Desmoid fibromatosis is more cellular and lacks the large elastic fibers of elastofibroma and elastofibroma does not infiltrate skeletal muscle.

Treatment and Prognosis. Elastofibroma is non-neoplastic and cured by simple excision. The recurrence rate is negligible.

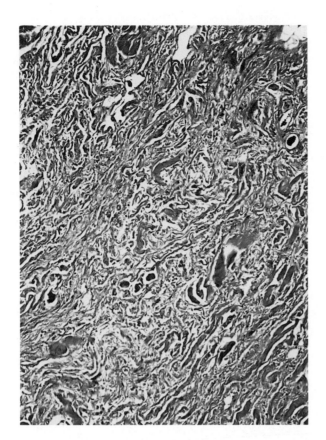 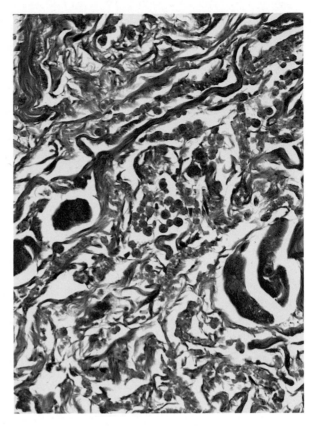

Figure 2-26
ELASTOFIBROMA
Left: Closer examination reveals thick, densely eosinophilic elastin bands admixed with collagen.
Right: The intact bands have serrated edges and are associated with detached globular elastin arranged like beads on a string.

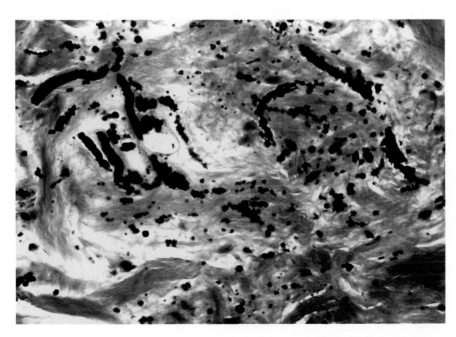

Figure 2-27
ELASTOFIBROMA
(VERHOEFF ELASTIN STAIN)
The elastin fibers are highlighted by this stain which accentuates the bead-like arrangement of the elastin globules.

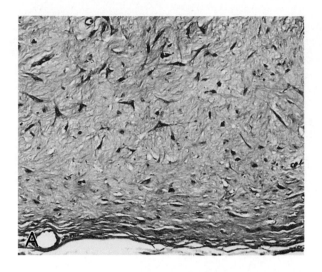

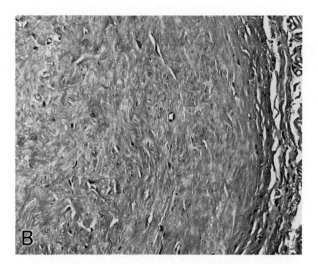

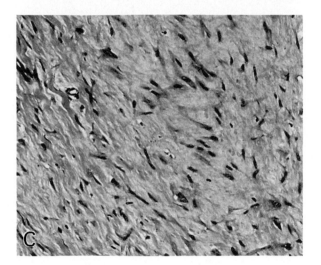

Figure 2-28
DESMOPLASTIC FIBROBLASTOMA
A: This typical field shows large, "reactive-appearing," spindled to stellate fibroblasts sparsely distributed in fibrous matrix.
B: Another area of the same example, demonstrating very low cellularity and densely collagenous background.
C: This is the greatest cellularity that was observed in Evans' series. The large "reactive-appearing" fibroblasts are characteristic.

Desmoplastic Fibroblastoma (Collagenous Fibroma)

Definition. Desmoplastic fibroblastoma is a recently described benign soft tissue fibrous lesion characterized by low cellularity, abundant collagen, and medium-sized to large fibroblasts with a "reactive" appearance (51–53).

Clinical Features. The lesions have all been located in soft tissue, with some subcutaneous and others intramuscular. Sites involved include the neck, upper arm, forearm, shoulder, hand, lateral thigh, abdominal wall, and ankle and foot. Lesions ranged from 1 to 20 cm. Size did not clearly correlate with depth.

Pathologic Findings. Grossly, desmoplastic fibroblastomas are firm masses that appear well circumscribed and are white to gray to tan on cut section. Microscopically, they are typified by moderately low to very low cellularity and a fibromyxoid to densely fibrous background populated by medium-sized to large spindled to stellate fibroblasts (fig. 2-28). These fibroblasts have a "reactive" appearance, with relatively large, normochromatic nuclei, often easily visible nucleoli, and amphophilic cytoplasm. Mitotic figures are rare or entirely absent, tumor necrosis is not a feature of these lesions, and blood vessels are sparse. The border is most often well delineated, although interdigitation with adjacent fat or muscle can be observed focally in some cases.

Special Studies. In one study, six desmoplastic fibroblastomas were analyzed immunohistochemically with the following results: all were diffusely positive for vimentin, one tumor showed diffuse staining for smooth muscle actin, two tumors were focally positive for that antibody, two were faintly positive for S-100 protein, and all were negative for desmin, keratin, and CD34 (53). Another study reported faint focal staining for keratin but otherwise confirmed these results (52). Ultrastructural examination shows the constituent cells to resemble myofibroblasts and fibroblasts (53). Two tumors have had clonal abnormalities involving the long arm of chromosome 11, an abnormality shared with a single case of fibroma of tendon sheath (53a).

Differential Diagnosis. The most important differential diagnostic consideration is desmoid fibromatosis because of its local aggressiveness and at least partial histologic similarity to desmoplastic fibroblastoma. However, desmoid tumors differ by their higher cellularity, greater number of blood vessels, many of which are slit-like, and larger and more obvious areas of infiltration, most often of skeletal muscle, at their periphery. Moreover, stellate-shaped cells are not usually a feature of desmoids. Other differential diagnostic considerations, less important because they are benign, include hyalinized nodular fasciitis, fibroma of tendon sheath, nuchal fibroma, and calcifying fibrous tumor/pseudotumor. The constituent cells of nodular fasciitis and fibroma of tendon sheath may resemble those in desmoplastic fibroblastoma, but nodular fasciitis is more cellular and typically has a loose, "tissue culture-like" appearance. Characteristically, "burnt-out" nodular fasciitis features central microcystic changes. Fibroma of tendon sheath is almost always acral in location; unlike desmoplastic fibroblastoma, it is characteristically lobulated and has numerous vessels. The fibroblasts in nuchal fibroma are smaller and do not feature large nuclei. Calcifying fibrous tumor/pseudotumor is also composed of smaller, more mature fibroblasts and fibrocytes, and focal calcification and prominent chronic inflammation are constant features. Furthermore, it usually occurs in younger individuals than does desmoplastic fibroblastoma. Low-grade fibromyxoid sarcoma is generally more cellular than desmoplastic fibroblastoma, and the constituent cells are usually smaller and have denser chromatin than do the "reactive-appearing" fibroblasts of desmoplastic fibroblastoma. Moreover, low-grade fibromyxoid sarcomas feature contrasting fibrous and myxoid zones, and a swirling, whorled growth pattern in at least a portion of the tumor.

Treatment and Prognosis. In the series thus far reported, there has been no recurrence after excision.

Calcifying Fibrous Tumor/Pseudotumor

Definition. Calcifying fibrous tumor/pseudotumor is a rare, benign, fibrous soft tissue lesion occurring in children and young adults that is characterized by low cellularity, dense collagen, focal calcifications, and a patchy lymphoplasmacytic chronic inflammatory infiltrate.

Clinical Features. Calcifying fibrous tumor/pseudotumor occurs predominantly in children and teenagers but sometimes in young adults (54,54a). Reported examples have involved a variety of soft tissue locations, without a clear predilection for any particular site. Occurrence in the pleura has been observed, and we have seen a case in the adrenal gland. The lesion may be found in either subcutaneous or deeper soft tissue. The maximum dimension has ranged from 2.5 cm up to 15 cm; more than half the published cases have measured over 5 cm.

Pathologic Findings. Grossly, calcifying fibrous tumor/pseudotumor is firm and fibrous, and white to tan to gray on cut section. The calcification sometimes imparts a gritty texture. In reported cases, the border of the lesion has varied from well circumscribed to somewhat infiltrative. Microscopically, there is a paucicellular proliferation of relatively small, inconspicuous, mature fibrocytes set in a densely collagenous background (fig. 2-29A,B). A characteristic feature is the presence of small calcifications that range from psammomatous to irregular, structureless, and dystrophic. Another typical finding is a patchy lymphoplasmacytic chronic inflammatory infiltrate that may include germinal centers and in some cases includes occasional eosinophils or mast cells (fig. 2-29C). There is usually some degree of infiltration into adjacent tissues at the lesional edge, even when the border seems grossly well circumscribed.

Differential Diagnosis. Most fibrous tumors and proliferations are unlikely to be confused with calcifying fibrous tumor/pseudotumor because they are more cellular and lack calcifications and abundant patchy chronic inflammation.

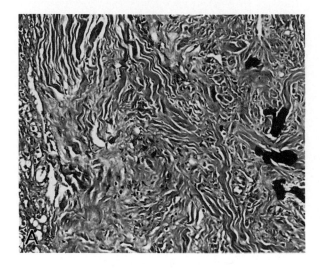

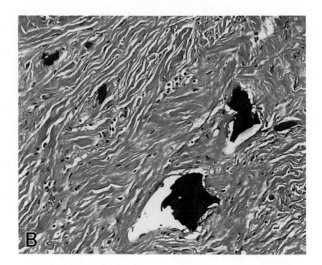

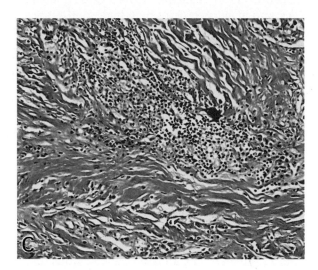

Figure 2-29
CALCIFYING FIBROUS TUMOR/PSEUDOTUMOR
A: This example involved the adrenal gland. The lesion consists of a paucicellular fibrous proliferation with focal microcalcifications.
B: Microcalcifications of varying size are typical.
C: Another characteristic feature is patchy lymphoplasmacytic chronic inflammation.

Desmoplastic fibroblastoma has low cellularity, but its larger, more prominent fibroblasts, lack of microcalcifications, and inconspicuous or absent chronic inflammatory infiltrate allow it to be distinguished from calcifying fibrous tumor/pseudotumor. Moreover, desmoplastic fibroblastoma occurs in an older age group. Calcifying aponeurotic fibroma demonstrates calcifications; however, it is more cellular than calcifying fibrous tumor/pseudotumor, usually occurs in a more distal location, and is almost always smaller. Inflammatory myofibroblastic tumor (inflammatory fibrosarcoma) is another lesion with a similar age incidence and one that typically contains chronic inflammation, but it has considerably greater cellularity than calcifying fibrous tumor/pseudotumor and usually does not exhibit calci-

fications. The presence of plasma cells and Russell bodies may raise the possibility of amyloid tumor but no foreign body giant cells are present and no amyloid can be demonstrated.

Treatment and Prognosis. Recurrences after excision are rare and if they do occur they are not destructive. Multiple recurrences have been observed.

Nuchal Fibroma

This rare lesion, which may well be reactive, was first described by Enzinger and Weiss in their textbook *Soft Tissue Tumors* and nine more examples were reported by Balachandran et al. in 1995 (55,56). More recently, 52 cases were reported by Michal and colleagues including examples from

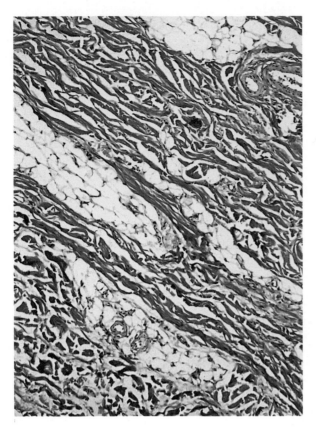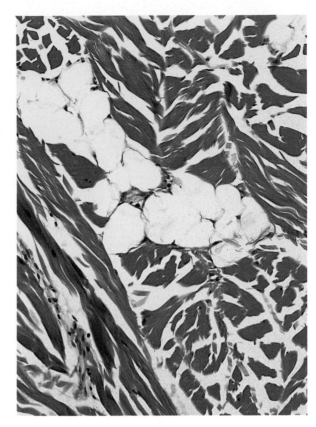

Figure 2-30
NUCHAL FIBROMA
Left: Strands of acellular collagen are admixed with mature fat.
Right: The striking low cellularity of this lesion serves to separate it from desmoid fibromatosis.

extranuchal sites (56a). It occurs most commonly in the subcutaneous tissue of the neck, occipital area, and over the dorsum of the spine but rare examples are found in other sites. The tumor is poorly circumscribed and consists of broad bundles of almost acellular collagen containing a small number of small mature fibrocytes, with a variable number of adult fat cells probably trapped by the advancing collagenous tissue (fig. 2-30). Nerve twigs are often entrapped and large nerves with perineural fibrosis may be seen in the lesion.

The differential diagnosis includes fibrolipoma. Distinction between the two rests on the characteristic location, lack of circumscription, and large amount of extremely hypocellular collagen in nuchal fibroma whereas collagen is usually focal in fibrolipoma. Since both lesions are benign, the distinction is of no great clinical relevance. However, distinguishing nuchal fibroma from desmoid is important. Desmoids are tumors of the deep soft tissues not the subcutaneous tissue, are more cellular, and are not common in the areas where nuchal fibroma occurs. Solitary fibrous tumor also features hyalinized collagen, at least focally, but its constituent cells are commonly arranged in bundles rather than being sheet-like and the lesion is much more cellular than nuchal fibroma. Moreover, 80 to 90 percent of solitary fibrous tumors contain CD34-positive cells. Nuchal fibroma lacks the abundant abnormal elastic fibers of elastofibroma.

Nuchal fibroma can recur, but all recurrences have been controlled by re-excision (56,56a).

Pleomorphic Fibroma of Skin

This uncommon, benign, nonrecurring cutaneous fibroblastic proliferation of the skin occurs in adults and is virtually identical to the ordinary fibroepithelial polyp except that it features

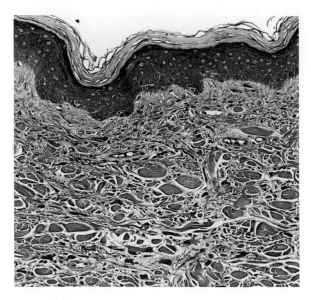 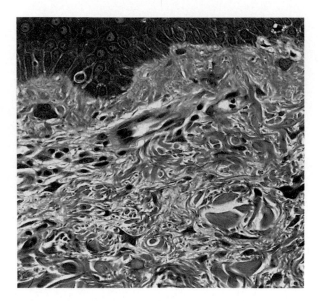

Figure 2-31
PLEOMORPHIC FIBROMA

Left: At low power the impression is of large, pleomorphic cells widely separated by collagen.
Right: The atypical cells have smudged chromatin and there are either no mitotic figures or they are very difficult to find. In contrast, the malignant proliferations with which this lesion may be confused feature easily found mitotic figures (some of which are abnormal) and abnormal nuclei that do not have a smudged degenerative appearance.

cells with enlarged, bizarre, smudged, hyperchromatic nuclei and rare mitotic figures (57). The cells are reminiscent of the enlarged atypical cells found in pleomorphic lipoma and ancient schwannoma.

The lesions are typically either polypoid or dome-shaped solitary lesions that range in size from a few millimeters up to 1.6 cm. Histologically, they feature thick bundles of collagen which replace the dermis. Markedly atypical cells with enlarged, hyperchromatic nuclei are scattered between the collagen bundles (fig. 2-31). Rare mitotic figures may be encountered, some of which may be abnormal. A myxoid variant has been described.

The differential diagnosis of this cutaneous lesion includes atypical fibroxanthoma, dermatofibroma with monster cells (atypical dermal fibrous histiocytoma), giant cell fibroblastoma, desmoplastic melanoma, and desmoplastic Spitz's nevus. An S-100 protein stain is often useful to exclude the latter two. Atypical fibroxanthoma is more cellular than pleomorphic fibroma and mitotic figures, both normal and abnormal, are more frequent in atypical fibroxanthoma. Dermatofibroma with monster cells is more cellular than pleomorphic fibroma, and contains foam cells and

hemosiderin-laden macrophages. Giant cell fibroblastoma resembles pleomorphic fibroma in that both contain atypical fibroblastic cells, but giant cell fibroblastoma is usually a pediatric lesion, is characterized by infiltrative growth, and features sinusoidal structures lined by atypical cells, features not seen in pleomorphic fibroma. Desmoplastic Spitz's nevus has at least some areas of obvious melanocytic differentiation and the constituent cells, unlike those in pleomorphic fibroma, are S-100 protein positive.

Solitary Fibrous Tumor of the Soft Tissues

Definition. Solitary fibrous tumor (SFT) is a spindle cell fibrous and myofibroblastic proliferation in which the constituent cells are not arranged in consistent patterns but, at least focally, are almost always separated by strip-like bands of collagen; frequently, a pericytic vascular pattern is present. The tumor cells are almost always CD34 positive.

General Considerations. SFTs most frequently occur on the pleura but over the past few years there has been an ever-increasing number reported in extrapleural sites including the soft

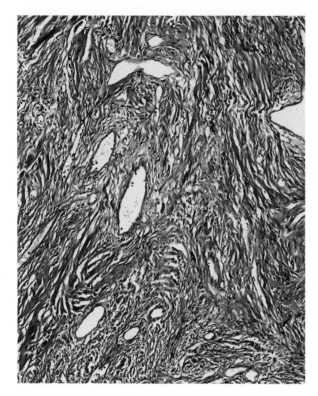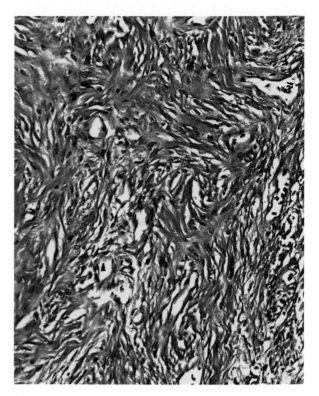

Figure 2-32
SOLITARY FIBROUS TUMOR OF THE SOFT TISSUES
Left: The proliferation has a moderately cellular fibroblastic appearance at low-power microscopy.
Right: Parallel arrays of collagen separated by fibroblastic nuclei are evident at medium power.

tissue (58,60–68,70,71). Undoubtedly, the list of sites will expand over the next few years. The constituent cells of pleural SFTs have myofibroblastic ultrastructural features but very few of the tumor cells are actin positive when paraffin-embedded tissues are stained and it is rare for the cells to express desmin (69). This apparent contradiction is explained by the observation that there are at least four different myofibroblastic phenotypes including ones in which alpha-smooth muscle actin is absent. Of great diagnostic significance is the observation that over 90 percent of SFTs contain cells that express an antigen recognized by CD34 and a significant number are CD99 positive (62,63).

Histologically bland SFTs very rarely may metastasize, so these lesions are better placed in the intermediate tumor category IIc (see Table 1-10) than among the benign tumors. We have left them in the benign category until more information about the frequency of metastases is known. As noted in the Pathologic Features section below, SFTs rarely may have malignant features and when they do, there is a significant incidence of recurrence and metastasis (66,68). As a result, a category of malignant SFT has been added (see Table 2-1) (68).

Clinical Features. Extrapleural SFTs are most often asymptomatic and are found by chance or by the discovery of a mass. The patients are almost exclusively adults, usually middle-aged or older. The most common extrapleural sites are the peritoneum, retroperitoneum, mediastinum, and orbit, although they also occur throughout the soft tissues.

Pathologic Findings. Grossly, SFTs are usually well circumscribed; larger examples may be lobulated. On cut section they are composed of white to brown, whirled, fibrous-appearing tissue. They vary from less than 1 cm to over 20 cm. Microscopically, SFT is composed of spindle cells with either elongate, thin, dense nuclei or vesicular nuclei with inconspicuous nucleoli (figs. 2-32, 2-33). Cytoplasm is scant, indistinct,

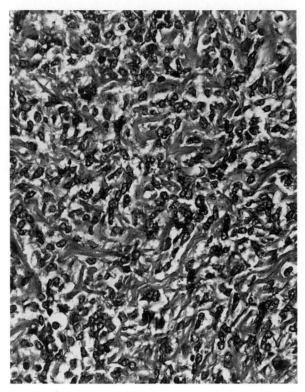

Figure 2-33
SOLITARY FIBROUS TUMOR
A more cellular variant is composed of cells with scanty cytoplasm and uniform spindled nuclei. Note the thin bands of intercellular collagen.

and palely eosinophilic. The cells may be arranged in sheets, short fascicles, or whirling or storiform patterns or they may grow randomly. Although it may not be prominent in more cellular areas of the tumor, somewhere most SFTs feature often parallel thin bands of collagen between the constituent cells. This distinctive pattern of collagen formation serves as a hallmark of the lesion. Areas of myxoid stroma may also be detected in some tumors as well as focal sheet-like hyalinization and dystrophic calcification. Rarely, a myxoid stroma may predominate (57a). The vessels may be hyalinized, plexiform, or pericytic, sometimes with a condensation of cells around gaping vessels. A pericytic vascular pattern is often prominent, at least focally.

Although the cells in most SFTs are bland and uniform, a minimal degree of pleomorphism is not uncommon and does not predict malignant behavior. However, like their counterparts on the pleura, a few SFTs of the soft tissue demonstrate histo-

logic evidence of malignancy including pleomorphism, high cellularity, numerous mitotic figures, both normal and abnormal, and tumor cell necrosis (59,68). These histologic features, particularly a mitotic index of more than 4 mitotic figures per 10 high-power fields, predict an increased incidence of recurrence and metastasis, and such tumors should be considered malignant (68).

The most important clues for recognizing the usual SFT are bland spindled cells associated with parallel, relatively thin, strip-like bands of collagen and a pericytic vascular pattern. As noted in the next paragraph, the diagnosis can almost always be confirmed with a stain for CD34.

Special Studies. At least 80 to 90 percent of SFTs are CD34 positive and at least half are CD99 positive (69,70); bcl-2 is also commonly positive. SFTs do not stain for keratin, S-100 protein, or epithelial membrane antigen and are usually actin and desmin negative.

Ultrastructurally, the cells in pleural SFTs have features of myofibroblasts.

Differential Diagnosis. Hemangiopericytoma shares a common vascular pattern with SFT and cells that resemble those in SFT, although they are seldom in fascicles or between bands of collagen; rather, they are usually haphazardly arranged. About half of hemangiopericytomas contain CD34-positive cells. In fact, hemangiopericytoma and SFT are related, either the same tumor or different parts of the same tumor spectrum (see section on hemangiopericytoma), and distinction between the two is probably not important. What is important is to realize that the same histologic features predict malignant potential in both hemangiopericytomas and SFTs: tumor cell necrosis, high cellularity, mitotic counts above 4 mitotic figures per 10 high-power fields, pleomorphism, and nuclear atypia. Smooth muscle tumors contain cells with more abundant cytoplasm which may be desmin and actin positive. These antibodies are rarely diffusely positive in SFT. Smooth muscle cells are often arranged in long fascicles rather than the short fascicles, whirling patterns, or random patterns often seen in SFT. Benign neural tumors are S-100 protein positive and SFT is S-100 protein negative. Benign and low-grade fibrous histiocytomas do not demonstrate the type of collagen seen in SFT and they contain histiocyte-like cells in addition to spindled cells. Sarcomas usually

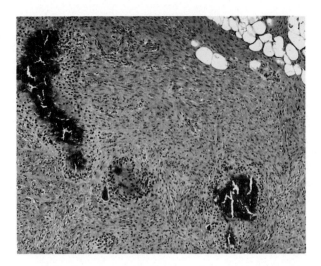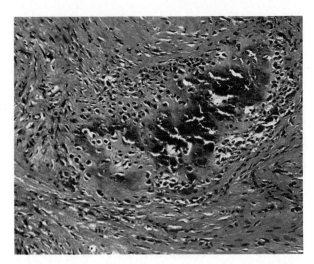

Figure 2-34
CALCIFYING APONEUROTIC FIBROMA
Left: This lesion is a poorly circumscribed fibroproliferative process with scattered, linear, calcified zones.
Right: Amorphous calcification delimited by palisaded cells can be seen. The low-power appearance may suggest a rheumatoid nodule or soft tissue manifestation of a crystalopathy.

have pleomorphism and increased mitotic activity not present in the soft tissue SFTs thus far reported. CD34 staining should be helpful whenever there is any doubt.

Treatment and Prognosis. The treatment for SFT is complete excision. Bland tumors are usually cured by the surgical procedure but may recur and very rarely metastasize (68). There is no way to recognize these outliers. Those that demonstrate pleomorphism, high cellularity, increased mitotic activity, and tumor cell necrosis can metastasize and should be considered to be malignant. Experience with a small number of such tumors indicates that about half will recur or metastasize.

Calcifying Aponeurotic Fibroma

Definition. Calcifying aponeurotic fibroma (CAF) is a fibroblastic lesion, usually of children, in which large numbers of plump fibroblasts cluster around nodules of calcium or cartilage; rarely, bone may be present. The lesion is benign but has a high incidence of nondestructive recurrence.

Clinical Features. CAF is a very uncommon lesion and almost always occurs in children and teenagers; the median age at diagnosis is about 12 years (72); however, the reported age range in the literature is from birth to 64 years (73). Almost all the lesions occur in the hands and feet, with over three fourths in the hands (72,73). Fingers, palm, and wrist are well-known sites of involvement; the toes are an unusual site since most CAFs involving the foot occur in the plantar and ankle regions. Exceptionally, CAF has been found in other sites including the arms, legs, and back (72a). Patients usually complain of a mass, but not always one that is ill-defined and painless. Destructive growth is not a feature of CAF and nearly all examples are less than 3 cm in diameter. However, in sites outside the hands and feet, the tumors may grow to a larger size. Radiographs usually demonstrate the calcification which marks these tumors.

Pathologic Findings. Grossly, the cut surface of CAF appears gray-white and may feel gritty. At low magnification, the typical case presents a unique pattern of multiple cellular nodules composed of fibroblasts surrounding central punctate areas of calcium or cartilage (fig. 2-34). The nodules seem to arise out of dense, often paucicellular fibrous tissue. At higher magnification it can be seen that the cells forming the nodules tend to line up in parallel rows or palisade as they circle around the areas of calcification and the nests of cartilage (fig. 2-35). These cells have distinctive plump, oval nuclei with vesicular chromatin that frequently is condensed immediately beneath the nuclear membrane. The

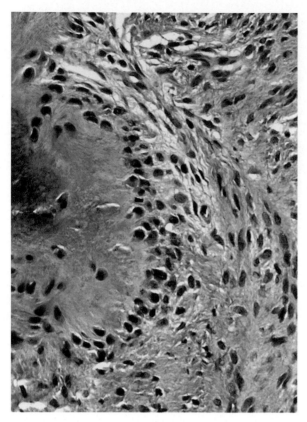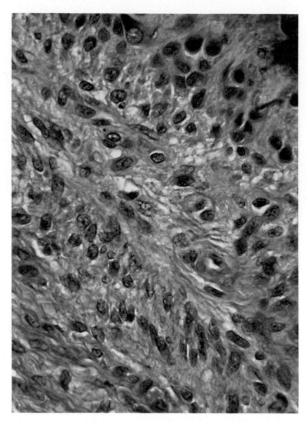

Figure 2-35
CALCIFYING APONEUROTIC FIBROMA

Left: The typical zonation pattern of this lesion consists of cellular, plump fibroblastic cells palisaded around a hyalinized collagenous zone, which in turn surrounds the calcification.

Right: The cells immediately adjacent to the hyalinized layer are commonly more rounded. Fully developed cartilage may sometimes be seen.

cytoplasm is usually discernible, although cell margins are often difficult to find.

These cytologic features are in striking contrast to the dense, evenly dispersed chromatin that characterizes the elongate, smaller, mature fibrocytes that make up the intervening stroma between the nodules. Rays of fibrous tissue extend from the main lesion into the surrounding tissue and may infiltrate muscle or nerves. Calcification is present in the centers of the nodules except in lesions removed from infants and very young children. The pattern of calcium deposition varies from amorphous masses to granular elongate lines. Nuclei are often present within the calcified areas. Occasionally, multinucleated giant cells are encountered. Toward the center of some nodules, the stroma may take on a chondroid appearance, and sometimes mature

cartilage with variable degrees of calcification is present (fig. 2-36). The cellularity of CAF varies from lesion to lesion and within the same lesion; however, the most common situation is for the areas adjacent to the cartilage and calcium to be cellular and those away from these centers to be paucicellular. Mitotic figures are characteristically difficult to find. Transformation of the histologic features of CAF to a more mitotically active cellular lesion identical to fibrosarcoma has been observed but is extremely rare.

Overall, the histologic pattern of nodules with central punctate calcification surrounded by cells with plump nuclei within a hyaline cartilage-like stroma or a cartilaginous stroma should cause the observer to think of CAF, particularly if the lesion is in the distal extremity of a child or young adult.

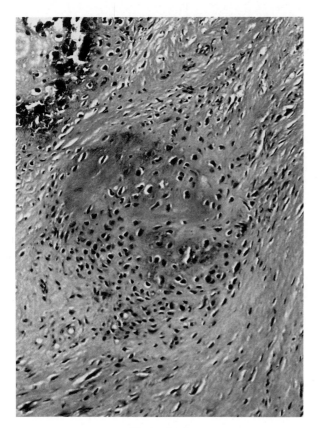

Figure 2-36
CALCIFYING APONEUROTIC FIBROMA
A chondroid area (top left) is adjacent to a calcified zone.

Differential Diagnosis. Because the fibroblasts in fibrous hamartoma of infancy (FHI) can resemble those that form CAF, because CAF in infants and young children may contain little or no calcium, and because CAF often infiltrates fat in a way that can cause the observer to wonder if the fat is part of the lesion, FHI enters into the differential diagnosis of CAF. However, FHI also contains immature mesenchyme not found in CAF and fibroblasts arranged in trabeculae rather than in parallel rows around calcified nodules. Moreover, neither cartilage nor calcification are found in FHI and FHI does not occur in the hands and feet, the most frequent site of occurrence of CAF. Infantile desmoid fibromatosis practically never occurs in the hands and feet, is not calcified or nodular, and does not have cartilaginous features. Typically, large amounts of fat are present within the center of infantile desmoid tumors, whereas CAF infiltrates fat, so fat cells are present only at the periphery.

Palmar fibromatosis in patients is rare under the age of 20, does not infiltrate muscle and nerves as does CAF, is not associated with calcification, and rarely demonstrates cartilage or chondroid. The constituent cells are more slender and often have denser nuclei than those in CAF. Soft tissue chondromas, while they may calcify, are not associated with nodules of cellular fibrous tissue and are mostly found in adults, a group in which CAF is rare. Chondromas are also lobulated and have a less infiltrating pattern. In rare cases, distinction of a calcified chondroma from CAF may be problematic, but fortunately, the worst that can happen as a result of either lesion is nondestructive recurrence, so distinction is not critical. Chondrosarcoma of the hands is extremely rare, is a tumor exclusively found in adults, and practically always originates in bone, a feature that can be appreciated in radiographs. Fibro-osseous pseudotumor of the digits with scant bone and osteoid may contain cells that resemble those in CAF, but does not display cellular nodules arising in a background of paucicellular collagen, rather it closely resembles nodular fasciitis.

Treatment and Prognosis. About half the patients with CAF experience a recurrence, but the recurrences are not destructive and the lesion does not metastasize (72,72a,73). The incidence of recurrence decreases with age and a conservative approach to therapy that does not impair function is indicated for patients of all ages. Recurrences are often cured by simple removal of the recurrent lesion. A single case has been reported to metastasize after transformation to fibrosarcoma and we have seen a similar case (74).

Fibromatosis Colli

Definition. Fibromatosis colli denotes partial replacement of the sternocleidomastoid muscle by fibrous tissue; it is often complicated by muscular torticollis or wryneck. It occurs exclusively in infants and children, almost always after the first 2 weeks of life, and is to be distinguished from the unrelated acquired torticollis that results from muscle spasm or injury of some sort and occurs in older individuals.

Clinical Features. In the usual situation, a lump is noticed within the lower portion of the sternocleidomastoid muscle 2 to 6 weeks after birth (75). It can develop in older children, but has not been reported in adults and does not affect other muscles or the overlying skin. After an initial phase of fairly rapid growth, the mass characteristically stabilizes and, in most cases, slowly regresses over a period of several years. When this fibrous proliferative process is growing, it may cause torticollis but characteristically the most marked rotation of the head occurs after the lesion has been present for several years and has stopped growing. Torticollis is, of course, not limited to patients with a fibrous mass within the sternocleidomastoid, and in fact, torticollis acquired as a result of injury or muscle spasm is not associated with fibrosis of the sternocleidomastoid muscle. Many patients with fibromatosis colli have a history of a complicated birth (81). Rare familial cases have been reported (82).

Pathologic Findings. The fibrous mass is white and rarely exceeds 2 to 3 cm. Microscopically, the characteristic feature is fibrous tissue of variable cellularity coursing in and among residual muscle fibers (fig. 2-37). Although the cellularity is variable, most lesions tend to be paucicellular and the constituent nuclei are uniform. Many of the surrounding skeletal muscle fibers display evidence of injury in the form of regressive or regenerative changes, such as nuclear enlargement, nuclear hyperchromasia, multinucleation, loss of cross-striations, and atrophy. The stroma within the lesion is predominantly collagenous (fig. 2-38). Mitotic figures are usually sparse and never abnormal.

Differential Diagnosis. The distinctive patient age, tumor location, and histologic pattern of muscle fibers surrounded by fibrous tissue limits the entities in the differential diagnosis. Infantile desmoid fibromatosis destroys all the muscle fibers in its path except at its periphery and it practically never occurs in the sternocleidomastoid muscle. Neither does proliferative myositis, which also features residual muscle fibers within the lesion. In addition, proliferative myositis does not have a collagenous stroma; rather, the constituent fibroblasts and stroma that surround the muscle fibers resemble those found in granulation tissue. Myositis with fibrosis features inflammatory cells. Fibrodysplasia ossificans progressiva, while it leaves residual muscle fibers, always involves sites other than the sternocleidomastoid muscle; most notably, there are malformations of the hand. Moreover, the older le-

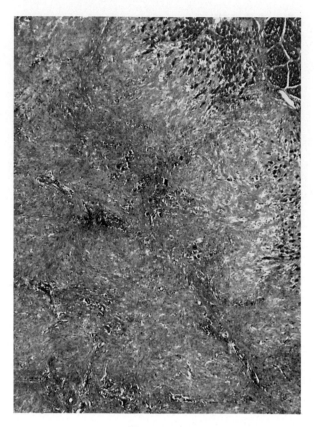

Figure 2-37
FIBROMATOSIS COLLI
A multinodular proliferation of relatively acellular collagenized tissue replaces part of the sternocleidomastoid muscle.

sions contain bone in addition to fibrous tissue, which is not a feature of fibromatosis colli.

Treatment and Prognosis. Nearly two thirds of lesions spontaneously resolve so surgical intervention is used only when there are complications from the torticollis (76–80). Therefore, it is unusual to receive a specimen of fibromatosis colli in the surgical pathology laboratory. The lesion is never aggressive and does not recur.

Fibrous Hamartoma of Infancy

Definition. This is a pediatric, benign, superficial soft tissue mass featuring a mixture of three different tissue types: 1) closely approximated spindle cells arranged in trabeculae within a collagenous matrix; 2) myxoid stroma containing small, round, primitive cells; and 3) mature fat.

Clinical Features. Fibrous hamartoma of infancy (FHI) may be discovered at birth, but the majority of lesions come to light within the first

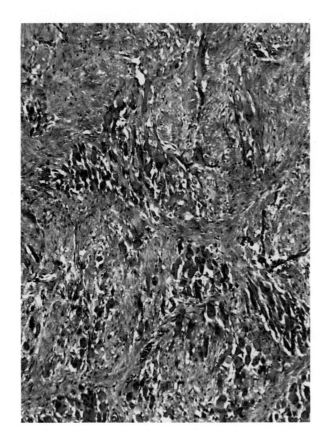 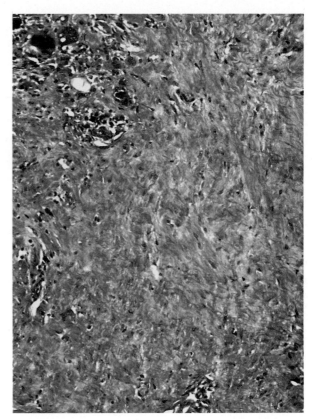

Figure 2-38
FIBROMATOSIS COLLI
Left: Skeletal muscle fibers are trapped at the advancing edge of this lesion.
Right: Scattered, cytologically bland fibrocytes are widely separated by dense collagen.

year of life (83,83a,84,89). FHI is practically never diagnosed past the age of 3 or 4 years and apparently does not occur at all after puberty. It occurs most frequently in the area of the axilla, followed by the upper arm and shoulder, thigh, inguinal area, back, and forearm. However, all superficial soft tissue sites in the body may be affected except the hands. The usual history is of a rapidly growing, freely movable, apparently painless, dermal-subcutaneous mass. Attachment to muscle or fascia does occur, but is distinctly unusual. Most lesions are under 5 cm, but rare examples have reached 20 cm in size (83). It is more common in males but there is no evidence that FHI is a familial disease.

Pathologic Findings. FHI is usually not circumscribed and, on cut section, one often finds gray-white tissue alternating with yellow fat. The fat can be inconspicuous but is usually prominent and may at times constitute the bulk

of the lesion. This gross appearance is distinctive and when found in a lesion removed from an infant or child should always cause the observer to think of fibrous hamartoma. Histologically, the three distinct components of FHI make recognition easy (figs. 2-39, 2-40). The spindled fibrous component varies from loosely cellular to densely fibrotic and the constituent fibroblasts and myofibroblasts are arranged in bundles that intersect each other at variable angles. Interspersed among and around the bundles of spindle cells are islands of small, primitive, undifferentiated cells with regular nuclei and scant cytoplasm embedded in a myxoid matrix. Mature fat completes the triad of required tissue types. Even though one or the other component can be inconspicuous, all three are present in every lesion although extensive sectioning may be needed to identify all of them. Occasionally, particularly in older children, hyalinized dense collagenous tissue

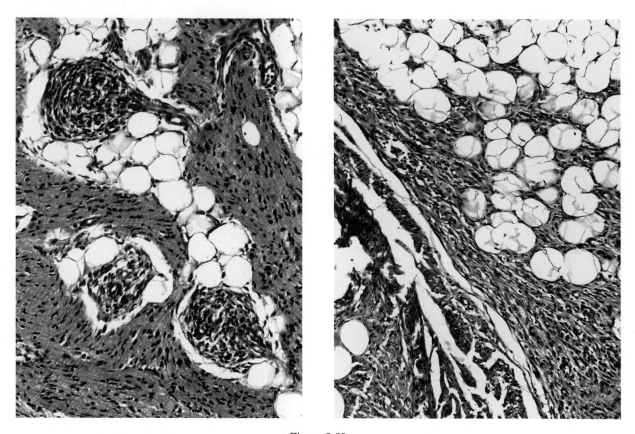

Figure 2-39
FIBROUS HAMARTOMA OF INFANCY

Left: The hallmark of this lesion is a triphasic pattern: fibrous spindle cell areas delimiting islands of the two other components, mature fat and primitive spindled cells.

Right: The primitive spindled cells may infiltrate the adult adipose tissue.

Figure 2-40
FIBROUS HAMARTOMA
OF INFANCY

The primitive spindled cells are cytologically bland and monomorphous, and mitotic figures are difficult to find. This is also true of the cells in the fibrous areas.

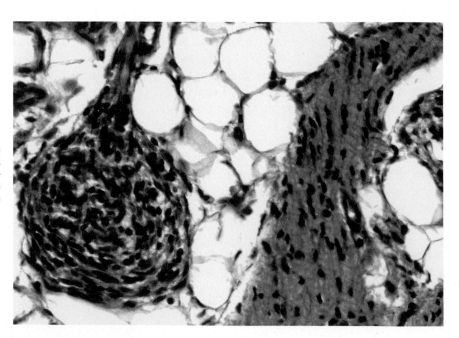

somewhat resembling ancient neurofibroma can replace much of the tumor. Mitotic figures are unusual and if present are normal.

Special Studies. Ultrastructurally there are no surprises. Where mature adipose tissue is expected it is found; the fibroblastic areas are composed of fibroblastic and myofibroblastic cells (86–88), while the myxoid areas contain primitive mesenchymal cells with slender cytoplasmic processes. Immunohistochemical analysis reveals vimentin positivity of the fibroblastic and primitive cells and S-100 protein positivity of the fat; desmin, cytokeratin, factor VIII-related antigen, and myoglobin are all negative (85,88). Actin is positive in some of the collagen forming cells (88).

Differential Diagnosis. The age of the patient, the location of the lesion, and the distinctive organoid histologic pattern all contribute to making the diagnosis of most fibrous hamartomas an easy task. The cellularity of the spindled component may give rise to an initial concern for a sarcoma, but the blandness of the cells, the uniformity of their nuclei, and the other components almost always allow for a correct diagnosis. Infantile desmoid fibromatosis may involve the subcutaneous tissue and may have a mixture of primitive cells, fibroblasts, and fat, but it is centered in skeletal muscle and the three components are randomly arranged rather than discretely organized. While the spindled areas of FHI may resemble those in infantile fibrosarcoma, the latter lacks intralesional fat and primitive mesenchymal cells. The same can be said for leiomyomas and neurofibromas. The latter are also S-100 protein positive while the cells in FHI are not. As noted, a heavily hyalinized fibrous hamartoma can superficially resemble a neural tumor but a search for more characteristic areas and a S-100 protein stain are usually sufficient to make the correct interpretation. Calcifying aponeurotic fibroma before it calcifies may demonstrate fascicles of spindle cells as well as fat, but it lacks primitive undifferentiated cells within a myxoid stroma and it occurs almost exclusively on the hands, a site where FHI has never been reported. Myofibromas are composed of fibroblasts and myofibroblasts plus primitive undifferentiated cells and these two components may suggest FHI. However, the primitive undifferentiated cells of myofibroma are accompanied by a prominent hemangio-pericytoma-like vascular pattern and fat is not found in the central portions of the lesion.

Treatment and Prognosis. FHI is benign and almost always cured by local excision. The rare recurrences (about 10 percent of cases are reported to recur) are not destructive and are cured by reexcision.

Inclusion Body (Digital) Fibromatosis

Definition. This is a fibrous and myofibroblastic recurring proliferation that occurs almost exclusively on the fingers and toes, most commonly in infants, in which some of the constituent cells contain intracytoplasmic eosinophilic actin inclusions.

General Considerations. Initially it was reported that this lesion occurred exclusively in the fingers and toes of infants, hence its original name *infantile digital fibromatosis* (98). Later it became apparent that older children and, rarely, adults, could develop this lesion, and it also has been reported in sites other than the fingers (91, 93,97). Consequently, "infantile" and "digital" are not entirely appropriate labels for this lesion and we think a better term is inclusion body fibromatosis, a name that emphasizes its defining histologic features.

Clinical Features. The lesion presents as a painless, dome-shaped nodule almost always within the first year of life, and a third are present at birth. The third, fourth, and fifth digits are most frequently involved, while the thumb and great toe are not known to be sites of occurrence. Not infrequently, the lesions involve multiple sites including both hands and feet. Multiple lesions may be synchronous or asynchronous. Sometimes the lesions cause functional problems or joint abnormalities. Inclusion-body fibromatosis is practically always under 2 cm in diameter and there is no evidence it is familial.

Pathologic Findings. Grossly, the lesions are nodular and on cut section they look like white fibrous tissue. On microscopic examination, the lesion is cellular and composed of myofibroblasts with enlarged vesicular nuclei arranged in randomly placed bundles. The stroma is collagenized (figs. 2-41, 2-42). Variable numbers of the constituent cells contain small, round, often perinuclear eosinophilic inclusions within their cytoplasm (fig. 2-43). These most closely

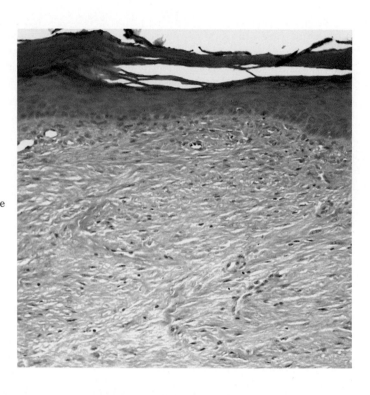

Figure 2-41
INCLUSION BODY FIBROMATOSIS
The proliferation extends from the epidermis to the deep dermis or subcutis.

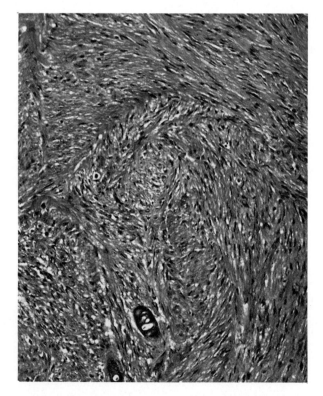
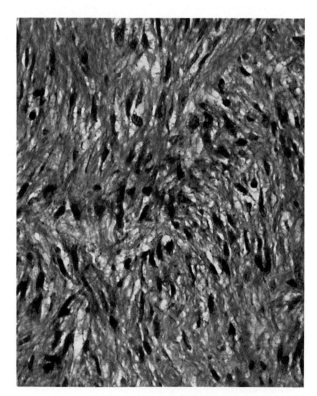

Figure 2-42
INCLUSION BODY FIBROMATOSIS
Left: A cellular proliferation of fibroblastic cells swirls around and engulfs an eccrine duct.
Right: The constituent cells are monomorphous and cytologically bland.

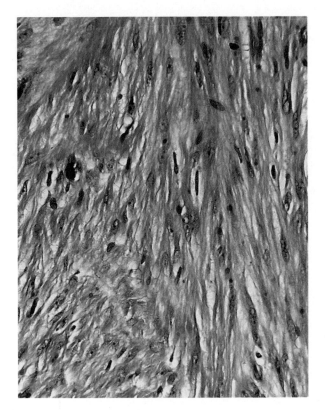

Figure 2-43
INCLUSION BODY FIBROMATOSIS
The distinctive inclusions of this lesion are present in several cells (center field) and can be compared with the scattered red blood cells in the field.

resemble intracytoplasmic erythrocytes and are the distinctive feature of this proliferation. The eosinophilic inclusions may be difficult to find on H&E-stained sections, so it is useful to know they stain red with the trichrome stain and black with iron hematoxylin while they are negative for periodic acid–Schiff (PAS) and Alcian blue. However, in some tumors the inclusions are so numerous as to be difficult to overlook. Mitotic figures are usually present, but are normal. Characteristically, the lesion extends from the overlying, often flattened epidermis to, or into, the subcutaneous tissue.

Special Studies. The inclusions react positively with antibodies against actin (90,93,94,96,99, 100). Ultrastructurally, the constituent cells have the features of myofibroblasts. The inclusions are composed of 5 to 7 nm intermediate filaments with dense bodies identical to the actin-myosin filaments found in normal myofibroblasts and smooth muscle cells (90,92,94,95,99,100).

Differential Diagnosis. When the lesion occurs on the finger or toe of an infant or child and the inclusions are identified histologically, ultrastructurally, or immunohistochemically, the diagnosis should not be in doubt. Infantile fibrosarcoma is more cellular, the nuclei contain denser and more irregular chromatin, mitotic figures are more numerous and, of course, inclusions are absent. Fibrosarcoma is almost always over 2 cm in diameter and is very rare on the fingers and toes. Infantile desmoid fibromatosis and inclusion body fibromatosis share some histologic similarities, but the location and the size of the two lesions are quite different. Infantile desmoid tumors rarely occur in the hand and they are more often than not over 2 cm. Palmar fibromatosis does not occur in the fingers and the cells do not contain inclusions. Myofibromatosis is discussed in the next section. The constituent cells of that lesion do not contain cytoplasmic inclusions, there are areas of primitive cells with a pericytic vascular pattern, and the fingers are an unusual site of involvement. The cells of leiomyoma have more abundant cytoplasm and do not contain inclusions. Neurofibroma can be distinguished from digital fibromatosis on the basis of the S-100 protein–positive cells in the former and the inclusions in the latter. The cells in nodular fasciitis do not contain intracytoplasmic inclusions and nodular fasciitis practically never occurs on the fingers or toes. The cells of fibroma of tendon sheath do not contain inclusions, the stroma is usually extensively hyalinized, and most lesions occur in adults.

Treatment and Prognosis. Nearly 60 percent of patients with inclusion-body fibromatosis have a recurrence and some have more than one. However, recurrences are not destructive, although the primary tumor and recurrences may be associated with contractures and deviation deformities. Some patients with one lesion subsequently develop digital fibromatosis on other fingers or toes. Some lesions regress spontaneously, often after an initial growth spurt. Treatment should consist of no more than a minimal excision, because recurrences are not destructive and metastases do not occur. Because spontaneous regression occurs, observation is also an option, but is probably best reserved for patients with multiple lesions after the diagnosis has been established by excision of one lesion.

Myofibroma, Solitary and Multicentric (Myofibromatosis)

Definition. Myofibroma is a unifocal or multifocal, typically pediatric fibroblastic/myofibroblastic proliferation. The lesions characteristically exhibit a biphasic pattern featuring nodules of spindle cells having an appearance reminiscent of smooth muscle and less differentiated cells with small, round, basophilic nuclei associated with a hemangiopericytic vascular pattern. Characteristically, the former surround a central zone containing the latter. Sometimes the less differentiated basophilic cells are absent or inconspicuous.

General Considerations. The literature dealing with myofibroma and myofibromatosis is confusing. These proliferations are rare, may be single or multiple, may or may not be fatal, and have been reported under a large number of different terms. The most common labels used to describe this lesion include *congenital generalized fibromatosis, congenital mesenchymal hamartomas,* and *infantile myofibromatosis* (102–104, 106,107,110,113,115,117). The latter term was chosen by Chung and Enzinger (103) in their report of 61 cases in 1981 because many of the constituent cells are myofibroblasts. Since rare cases have been reported in adults, the modifier "infantile" has been dropped from the label in the latest WHO classification and the lesion is now named "myofibroma, solitary and multicentric." Fletcher and colleagues (102) have pointed out that myofibroma and infantile hemangiopericytoma share many features and should probably be regarded as the same (or very closely related) lesion(s). Most recently these authors have also pointed out similar overlap between adult cases of myofibroma and tumors showing differentiation towards perivascular contractile cells (107a) and they have suggested that myofibromas are truly pericytic lesions (in other words a type of "true" hemangiopericytoma; see chapter 8).

Clinical Features. In almost 90 percent of cases, myofibroma is discovered before the patient is 2 years of age; in fact, nearly two thirds of the lesions are present at birth or become apparent shortly thereafter. Most of the remainder are diagnosed in children, although rare examples have been reported in adults (107a). Multicentricity is a well-known characteristic of myofibroma, but 70 to 80 percent are single

masses (103,111). The most common sites of involvement are the skin, subcutaneous tissue, and skeletal muscle, usually of the head and neck and trunk, but any site, including bones and other organs, may be affected (116). Multicentric tumors are particularly prone to involve bone and internal organs, including the lungs, kidney, pancreas, and gastrointestinal tract, while solitary lesions tend to be in the superficial soft tissues. Patients with multicentric disease may have just a few nodules or one hundred or more lesions in many different sites. The situation in which there are dozens of lesions has been termed generalized disease. Myofibroma in adults is usually solitary but may be multifocal and superficial, rarely recurs, and most commonly develops in the head and neck or upper trunk (107a,108,114).

The occurrence of myofibromas in several members of families has been reported and the pattern of inheritance is that of autosomal dominance (101,109). Associated congenital abnormalities occur but no consistent set of associated defects has emerged (115).

Myofibromas are reportedly not painful unless they are squeezed, but the symptoms are somewhat uncertain since so many patients are infants. Some skin lesions have a purplish hue and thus resemble hemangiomas, while others present as white nodules or masses. Occasionally, the only gross manifestation is what appears to be a small scar. The lesions vary from a few millimeters to many centimeters, with most in the 1 to 5 cm range. Deeper masses tend to be larger. The lesions usually grow after birth, but many tend to stabilize during childhood. Radiographically, the soft tissue lesions often contain foci of calcification, while the bony lesions are lytic and appear cystic. Among bones, the skull, vertebrae, ribs, femur, and tibia are most often affected.

Pathologic Findings. Grossly, the tumor nodules are usually firm and white. Microscopically, more superficial lesions tend to be circumscribed, while deeper ones are more often diffuse or infiltrative. Lobulation is common. The microscopic picture is sometimes characterized by a zonation phenomenon, in which bundles of myofibroblasts with uniform, most often vesicular nuclei and easily seen eosinophilic or clear cytoplasm with easily discerned cell margins congregate at the periphery of nodules while toward the

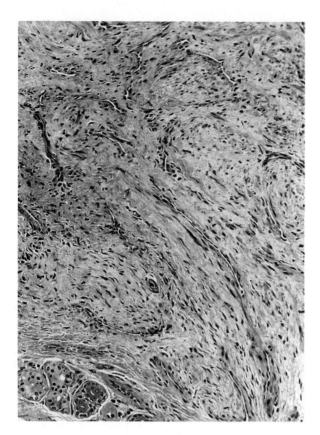 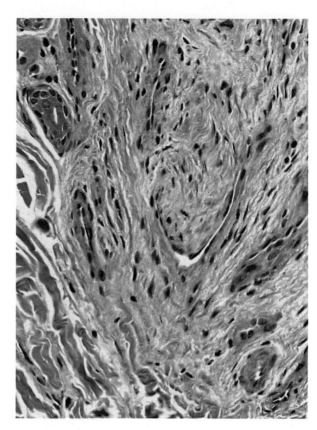

Figure 2-44
MYOFIBROMA AND MYOFIBROMATOSIS

Left: A solitary cutaneous lesion features zones of fibrous tissue in which bundles of myofibroblastic cells are dispersed. Note the prominent thin-walled vessels.

Right: A higher power view of the same case shows the interface of the process with normal collagen.

center the cells have less cytoplasm and the nuclei are distinctly basophilic (figs. 2-44–2-46). The cytoplasm of the latter cells is in fact most often sparse, cell margins are indistinct, and the nuclei are oval to elongate. It is among these cells that a hemangiopericytoma-like vascular pattern develops. The peripheral myofibroblasts are typically arranged in bundles and merge imperceptibly with the less differentiated, more primitive-appearing cells that lie toward the center. In some myofibromas, particularly those found in adults, this zonation is not apparent; rather, the two types of cells are intertwined or clusters of the two types of cells are mixed throughout the tumor. In this situation, the pericytic vascular pattern may be present peripherally and the morphologic features overlap with those of hemangiopericytoma (107a). Sometimes the less differentiated cells are sparse or absent. Mild to moderate nuclear pleomorphism can be found, at

least focally, in most lesions. Normal mitotic figures are common and may be quite numerous, but abnormal forms should not be present. Sometimes, cyst formation is seen and hyalinization in the areas of myofibroblastic differentiation can be prominent. Necrosis can be present, particularly near the center of the lesion, but is essentially limited to myofibromas in children and adults. Calcification is a not uncommon feature and a collagenous stroma may be found anywhere within the lesion. At the edge, the cells that form myofibromas often appear to infiltrate into the surrounding tissue. Occasionally, chronic inflammatory cells are mixed with lesional cells, particularly at the periphery. Visceral and bony lesions tend to contain more of the undifferentiated cells while lung lesions often feature large areas of well-differentiated myofibroblasts. Intravascular growth is common but does not affect the prognosis.

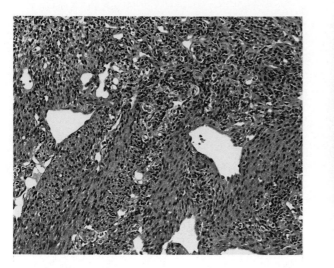
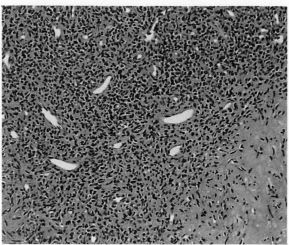

Figure 2-45
MYOFIBROMA AND MYOFIBROMATOSIS
Left: Biphasic pattern features immature cells arranged in a hemangiopericytoma pattern associated with bundles of myofibroblastic cells.
Right: The central hemangiopericytic area is rimmed by a hyalinized myofibroblastic area.

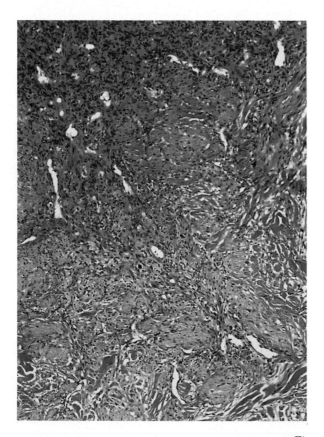
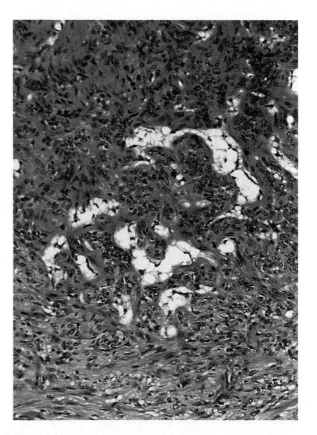

Figure 2-46
MYOFIBROMA AND MYOFIBROMATOSIS
Left: The junction between myofibroblastic cells and immature spindled cells is seen.
Right: Higher power view shows myofibroblastic spindled cells and immature cells arranged in a hemangiopericytic pattern.

Special Studies. Ultrastructurally, the constituent cells of myofibroma are either undifferentiated or have the features of myofibroblasts (111). Both cell types stain for alpha smooth muscle actin and are S-100 protein and cytokeratin negative. In addition, most workers report desmin negativity thus supporting the impression that the constituent cells are myofibroblasts (101,105).

Differential Diagnosis. The initial impression when examining myofibroma is often that of a smooth muscle tumor, but the areas of undifferentiated cells associated with a hemangiopericytoma-like vascular pattern should raise the question of myofibroma, either solitary or multicentric, particularly when the patient is an infant or child. There is some importance in accurately distinguishing between leiomyoma and myofibroma, because patients with what appears to be a solitary myofibroma may actually have multiple lesions, including visceral and bony tumors, that are not apparent at the initial examination. Smooth muscle tumors in the soft tissue are almost always single and do not usually show zonation with a pericytic vascular pattern. Desmin staining is of little value in making this distinction because the staining profile of myofibroblasts and smooth muscle cells overlaps considerably. If there is any doubt, the patient should have imaging studies to exclude other lesions. Inflammatory myofibroblastic tumors occur in children and young adults as a mass lesion but they feature a prominent inflammatory infiltrate including plasma cells and they do not contain the primitive cells with a pericytic vascular pattern that characterize myofibroma.

Infantile hemangiopericytoma figures prominently in the differential diagnosis because the pattern of primitive cells associated with a pericytic vascular pattern is indistinguishable from that of infantile hemangiopericytoma. Indeed, Fletcher and associates (112) have pointed out that myofibroblastic cells can be seen in examples of infantile hemangiopericytoma, so it is reasonable to conclude that these supposedly different tumors are one and the same with different proportions of hemangiopericytic areas.

The lesions of hyaline fibromatosis are usually limited to the skin and the stroma is eosinophilic and hyalinized. The remainder of the differential diagnosis for myofibroma is the same as that for digital fibromatosis above.

Treatment and Prognosis. The clinical outcome for young patients depends on whether the process is solitary or multicentric and its site. Patients with solitary or multicentric lesions confined to the skin, soft tissues, and bones are cured by a diagnostic procedure or minimal excision. Spontaneous resolution of such lesions is common (103,107,113,117). On the other hand, infants with multicentric visceral lesions have symptoms relating to the distribution of lesions and may die of their disease, although the lesions in some affected individuals spontaneously resolve (95,96,99,109). Adult lesions are solitary, superficial, and cured by excision although rare examples may recur nonaggressively.

Hyaline Fibromatosis

Definition. This hereditary condition is first manifest in childhood and consists of cutaneous and subcutaneous lesions composed of nodules of spindled fibroblasts set within a hyalinized stroma.

Clinical Features. Juvenile hyaline fibromatosis is very rare and almost always manifests in children (118,119). Classically, patients present with multiple, painless skin and subcutaneous nodules. The nodules vary from a few millimeters to around 5 cm in diameter. Sites of predilection include the head and neck, back, and lower extremities. Other affected areas include the gums, joints, tongue, intestinal tract, and lymph nodes. In fact, gingival lesions and flexion deformities are the first manifestations of the disease in a few patients.

Pathologic Findings. The tumor nodules are formed by bland fibroblasts with dense thin nuclei, set in variously abundant, eosinophilic, hyalinized stroma that does not contain mature collagen fibers or elastic fibers.

Differential Diagnosis. The youth of the patients and the striking clinical picture of multiple cutaneous and subcutaneous nodules is distinctive and sharply limits the differential diagnostic possibilities. The constituent spindle cells of multicentric myofibromas (infantile myofibromatosis) bear a stronger resemblance to smooth muscle cells than the fibroblastic cells of hyaline fibromatosis. In addition, hyaline fibromatosis does not feature the areas of undifferentiated cells with a pericytic vascular pattern characteristic of myofibroma. Gingival fibromatosis is limited to the gums and is characterized histologically by collagen-rich fibrous tissue rather than hyaline without collagen fibers. Winchester's syndrome is a rare autosomal disease that features severe joint and bone abnormalities. The cutaneous nodules that occur in this disorder are composed of collagenous fibrous tissue but with no hyaline matrix. Neurofibromas may have a hyalinized stroma but the nuclei tend to undulate, and they are positive for S-100 protein in contrast to the negativity of hyaline fibromatosis.

Treatment and Prognosis. Unless they interfere with joint function the lesions are harmless and most are removed for cosmetic reasons. The nodules formed in childhood tend to persist unless they are removed, and new nodules may form well into adulthood. Surgical removal is usually successful and cosmetically rewarding although excision of digital lesions may lead to deformity.

INTERMEDIATE FIBROUS AND MYOFIBROBLASTIC TUMORS (MANAGERIAL GROUPS IIa AND IIc, TABLE 1-10)

SUPERFICIAL FIBROMATOSES

Palmar Fibromatosis (Dupuytren's Contracture)

Definition. Palmar fibromatosis is a nodular, fibroproliferative process that affects the palmar aponeurosis and surrounding subcutaneous fat, and sometimes the dermis. The constituent cells are a mixture of fibroblasts, myofibroblasts, and fibrocytes with uniform nuclear features.

Clinical Features. Palmar fibromatosis is very common and the usual clinical description is "Dupuytren's contracture." It can be familial but there is reasonable evidence to suggest that some cases are the result of repeated episodes of microtrauma. However, not all individuals so exposed develop the lesion, so other factors may play a role. About half the cases are bilateral. Palmar fibromatosis is rare under the age of 20 and its incidence rises with increasing age, reaching a peak in the seventh and eighth decades (122).

The initial manifestation of the process in many patients is the appearance of a nodule that typically protrudes into the palm. This is usually followed by the development of more nodules. Pain may be mild at first, but later can be signif-

icant. Disease progression is marked by the formation of cords of fibrous tissue bridging the palmar nodules and the tendons of the fingers, resulting in flexion contractures. Rarely, the extensor fascia is involved, causing hyperextension of the fingers. The extent of progression and the degree of functional impairment varies from patient to patient.

Around 10 to 20 percent of patients with palmar fibromatosis develop plantar fibromatosis and about 1 percent develop penile fibromatosis. Knuckle pads are also more common in patients with palmar fibromatosis. Other diseases that have been reported to be present in a higher than expected incidence in patients with palmar fibromatosis are epilepsy, cirrhosis, alcoholism, and diabetes.

Pathologic Findings. Most specimens of palmar fibromatosis are obtained by a fasciectomy and when this is the case a fragment of the palmar aponeurosis and attached fat will be received in the laboratory. Most often, the fascia is dotted by firm, gray-white nodules of varying size, measuring up to about 1 cm, but occasionally a specimen with a dominant nodule is received. Microscopically, the diagnosis of palmar fibromatosis is usually straightforward when the location of the lesion, the gross appearance, and the clinical findings are known. The lesion is characterized by nodules composed of fibroblasts and myofibroblasts, with uniform vesicular to dense nuclei set within a collagenous stroma (fig. 2-47) (120,121). The degree of cellularity of the nodules is variable, and some lesions are quite cellular. Older lesions tend to be less cellular, and in these the cells characteristically are mature fibrocytes with small, regular, dense nuclei. Not infrequently, normal mitotic figures are identified, sometimes in large numbers; however, abnormal forms are not present. The cords between the cellular nodules and the tendons of the fingers are composed of dense collagen that is usually less cellular than the nodules. Rarely, foci of metaplastic bone or cartilage are found and some lesions may be associated with chronic inflammation or hemosiderin deposits. Palmar fibromatosis does not infiltrate surrounding tissue beyond the nearby subcutaneous fat but, in some cases, the nodules are attached to the lower dermis. In this situation, skin may be part of the specimen. The dermal involvement sometimes seen is thought

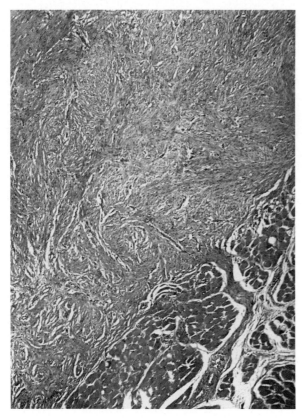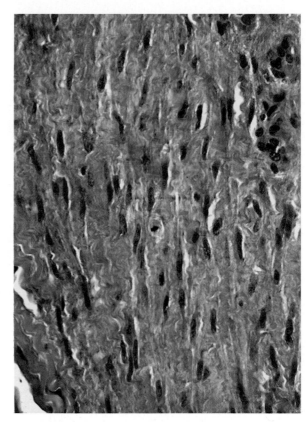

Figure 2-47
PALMAR FIBROMATOSIS

Left: A nodule of variably cellular fibroblastic tissue infiltrates aponeurosis. Cytologically bland, uniform spindled cells are set within dense hyalinized collagen.

Right: Mitotic figures may be seen in proliferating, cellular regions of fibromatosis but are never atypical.

by some to represent recruitment of local dermal fibroblasts rather than invasion of the dermis.

Differential Diagnosis. Because palmar fibromatosis is so common and the clinical presentation so characteristic, the diagnosis is seldom in doubt. The cellularity and mitotic activity of some nodules may raise concern about fibrosarcoma, but this can be quickly dispelled when it is realized that fibrosarcoma presents as a single large mass, not multiple small nodules; is located in the deep soft tissues, not in the palmar fascia; is composed of cells that have chromatin abnormalities; and has cells arranged in intersecting bundles. Moreover, sarcomas, including fibrosarcoma, are extremely rare in the hands. The one exception to this rule is epithelioid sarcoma; unfortunately, the nodular growth of epithelioid sarcoma can resemble the nodular growth of palmar fibromatosis and spindled cells

may be present or even predominate. However, at least some of the constituent cells of most epithelioid sarcomas have a distinctly epithelial appearance and easily visible, brightly eosinophilic cytoplasm. Moreover, the collagen in epithelioid sarcoma is usually more eosinophilic than that in palmar fibromatosis and necrosis is common, whereas it does not occur in palmer fibromatosis. Whenever there is any doubt, keratin and CD34 stains should clarify the situation because the cells in epithelioid sarcoma react with one or both of these antibodies in a very high percentage of cases while the cells in palmar fibromatosis are nonreactive.

Desmoid tumors rarely occur in the hand, but when they do distinction from palmar fibromatosis is critical because the former can be destructive (123). Desmoids present as a dominant mass, not small nodules limited to the palmar fascia and dermis, and desmoids almost always infiltrate skeletal muscle. The nodules of palmar fibromatosis are often more cellular than a desmoid lesion.

Rare cases of palmar fibromatosis may undergo cartilaginous metaplasia, raising the possibility of calcifying aponeurotic fibroma (CAF). However, the chondroid areas of that lesion almost always are calcified, a feature not found in palmar fibromatosis, and CAF is rare after 20 years of age, while palmar fibromatosis is rare before this age. Other distinguishing features between the two are presented in the differential diagnosis of CAF.

Treatment and Prognosis. The lesions of palmar fibromatosis may recur, but they don't recur aggressively. However, pain and contractures can cause considerable patient discomfort and functional disability. Some lesions spontaneously regress after being present for long periods of time.

Plantar Fibromatosis

Definition. Plantar fibromatosis is a nodular, fibroproliferative process that affects the plantar aponeurosis and subcutaneous fat. The constituent cells are a mixture of uniform cells with the differentiated features of fibroblasts, myofibroblasts, and fibrocytes.

Clinical Features. Plantar fibromatosis occurs at an earlier age than palmar fibromatosis; one third of the patients are younger than 30, and occasionally children are affected (124,125,127). The initial complaint is usually of single plantar nodule that becomes painful after walking or standing for long periods of time. Unlike palmar fibromatosis, more often than not, the nodule is single rather than multiple. One or both feet may be affected. Flexion contractures of the toes rarely develop (126). There is an association with palmar fibromatosis and penile fibromatosis, so when nodules are discovered in the foot or feet of a patient who has or has had palmar fibromatosis, penile fibromatosis, or knuckle pads, they almost always turn out to be plantar fibromatosis. Traumatic ulceration may occur and raise the possibility of malignancy (128).

Pathologic Findings. The nodule or nodules of plantar fibromatosis are usually in the range of 2 to 3 cm and they tend to blend into the surrounding fascial connective tissue. Sometimes, what appears to be a single mass will, on closer inspection, be multinodular. On cut section, the nodules are dull gray-white, in striking contrast to the glistening fascia. Histologically, the changes are identical to those of palmar fibromatosis, i.e., nodules of fibroblasts, myofibroblasts, and fibrocytes set within a collagenous stroma. The nuclei of the constituent cells are uniform and normal mitotic figures may be numerous. The nodules vary in cellularity from those so cellular as to raise concern about sarcoma to lesions that are mainly fibrotic, although extensive fibrosis is less common in plantar lesions than in palmar ones. There can be variation in the degree of cellularity within the same nodule. Almost all nodules, however, are more cellular than the surrounding fascia. Chronic inflammatory cells may be prominent and hemosiderin is seen in some lesions. Osseous and cartilaginous metaplasia may develop, although this is rare.

Although most of the lesions of plantar fibromatosis are discrete without involvement of other tissues except the overlying skin, occasional cases, especially recurrent tumors, infiltrate surrounding tissue. However, the cords that extend from the nodules to the tendons of the digits, so frequent in palmar fibromatosis, are largely absent in plantar fibromatosis.

Differential Diagnosis. The differential diagnosis includes monophasic synovial sarcoma, fibrosarcoma, desmoid fibromatosis, and calcifying aponeurotic fibroma; features that are helpful in distinguishing among these are discussed in the Differential Diagnosis section of palmar fibromatosis above. It is particularly important to distinguish desmoid fibromatosis from plantar fibromatosis because desmoids are destructive and may also extend into more proximal portions of the leg. An infiltrating, bland fibrous proliferation in the foot that is over 2 to 3 cm in size, particularly if it is away from the plantar fascia, may well be a desmoid and if the lesion infiltrates skeletal muscle it is even more likely to be a desmoid. If there is uncertainty whether a bland fibrous proliferation in the foot is plantar fibromatosis or a desmoid, the possibility of the latter should be mentioned in the pathology report. In some examples of plantar fibromatosis, the nodules may be densely fibrotic and paucicellular, resembling a scar. Any lesion resembling scar that involves the plantar fascia or infiltrates surrounding tissue should be interpreted with caution, particularly if it is nodular or multinodular, because it may be plantar fibromatosis which has recurring potential.

Acral lentiginous melanoma and clear cell sarcoma both may contain spindle cells but practically never are localized to the plantar fascia. An S-100 protein stain can be performed in cases where there is concern about these entities.

Treatment and Prognosis. Plantar fibromatosis can recur but does not do so destructively. If a fibroproliferative process recurs as a large mass or is destructive, consideration should be given to either a sarcoma or desmoid fibromatosis.

DEEP FIBROMATOSES

The deep fibromatoses are fibroproliferative processes with the capacity for infiltration and recurrence, which may be uncontrollable and destructive, but do not metastasize. As the name suggests, the deep fibromatoses do not originate from the subcutaneous tissue or the skin, although these structures may be involved secondarily. The deep fibromatoses are traditionally divided on the basis of anatomic location into those that arise in the abdominal wall (labeled either *abdominal fibromatosis* or *abdominal desmoid*), those found within the abdominal cavity and pelvis (*pelvic fibromatosis, mesenteric fibromatosis,* and *retroperitoneal fibromatosis*), and those that develop within the deep soft tissues outside the abdomen and the abdominal wall (variably classified as either *extra-abdominal fibromatosis* or *extra-abdominal desmoid*). In addition, the deep fibromatoses are further divided in accordance with the age of the patient into those that occur in infants and children under 5 (*infantile fibromatosis*) and those that occur in postpubertal individuals.

Recognition of the deep fibromatoses is critical because of their nonmetastasizing but potentially recurring behavior. The usual problem is to distinguish them on the one hand from benign conditions, such as scar, nodular fasciitis, and benign fibrous histiocytoma, and on the other hand from fibrosarcoma. This is discussed in detail in the Differential Diagnosis sections below. However, as a general rule, the deep fibromatoses are usually larger at the time of diagnosis than most benign conditions and are less cellular and mitotically active than fibrosar-

coma. It is also useful to know that they are more common than fibrosarcoma.

The recurrence rate varies depending on their location, the age of the patient, and the type of therapy. Occasionally, a deep fibromatosis will undergo spontaneous resolution, but it is impossible to predict on the basis of the pathologic or clinical features which tumor will undergo this happy event. There are reports of deep fibromatoses evolving into fibrosarcoma; one wonders whether such lesions were sampled well enough to rule out sarcoma. In any event this phenomenon is so rare that it need not be taken into account when planning therapy or estimating prognosis.

Extra-abdominal Fibromatosis (Extra-abdominal Desmoid Fibromatosis)

Definition. This is an infiltrating fibroproliferative process that develops in the soft tissues deep to the subcutaneous tissue and is composed of fibrocytes, fibroblasts, and myofibroblasts set within a collagenous to myxoid stroma that possess uniformly bland nuclear features. Infiltration of skeletal muscle is so common as to be practically definitional. The proliferations cannot be more than moderately cellular, and morphologically identical lesions arising in the abdominal wall, within the abdominal cavity, and in infants and children are excluded from the category.

General Considerations. The clinical importance of extra-abdominal fibromatosis (EAF) derives both from its relative frequency among soft tissue tumors and its recurring potential in spite of bland histology. It should be in the differential diagnosis of any fibroproliferative process and often when a diagnosis of fibrous histiocytoma is considered. The inexperienced pathologist may be tempted to interpret EAF as a "fibroma" because of its bland histology, a mistake that is dangerous to the patient and another good reason why "fibroma" should never be used as a diagnosis for any soft tissue lesion (144). In this chapter we conform to the WHO classification in using the term extra-abdominal fibromatosis; however, this lesion is widely known as *desmoid fibromatosis* or, alternatively, *extra-abdominal desmoid fibromatosis,* terms which are equally acceptable.

Clinical Features. Most patients with EAF go to a physician because they detect a mass or because of pain. Less commonly, patients may experience functional disability. The majority of patients are between the ages of 15 to 40 years at the time of diagnosis, although this lesion has been found in individuals from age 5 to those in their ninth decade. Definitionally, EAF in individuals under the age of 5 is categorized as infantile fibromatosis, but EAF is rare in individuals under the age of 12. EAF can occur at any nonabdominal site, but the most commonly involved areas are the shoulder girdle and upper arm, the thigh, the buttock, and the trunk (134–136,151,153). It is rare for EAF to occur in the feet and hands (152). Around 10 percent occur in the head and neck area (132,137,146,154). This incidence varies in different series, presumably because lesions that begin in the shoulder have easy access to the neck and may be counted as having originated there. About 10 percent of EAFs are multicentric, and when this occurs the tumors almost always involve the same extremity or girdle area, although rarely, multiple tumors occur in unrelated sites (130,155,156). Recurrences may develop in more proximal areas of an extremity than the site of the original tumor. There is a general assumption that multiple EAFs or recurrences in the more proximal site do not represent metastasis; rather, they are considered to be multicentric primary neoplasms. The gender distribution of EAF varies from series to series, but most indicate a slight female predominance. About 20 percent of patients report antecedent trauma (137).

CT scans and MRI are often useful in confirming a mass and MRI may be utilized to determine the extent of the lesion. EAFs are almost always located within muscle and the overlying fascia, although large tumors can extend into the subcutaneous tissue.

Pathologic Findings. Most examples of EAF are large, with an average size of 5 to 10 cm. Huge tumors of 15 to 20 cm can be encountered but it is unusual for EAF to be diagnosed when it is under 3 cm. Although EAF can look deceptively circumscribed grossly, skeletal muscle infiltration is present in almost all tumors and sometimes residual muscle can be detected grossly as reddish areas toward the periphery of the tumor. Since muscle infiltration is an important feature that helps distinguish EAF from some of its mimics, areas grossly suggestive of muscle infiltration should be sampled (fig. 2-48). Even if

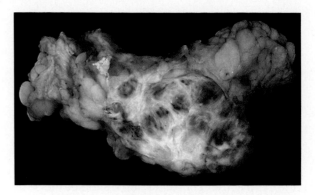

Figure 2-48
EXTRA-ABDOMINAL FIBROMATOSIS
Dense, white, trabeculated fibrous tissue invades skeletal muscle to produce this cross section of alternating white and red patches.

infiltration is not seen grossly, sections always should be taken at the junction of tumor and muscle. When incised, most examples of EAF appear to be composed of glistening white, gristle-like fibrous tissue, although myxoid areas may be noted grossly.

Microscopically, EAF is a no more than moderately cellular lesion composed of elongate, uniform, bland fibroblasts and myofibroblasts loosely arranged in sweeping bundles (figs. 2-49–2-52). The constituent cells are set within a collagenous to myxoid matrix causing the lesion to closely resemble normal cellular fibrous tissue or scar. Infiltration of skeletal muscle by bland lesional fibrous tissue is almost invariably limited to the periphery, although rarely, residual muscle may be found within the more central parts of the lesion. The muscle fibers at the muscle-tumor interface are surrounded by lesional fibroblasts and often display evidence of atrophy or muscle injury (fig. 2-50, right). Some damaged fibers may be multinucleated with enlarged dense nuclei and this change can cause concern for sarcoma; however, the even distribution of chromatin, the paucity of mitotic figures, and the bland appearance of the rest of the neoplasm provide assurance that the enlarged cells are degenerating skeletal muscle cells.

There is little variation on this basic theme from lesion to lesion. The uniform fibroblastic or myofibroblastic nuclei may be slightly enlarged and vesicular or they may be smaller and have denser chromatin. However, significant nuclear

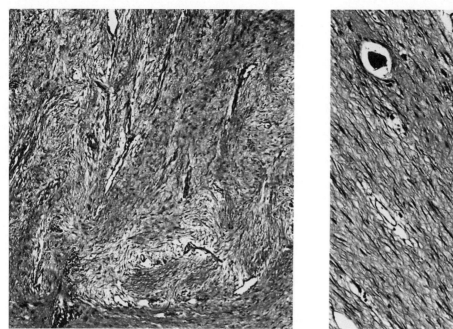
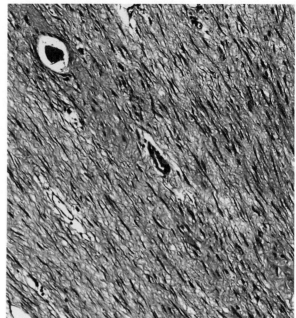

Figure 2-49
EXTRA-ABDOMINAL FIBROMATOSIS

Left: The low-power appearance is that of paucicellular fibrous proliferation arranged in long fascicles. Note the numerous slit-like vessels characteristic of desmoid fibromatosis.

Right: The constituent fibroblasts possess spindled, dense, wavy nuclei and little visible cytoplasm.

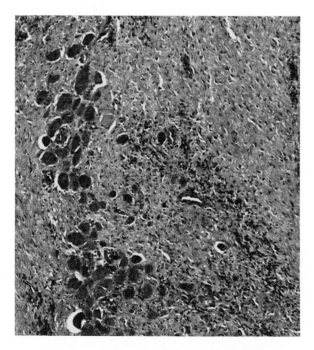
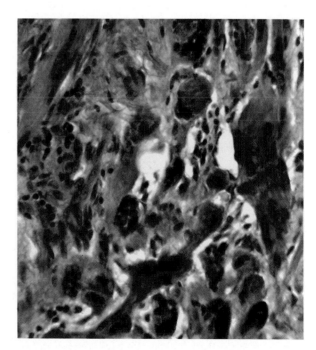

Figure 2-50
EXTRA-ABDOMINAL FIBROMATOSIS

Left: The margin of the lesion shows infiltration of skeletal muscle by the fibromatosis. This is a very common feature of musculoaponeurotic fibromatosis.

Right: Damaged atrophic and regenerating muscle fibers at the edge of the lesion may be confused with rhabdomyoblasts.

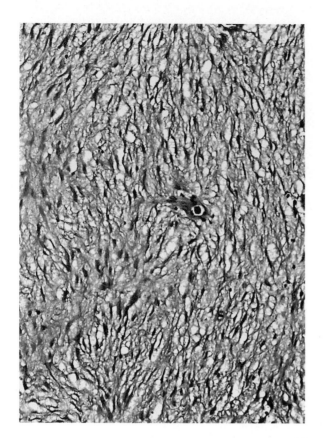 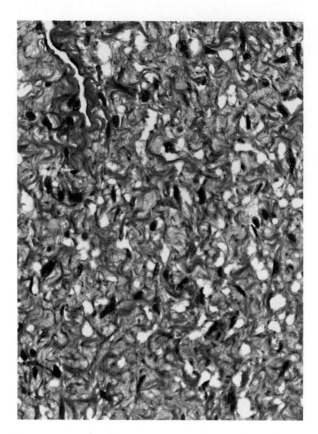

Figure 2-51
EXTRA-ABDOMINAL FIBROMATOSIS

Left: Some fibromatoses may have a myxoid appearance.
Right: The cells are uniformly bland, unlike the cells in malignant myxoid proliferations with which this lesion might be confused.

pleomorphism, abnormal chromatin patterns, and nuclear membrane irregularity are not seen. Most lesions are paucicellular but up to moderate cellularity is acceptable in EAF (fig. 2-52, left). The often wavy collagenous stroma gives way in some tumors to a myxoid background in which the collagen fibers and the cells are pushed aside by acid mucopolysaccharide (fig. 2-51). In some tumors, the smaller stromal collagen fibers are replaced by enlarged, keloid-like collagen bundles (fig. 2-52, right).

Mitotic figures are characteristically difficult to find and abnormal forms are definitionally not present. Occasionally, normal mitotic figures are quite numerous, with up to, but rarely surpassing, 5 mitotic figures per 10 high-power fields. When the mitotic activity is greater than 10 per 10 high-power fields, we think the possibility of sarcoma should be raised. Arteries are characteristically thick-walled and most tumors con-

tain numerous thin-walled vessels, some of which become compressed and appear slit-like. Perivascular microhemorrhages and extravasation of red blood cells are seen in some tumors. Focal collections of lymphocytes are usual, particularly at the periphery, and rarely calcification or metaplastic bone or cartilage is found. Foam cells and hemosiderin deposits are rare. Nerves may be encased by tumor.

Special Studies. Because the differential diagnosis of EAF mainly concerns other lesions composed of fibroblasts and myofibroblasts, electron microscopy and immunohistochemistry are of limited diagnostic utility. Immunohistochemical studies reveal the cells in EAF to be actin positive, and in some tumors desmin positive, but usually only focally (138). Epithelial membrane antigen, cytokeratin, S-100 protein, and CD34 are negative. Bridge and coworkers (133) cytogenetically analyzed 26 desmoid tumors from both abdominal and

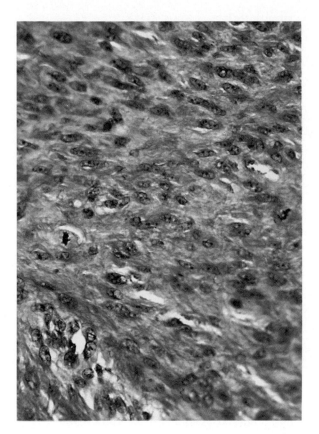
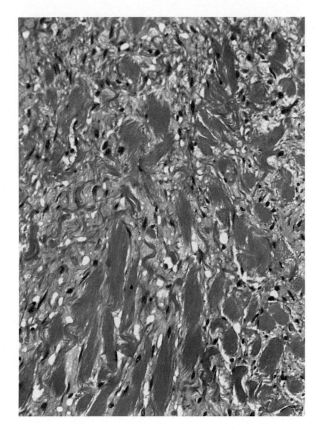

Figure 2-52
EXTRA-ABDOMINAL FIBROMATOSIS
Left: In this more cellular example of fibromatosis, scattered mitotic figures were encountered.
Right: A keloid-like pattern may be observed in some areas of deep fibromatoses.

extra-abdominal sites. They found clonal abnormalities involving the long arm of chromosome 5 in 7 tumors and random abnormalities of chromosome 5 in 14 cases. Five cases demonstrated teleometric fusion and chromosome Y was deleted in 2 tumors. Interestingly, the familial adenomatous polyposis syndrome and Gardner's syndrome, diseases in which intra-abdominal fibromatosis may be a part, are inherited by a heterozygous mutation of a gene also localized on the long arm of chromosome 5, the APC gene (148,161).

Differential Diagnosis. The differential diagnosis of EAF initially involves distinguishing it from benign fibrous proliferations on the one hand and from fibrosarcoma on the other. Hypertrophic scar is always a major consideration when considering a diagnosis of EAF because the two have many similarities. However, in most scars the healing process is in different stages in different areas of the mass so that granulation tissue and extensive hemorrhage may be seen in some areas while EAFs most often have a uniform collagenous or myxoid appearance throughout. Hemosiderin deposits and hemosiderin macrophages are common in scar and rare in EAFs. The characteristic peripheral infiltration of skeletal muscle found in almost all EAFs can be present in scars but is unusual. Finally, EAFs are almost always larger than scars.

The cells in the myxoid areas in EAF can be identical to those in nodular fasciitis, but elsewhere there will be a collagenous stroma in EAF which is absent or only focally present in nodular fasciitis. Large numbers of normal mitotic figures are expected in nodular fasciitis while mitotic figures are usually sparse in EAFs and, of course, EAFs are usually over 5 cm and nodular fasciitis rarely attains that size. Proliferative myositis characteristically features interdigitation of lesional cells with normal skeletal muscle fibers, producing the characteristic repetitive "checkerboard" pattern, while muscle fibers are almost always destroyed and replaced by fibrous tissue within EAF. Moreover, ganglion-like cells, the hallmark of proliferative myositis, are absent in EAFs. Desmoplastic fibroblastoma is less cellular than EAF, does not infiltrate as widely, and has few or no slit-like vessels of the type seen in EAF. Nuchal fibroma occurs in the subcutaneous tissue and is less cellular than EAF. Palmar and plantar fibromatoses grow as small nodules on the palmar or plantar fascia and within the dermis, while EAFs are larger masses that infiltrate widely. The two can be indistinguishable histologically, so knowledge of the operative findings and gross appearance is important. This differential is further discussed above in the sections allocated to palmar and plantar fibromatoses. The childhood fibromatoses can be distinguished from EAF on the basis of the age of the patient, and the lesion's location, size, and histologic pattern.

Fibrosarcomas generally are more cellular than EAF and the tumor cell nuclei typically have grainier chromatin. However, the interface between grade I fibrosarcoma (tumors which on occasion can metastasize) and EAF (tumors which do not metastasize) is blurred; grade I fibrosarcomas are only moderately cellular, often do not contain abnormal mitotic figures, and the constituent cells may display only minor nuclear chromatin abnormalities. In EAFs cellular enough to raise the issue of grade I fibrosarcoma, we evaluate the mitotic index. More than 5 mitotic figures per 10 high-power fields in a tumor that is otherwise a moderately cellular EAF composed of uniform fibroblasts prompts us to alert the clinician to the possibility of metastasis and we employ either the label "borderline" or "uncertain malignant potential" to highlight this concern. More than 10 figures per 10 fields probably means the tumor has at least low metastatic capacity and warrants the label grade I fibrosarcoma, although these criteria have never been adequately tested in a clinicopathologic study. Significant chromatin abnormalities, abnormal mitotic figures, and high cellularity are features of fibrosarcoma. Fibrosarcomas can possess paucicellular collagenous areas that mimic desmoids, a problem in small biopsies. The distinction of low-grade fibromyxoid sarcoma from EAF is discussed in the section on that neoplasm.

Because EAF can be focally myxoid, intramuscular and juxta-articular myxomas may be considered, but these latter two are usually extremely paucicellular and do not have the collagenous stroma required for a diagnosis of EAF. Myxoid MFH (myxofibrosarcoma) is more pleomorphic than EAF, at least focally, and does not have a collagenous stroma. Benign neural tumors are almost always S-100 positive, a reaction that is negative in EAFs. Malignant peripheral nerve sheath tumors are more cellular and mitotically active than EAFs. They arise from a nerve or a neurofibroma and about half are S-100 protein positive. Monophasic synovial sarcoma is far more cellular than any EAF and the stippled chromatin of the nuclei of the constituent cells is not present in the cells of EAF. Desmoplastic malignant melanomas can closely mimic EAF and S-100 protein staining is useful for any lesion involving the dermis that looks like EAF, particularly if that lesion arises in the head or neck. Benign and recurring fibrous histiocytomas contain histiocyte-like cells not found in EAFs, and this usually allows them to be distinguished from EAFs. However, such cells may be sparse in plexiform fibrous histiocytoma and the spindled areas can closely resemble EAF. The superficial location, plexiform architecture, and nodules of giant cells and histiocyte-like cells allow recognition of plexiform fibrous histiocytoma. Pleomorphic MFH displays more pleomorphism than is allowed in EAF and abnormal mitotic figures are often found.

Treatment and Prognosis. EAF has the potential for recurrence, which can be destructive and uncontrolled (135,143,150,153,157). The older literature suggests that the crude overall recurrence rate is 40 to 60 percent, but this rate depends on the size of the lesion, its location, the age of the patient, and the treatment. Larger lesions are more prone to recur as are those not excised with a surgical margin grossly free of tumor. EAFs in areas where complete excision is difficult, such as the shoulder girdle and neck, are more likely to recur, and the younger the patient the more likely is tumor recurrence. More recent studies have emphasized the importance of grossly free surgical margins on the recurrence rate: when the margins are free of involvement grossly, the recurrence rate is reduced to 20 to 40 percent, even though the margins may be involved microscopically.

Radiation therapy is effective in controlling the growth of EAFs and postoperative radiotherapy is generally recommended for patients whose tumor margins are grossly involved (129,131,139,140, 142,147). Some recommend postoperative radiotherapy for patients whose margins are histologically involved (146); others advocate delaying additional therapy until a recurrence is observed (147).

Most observers have failed to find any histologic features that correlate with frequency of recurrence. Two different groups of investigators have reported that tumors which recur have a larger number of slit-like vascular spaces and more extensive myxoid areas than those that do not, but we think these results need to be confirmed and analyzed in a multivariate fashion before they are utilized for patient management.

Because EAF does not metastasize, a generally accepted treatment philosophy has evolved that limits the extent of surgical procedures to those that will not interfere with function or cause disfigurement. More extensive surgery is restricted to those cases in which the tumor has already destroyed function or threatens vital structures such as the trachea or major vessels. Radiotherapy as the primary treatment has also been recommended for those patients in whom a disabling or deforming operation would be necessary to achieve a tumor-free margin (146). As noted, only 20 to 40 percent of patients with grossly uninvolved margins have a recurrence and even when gross tumor is left behind radiation therapy often achieves control (146).

The cells in some EAFs contain estrogen receptors and this has prompted the use of various hormonal treatments including tamoxifen, progestogens, and testosterone. These have been reported to be successful in controlling some inoperable tumors (141,158,159). Paradoxically, there is little or no correlation between the presence of tumor cell receptors and response to hormonal therapy; consequently, negative receptor status is not a reason for denying patients hormonal therapy. Tumor regression has also been reported in patients treated with nonsteroidal anti-inflammatory drugs, presumably because they interfere with the prostaglandin system. Chemotherapy has been used with some success in patients with uncontrolled recurrences, particularly pediatric patients (149). Rarely, EAFs regress spontaneously.

Patients rarely die as a result of their tumors. Those that do have uncontrolled recurrences that involve vital structures.

Abdominal Fibromatosis (Abdominal Desmoid Fibromatosis)

Definition. This is an infiltrating fibroproliferative process composed of fibroblasts and myofibroblasts with uniformly bland nuclear features which develops deep to the subcutaneous tissue in the fascia and muscles of the abdominal wall. Infiltration of skeletal muscle is present in nearly all cases and the lesions cannot be more than moderately cellular. Identical tumors in extra-abdominal sites, within the abdominal cavity, and in infants and children are excluded.

General Considerations. Except for its location, its predilection to occur in women in the childbearing years during or shortly after pregnancy, and its somewhat less aggressive potential, this tumor is pathologically and clinically identical to extra-abdominal fibromatosis.

Clinical Features. Approximately 70 to 90 percent of cases occur in women during the reproductive years; the majority of these patients are 20 to 30 years of age (163). Sporadic cases do occur in males and in children of both sexes. Almost all patients come to a physician because they notice a mass in the abdominal musculature. The tumor is usually confined to the abdominal wall but can extend into the pelvis or abdomen. In the latter circumstance, as long as the abdominal wall muscle or fascia appears to be the primary site, the tumor is considered to be abdominal fibromatosis. Abdominal fibromatosis tends to be smaller when discovered than extra-abdominal fibromatosis; its average size is 3 to 7 cm. Rarely, abdominal fibromatosis occurs in patients with familial polyposis syndrome or Gardner's syndrome, however, the more common location of the fibromatosis in patients with these syndromes is intra-abdominal (see below).

Pathologic Findings. The gross and microscopic features are identical to those of extra-abdominal fibromatosis described above.

Differential Diagnosis. The same lesions in the differential diagnosis of extra-abdominal fibromatosis (see above) and mesenteric fibromatosis (see below) are in the differential for abdominal fibromatosis.

Treatment and Prognosis. The overall recurrence rate for abdominal fibromatosis is between 20 and 30 percent, which is somewhat lower than that for extra-abdominal fibromatosis but comparable to the recurrence rate of EAF with clear margins (162). This probably is the result of both the smaller size of the lesion when discovered and a location more amenable to complete excision. The management of patients with abdominal fibromatosis is the same as for those with the extra-abdominal type (see above).

Intra-abdominal Fibromatosis: Pelvic, Retroperitoneal, and Mesenteric

This category includes fibromatosis in three different locations: pelvic, retroperitoneal, and mesenteric. Pelvic fibromatosis is very similar to, if not an extension of, abdominal fibromatosis. It occurs predominantly in young women in the reproductive years but differs from abdominal fibromatosis in that most patients have not have a recent pregnancy. Because of its location, however, pelvic fibromatosis often grows to a large size before detection and is close to vital structures which can be destroyed by tumor infiltration. The pathologic features, differential diagnosis, course, prognosis, and management are identical to those for the extra-abdominal and abdominal fibromatoses described above.

Retroperitoneal fibromatosis may be localized to the retroperitoneum, in which case it is pathologically and clinically identical to pelvic and extra-abdominal fibromatosis. More commonly, fibromatosis in the retroperitoneum is an extension of mesenteric fibromatosis.

Mesenteric Fibromatosis

Definition. Mesenteric fibromatosis is an infiltrating fibroproliferative process composed of fibroblasts and myofibroblasts with uniformly bland nuclear features. It develops in the mesentery and retroperitoneum, and occasionally in the omentum or other intra-abdominal sites.

Clinical Features. Most intra-abdominal fibromatoses arise in the mesentery, most commonly the mesentery of the small bowel including the ileo-cecal area, although fewer tumors are found in the mesocolon, the root of the mesentery, and the omentum, and a few have been reported in the ligamentum teres. Even though mesenteric fibromatosis is the most common type of intra-abdominal fibromatosis, it is still a rare tumor. In fact, we are aware of only one large series of these tumors in the literature and much of the following information is obtained from this study by Burke et al. (164). About 10 to 15 percent of patients with mesenteric fibromatosis have the familial adenomatous polyposis syndrome (FAP) or Gardner's syndrome (colonic polyposis, desmoids, keratinous cysts of the skin, and osteomas). Patients with FAP syndrome also develop other types of tumors in other organs, most commonly gastric and duodenal polyps, thyroid neoplasms, and adrenal cortical tumors. About 8 to 12 percent of patients with FAP have or develop abdominal or intra-abdominal fibromatosis, often following an abdominal operation. Therefore, patients found to have an abdominal or intra-abdominal fibromatosis should be evaluated for the other features of the FAP syndrome and patients with the FAP syndrome should be evaluated for other tumors, including extra-abdominal fibromatosis and the tumors that make up Gardner's syndrome. If patients with FAP have an abdominal surgical procedure, they should be expectantly observed to be sure there is early recognition of mesenteric fibromatosis if it occurs. This interesting relationship between colonic polyps and mesenteric fibromatosis notwithstanding, the majority of patients with mesenteric fibromatosis do not have FAP or Gardner's syndrome.

The age of patients with mesenteric fibromatosis varies from around 10 years to the eighth decade, with a mean of 40 years. Apparently, the lesion does not develop in infants and young children. For the most part patients see a physician because of a mass, abdominal pain, or gastrointestinal bleeding. Not surprisingly, the majority of the tumors are large when discovered, averaging 15 cm in diameter. Although many examples of mesenteric fibromatosis are slowly growing, a history of amazingly rapid growth is not uncommon. Ten to 15 percent of the tumors are multiple and rare patients have both abdominal, i.e., abdominal wall, and mesenteric fibromatoses either concomitantly or sequentially.

Although most patients with FAP who develop mesenteric fibromatosis do so following a surgical procedure, usually a colectomy, only a small fraction (approximately 10 percent) of patients with mesenteric fibromatosis unassociated with FAP (sporadic mesenteric fibromatosis) have had prior abdominal surgery.

Pathologic Findings. Most often, mesenteric fibromatosis grows as a circumscribed mass; a minority are grossly infiltrating (fig. 2-53). The tumors are white and range from hard and fibrous to soft and myxoid. Microscopically, the fibroblasts and myofibroblasts that compose mesenteric fibromatosis have elongate, regular and uniform nuclei, with vesicular to dense chromatin and scant cytoplasm (figs. 2-54, 2-55). Some tumors have stromal features very similar to extra-abdominal fibromatosis; that is, the constituent cells are arranged in sweeping bundles and set in a collagenous to myxoid matrix. However, in contrast to extra-abdominal fibromatosis, mesenteric fibromatosis tends to have extensive myxoid areas, and in some tumors the myxoid stroma predominates to the extent that

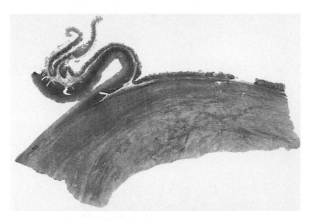

Figure 2-53
MESENTERIC FIBROMATOSIS
The mass appears to be extrinsic to the muscularis propria of the bowel, an important low-power feature that distinguishes gastrointestinal stromal tumors from mesenteric fibromatosis.

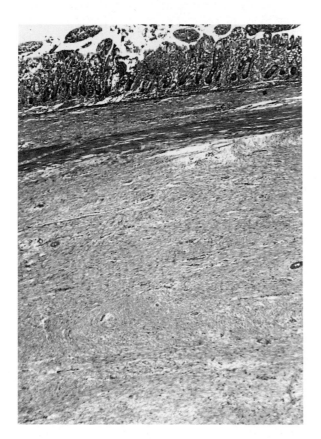
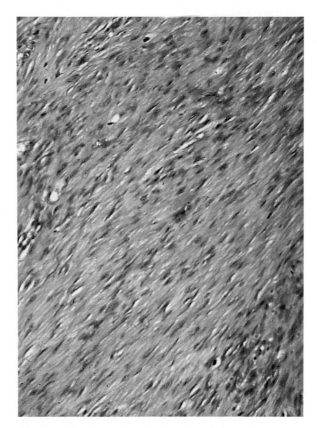

Figure 2-54
MESENTERIC FIBROMATOSIS
Left: A trichrome stain highlights the collagen in the fibromatosis and serves to distinguish this proliferation from the overlying normal muscularis propria.
Right: The fibromatosis is paucicellular and composed of relatively uniform, bland, spindled cells.

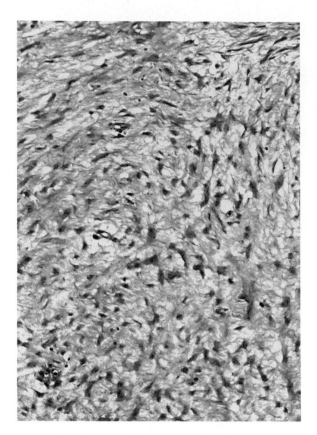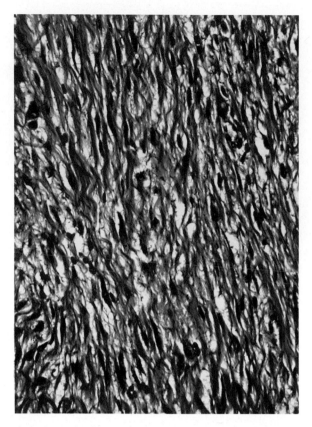

Figure 2-55
MESENTERIC FIBROMATOSIS
Left: Bland, mitotically active, uniform cells are set in a myxoid background.
Right: Less commonly, these uniform, bland, spindled cells are embedded between collagen bundles.

collagenous areas are difficult to find. Such tumors are easily confused with other myxoid neoplasms. A storiform pattern may also be present focally. The margins of mesenteric fibromatosis, although often grossly circumscribed, are microscopically infiltrating and this can be best seen where the tumor infiltrates the muscularis of the bowel. Other morphologic features that are prominent are thick-walled arteries, thin-walled dilated vessels with perivascular spaces, perivascular microhemorrhages, and thick keloid-like collagen fibers. Small numbers of normal mitotic figures are not uncommon but mitotic counts greater than 10 per 10 high-power fields should arose suspicion for sarcoma. Cellularity should not be more than moderate, pleomorphism is essentially never present, and abnormal mitotic figures are not found.

Special Studies. As would be expected, the ultrastructural features and immunohistochem-

ical profile of mesenteric fibromatosis are identical to those found in extra-abdominal fibromatosis. It is important to note that in our experience the cells in mesenteric fibromatosis are CD34 and CD117 negative (171a), a feature which is very helpful in distinguishing this process from gastrointestinal stromal tumors (see below). Clonal chromosomal abnormalities have been observed in some tumors, mainly deletions on the long arm of chromosome 5 in the region of the APC gene, which is also inactivated in patients with familial adenomatous polyposis (169,175).

Differential Diagnosis. The most frequent differential diagnostic problem is distinguishing mesenteric fibromatosis from a gastrointestinal (GI) stromal tumor (GI smooth muscle tumor). When GI stromal tumors are composed of cells with smooth muscle features or cells with an epithelioid phenotype, they are easy to recognize. However, many GI stromal tumors are composed of undifferentiated spindle cells that closely resemble those that form mesenteric fibromatosis. Location is sometimes helpful: although both processes can involve the bowel wall, a mass centered in the muscularis with ulceration of the mucosa favors GI stromal tumor, while a lesion predominantly in the mesentery favors fibromatosis. A predominantly myxoid stroma also favors fibromatosis while organization of the cells into fascicles favors GI stromal tumor. The cells in both tumors may express actin; desmin, which might be expected to be helpful because it is rarely present in the cells of mesenteric fibromatosis, is often not expressed by GI stromal tumors. However, antigens recognized by CD34 and CD117 are expressed by the cells in over 80 percent of GI stromal tumors and these antigens are not known to be expressed by the cells in mesenteric fibromatosis (171a). Both processes can recur aggressively and spread locally, but only malignant GI stromal tumors metastasize so distinguishing the two is important.

Because mesenteric fibromatosis can have an extensive myxoid stroma, neural tumors, myxoid MFH, and myxoid liposarcoma enter the differential diagnosis. Myxoid liposarcoma practically never occurs within the abdomen and lipoblasts are absent in mesenteric fibromatosis. Unlike benign neural tumors, mesenteric fibromatosis is S-100 protein negative. The diagnosis of myxoid MFH (myxofibrosarcoma) requires a greater degree of nuclear pleomorphism than is allowed in mesenteric fibromatosis and this is also true of the other types of MFH. The storiform pattern seen in some examples of mesenteric fibromatosis can cause the observer to think of pleomorphic MFH, but for that diagnosis significant pleomorphism must be present in some area of the tumor. Atypical lipomatous tumor (well-differentiated liposarcoma) can have extensive myxoid areas, but somewhere in this tumor fat cells and the characteristic cells with enlarged nuclei and smudged chromatin can be found. Immunohistochemistry can help exclude spindle cell carcinoma and spindle cell melanoma.

Mesenteritis (retractile mesenteritis) is an inflammatory process associated with fat necrosis, foam cells, pseudocysts, hemorrhage, and cholesterol clefts and in the healing stage, fibrosis (171). Inflammatory cells are a focal minor feature of mesenteric fibromatosis, if they are present at all, and fat necrosis is absent unless there has been prior trauma.

Retroperitoneal fibromatosis must be distinguished from idiopathic retroperitoneal fibrosis (Ormond's disease) which is an inflammatory, fibrosing, plaque-like lesion in the midline retroperitoneum that is frequently associated with bilateral medial ureteral deviation. It has been associated with a number of infectious agents and the use of a variety of drugs. Histologically, there is fibrosis and perivascular chronic inflammation. In contrast, mesenteric fibromatosis grows as a mass, does not often involve both ureters, and contains at most only a few inflammatory cells. Inflammatory myofibroblastic tumor has a triphasic pattern of myofibroblastic proliferation, fibrosis, and prominent inflammation containing large numbers of plasma cells. It occurs predominantly in children.

Low-grade fibromyxoid sarcoma usually occurs in the extremities and the trunk rather than the abdominal cavity and often has more extensive storiform areas than mesenteric fibromatosis. In addition, in mesenteric fibrosis the cells have a more reactive fibroblastic appearance and a more mature fibrocytic appearance. Thinner, denser nuclei are seen in low-grade fibromyxoid sarcoma.

Treatment and Prognosis. Although patients with sporadic mesenteric fibromatosis can have recurrences, these are almost always controlled by reexcision and, if necessary, postoperative radiation, steroid therapy, or therapy with nonsteroidal anti-inflammatory drugs (167,172–174). It is rare for patients with sporadic tumors to die as a result of their fibromatosis. In contrast, patients with mesenteric fibromatosis and familial adenomatous polyposis (FAP) or Gardner's syndrome have a significantly higher risk of recurrence, have recurrences that are more difficult to control, and more commonly die from fibromatosis (164–166,168,170). Moreover, patients with FAP and Gardner's syndrome whose tumors are unresectable respond less well to the therapies listed above. The size of the lesions, whether or not the tumor is grossly circumscribed, and the morphologic features including the level of mitotic activity have not been found to correlate well with outcome for either group of patients.

Infantile Fibromatosis
(Infantile Desmoid Fibromatosis)

Definition. Infantile fibromatosis is a fibrous proliferative process affecting individuals under the age of 10 in which the constituent cells vary from primitive mesenchymal cells to uniform fibroblasts/myofibroblasts set within a collagenous stroma. The process involves skeletal muscle and anatomically may be completely confined to that site.

General Considerations. Infantile fibromatosis is a very rare condition; the literature consists of sporadic case reports or small series (176, 177,180). The largest series, 85 cases from the Armed Forces Institute of Pathology (AFIP), forms the basis of the discussion of this entity in the Enzinger and Weiss textbook on soft tissue tumors (178), and also forms the basis of the discussion below.

Developing a clear notion of the clinicopathology of this entity is hampered not only by its rarity but also by the definitional problems that abound in this area. These chiefly relate to histology and the age of patients at diagnosis. Histologically, the reported cellular examples of this entity overlap considerably with infantile fibrosarcoma while the paucicellular tumors overlap with adult extra-abdominal fibromatosis. The age range of patients with this lesion is variously reported: some feel that infantile fibromatosis rarely occurs past the age of 5 years; this may be so, in part, because this possibility has been defined out of existence. Specifically, tumors that occur in individuals over the age of 5 and that are histologically indistinguishable from adult extra-abdominal fibromatosis are assigned by some pathologists to that group rather than the infantile fibromatosis group. Similarly, the subset of infantile fibromatosis which is cellular and in which primitive mesenchymal cells form most or all of the tumor, while very unusual in individuals older than 5 years, has been reported and accounts for some of the cases in children over 5 years of age. In any case, 10 years seems to be the accepted upper age limit for infantile fibromatosis.

Clinical Features. Usually, patients are brought to a physician because a soft tissue mass has been found, although larger lesions may interfere with function and not be palpable. Almost all patients are under 5 years of age (see General Considerations above). The most common sites are the muscles and fascia of the shoulder girdle, head and neck, and thigh. In the head and neck, there is a predilection for the tongue, the areas around the mandible, and the mastoid process. Bowing of the long bones may be associated with lesions in the leg, and in the head area bone may invaded.

Pathologic Findings. Grossly, the lesion infiltrates skeletal muscle and most often is a firm mass with irregular borders. Microscopically, there are two basic patterns, both of which may be present in the same tumor. One is labeled as the immature or diffuse pattern and is characterized by regular, uniform cells with oblong nuclei and scant cytoplasm set within a delicate myxoid stroma. The cells always infiltrate in and between skeletal muscle fibers, leaving some fibers intact in a pattern reminiscent of the "checkerboard" pattern found in proliferative myositis. Variable amounts of fat accompany the infiltrating cells and scattered chronic inflammatory cells may be present. The second pattern is histologically indistinguishable from adult extra-abdominal fibromatosis, but occurs in children under the age of 5. Metaplastic bone is found in some lesions (179).

Differential Diagnosis. The major differential diagnostic difficulty is distinguishing cellular infantile fibromatosis from infantile fibrosarcoma involving skeletal muscle. The claimed clinical distinction is that cellular infantile fibromatosis recurs but does not metastasize while infantile fibrosarcoma both recurs and, in less than 10 percent of cases, will eventually metastasize. Clearly, developing criteria that would effectively separate these two processes is difficult given the low metastatic rate of infantile fibrosarcoma and the rarity of these neoplasms. Be that as it may, the usual convention is to consider moderately to highly cellular fibrous proliferations that have cells with chromatin abnormalities, little in the way of collagenous stroma, and an infiltrating pattern that obliterates skeletal muscle to be fibrosarcoma. Cellular infantile fibromatosis may have a more collagenous stroma, at least focally, and chromatin abnormalities are muted. The diffuse form of infantile fibromatosis also leaves some muscle fibers intact within the center of the lesion and is associated with fat whereas fibrosarcoma obliterates muscle and intralesional fat is very rare.

The fibroblasts in the diffuse type of infantile fibromatosis may be associated with fat cells which could raise the question of lipoblastomatosis, but in the latter the fat is often arranged in a lobular pattern, although this may be lost in the diffuse type of lipoblastomatosis. This differential is further discussed in the lipoblastomatosis section of chapter 4. Myxoid liposarcoma practically never occurs in children under 10. Embryonal rhabdomyosarcoma enters the differential diagnosis of the diffuse type of infantile fibromatosis, but the former is very rare in skeletal muscle and does not feature intralesional fat. A desmin stain may be helpful. Distinction of infantile fibromatosis from fibrous hamartoma of infancy has been discussed with the latter.

Treatment and Prognosis. Infantile fibromatosis can recur but does not metastasize, so as complete an excision as possible, without interfering with function or causing disfigurement, is the general treatment philosophy. Schmidt et al. (181) suggest that the more undifferentiated the tumor is and the greater number of slit-like blood vessels there are, the more aggressive the lesion. There is some data to suggest that radiation therapy, hormonal manipulation, and treatment with nonsteroidal anti-inflammatory drugs are as effective for patients with infantile fibromatosis as they are for older patients with deep fibromatosis.

Extrapulmonary Inflammatory Myofibroblastic Tumor (Extrapulmonary Inflammatory Pseudotumor, Inflammatory Fibrosarcoma)

Definition. Inflammatory myofibroblastic tumor (inflammatory pseudotumor, inflammatory fibrosarcoma) is a predominantly pediatric, myofibroblastic proliferative process invariably associated with a prominent infiltration of inflammatory cells, predominantly plasma cells and lymphocytes.

General Considerations. Within the last two decades it has become apparent that the lesion originally described as inflammatory pseudotumor occurs in the soft tissues as well as in the lungs and other organs, and that the main noninflammatory cellular constituent of inflammatory pseudotumor is the myofibroblast. As a result of the latter observation, there has been a trend toward classifying inflammatory pseudotumors as inflammatory myofibroblastic tumors, at least in extrapulmonary sites. Inflammatory myofibroblastic tumors can recur and occasionally the recurrences can be uncontrolled. In 1991, Meis and Enzinger (183) reported lesions that appeared to be histologically similar or identical to extrapulmonary inflammatory myofibroblastic tumors as inflammatory fibrosarcoma because they concluded that three (11 percent) of the patients in their study developed metastases. However, inflammatory myofibroblastic tumor can be multifocal and it is sometimes difficult to determine whether lesions involving multiple sites are separate lesions or metastases. In spite of that, there are rare examples (less than 5 percent) which do metastasize. Unless it is confirmed that these lesions have a higher metastatic rate, we agree with Coffin and associates (182, 182a) that they should be considered intermediate tumors (group IIc, Table 10-1) with the potential to recur but with rare metastatic potential rather than sarcomas and that inflammatory myofibroblastic tumor rather than inflammatory fibrosarcoma is the best diagnostic label.

Clinical Features. Most patients are infants and children under the age of 14 years but a few adults, particularly young adults, develop this lesion. It is very rare for extrapulmonary inflammatory myofibroblastic tumor to present in individuals over the age of 30. Patients may come to the attention of a physician because of a mass, but it is also common for them to seek medical assistance because of unexplained fever, pain, or malaise. A significant number are anemic. Over half the tumors develop within the abdomen, particularly in the mesentery, but they are also found in the bladder, the mediastinum, and rarely, in the soft tissues inside and outside the abdomen including the extremities and the head and neck area.

Pathologic Findings. Grossly, inflammatory myofibroblastic tumors are usually circumscribed, white to tan masses that may be nodular; sometimes they have infiltrating margins and a few infiltrate widely. A focal myxoid appearance is not unusual, and some contain scar-like areas. Microscopically, inflammation is constant and accompanies three different patterns of myofibroblastic proliferation (figs. 2-56–2-58). The

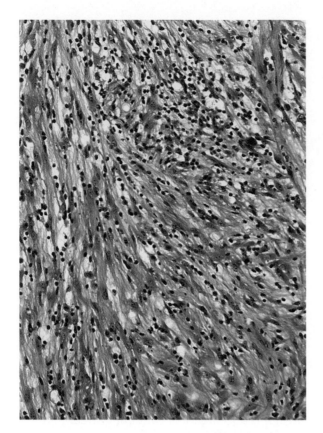 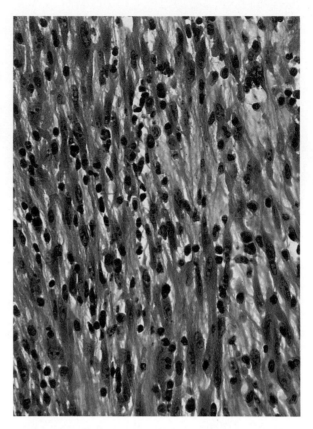

Figure 2-56
INFLAMMATORY MYOFIBROBLASTIC TUMOR

Left: This is the usual appearance of this proliferation, featuring spindled myofibroblastic cells broken up by an inflammatory infiltrate.

Right: Higher power view.

proportion of these patterns is variable from tumor to tumor and from area to area within a tumor. One pattern, which closely resembles granulation tissue or nodular fasciitis, is marked by elongate myofibroblasts with variably abundant eosinophilic cytoplasm and large vesicular nuclei set within a loose or myxoid stroma. The predominant inflammatory cells in these areas are neutrophils, lymphocytes, and eosinophils. Typically, there are only small numbers of plasma cells. The second pattern is more cellular with closely approximated spindled fibroblasts and myofibroblasts set within a compact stroma. These cells may be arranged as islands surrounded by myxoid or hyalinized stroma, and normal mitotic figures may be numerous. Plasma cells are present and tend to be the predominant cell type, although lymphocytes are usually numerous and sometimes are arranged in follicles. In the third pattern, the stroma

is densely hyalinized and paucicellular, with a few plasma cells and lymphocytes caught up in the stroma (fig. 2-58). In some tumors, large "histiocyte-like" or "ganglion cell-like" cells are present, and rarely they may form the predominant cellular population. These cells have large, round, vesicular nuclei with prominent nucleoli and can be considerably pleomorphic. Such cells may be more prominent in recurrences, but their presence does not seem to affect patient outcome.

Special Studies. Immunohistochemically, more than 90 percent of inflammatory myofibroblastic tumors contain cells that are smooth muscle actin, muscle-specific actin, and vimentin positive. Coffin and associates (182a) reported that two thirds of the tumors contained desmin-positive cells, but desmin staining was negative in the tumors reported by Meis and Enzinger (183) as inflammatory fibrosarcoma. Both groups of

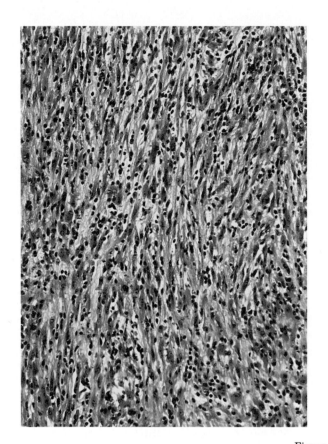
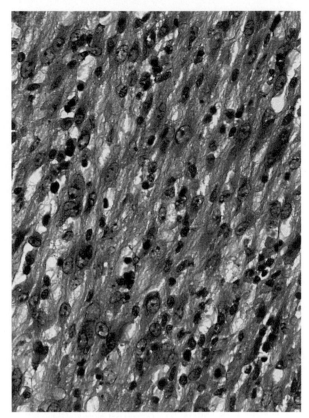

Figure 2-57
INFLAMMATORY MYOFIBROBLASTIC TUMOR
Left: Inflammation obscures the underlying myofibroblastic proliferation.
Right: Higher power view shows the constituent spindled cells.

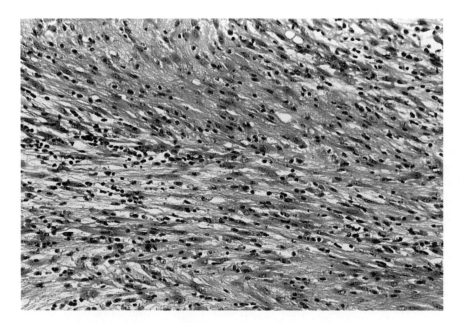

Figure 2-58
INFLAMMATORY
MYOFIBROBLASTIC TUMOR
This example of inflammatory
myofibroblastic tumor has a more
fibrous stroma.

investigators reported keratin to be positive in a third or more of the lesions while CD68 staining varied from 24 percent of the tumors in the Coffin et al. series to 93 percent in the other. ALK rearrangements at chromosome 2p23 are present in some lesions and some are ALK positive immunohistochemically (182b,183b)

Differential Diagnosis. Diffuse sclerosing lesions such as sclerosing mesenteritis and retroperitonitis (retroperitoneal fibrosis), sclerosing mediastinitis, and sclerosing cholangitis all are fibroblastic and myofibroblastic proliferative disorders associated with variable degrees of inflammation, but they are more diffuse processes and do not commonly occur in children. When myofibroblasts are set in a loose or myxoid stroma in inflammatory myofibroblastic tumor the resulting histologic pattern can be indistinguishable from that found in nodular fasciitis. However, inflammatory myofibroblastic tumors are generally larger than nodular fasciitis and tend to occur primarily in a younger age group. Moreover, nodular fasciitis lacks the other two histologic patterns and the striking inflammatory infiltrate characteristically present in inflammatory myofibroblastic tumor. The solid pattern of inflammatory myofibroblastic tumor can mimic fibrous histiocytoma, a smooth muscle tumor, fibromatosis, and other spindle cell proliferations. Indeed, inflammatory myofibroblastic tumor has undoubtedly been classified as one or more of these tumors in the past. Knowing the age of the patient, looking for more than one histologic pattern, paying attention to an inflammatory infiltrate if present, and making judicious use of immunohistochemistry should allow proper classification.

When inflammatory myofibroblastic tumor contains enlarged histiocyte-like (ganglion cell-like) cells, inflammatory MFH is a consideration but is excluded by the absence of a "sea" of neutrophils which is a marker of the latter. Lymphoma can be a consideration and should be excluded by appropriate immunohistochemical studies if necessary. Myofibromatosis is composed in part of myofibroblasts but it also usually features areas of small cells with basophilic nuclei which are associated with a pericytic vascular pattern. Necrosis may be present but the characteristic plasma cell–lymphoid infiltrate of inflammatory myofibroblastic tumor is lacking or muted in myofibromas.

Treatment and Prognosis. Most patients with inflammatory myofibroblastic tumor are cured by simple excision. Occasional tumors recur and rarely these lesions can cause patient death by uncontrolled local growth. None of the 84 patients in the series of Coffin et al. (182a) developed metastases and most patients were well after excision. Some tumors recurred but this was related to difficulty in removing all of it because of location. Patients in this series who died did so because of uncontrolled local growth. Meis and Enzinger (183) reported metastasis in three patients: two to the lung and one to the brain, and rare examples have been observed by some of the authors of this Fascicle. However, it appears that the metastatic rate is less than 5 percent. This is also discussed in the General Considerations section above. There have been no documented benefits from radiation or chemotherapy.

Inflammatory Myxohyaline Tumor of Distal Extremities (Acral Myxoinflammatory Fibroblastic Sarcoma)

Definition. Inflammatory myxohyaline tumor of the distal extremities is a neoplasm of low malignant potential characterized by enlarged ganglion cell–like cells, myxoid nodules, and a variably cellular to hyalinized stroma that is inflamed.

General Considerations. To date there are two reports of this neoplasm, both published in 1998, that contain significant numbers of patients (183c,183d). One group of investigators labeled the tumors "inflammatory myxohyaline tumor of distal extremities" (183d) while the other proposed the term "acral myxoinflammatory fibroblastic sarcoma" (183c). Although the label "sarcoma" has been appended to this neoplasm by the latter investigators, no distant metastases have been documented among the 63 patients with follow-up and only 1 patient has developed regional lymph node metastasis (or tumor transport). However, two thirds of the patients in one report and one fifth in the other had recurrence. Consequently, we think the tumor belongs in the intermediate group of neoplasms rather than the sarcoma group, and for this reason prefer the label inflammatory myxohyaline tumor (IMHT).

Clinical Features. The age of patients with this lesion has ranged from childhood to the

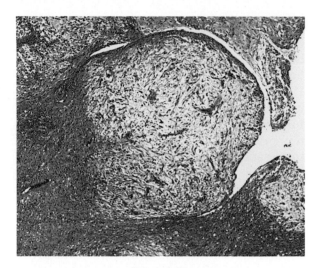

Figure 2-59
INFLAMMATORY MYXOHYALINE TUMOR
The myxoid nodules are surrounded by inflamed, more solid tissue that characterizes this tumor. When the tumor infiltrates synovium, as in this photomicrograph, the histologic pattern may simulate tenosynovitis.

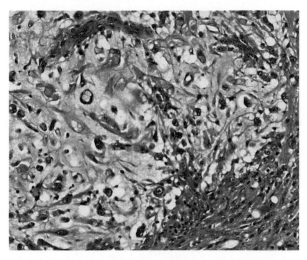

Figure 2-60
INFLAMMATORY MYXOHYALINE TUMOR
A higher power view demonstrates a myxoid nodule containing cells with vacuolated cytoplasm. A more solid cell area can be seen on the lower right.

ninth decade but most are in their fifth and sixth decades. Almost all lesions developed in the hands (two thirds), feet, ankle, and wrists while a few involved the lower legs or arms. None have been found in the trunk, body cavities, pelvis, or head and neck. Patients report a slowly growing, 1 to 8 cm mass (median, 3 to 4 cm), most often in the subcutaneous tissue. The clinical diagnosis is usually ganglion cyst or localized tenosynovial tumor (giant cell tumor of the tendon sheath).

Pathologic Findings. Grossly, the lesions are white and multinodular, and often gelatinous focally. They frequently infiltrate synovium, subcutaneous fat, and dermis, however, epidermal and bone invasion has not been reported. Microscopically, the most prominent features are nodules of myxoid tissue surrounded by cellular to hyalinized stroma, variable numbers of inflammatory cells, and enlarged atypical cells with prominent nucleoli (figs. 2-59, 2-60). The latter often have bizarre shaped nuclei and their appearance spans a spectrum from ganglion-like cells resembling those found in proliferative myositis to Reed-Sternberg–like cells to cells mimicking lipoblasts. The ganglion-like cells usually have a single, large, irregularly vesicular, sometimes irregularly shaped nucleus and a huge nucleolus (fig. 2-61). Their cytoplasm

is prominent and spindled forms are not uncommon. Sometimes they are binucleate and come to resemble Reed-Sternberg cells. These cells are interspersed throughout both the nonmyxoid stroma and the paucicellular myxoid tissue. The multivacuolated lipoblast-like cells are usually found in the myxoid areas and feature hyperchromatic, enlarged, sometime indented nuclei in addition to cytoplasmic vacuoles (183c). Occasionally scattered multinucleated giant cells are identified. The stroma outside the myxoid nodules alternates from cellular to hyalinized. In the former the cells vary from spindled to epithelioid and except for the enlarged bizarre cells demonstrate mild to moderate nuclear atypia (fig. 2-60). Mitotic figures, including abnormal forms, may be present but usually are difficult to find. The hyalinized areas, prominent in many tumors, contain only a few tumor cells and thick-walled vessels. Hemosiderin is present in some tumors.

Completing the histologic pattern of these tumors are the inflammatory cells, which are most prominent in the nonmyxoid cellular areas. These can be so numerous as to partially obscure the larger atypical cells. The inflammatory cell population is composed of lymphocytes, plasma cells, polymorphonuclear leukocytes (particularly in the myxoid areas), and eosinophils. The

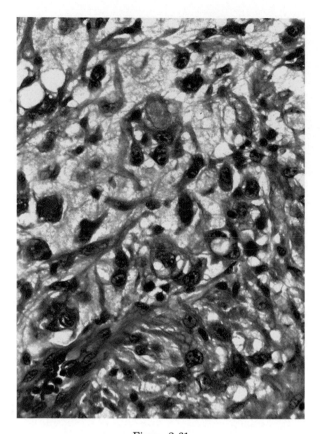

Figure 2-61
INFLAMMATORY MYXOHYALINE TUMOR
This myxoid nodule contains the ganglion-like cells with prominent nucleoli that are characteristic of this tumor.

key features, then, of IMHTs are the location on the distal extremities, myxoid nodules scattered through a hyalinized to cellular stroma, enlarged often bizarre ganglion cell–like or lipoblast-like cells, and a mixed, usually heavy, inflammatory cell infiltrate.

Special Studies. Immunohistologic examination of 35 cases demonstrated staining for vimentin in all of the atypical cells (183c,183d). Variable numbers of atypical cells have stained for CD68 and CD34. Smooth muscle actin and keratin stains have been reported to be focally and weakly positive in a few cases, while S-100 protein, leukocyte common antigen, and epithelial membrane antigen (EMA) stains have been negative.

Differential Diagnosis. The prominent inflammatory component as well as the paucicellular nature of the myxoid areas in IMHT can lead to consideration of tenosynovitis, particularly when the inflammatory infiltrate is so

heavy it obscures the enlarged atypical cells. Careful search for these cells in cases thought to be tenosynovitis should avoid this error. The inflammation and the spindle cell component of IMHT may raise the question of inflammatory myofibroblastic tumor (inflammatory pseudotumor), however, the bizarre cells of IMHT are not present in inflammatory myofibroblastic tumor and inflammatory myofibroblastic tumors practically never occur in the distal extremities. Ganglion cysts and juxta-articular myxomas do not contain the enlarged atypical cells found in IMHT. In addition, juxta-articular myxomas almost always involve large joints rather than the joints of the distal extremity, and are not nearly as cellular as IMHT is at least focally. The ganglion-like cells of IMHT are much more atypical than the ganglion-like cells of proliferative fasciitis, which also lacks marked inflammation. Benign neural tumors containing cells with enlarged nuclei may have a myxoid stroma but the constituent cells are S-100 protein positive while the cells in IMHT are S-100 protein negative. The lipoblast-like cells IMHT may lead to an erroneous impression of myxoid liposarcoma. Myxoid liposarcoma practically never occurs on the distal extremities and does not feature the enlarged atypical cells found in IMHT, and IMHT does not have the plexiform vascular network or the signet ring lipoblasts characteristically present in myxoid liposarcoma. Pleomorphic liposarcoma is extremely rare in acral locations and the enlarged multi-vacuolated cells of IMHT are not lipoblasts. The marked inflammation, fibrosis, and cellular atypia of IMHT are not features of extraskeletal myxoid chondrosarcoma. Atypical lipomatous tumor contains adult fat in addition to enlarged atypical cells.

Perhaps the most difficult lesions to distinguish from IMHT are myxofibrosarcoma (myxoid malignant fibrous histiocytoma [MFH]), and epithelioid sarcoma. Epithelioid sarcoma can be significantly inflamed, it can contain scattered atypical polygonal and spindle-shaped cells, and it often originates in the superficial tissues of the distal extremities. However, the majority of cells in epithelioid sarcoma are round cells with brightly eosinophilic cytoplasm and if enlarged atypical cells are present, they are strongly and diffusely cytokeratin positive while such cells are usually cytokeratin negative in IMHT. Even if keratin-positive cells are present in IMHT, they are focal and the staining is weak. Distinction of IMHT from myxofibrosarcoma (myxoid MFH) on purely histologic grounds is indeed problematic. However, presentation on the distal extremity, paucity of mitotic figures, ganglion-like or Reed Sternberg–like cells, and marked inflammation are features that are useful in recognizing IMHT.

Treatment and Prognosis. In the two series with significant numbers of patients with follow-up the recurrence rate was 22 percent and 67 percent (183c,183d). Some recurrences are multiple or aggressive enough to require amputation, and in one patient recurrence extended up the arm. Recurrences can occur more than a decade after the initial excision. Whether postoperative radiation therapy is effective is unknown and information about its efficacy will be difficult to obtain given the prolonged course of many of these tumors. Spread to a regional lymph node has been documented in one case, but distant metastases have not been documented. Thus IMHT appears to be a tumor with recurring potential but its metastatic capacity, as far as we know, is very low. In the series of Meis-Kindblom et al. (183c) 31 percent of the patients were known to have persistent disease, 64 percent were alive without disease, and 5 percent were dead of other causes. No patient had died at the last follow-up.

MALIGNANT FIBROUS AND MYOFIBROBLASTIC TUMORS (MANAGERIAL GROUP III, TABLE 1-10)

Fibrosarcoma

Fibrosarcoma is a cellular malignant neoplasm composed of a uniform population of spindled fibroblasts and myofibroblasts, organized into bundles that often intersect each other at acute angles. The cells, by definition, demonstrate neither significant pleomorphism nor other types of cellular differentiation.

Fibrosarcoma is divided into two major types: those that occur in adults and those that occur in infants and children. This division is in place because tumors with identical morphology have a significantly lower incidence of metastasis in children and infants than they do in adults. Unfortu-

nately, a sharp cut-off age has not been definitely established, but the largest study in the literature reported that tumors in patients 5 years and under have a metastatic rate of less than 10 percent, while nearly 50 percent of patients 10 years and older with fibrosarcoma develop metastases (200). Too few patients between 5 and 10 years of age have been studied to be sure about the metastatic potential of their fibrosarcomas, but there is evidence to suggest that their tumors behave more like those in individuals under 5 years than those in adults.

As conventionally defined, fibrosarcoma is an endangered species. The reasons for this are multiple. In the past, sarcomas composed of fibroblasts and myofibroblasts with histiocyte-like cells, giant cells, and significant pleomorphism were often classified as pleomorphic fibrosarcoma. Within the past two decades, most workers have reclassified these as pleomorphic MFH. The purpose of this taxonomic shift was to provide a sharper distinction between fibrosarcoma and MFH. As a result, fibrosarcomas definitionally cannot contain significantly pleomorphic cells. Second, the custom of labeling the deep fibromatoses as grade I fibrosarcoma has almost entirely stopped, further decreasing the number of fibrosarcomas. Third, the introduction first of electron microscopy and then immunohistochemistry has allowed spindle cell tumors composed of cells that resemble fibroblasts and myofibroblasts in H&E-stained sections, but with other than fibrous and myofibroblastic differentiated features, to be classified as other types of neoplasms. Finally, the widespread recognition of nodular fasciitis and other reactive fibrous proliferations has decreased the practice of erroneously placing them in the fibrosarcoma category. Inevitably, this trend has shifted and there are attempts to repopulate the ranks of fibrosarcoma by the addition of variants as described below.

In spite of these reshufflings, the borders of the fibrosarcoma group are not crisp. There is considerable uncertainty about what features to use to distinguish low-grade fibrosarcoma from cellular fibromatosis and there is considerable difference of opinion among pathologists in this area about what counts as evidence of fibroblastic and myofibroblastic differentiation. For example, the minimal features required before a cell is deemed to be of smooth muscle type rather than a myofibroblast

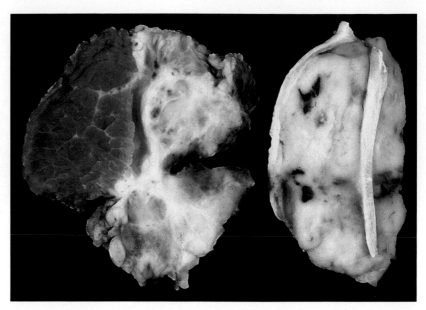

Figure 2-62
ADULT FIBROSARCOMA
Desmoid fibromatosis (left) is contrasted with high-grade fibrosarcoma (right). In contrast to the gristle-like consistency of fibromatosis, fibrosarcomas tend to be white, fleshy, necrotic neoplasms. A tendon lies over the mass. Of course, the better differentiated, collagen-rich fibrosarcomas will approximate the gross appearance of fibromatosis.

have never been sharply defined. In this gray zone, one pathologist's fibrosarcoma is another's leiomyosarcoma. The same problem exists for tumors with morphologic features at the border between fibrosarcoma and pleomorphic MFH with minimal pleomorphism and few histiocyte-like cells.

Adult Fibrosarcoma

Clinical Features. For the definitional reasons discussed above, adult fibrosarcoma is limited to individuals 10 years of age or older. Patients are most often between 40 and 55 years, although all permissible ages can be affected (184,186,189–191). Fibrosarcoma almost always develops in the deep soft tissues, most commonly in the lower extremities and trunk. However, any deep soft tissue site can be affected. Involvement of the retroperitoneum and mediastinum is extraordinarily rare except for the so called inflammatory subtype of fibrosarcoma, a lesion we think is better classified as inflammatory myofibroblastic tumor. Another exception is the development of fibrosarcoma as the dedifferentiated component in a retroperitoneal dedifferentiated liposarcoma. The subcutis rarely is the site of primary fibrosarcoma but it may become involved secondarily. However, dermatofibrosarcoma protuberans may dedifferentiate to fibrosarcoma. There are quite a few early reports of fibrosarcoma occurring in the head and neck, but

some of these tumors probably would be classified as another type of neoplasm today (185,187).

There is a considerable literature describing fibrosarcoma arising in radiated tissue and burn scars. The tumors in some of the older reports might be classified as pleomorphic MFH rather than fibrosarcoma today but there is no question fibrosarcoma can arise in these circumstances, although such a complication is very rare. Fibromatosis practically never dedifferentiates to fibrosarcoma.

Pathologic Findings. Grossly, fibrosarcomas vary from fleshy, focally necrotic and hemorrhagic deep soft tissue neoplasms to firm fibrous matter resembling fibromatosis. The former appearance is characteristic of high-grade lesions while the latter is typical of better differentiated collagenized neoplasms (fig. 2-62).

The basic diagnostic requirement for fibrosarcoma is the presence of elongate, fairly uniform cells with scant cytoplasm and no more than minimal pleomorphism, arranged in fascicles that may intersect at acute angles ("herringbone" pattern) or grow in a long, sweeping fashion (figs. 2-63–2-66). The amount of collagen in the stroma varies from abundant to nonexistent. Mitotic figures are always present and usually numerous, and abnormal forms are common. Chromatin is increased over that found in the cells in fibromatosis; it is usually granular and often abnormally distributed. Nucleoli, often multiple,

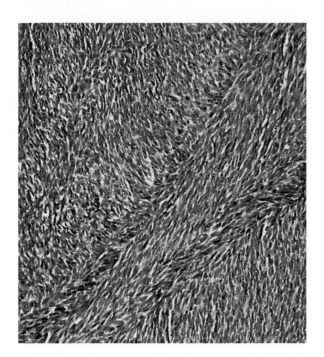 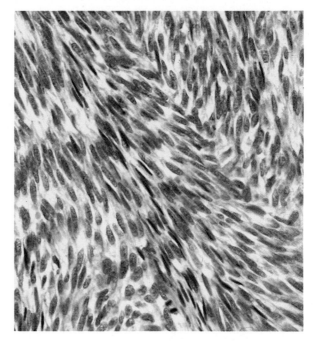

Figure 2-63
ADULT FIBROSARCOMA

Left: At low power, fibrosarcoma is composed of atypical but uniform cells which are arranged in a herring-bone pattern.
Right: The individual cells have coarse chromatin and although not pleomorphic they are clearly malignant.

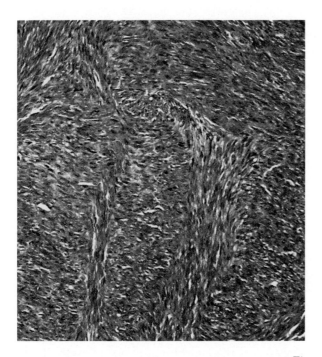 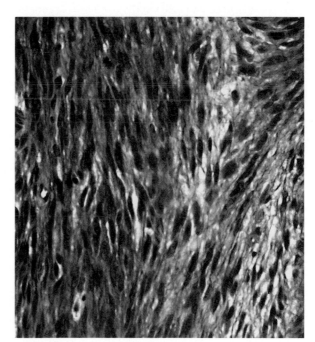

Figure 2-64
ADULT FIBROSARCOMA

Left: Grade I fibrosarcoma: there is minimal nuclear pleomorphism, the mitotic index is low, and the proliferation is more cellular than fibromatosis.
Right: Higher power view.

may be prominent. A cytologically malignant tumor composed of a uniform population of cells, with elongate nuclei that resemble fibroblasts and myofibroblasts, arranged in bundles or fascicles but which display no other line of differentiation, whether detected by electron microscopy, immunohistochemistry, or in H&E sections, is generally considered a fibrosarcoma, although this leaves considerable overlap with monophasic synovial sarcoma and leiomyosarcoma (see Differential Diagnosis section below). Fibrosarcomas with abundant collagenous stroma may contain areas of osseous and cartilaginous metaplasia.

Other histologic patterns may be encountered in what is otherwise a typical fibrosarcoma. In one variation, thick hyalinized collagen fibers dissect and separate the tumor, sometimes breaking up the fascicular arrangement. This has been called the "keloid-like" pattern. In a second, the fascicular arrangement of the cells is loose, and bundles are poorly formed and intersect each other only focally. A focally myxoid stroma in which the cells lose orientation is not uncommon. Another variation reported under the rubric "sclerosing epithelioid fibrosarcoma" is characterized by cells with round to ovoid nuclei and clear cytoplasm arranged in cords or clusters embedded in a dense eosinophilic hyalinized stroma that resembles osteoid (184a,188a). This appearance often causes the observer to think of lobular carcinoma of the breast. These areas must blend into more conventional areas of fibrosarcoma. Cartilaginous and osseous metaplasia is found in some sclerosing epithelioid fibrosarcomas and foci of myxoid stroma are not uncommon. Interestingly, Meis and Enzinger (188a) report that of 14 tumors of the epithelioid variant, 4 were keratin positive, 7 contained cells that were focally epithelial membrane antigen positive, and 4 contained cells that expressed S-100 protein focally. Whether this tumor is a form of fibrosarcoma is uncertain at this time.

The most controversial lesion reported as fibrosarcoma is the one labeled "inflammatory fibrosarcoma" by Meis and Enzinger (188). This tumor, which occurs mainly within the abdomen, including the retroperitoneum, mediastinum, and abdominal wall, and usually, but not exclusively, in children and adolescents, appears to be the same lesion reported in the past as extrapulmonary pseudotumor and more recently as inflammatory myofibroblastic tumor. For rea-sons discussed in the corresponding section above we think this lesion is better classified as inflammatory myofibroblastic tumor.

It is traditional to grade fibrosarcomas, but grading criteria have not been standardized (186,191). Since there seems to be reasonable correlation between the degree of chromatin abnormalities, the mitotic index, the extent of collagenized stroma (i.e., cellularity), the extent of tumor cell necrosis, the degree of fascicle formation, and outcome, we use these parameters to grade fibrosarcomas (figs. 2-65–2-67). Fibrosarcomas composed of cells with nuclei that are only a little larger, only slightly more abnormal than the fibroblasts that characterize fibromatosis, and set within an abundant collagenous stroma are classified as grade I, while those with closely packed cells with markedly dense granular chromatin and little or no collagenous stroma are grade III. Mitotic figures are numerous in the latter and abnormal forms may be found. Grade II tumors are intermediate between grade I and grade III. If there is a discrepancy between nuclear features and the degree of collagenization of the stroma, we use the nuclear features to grade the tumor. Necrosis and hemorrhage are common features of grades II and III but not grade I tumors. Focally, even high-grade fibrosarcoma may demonstrate areas indistinguishable from fibromatosis, so thorough sampling is necessary.

Special Studies. About half the fibrosarcomas tested in one study contained cells that expressed muscle actin, but desmin, CD34, and S-100 protein are generally reported to be negative (192). The immunohistochemical profile of the epithelioid variant has been described above. Ultrastructurally, fibrosarcomas exhibit both fibroblastic and myofibroblastic differentiation (192).

Differential Diagnosis. Because fibroblasts and myofibroblasts are present in many different types of tumors, the differential diagnosis of fibrosarcoma is extensive. The key definitional features of fibrosarcoma require that no other type of cell is allowed other than spindled fibroblastic or myofibroblastic cells, these cells must be arranged in fascicles, at least focally, and significant pleomorphism is not allowed. Thus, the differential diagnosis is essentially an exercise in sorting through monomorphous spindle cell neoplasms with uniform nuclei. For purposes of this discussion, these will be broken

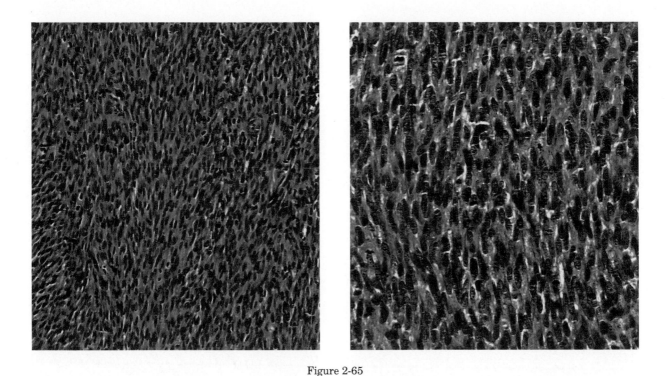

Figure 2-65
ADULT FIBROSARCOMA
Left: Grade II fibrosarcoma shows features intermediate between those in figures 2-61 and 2-63.
Right: Higher power view.

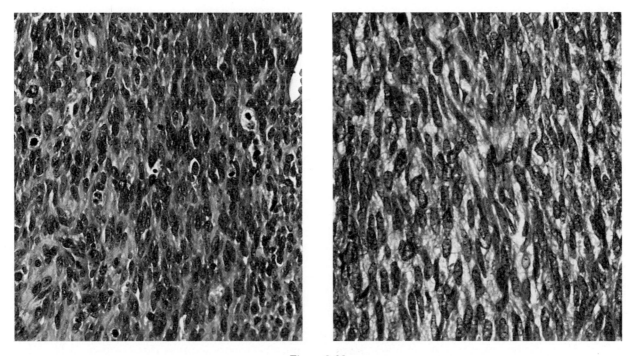

Figure 2-66
ADULT FIBROSARCOMA
Left: Grade III fibrosarcoma: high-grade nuclear atypia and high mitotic index.
Right: Higher power view.

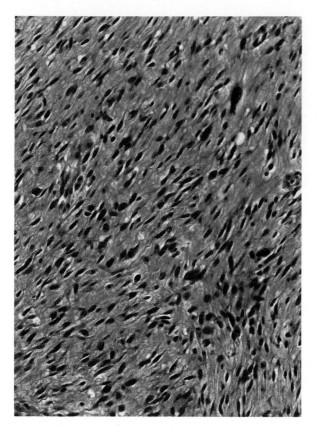 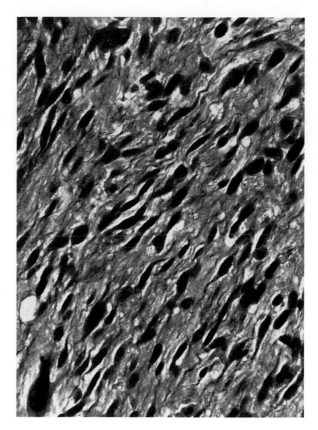

Figure 2-67
MALIGNANT FIBROUS HISTIOCYTOMA
Left: Fibrous variant of malignant fibrous histiocytoma. This degree of nuclear pleomorphism is not acceptable in the fibrosarcoma group.
Right: Higher power view.

down into the following groups: 1) other fibrous tumors, 2) fibrohistiocytic tumors, 3) smooth muscle tumors, 4) neural tumors, 5) monophasic synovial sarcoma, 6) miscellaneous spindled soft tissue tumors, 7) mesothelioma, and 8) spindle cell melanoma and carcinoma.

The features that aid in distinguishing fibrosarcoma from nodular fasciitis, cellular fibroma of tendon sheath, and desmoid fibromatosis have been discussed above in the sections devoted to those lesions. Fibrohistiocytic tumors contain round histiocyte-like cells, including foam cells and giant cells, in addition to the spindled cells (fig. 2-67). Such cells are not allowed in fibrosarcoma. Pleomorphism is a hallmark of MFH, while the cells in fibrosarcoma must be reasonably uniform. Smooth muscle tumors are among the most difficult to distinguish from fibrosarcoma because myofibroblasts and smooth muscle cells share

many cytologic features. Tumors composed of cells that populate the fibroblastic end of the spectrum are easily distinguished from those that contain classic smooth muscle cells. However, observer agreement on the assignment of tumors composed of cells in the midrange of this continuum is poor. Considerable pleomorphism is not uncommon in leiomyosarcoma and is not allowed in fibrosarcoma. Leiomyosarcoma is common in the retroperitoneum and pelvis, sites where fibrosarcoma is distinctly rare and fibrosarcoma is rare in the subcutis and dermis, locations where leiomyosarcoma is common. Desmin expression is common in leiomyosarcomas, in fact, the cells of most soft tissue smooth muscle tumors express this antigen, at least focally, whereas desmin is absent in fibrosarcoma. The cells in benign nerve sheath tumors express S-100 protein and about half of the nerve sheath sarcomas contain S-100 protein–positive cells. In addition, malignant peripheral nerve sheath tumors definitionally must arise from a nerve, a neurofibroma, or in an individual with von Recklinghausen's disease. The features that distinguish fibrosarcoma from monophasic synovial sarcoma are discussed in chapter 11. Hemangiopericytoma contains "staghorn," often gaping vessels, and the cells are not arranged in fascicles. About half of hemangiopericytomas contain CD34-positive cells and this stain is negative in fibrosarcoma. Likewise, almost all solitary fibrous tumors are CD34 positive. Spindle cell hemangioendothelioma occurs in young adults in the subcutaneous tissue or dermis, mainly of the distal extremities, an age and site in which fibrosarcoma is rare. It contains gaping vessels not present in fibrosarcoma and the cells are not organized into fascicles. The cells in dermatofibrosarcoma protuberans (DFSP) are arranged in a repetitive storiform pattern rather than in fascicles, and over 95 percent of tumors express an antigen recognized by CD34. However, fibrosarcoma can arise in a DFSP and the cells in such areas have been reported to express CD34. Finding a superficially located fibrosarcoma, particularly if it is CD34 positive, should always raise concern about DFSP. Spindled embryonal rhabdomyosarcoma occurs mainly in children and a desmin stain should be useful in diagnosing this tumor. Distinction of fibrosarcoma from a GI stromal tumor involves the same considerations as distinguishing mesenteric fibromatosis from GI stromal tumors (see above). Over 80 percent of GI stromal tumors contain cells that express CD34 and some are positive for desmin and S-100 protein. Fibrosarcoma lacks the hemorrhagic gross appearance of spindle cell hemangioma and the latter is associated with cavernous vascular spaces and slit-like spaces in the spindle cell areas, not present in the former.

For the sclerosing epithelioid type of fibrosarcoma, the differential diagnostic considerations are metastatic lobular carcinoma, sclerosing lymphoma, synovial sarcoma, clear cell sarcoma, alveolar rhabdomyosarcoma, granulocytic sarcoma, and ossifying fibromyxoid tumor.

Treatment and Prognosis. Almost all large series reporting outcome for adult patients with fibrosarcoma were published at least 15 to 20 years ago, so current information is in short supply (184,

186,189–191). However, grade seems to be very important (186,191). Patients with grade I fibrosarcoma have a prognosis very close to that of patients with desmoid type fibromatosis, the difference being the few grade I fibrosarcomas that metastasize. Grade II and particularly grade III fibrosarcomas behave as any other high-grade sarcomas, i.e., they have a recurrence rate of about 50 percent and a 40 to 50 percent patient mortality rate when the tumors are deep-seated and large. Metastases are mainly to the lungs and may occur a decade or more after the primary tumor is removed. Lymph node metastases are sufficiently rare in surgical series to warrant withholding lymph node dissection.

Infantile Fibrosarcoma

Definition. This is a cellular neoplasm occurring in individuals under the age of 10, and is composed of a uniform population of fibroblasts/myofibroblasts arranged in intersecting fascicles in a pattern similar to that of adult fibrosarcoma. Significant pleomorphism or any other type of cellular differentiation is not allowed.

General Considerations. When neoplasms that are morphologically indistinguishable from adult fibrosarcoma occur in infants and children, they are much less aggressive. In fact, under the age of 5, less than 10 percent metastasize, while probably a quarter recur. Some have argued that in this age group the designation "sarcoma" should not be used (194). Although the category of infantile fibrosarcoma has been expanded by some authors by the inclusion of tumors with round cells and those that lack a fascicular pattern, it remains true that the usual infantile fibrosarcoma must have, at least focally, morphologic features essentially identical to grade II or grade III adult fibrosarcoma. Unlike adult fibrosarcomas, infantile fibrosarcomas frequently involve the subcutaneous tissue.

Clinical Features. In several series, almost 90 percent of infantile fibrosarcomas developed before the end of the first year of life, and in a significant number of cases the tumor was present at birth (193,197,200). In almost all series, the vast majority of patients are under the age of 5 years. Most of the tumors develop in the extremities, but the trunk and head and neck areas are also affected. Tumor growth can be

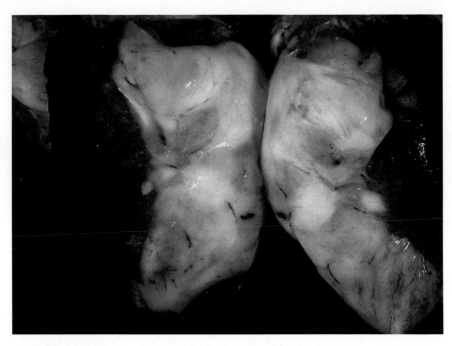

Figure 2-68
INFANTILE AND
CHILDHOOD
FIBROSARCOMA
Gross picture showing a fleshy white mass similar to an adult fibrosarcoma.

rapid and tumor size varies from a few centimeters to gigantic tumors that involve an entire extremity; bones may be bowed or invaded.

Pathologic Findings. Grossly, the tumors are gray-white, except where there is necrosis and hemorrhage, which is common in large tumors (fig. 2-68). Except for the rather common presence of a diffuse chronic inflammatory infiltrate, the usual infantile fibrosarcoma is histologically very similar to grade II to grade III fibrosarcoma in adults as described above (figs. 2-69–2-72). Consequently, collagen may be inconspicuous or absent and the tumors are cellular. Other features found in infantile fibrosarcoma are large numbers of dilated, blood-filled vessels, hemangiopericytic areas, and round cell areas. In some areas, the stroma may become myxoid and the cells lose their elongate shape and fascicular arrangement. Tumors that contain round cell areas or myxoid areas should also have areas of classic fibrosarcoma if they are to be classified as fibrosarcoma. Some have reported that recurrences of infantile fibrosarcoma have the same appearance as the primary lesion (195); others have reported a loss of differentiation in recurrent tumors (198).

Special Studies. The ultrastructural features of infantile fibrosarcoma are those of embryonic fibroblasts (196). Immunohistochemically, the tumor cells express vimentin, but are negative for S-100 protein and desmin. Rare tumor cells are CAM5.2 and actin positive. Almost all infantile fibrosarcomas contain cells with nonrandom gains in chromosomes 8, 11, 17, and 20 (199). One of three cellular fibromatoses in one study also demonstrated identical chromosome gains; however, these gains were not seen in less cellular fibromatosis or fibrosarcoma in older individuals (199). The DNA content of the cells has been reported to be diploid or near diploid in most tumors (194).

Differential Diagnosis. Because of the age of the patients, the differential diagnosis of infantile fibrosarcoma mainly involves infantile desmoid fibromatosis, other childhood fibromatoses, and, because round cells can be present, small round cell tumors. Distinction from fibromatosis is mainly on the basis of cellularity as described in the Infantile Desmoid Fibromatosis section above. Other childhood fibromatoses are not as cellular or as large as fibrosarcoma and rarely are they as mitotically active. Moreover, the chromatin abnormalities present in infantile fibrosarcoma are generally absent in the other forms of childhood fibromatosis. Stains for desmin can help exclude embryonal rhabdomyosarcoma, and CD99 stains are essentially always positive in primitive neuroectodermal tumors and Ewing's sarcoma. Although hemangiopericytoma-like areas can be

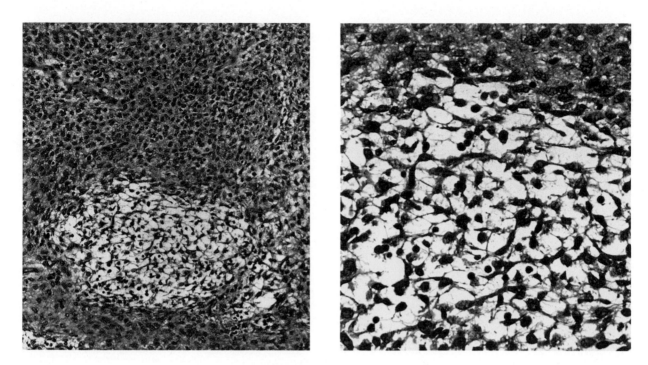

Figure 2-69
INFANTILE AND CHILDHOOD FIBROSARCOMA
Left: Biphasic pattern, with fibroblastic areas adjacent to cellular myxoid areas.
Right: Higher power view of myxoid areas.

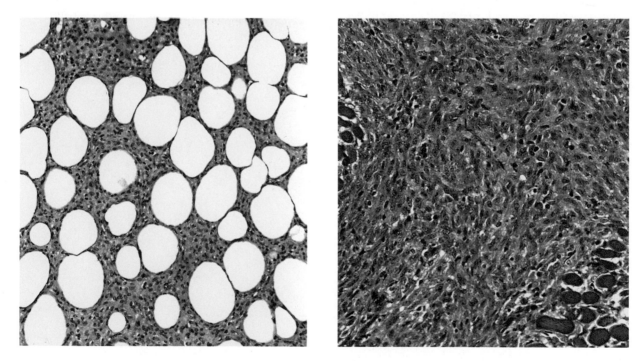

Figure 2-70
INFANTILE AND CHILDHOOD FIBROSARCOMA
Left: Fibrosarcoma infiltrating fat.
Right: Infiltration of muscle by fibrosarcoma.

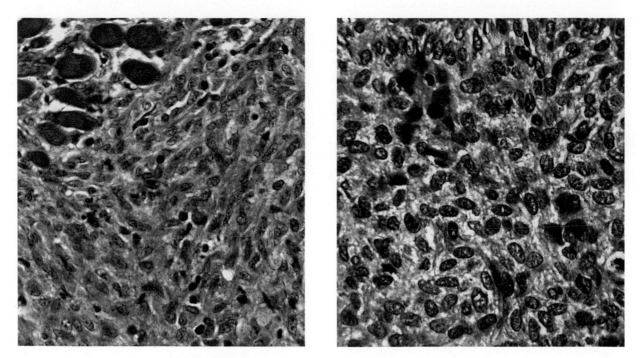

Figure 2-71
INFANTILE AND CHILDHOOD FIBROSARCOMA
Left: Spindled cells.
Right: Plump cells with granular chromatin.

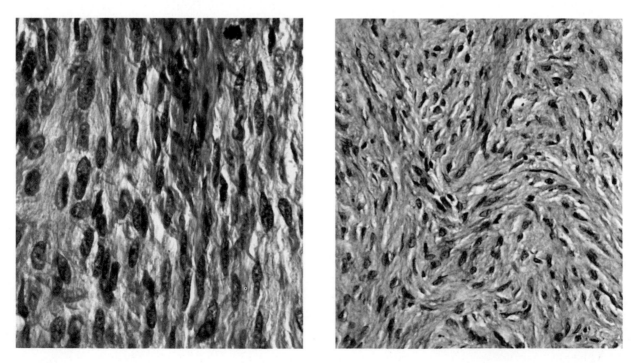

Figure 2-72
INFANTILE AND CHILDHOOD FIBROSARCOMA
Less cellular example which overlaps morphologically with infantile fibromatosis. Lesions with this degree of cellularity practically never metastasize.

found, somewhere a fascicular pattern must be identified in order to confirm the tumor is fibrosarcoma. Distinction of infantile fibrosarcoma with a pericytic vascular pattern from myofibroma(tosis) depends on finding a cellular fascicular area somewhere in the fibrosarcoma rather than the randomly arranged myofibroblasts with abundant cytoplasm found in myofibroma. The distinction of fibrosarcoma from MFH, malignant peripheral nerve sheath tumor, and smooth muscle tumors is discussed in the Adult Fibrosarcoma section above.

Treatment and Prognosis. Because infantile fibrosarcoma rarely metastasizes, can grow to great size, distorting limbs and interfering with function, and can regress spontaneously, and because radical surgery is particularly traumatic for infants and children, treatment decision making for patients with this tumor can be daunting. Unfortunately, there are no morphologic or other parameters that predict which tumors will recur or the very rare tumors that will metastasize. Certainly, if complete excision can be done without interfering with function or causing disfigurement, this is the best course of treatment. When complete excision will leave a functional deficit, treatment decisions become particularly difficult because there is insufficient information to know the risk that attaches to leaving tumor behind and watching the patient. There are preliminary reports that chemotherapy has been successful in eradicating inoperable tumor. Amputation is used when the limb has been rendered useless by the tumor mass.

Low-Grade Fibromyxoid Sarcoma

Definition. Low-grade fibromyxoid sarcoma is a histologically bland but clinically low-grade malignant fibromyxoid soft tissue neoplasm in which deceptively benign-appearing spindle cells are set within alternating areas of fibrous and myxoid stroma. The tumor has a swirling, whorled growth pattern, at least focally.

Clinical Features. Low-grade fibromyxoid sarcoma occurs predominantly in young adults, sometimes in middle-aged persons, and occasionally in teenagers and children. It is rare in the elderly. Although only about 25 cases have been reported thus far, the most common locations appear to be the thigh and the trunk and shoulder area, but other sites may be involved (201–203). Most low-grade fibromyxoid sarcomas develop in the deeper soft tissues, although subcutaneous examples have been reported. The neoplasms are often large at discovery; the median size (maximum dimension) was 9.5 cm in Evans' series and 6.5 cm in the series of Goodlad et al. (202,203). Some patients relate a long history of a slowly growing mass.

Pathologic Findings. Grossly, the usual low-grade fibromyxoid sarcoma is a seemingly well-circumscribed mass with a fibrous to myxoid cut surface; however, infiltration may be apparent grossly and we have observed two cases in which the femoral artery was surrounded by tumor.

Microscopically, the neoplasm is typified by small, bland, regular fibroblastic spindle cells growing in a variably fibrous to myxoid stroma (figs. 2-73–2-77). In at least a portion of the tumor, a swirling, whorled, or even at times storiform architectural pattern is apparent (figs. 2-73–2-77). Cellularity is generally low to moderate, mitotic figures are uncommon, and blood vessels are usually inconspicuous. Slight nuclear pleomorphism may be seen, but more pronounced pleomorphism is unusual, of no more than moderate degree, and focal in extent when observed. In some cases, there are zones with a straighter, more linear cell arrangement in addition to the whorled areas (fig. 2-78). The apparent gross circumscription of low-grade fibromyxoid sarcoma is often belied by microscopic evidence of extension into adjacent tissues, particularly skeletal muscle, although in some tumors the borders are microscopically well-defined. Focal findings in some low-grade fibromyxoid sarcomas include zones of increased cellularity, especially around vessels (fig. 2-79), and a rich capillary vascular network in myxoid areas (fig. 2-80). Cellularity, and to some degree mitotic activity, may be increased in recurrent and metastatic tumors (fig. 2-81), although the overall histologic appearance is typically maintained and it is most common for recurrences and metastases to closely resemble the primary neoplasm (fig. 2-82). Foci of at most moderate nuclear pleomorphism are more frequent in recurrences (fig. 2-83). A distinctive finding in pulmonary metastases is "balls" of paucicellular, heavily collagenized neoplasm filling alveolar spaces. We have seen one low-grade fibromyxoid sarcoma

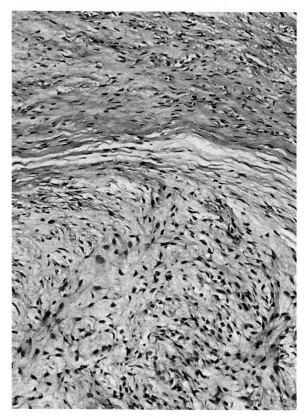

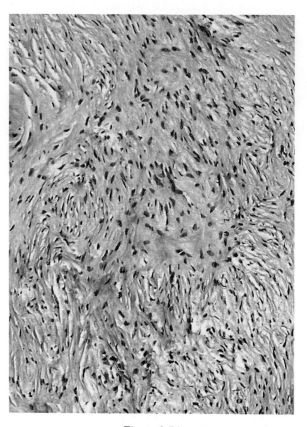

Figure 2-73
LOW-GRADE FIBROMYXOID SARCOMA

This photomicrograph shows characteristic features: contrasting fibrous and myxoid areas, regular, bland-appearing cells with minimal nuclear pleomorphism, low to moderate cellularity, and a swirling, whorled growth pattern.

Figure 2-74
LOW-GRADE FIBROMYXOID SARCOMA

The swirling, whorled growth pattern takes on an almost storiform character in this fibrous area from the case seen in figure 2-73.

Figure 2-75
LOW-GRADE
FIBROMYXOID SARCOMA

Cytologic regularity and swirling, whorled growth are notable. The background matrix ranges from fibromyxoid to densely fibrous. (Figures 2-75, 2-76, 2-81, and 2-82 are from the same case.) (Fig. 2 from Evans HL. Low-grade fibromyxoid sarcoma. A report of 12 cases. Am J Surg Pathol 1993;17:595–600.)

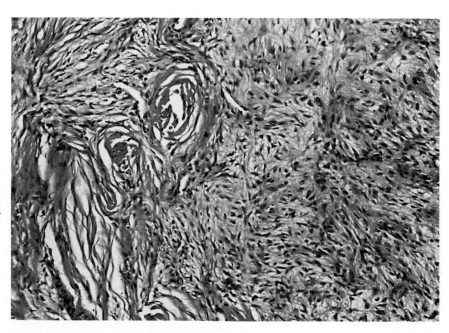

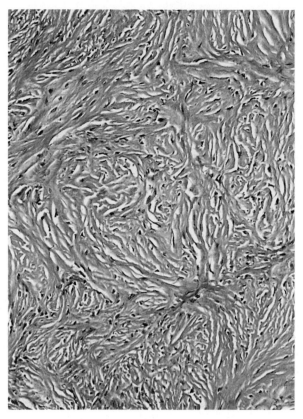

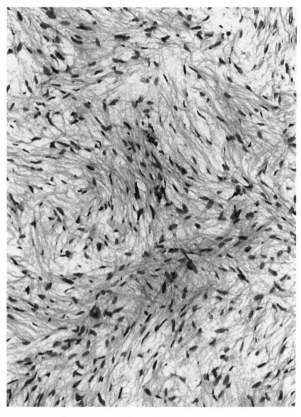

Figure 2-76
LOW-GRADE FIBROMYXOID SARCOMA
In this very hypocellular, heavily collagenized area the swirling, whorled growth pattern can still be seen. (Fig. 3 from Evans HL. Low-grade fibromyxoid sarcoma. A report of 12 cases. Am J Surg Pathol 1993;17:595–600.)

Figure 2-77
LOW-GRADE FIBROMYXOID SARCOMA
This myxoid zone shows typical cytologic features and swirling, whorled growth. (Fig. 4 from Evans HL. Low-grade fibromyxoid sarcoma. A report of 12 cases. Am J Surg Pathol 1993;17:595–600.)

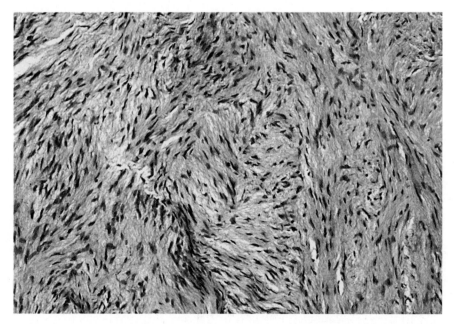

Figure 2-78
LOW-GRADE
FIBROMYXOID SARCOMA
There is a relatively linear cell arrangement in this area. Other areas of the tumor had the characteristic swirling, whorled pattern.

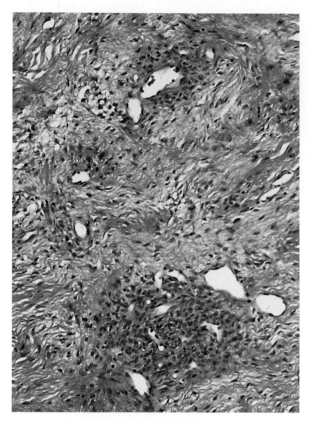

Figure 2-79
LOW-GRADE FIBROMYXOID SARCOMA
In this example, there were zones with increased cellularity around vessels. (Fig. 5 from Evans HL. Low-grade fibromyxoid sarcoma. A report of 12 cases. Am J Surg Pathol 1993;17:595–600.)

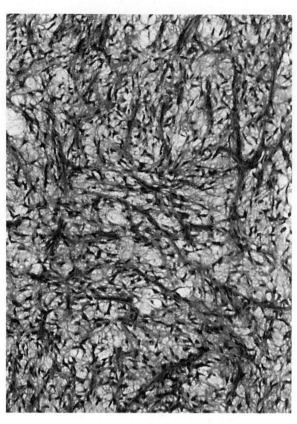

Figure 2-80
LOW-GRADE FIBROMYXOID SARCOMA
Sometimes in myxoid areas there is a rich capillary vascular network. Typical cytologic regularity is apparent. (Fig. 6 from Evans HL. Low-grade fibromyxoid sarcoma. A report of 12 cases. Am J Surg Pathol 1993;17:595–600.)

Figure 2-81
LOW-GRADE
FIBROMYXOID SARCOMA
Cellularity is increased in this late recurrence; however, cytologic regularity is retained. (Fig. 8 from Evans HL. Low-grade fibromyxoid sarcoma. A report of 12 cases. Am J Surg Pathol 1993;17:595–600.)

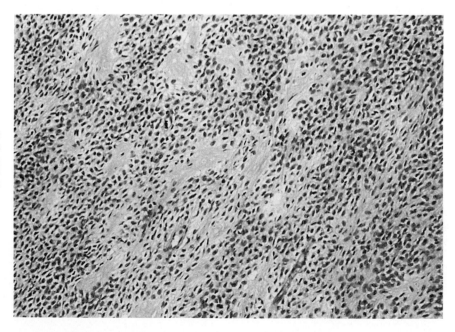

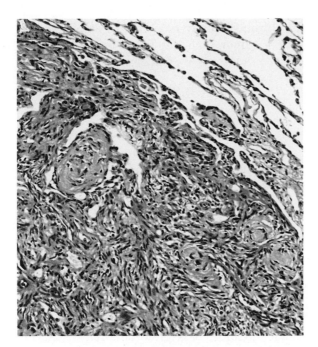

Figure 2-82
LOW-GRADE FIBROMYXOID SARCOMA
Lung metastasis of low-grade fibromyxoid sarcoma. The features are similar to those of the primary neoplasm (fig. 2-75). (Fig. 9 from Evans HL. Low-grade fibromyxoid sarcoma. A report of 12 cases. Am J Surg Pathol 1993;17:595–600.)

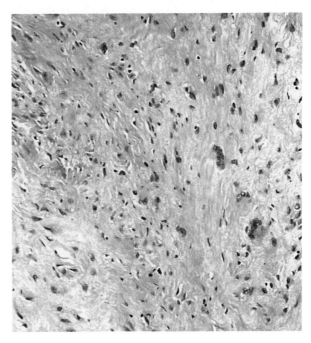

Figure 2-83
LOW-GRADE FIBROMYXOID SARCOMA
This recurrent neoplasm exhibited focal moderate nuclear pleomorphism. Pleomorphism was much less in other portions of the specimen. (Fig. 7 from Evans HL. Low-grade fibromyxoid sarcoma. A report of 12 cases. Am J Surg Pathol 1993;17:595–600.)

that "dedifferentiated" to an anaplastic round cell sarcoma after repeated recurrences extending over many years.

Recently, 19 examples of a tumor very similar to low-grade fibromyxoid sarcoma but with rosette-like structures have been reported with the label of hyalinizing spindle cell tumor with giant rosettes (204). In addition to the rosettes other histologic features included areas of dense hyalinization, cellular spindled stroma, and myxoid areas. There are documented examples of hyalinizing spindle cell tumors that have metastasized, further emphasizing the probable close relationship to low-grade fibromyxoid sarcoma (202a,204a)

Immunocytochemically, low-grade fibromyxoid sarcoma demonstrates diffuse staining for vimentin and focal, weak, or absent staining for smooth muscle actin, HHF-35, desmin, keratin, S-100 protein, CD34, and epithelial membrane antigen. S-100 protein may be positive in the rosette-like areas of the hyalinizing spindle cell tumor with giant rosettes (204).

Differential Diagnosis. The neoplasms most likely to be confused with low-grade fibromyxoid

sarcoma are desmoid fibromatosis, neurofibroma, and low-grade myxoid MFH (low-grade myxofibrosarcoma). Desmoids are distinguished by a straighter alignment of the constituent cells, and many of the cells are somewhat reminiscent of reactive fibroblasts, unlike the cells that constitute low-grade fibromyxoid stroma. Distinctive slit-like vessels are a feature of desmoid tumors but not low-grade fibromyxoid sarcoma. Neurofibroma typically contains cells whose nuclei demonstrate greater waviness than do those of low-grade fibromyxoid sarcoma, and neurofibroma often has thick collagen bundles coursing across a myxoid background. The cells of neurofibroma essentially always express S-100 protein diffusely while S-100 protein–positive cells are rare, or more commonly absent, in low-grade fibromyxoid sarcoma. Schwannomas are also uniformly and diffusely S-100 positive.

Pleomorphic MFH demonstrates much greater cellularity, nuclear pleomorphism and hyperchromatism, and mitotic activity than low-grade fibromyxoid sarcoma. The myxoid areas in myxoid MFH (myxofibrosarcoma) may resemble the myxoid areas in low-grade fibromyxoid sarcoma but the nuclear pleomorphism and hyperchromatism is greater than that present in low-grade fibromyxoid sarcoma. Moreover, abnormal mitotic figures and bizarrely enlarged nuclei are common in myxoid MFH and absent in low-grade fibromyxoid sarcoma. MFH, myxoid and otherwise, usually occurs in an older age group. Although some low-grade fibromyxoid sarcomas have been included diagnostically under the general rubric of fibrosarcoma in the past, fibrosarcomas as currently defined are more cellular and have cells arranged in intersecting bundles instead of whorled patterns. Low-grade fibromyxoid sarcoma shares many features with but must be sharply distinguished from other low-grade bland myxoid lesions of the soft tissues. Distinction is based on the alternating fibrous and myxoid areas and the swirling or storiform arrangement of the cells in low-grade fibromyxoid sarcoma as opposed to the uniformly myxoid stroma in tumors that have only recurring potential (see Myxoid Lesions, chapter 11). Intramuscular and juxtaarticular myxomas are distinctly less cellular than low-grade fibromyxoid sarcoma and do not feature a whorled arrangement of the cells or alternating fibrous and myxoid areas. Aggressive angiomyxomas are uniformly myxoid, have large prominent vessels, and occur in the genitalia, pelvis, and perineum.

Treatment and Prognosis. Low-grade fibromyxoid sarcoma is a slowly growing tumor but one that has a disposition toward both local recurrence and distant metastasis. Currently, the only effective therapy is complete excision. Local recurrence may be repeated and extend over many years, especially when the aggressive capacity of the neoplasm is not appreciated and surgical treatment is inadequate. Seven of the 12 patients in Evans' series (202) developed metastases, most frequently to the lungs and pleura. Metastases may be noted at the time of initial diagnosis or identified years later; in either event, patients often live for long periods with known metastatic tumor. In Evans' study, patients who died of tumor survived for periods varying from 8 to 31 1/2 years, and those who were alive with uncontrolled locally recurrent or distantly metastatic tumor at latest follow-up had survival periods ranging from 6 1/2 to 50 years.

Myofibrosarcoma

Through the years a small number of tumors have been reported as myofibrosarcoma, usually on the basis of ultrastructural examination or immunohistochemistry which reveal cells differentiated as myofibroblasts. On the basis of the described histologic features, most of these tumors could have been just as well classified as either fibrosarcoma or MFH, because myofibroblasts can be found in both. Unless a well-defined group of sarcomas composed predominantly of myofibroblasts is described that has distinctly different histologic patterns from fibrosarcoma or pleomorphic MFH or has a significantly different outcome, it is preferable not to use the term myofibrosarcoma diagnostically. One group of tumors that may meet this requirement is the six myofibrosarcomas of the head in neck in children reported by Smith and associates (206). Although these tumors had histologic features similar to fibrosarcoma or pleomorphic MFH (or even possibly a reactive myofibroblastic process in the case of the lower grade lesions), the clinical presentation of the tumors and the age of the patients were distinctive. Another tumor that meets the requirement is the low-grade myofibroblastic sarcoma recently described by Mentzel and colleagues (205). These are composed of spindle-shaped cells arranged mainly in fascicles set in an often-hyalinized collagenous stroma. The tumor cells have pale inconspicuous cytoplasm and fusiform nuclei that resemble those of smooth muscle cells. Immunohistochemically all stained for at least one myogenous marker: 12 cases were desmin positive, 11 were alpha smooth muscle actin positive, and 6 were positive for muscle actin (HHF-35). Two of the 11 patients with follow-up had local recurrence and one other patient developed metastasis.

Mentzel and Fletcher (205a) have recently summarized the current status of myofibroblasts in soft tissue neoplasia.

REFERENCES

Introduction

1. Coffin CM, Watterson J, Priest JR, Dehner LP. Extrapulmonary inflammatory myofibroblastic tumor (inflammatory pseudotumor). A clinicopathologic and immunohistochemical study of 84 cases. Am J Surg Pathol 1995;19:859–72.

1a. Dahl I, Angervall L. Pseudosarcomatous lesions of the soft tissues reported as sarcoma during a 6-year period (1958–1963). Acta Pathol Microbiol Scand [A] 1977;85:917–30.

2. Dahl I, Angervall L. Pseudosarcomatous proliferative lesions of soft tissue with or without bone formations. Acta Pathol Microbiol Scand [A] 1977;85:577–98.

3. Mackenzie D. Fibroma: a dangerous diagnosis. Br J Surg 1964;51:607–14.

4. Mentzel T, Fletcher CD. The emerging role of myofibroblasts in soft tissue neoplasia. Am J Clin Pathol 1997;107:2–5.

Nodular Fasciitis

5. Allen PW. Nodular fasciitis. Pathology 1972;4:9–29.

6. Bernstein KE, Lattes R. Nodular (pseudosarcomatous) fasciitis, a nonrecurrent lesion: clinicopathologic study of 134 cases. Cancer 1982;49:1668–78.

7. Daroca PJ, Pulitzer DR, LoCicero JB. Ossifying fasciitis. Arch Pathol Lab Med 1982;106:682–5.

8. el-Jabbour J, Wilson GD, Bennett MH, Burke MM, Davey AT, Eames K. Flow cytometric study of nodular fasciitis, proliferative fasciitis, and proliferative myositis. Hum Pathol 1991;22:1146–9.

9. Goodlad JR, Fletcher CD. Intradermal variant of nodular "fasciitis." Histopathology 1990;17:569–71.

10. Hutter R, Foote F, Francis K, et al. Parosteal fasciitis. A self-limited benign process that simulates a malignant neoplasm. Am J Surg 1962;104:800–12.

11. Konwaler B, Keasbey L, Kaplan L. Subcutaneous pseudosarcomatous fibromatosis (fasciitis). Am J Clin Pathol 1955;25:241–52.

12. Kwittken J, Branche M. Fasciitis ossificans. Am J Clin Pathol 1969;51:251–5.

13. Lauer DH, Enzinger FM. Cranial fasciitis of childhood. Cancer 1980;45:401–6.

14. Meister P, Buckmann FW, Konrad E. Nodular fasciitis (analysis of 100 cases and review of the literature). Pathol Res Pract 1978;162:133–65.

15. Montgomery EA, Meis JM. Nodular fasciitis. Its morphologic spectrum and immunohistochemical profile. Am J Surg Pathol 1991;15:942–8.

16. Patchefsky AS, Enzinger FM. Intravascular fasciitis: a report of 17 cases. Am J Surg Pathol 1981;5:29–36.

17. Patterson JW, Moran SL, Konerding H. Cranial fasciitis. Arch Dermatol 1989;125:674–8.

18. Price E, Silliphant W, Shuman R. Nodular fasciitis: a clinicopathologic analysis of 65 cases. Am J Clin Pathol 1961;35:122–36.

19. Shimizu S, Hashimoto H, Enjoji M. Nodular fasciitis: an analysis of 250 patients. Pathology 1984;16:161–6.

20. Weiss SW. Proliferative fibroblastic lesions. From hyperplasia to neoplasia. Am J Surg Pathol 1986;10(Suppl.):14–25.

Proliferative Myositis

21. el-Jabbour J, Wilson GD, Bennett MH, Burke MM, Davey AT, Eames K. Flow cytometric study of nodular fasciitis, proliferative fasciitis, and proliferative myositis. Hum Pathol 1991;22:1146–9.

22. el-Jabbour JN, Bennett MH, Burke MM, Lessells A, O'Halloran A. Proliferative myositis. An immunohistochemical and ultrastructural study. Am J Surg Pathol 1991;15:654–9.

23. Enzinger FM, Dulcey F. Proliferative myositis. Report of thirty-three cases. Cancer 1967;20:2213–23.

24. Kern W. Proliferative myositis: a pseudosarcomatous reaction to injury. Arch Pathol 1960;69:209–15.

25. Lundgren L, Kindblom LG, Willems J, Falkmer U, Angervall L. Proliferative myositis and fasciitis. A light and electron microscopic, cytologic, DNA-cytometric and immunohistochemical study. APMIS 1992;100:437–48.

26. Meis JM, Enzinger FM. Proliferative fasciitis and myositis of childhood. Am J Surg Pathol 1992;16:364–72.

27. Navas-Palacios J. The fibromatoses. An ultrastructural study of 31 cases. Pathol Res Pract 1983;176:158–75.

28. Rose AG. An electron microscopic study of the giant cells in proliferative myositis. Cancer 1974;33:1543–7.

Proliferative Fasciitis and Ischemic Fasciitis

29. Chung EB, Enzinger FM. Proliferative fasciitis. Cancer 1975;36:1450–8.

30. Diaz-Flores L, Martin HA, Garcia MR, Gutierrez GR. Proliferative fasciitis: ultrastructure and histogenesis. J Cutan Pathol 1989;16:85–92.

31. el-Jabbour J, Wilson GD, Bennett MH, Burke MM, Davey AT, Eames K. Flow cytometric study of nodular fasciitis, proliferative fasciitis, and proliferative myositis. Hum Pathol 1991;22:1146–9.

32. Lundgren L, Kindblom LG, Willems J, Falkmer U, Angervall L. Proliferative myositis and fasciitis. A light and electron microscopic, cytologic, DNA-cytometric and immunohistochemical study. APMIS 1992;100:437–48.

33. Meis JM, Enzinger FM. Proliferative fasciitis and myositis of childhood. Am J Surg Pathol 1992;16:364–72.

34. Montgomery EA, Meis JM, Mitchell MS, Enzinger FM. Atypical decubital fibroplasia. A distinctive fibroblastic pseudotumor occurring in debilitated patients. Am J Surg Pathol 1992;16:708–15.

35. Navas-Palacios J. The fibromatoses. An ultrastructural study of 31 cases. Pathol Res Pract 1983;176:158–75.

36. Perosio PM, Weiss SW. Ischemic fasciitis: a juxta-skeletal fibroblastic proliferation with a predilection for elderly patients. Mod Pathol 1993;6:69–72.

37. Weiss SW. Proliferative fibroblastic lesions. From hyperplasia to neoplasia. Am J Surg Pathol 1986;1:14–25.

Fibroma of Tendon Sheath

38. Azzopardi JG, Tanda F, Salm R. Tenosynovial fibroma. Diagn Histopathol 1983;6:69–76.
39. Chung EB, Enzinger FM. Fibroma of tendon sheath. Cancer 1979;44:1945–54.
40. Lundgren LG, Kindblom LG. Fibroma of tendon sheath. A light and electron–microscopic study of 6 cases. Acta Pathol Microbiol Immunol Scand [A] 1984;92:401–9.
41. Pulitzer DR, Martin PC, Reed RJ. Fibroma of tendon sheath. A clinicopathologic study of 32 cases. Am J Surg Pathol 1989;13:472–9.

Elastofibroma

42. Benisch B, Peison B, Marquet E, Sobel HJ. Pre-elastofibroma and elastofibroma (the continuum of elastic-producing fibrous tumors). A light and ultrastructural study. Am J Clin Pathol 1983;80:88–92.
43. Fukuda Y, Miyake H, Masuda Y, Masugi Y. Histogenesis of unique elastinophilic fibers of elastofibroma: ultrastructural and immunohistochemical studies. Hum Pathol 1987;18:424–9.
44. Govoni E, Severi B, Laschi R, Lorenzini P, Ronchetti IP, Baccarani M. Elastofibroma: an in vivo model of abnormal neoelastogenesis. Ultrastruct Pathol 1988;12:327–39.
45. Jarvi OH, Saxen AE, Hopsu HV, Wartiovaara JJ, Vaissalo VT. Elastofibroma—a degenerative pseudotumor. Cancer 1969;23:42–63.
46. Kindblom LG, Spicer SS. Elastofibroma. A correlated light and electron microscopic study. Virchows Arch [Pathol Anat] 1982;396:127–40.
47. Kransdorf MJ, Meis JM, Montgomery E. Elastofibroma: MR and CT appearance with radiologic–pathologic correlation. Am J Roentgenol 1992;159:575–9.
48. Kumaratilake JS, Krishnan R, Lomax SJ, Cleary EG. Elastofibroma: disturbed elastic fibrillogenesis by periosteal-derived cells? An immunoelectron microscopic and in situ hybridization study. Hum Pathol 1991;22:1017–29.
49. Machens HG, Mechtersheimer R, Gohring U, Schlag PN. Bilateral elastofibroma dorsi. Ann Thorac Surg 1992;54:774–6.
50. Nagamine N, Nohara Y, Ito E. Elastofibroma in Okinawa. A clinicopathologic study of 170 cases. Cancer 1982;50:1794–805.

Desmoplastic Fibroblastoma

51. Evans HL. Desmoplastic fibroblastoma. A report of seven cases. Am J Surg Path 1995;19:1077–81.
52. Miettinen W, Fetsch JF. Collagenous fibroma (desmoplastic fibroblastoma): a clinicopathologic study of 63 cases of a distinctive soft tissue lesion with stellate-shaped fibroblasts. Hum Pathol 1998;29:676–82.
53. Nielsen GP, O'Connell JX, Dickersin R, Rosenberg AE. Collagenous fibroma (desmoplastic fibroblastoma): a report of seven cases. Mod Pathol 1996;9:781–5.
53a. Sciot R, Samson I, van den Berghe H, Van Damme B, Dal Cin P. Collagenous fibroma (desmoplastic fibroblastoma): genetic link with fibroma of tendon sheath? Mod Pathol 1999;12:565–8.

Calcifying Fibrous Tumor/Pseudotumor

54. Fetsch JF, Montgomery EA, Meis JM. Calcifying fibrous pseudotumor. Am J Surg Pathol 1993;17:502–8.
54a. Rosenthal NS, Abdul-Karim FW. Childhood fibrous tumor with psammoma bodies. Arch Pathol Lab Med 1988;112:798–800.

Nuchal Fibroma

55. Balachandran K, Allen PW, MacCormac LB. Nuchal fibroma. A clinicopathological study of nine cases. Am J Surg Pathol 1995;19:313–7.
56. Enzinger FM, Weiss SW. Soft tissue tumors. 3rd ed. St Louis: Mosby, 1995:186–2.
56a. Michal M, Fetsch JF, Hes O, Miettinen M. Nuchal-type fibroma: a clinicopathologic study of 52 cases. Cancer 1999;85:156–63.

Pleomorphic Fibroma of Skin

57. Kamino H, Lee JY, Berke A. Pleomorphic fibroma of the skin: a benign neoplasm with cytologic atypia. A clinicopathologic study of eight cases. Am J Surg Pathol 1989;13:107–13.

Solitary Fibrous Tumor of the Soft Tissues

57a. de Saint Aubain SN, Rubin BP, Fletcher CD. Myxoid solitary fibrous tumor: a study of seven cases with emphasis on differential diagnosis. Mod Pathol 1999;12:463–7.
58. Dorfman DM, To K, Dickersin GR, Rosenberg AE, Pilch BZ. Solitary fibrous tumor of the orbit. Am J Surg Pathol 1994;18:281–7.
59. England DM, Hochholzer L, McCarthy MJ. Localized benign and malignant fibrous tumors of the pleura. A clinicopathologic review of 223 cases. Am J Surg Pathol 1989;13:640–58.
60. Flint A, Weiss SW. CD-34 and keratin expression distinguishes solitary fibrous tumor (fibrous mesothelioma) of pleura from desmoplastic mesothelioma. Hum Pathol 1995;26:428–31.

61. Fukunaga M, Naganuma H, Nikaido T, Harada T, Ushigome S. Extrapleural solitary fibrous tumor: a report of seven cases. Mod Pathol 1997;10:443–50.
62. Goodlad JR, Fletcher CD. Solitary fibrous tumour arising at unusual sites: analysis of a series. Histopathology 1991;19:515–22.
63. Hanau CA, Miettinen M. Solitary fibrous tumor: histological and immunohistochemical spectrum of benign and malignant variants presenting at different sites. Hum Pathol 1995;26:440–9.
64. Ibrahim NB, Briggs JC, Corrin B. Double primary localized fibrous tumours of the pleura and retroperitoneum. Histopathology 1993;22:282–4.
65. Mentzel T, Bainbridge TC, Katenkamp D. Solitary fibrous tumour: clinicopathological, immunohistochemical, and ultrastructural analysis of 12 cases arising in soft tissues, nasal cavity and nasopharynx, urinary bladder and prostate. Virchows Arch 1997;430:445–53.
66. Nielsen GP, O'Connell JX, Dickersin GR, Rosenberg AE. Solitary fibrous tumor of soft tissue: a report of 15 cases, including 5 malignant examples with light microscopic, immunohistochemical, and ultrastructural data. Mod Pathol 1997;10:1028–37.
67. Suster S, Nascimento AG, Miettinen M, Sickel JZ, Moran CA. Solitary fibrous tumors of soft tissue. A clinicopathologic and immunohistochemical study of 12 cases. Am J Surg Pathol 1995;19:1257–66.
68. Vallat-Decouvelaere A, Dry SM, Fletcher CD. Atypical and malignant solitary fibrous tumors in extra-thoracic locations: evidence of their comparability to intrathoracic tumors. Am J Surg Pathol 1998;22:1501–11.
69. van de Rijn M, Lombard CM, Rouse RV. Expression of CD34 by solitary fibrous tumors of the pleura, mediastinum, and lung. Am J Surg Pathol 1994;18:814–20.
70. Westra WH, Gerald WL, Rosai J. Solitary fibrous tumor. Consistent CD34 immunoreactivity and occurrence in the orbit. Am J Surg Pathol 1994;18:992–8.
71. Witkin GB, Rosai J. Solitary fibrous tumor of the mediastinum. A report of 14 cases. Am J Surg Pathol 1989;13:547–57.

Calcifying Aponeurotic Fibroma

72. Allen PW, Enzinger FM. Juvenile aponeurotic fibroma. Cancer 1970;26:857–67.
72a. Fetsch JF, Miettinen M. Calcifying aponeurotic fibroma: a clinicopathologic study of 22 cases arising in uncommon sites. Hum Pathol 1998;29:1504–10.
73. Goldman RL. The cartilage analogue of fibromatosis (aponeurotic fibroma). Further observations based on 7 new cases. Cancer 1970;26:1325–31.
74. Lafferty KA, Nelson EL, Demuth RJ, Miller SH, Harrison MW. Juvenile aponeurotic fibroma with disseminated fibrosarcoma. J Hand Surg [Am] 1986;11:737–40.

Fibromatosis Colli

75. Armstrong D, Pickrell K, Fetter B, Pitts W. Torticollis: an analysis of 271 cases. Plas Recon Surg 1965;35:14–25.
76. Binder H, Eng GD, Gaiser JF, Koch B. Congenital muscular torticollis: results of conservative management with long-term follow-up in 85 cases. Arch Phys Med Rehabil 1987;68:222–5.
77. Bredenkamp JK, Hoover LA, Berke GS, Shaw A. Congenital muscular torticollis. A spectrum of disease. Arch Otolaryngol Head Neck Surg 1990;116:212–6.
78. Canale ST, Griffin DW, Hubbard CN. Congenital muscular torticollis. A long-term follow-up. J Bone Joint Surg [Am] 1982;64:810–6.
79. Lawrence WT, Azizkhan RG. Congenital muscular torticollis: a spectrum of pathology. Ann Plast Surg 1989;23:523–30.
80. Morrison DL, MacEwen GD. Congenital muscular torticollis: observations regarding clinical findings, associated conditions, and results of treatment. J Pediatr Orthop 1982;2:500–5.
81. Suzuki S, Yamamuro T, Fujita A. The aetiological relationship between congenital torticollis and obstetrical paralysis. Int Orthop 1984;8:175–81.
82. Thompson F, McManus S, Colville J. Familial congenital muscular torticollis: case report and review of the literature. Clin Orthop 1986;193–6.

Fibrous Hamartoma of Infancy

83. Dickey GE, Sotelo-Avila C. Fibrous hamartoma of infancy: current review. Pediatr Dev Pathol 1999;2:236–43.
83a. Efem SE, Ekpo MD. Clinicopathological features of untreated fibrous hamartoma of infancy. J Clin Pathol 1993;46:522–4.
84. Enzinger F. Fibrous hamartoma of infancy. Cancer 1965;18:241–8.
85. Fletcher CD, Powell G, van Noorden S, McKee PH. Fibrous hamartoma of infancy: a histochemical and immunohistochemical study. Histopathology 1988;12:65–74.
86. Greco MA, Schinella RA, Vuletin JC. Fibrous hamartoma of infancy: an ultrastructural study. Hum Pathol 1984;15:717–23.
87. Groisman G, Lichtig C. Fibrous hamartoma of infancy: an immunohistochemical and ultrastructural study. Hum Pathol 1991;22:914–8.
88. Michal M, Mukensnabl P, Chlumska A, Kodet R. Fibrous hamartoma of infancy. A study of eight cases with immunohistochemical and electron microscopical findings. Pathol Res Pract 1992;188:1049–53.
89. Paller AS, Gonzalez CF, Sherman JO. Fibrous hamartoma of infancy. Eight additional cases and a review of the literature. Arch Dermatol 1989;125:88–91.

Inclusion Body (Digital) Fibromatosis

90. Battifora H, Hines JR. Recurrent digital fibromas of childhood. An electron microscope study. Cancer 1971;27:1530–6.

91. Beckett JH, Jacobs AH. Recurring digital fibrous tumors of childhood: a review. Pediatrics 1977;59:401–6.

92. Bhawan J, Bacchetta C, Joris I, Majno G. A myofibroblastic tumor. Infantile digital fibroma (recurrent digital fibrous tumor of childhood). Am J Pathol 1979;94:19–36.

93. Bittesini L, Dei Tos A, Doglioni C, Della LD, Laurino L, Fletcher CD. Fibroepithelial tumor of the breast with digital fibroma-like inclusions in the stromal component. Case report with immunocytochemical and ultrastructural analysis. Am J Surg Pathol 1994;18:296–301.

94. Choi KC, Hashimoto K, Setoyama M, Kagetsu N, Tronnier M, Sturman S. Infantile digital fibromatosis. Immunohistochemical and immunoelectron microscopic studies. J Cutan Pathol 1990;17:225–32.

95. Iwasaki H, Kikuchi M, Mori R, et al. Infantile digital fibromatosis. Ultrastructural, histochemical, and tissue culture observations. Cancer 1980;46:2238–47.

96. Mukai M, Torikata C, Iri H, Hata J, Naito M, Shimoda T. Immunohistochemical identification of aggregated actin filaments in formalin-fixed, paraffin-embedded sections. I. A study of infantile digital fibromatosis by a new pretreatment. Am J Surg Pathol 1992;16:110–5.

97. Purdy LJ, Colby TV. Infantile digital fibromatosis occurring outside the digit. Am J Surg Pathol 1984;8:787–90.

98. Reye R. Recurring digital fibrous tumors of childhood. Arch Pathol 1965;80:228–36.

99. Viale G, Doglioni C, Iuzzolino P, et al. Infantile digital fibromatosis-like tumour (inclusion body fibromatosis) of adulthood: report of two cases with ultrastructural and immunocytochemical findings. Histopathology 1988;12:415–24.

100. Yun K. Infantile digital fibromatosis. Immunohistochemical and ultrastructural observations of cytoplasmic inclusions. Cancer 1988;61:500–7.

Myofibroma, Solitary and Multicentric

101. Bracko M, Cindro L, Golouh R. Familial occurrence of infantile myofibromatosis. Cancer 1992;69:1294–9.

102. Briselli MF, Soule EH, Gilchrist GS. Congenital fibromatosis: report of 18 cases of solitary and 4 cases of multiple tumors. Mayo Clin Proc 1980;55:554–62.

103. Chung EB, Enzinger FM. Infantile myofibromatosis. Cancer 1981;48:1807–18.

104. Coffin CM, Neilson KA, Ingels S, Frank GR, Dehner LP. Congenital generalized myofibromatosis: a disseminated angiocentric myofibromatosis. Pediatr Pathol Lab Med 1995;15:571–87.

105. Daimaru Y, Hashimoto H, Enjoji M. Myofibromatosis in adults (adult counterpart of infantile myofibromatosis). Am J Surg Pathol 1989;13:859–65.

106. Fletcher CD, Achu P, Van NS, McKee PH. Infantile myofibromatosis: a light microscopic, histochemical and immunohistochemical study suggesting true smooth muscle differentiation. Histopathology 1987;11:245–58.

107. Goldberg NS, Bauer BS, Kraus H, Crussi FG, Esterly NB. Infantile myofibromatosis: a review of clinicopathology with perspectives on new treatment choices. Pediatr Dermatol 1988;5:37–46.

107a. Granter SR, Badizadegan K, Fletcher CD. Myofibromatosis in adults, glomangiopericytoma, and myopericytoma. A spectrum of tumors showing perivascular myoid differentiation. Am J Surg Pathol 1998;22:513–25.

108. Hogan SF, Salassa JR. Recurrent adult myofibromatosis. A case report. Am J Clin Pathol 1992;97:810–4.

109. Jennings TA, Duray PH, Collins FS, Sabetta J, Enzinger FM. Infantile myofibromatosis. Evidence for an autosomal-dominant disorder. Am J Surg Pathol 1984;8:529–38.

110. Kindblom LG, Termen G, Save-Soderbergh J, Angervall L. Congenital solitary fibromatosis of soft tissues, a variant of congenital generalized fibromatosis. 2 cases reports. Acta Pathol Microbiol Scand [A] 1977;85:640–8.

111. Liew SH, Haynes M. Localized form of congenital generalized fibromatosis. A report of 3 cases with myofibroblasts. Pathology 1981;13:257–66.

112. Mentzel T, Calonje E, Nascimento AG, Fletcher CD. Infantile hemangiopericytoma versus infantile myofibromatosis. Study of a series suggesting a continuous spectrum of infantile myofibroblastic lesions. Am J Surg Pathol 1994;18:922–30.

113. Roggli VL, Kim HS, Hawkins E. Congenital generalized fibromatosis with visceral involvement. A case report. Cancer 1980;45:954–60.

114. Speight PM, Dayan D, Fletcher CD. Adult and infantile myofibromatosis: a report of three cases affecting the oral cavity. J Oral Pathol Med 1991;20:380–4.

115. Spraker MK, Stack C, Esterly NB. Congenital generalized fibromatosis: a review of the literature and report of a case associated with porencephaly, hemiatrophy, and cutis marmorata telangiectatica congenita. J Am Acad Dermatol 1984;10:365–71.

116. Vigneswaran N, Boyd DL, Waldron CA. Solitary infantile myofibromatosis of the mandible. Report of three cases. Oral Surg Oral Med Oral Pathol 1992;73:84–8.

117. Wiswell TE, Davis J, Cunningham BE, Solenberger R, Thomas PJ. Infantile myofibromatosis: the most common fibrous tumor of infancy. J Pediatr Surg 1988;23:315–8.

Hyaline Fibromatosis

118. Finlay AY, Ferguson SD, Holt PJ. Juvenile hyaline fibromatosis. Br J Dermatol 1983;108:609–16.

119. Remberger K, Krieg T, Kunze D, Weinmann HM, Hubner G. Fibromatosis hyalinica multiplex (juvenile hyalin fibromatosis). Light microscopic, electron microscopic, immunohistochemical, and biochemical findings. Cancer 1985;56:614–24.

Palmar Fibromatosis

120. Allen PW. The fibromatoses: a clinicopathologic classification based on 140 cases. Am J Surg Pathol 1977;1:255–70.
121. Iwasaki H, Muller H, Stutte HJ, Brennscheidt U. Palmar fibromatosis (Dupuytren's contracture). Ultrastructural and enzyme histochemical studies of 43 cases. Virchows Arch [A] 1984;405:41–53.
122. Mikkelsen OA. Dupuytren's disease–initial symptoms, age of onset and spontaneous course. Hand 1977;9:11–5.
123. Ritter MA, Marshall JL, Straub LR. Extra-abdominal desmoid of the hand. A case report. J Bone Joint Surg 1969;51A:1641–4.

Plantar Fibromatosis

124. Allen R, Woolner L, Ghormley R. Soft-tissue tumors of the sole. J Bone Joint Surg 1955;37–A:14–27.
125. Aviles E, Arlen M, Miller T. Plantar fibromatosis. Surgery 1971;69:117–20.
126. Classen DA, Hurst LN. Plantar fibromatosis and bilateral flexion contractures: a review of the literature. Ann Plast Surg 1992;28:475–8.
127. Lee TH, Wapner KL, Hecht PJ. Plantar fibromatosis. J Bone Joint Surg Am 1993;75:1080–4.
128. Warthan TL, Rudolph RI, Gross PR. Isolated plantar fibromatosis. Arch Dermatol 1973;108:823–5.

Extra-abdominal (Desmoid) Fibromatosis

129. Acker JC, Bossen EH, Halperin EC. The management of desmoid tumors. Int J Radiat Oncol Biol Phys 1993;26:851–8.
130. Allen PW. The fibromatoses: a clinicopathologic classification based on 140 cases. Am J Surg Pathol 1977;1:255–70.
131. Bataini JP, Belloir C, Mazabraud A, et al. Desmoid tumors in adults: the role of radiotherapy in their management. Am J Surg 1988;155:754–60.
132. Batsakis JG, Raslan W. Extra-abdominal desmoid fibromatosis. Ann Otol Rhinol Laryngol 1994;103:331–4.
133. Bridge JA, Sreekantaiah C, Mouron B, Neff JR, Sandberg AA, Wolman SR. Clonal chromosomal abnormalities in desmoid tumors. Implications for histopathogenesis. Cancer 1992;69:430–6.
134. Dashiell TG, Payne WS, Hepper NG, Soule EH. Desmoid tumors of the chest wall. Chest 1978;74:157–62.
135. Enzinger FM, Shiraki M. Musculo-aponeurotic fibromatosis of the shoulder girdle (extra-abdominal desmoid). Analysis of thirty cases followed up for ten or more years. Cancer 1967;20:1131–40.
136. Enzinger FM, Weiss SW. Soft tissue tumors. 3rd ed. St Louis: Mosby, 1995.
137. Hayry P, Reitamo JJ, Totterman S, Hopfner HD, Sivula A. The desmoid tumor. II. Analysis of factors possibly contributing to the etiology and growth behavior. Am J Clin Pathol 1982;77:674–80.
138. Hayry P, Reitamo JJ, Vihko R, et al. The desmoid tumor. III. A biochemical and genetic analysis. Am J Clin Pathol 1982;77:681–5.
139. Karakousis CP, Mayordomo J, Zografos GC, Driscoll DL. Desmoid tumors of the trunk and extremity. Cancer 1993;72:1637–41.
140. Khorsand J, Karakousis CP. Desmoid tumors and their management. Am J Surg 1985;149:215–8.
141. Klein WA, Miller HH, Anderson M, DeCosse JJ. The use of indomethacin, sulindac, and tamoxifen for the treatment of desmoid tumors associated with familial polyposis. Cancer 1987;60:2863–8.
142. Leibel SA, Wara WM, Hill DR, et al. Desmoid tumors: local control and patterns of relapse following radiation therapy. Int J Radiat Oncol Biol Phys 1983;9:1167–71.
143. Lopez R, Kemalyan N, Moseley HS, Dennis D, Vetto RM. Problems in diagnosis and management of desmoid tumors. Am J Surg 1990;159:450–3.
144. Mackenzie D. Fibroma: a dangerous diagnosis. Brit J Surg 1964;51:607–14.
145. Masson JK, Soule EH. Desmoid tumors of the head and neck. Am J Surg 1966;112:615–22.
146. McCollough WM, Parsons JT, van der Griend R, Enneking WF, Heare T. Radiation therapy for aggressive fibromatosis. The experience at the University of Florida. J Bone Joint Surg [Am] 1991;73:717–25.
147. Miralbell R, Suit HD, Mankin HJ, Zuckerberg LR, Stracher MA, Rosenberg AE. Fibromatoses: from postsurgical surveillance to combined surgery and radiation therapy. Int J Radiat Oncol Biol Phys 1990;18:535–40.
148. Miyaki M, Konishi M, Kikuchi YR, et al. Coexistence of somatic and germ-line mutations of APC gene in desmoid tumors from patients with familial adenomatous polyposis. Cancer Res 1993;53:5079–82.
149. Patel SR, Evans HL, Benjamin RS. Combination chemotherapy in adult desmoid tumors. Cancer 1993;72:3244–7.
150. Reitamo JJ. The desmoid tumor. IV. Choice of treatment, results, and complications. Arch Surg 1983;118:1318–22.
151. Reitamo JJ, Hayry P, Nykyri E, Saxen E. The desmoid tumor. I. Incidence, sex, age, and anatomical distribution in the Finnish population. Am J Clin Pathol 1982;77:665–73.
152. Ritter MA, Marshall JL, Straub LR. Extra-abdominal desmoid of the hand. A case report. J Bone Joint Surg 1969;51A:1641–4.
153. Rock MG, Pritchard DJ, Reiman HM, Soule EH, Brewster RC. Extra-abdominal desmoid tumors. J Bone Joint Surg [Am] 1984;66:1369–74.
154. Rodu B, Weathers DR, Campbell WJ. Aggressive fibromatosis involving the paramandibular soft tissues. A study with the aid of electron microscopy. Oral Surg Oral Med Oral Pathol 1981;52:395–403.
155. Sanders R, Bennett M, Walton JN. A multifocal extra-abdominal desmoid tumour. Br J Plast Surg 1983;36:337–41.

156. Sundaram M, Duffrin H, McGuire MH, Vas W. Synchronous multicentric desmoid tumors (aggressive fibromatosis) of the extremities. Skeletal Radiol 1988;17:16–9.

157. Taylor LJ. Musculoaponeurotic fibromatosis. A report of 28 cases and review of the literature. Clin Orthop 1987;294–302.

158. Waddell WR, Gerner RE, Reich MP. Nonsteroid antiinflammatory drugs and tamoxifen for desmoid tumors and carcinoma of the stomach. J Surg Oncol 1983;22:197–211.

159. Waddell WR, Kirsch WM. Testolactone, sulindac, warfarin, and vitamin K1 for unresectable desmoid tumors. Am J Surg 1991;161:416–21.

160. Wilkins SA Jr, Waldron CA, Mathews WH, Droulias CA. Aggressive fibromatosis of the head and neck. Am J Surg 1975;130:412–5.

161. Yoshida MA, Ikeuchi T, Iwama T, et al. Chromosome changes in desmoid tumors developed in patients with familial adenomatous polyposis. Jpn J Cancer Res 1991;82:916–21.

Abdominal Fibromatosis

162. Reitamo JJ. The desmoid tumor. IV. Choice of treatment, results, and complications. Arch Surg 1983;118:1318–22.

163. Reitamo JJ, Hayry P, Nykyri E, Saxen E. The desmoid tumor. I. Incidence, sex, age, and anatomical distribution in the Finnish population. Am J Clin Pathol 1982;77:665–73.

Intra-abdominal Fibromatosis: Pelvic, Retroperitoneal, and Mesenteric

164. Burke AP, Sobin LH, Shekitka KM. Mesenteric fibromatosis. A follow-up study. Arch Pathol Lab Med 1990;114:832–5.

165. Burke AP, Sobin LH, Shekitka KM, Federspiel BH, Helwig EB. Intra-abdominal fibromatosis. A pathologic analysis of 130 tumors with comparison of clinical subgroups. Am J Surg Pathol 1990;14:335–41.

166. Khorsand J, Karakousis CP. Desmoid tumors and their management. Am J Surg 1985;149:215–8.

167. Klein WA, Miller HH, Anderson M, DeCosse JJ. The use of indomethacin, sulindac, and tamoxifen for the treatment of desmoid tumors associated with familial polyposis. Cancer 1987;60:2863–8.

168. Loccufier A, Vanhulle A, Moreels R, Deruyter L, Legley W. Gardner syndrome and desmoid tumors. Acta Chir Belg 1993;93:230–2.

169. Miyaki M, Konishi M, Kikuchi YR, et al. Coexistence of somatic and germ-line mutations of APC gene in desmoid tumors from patients with familial adenomatous polyposis. Cancer Res 1993;53:5079–82.

170. Patel SR, Evans HL, Benjamin RS. Combination chemotherapy in adult desmoid tumors. Cancer 1993;72:3244–7.

171. Remmele W, Muller LH, Paulus W. Primary mesenteritis, mesenteric fibrosis and mesenteric fibromatosis. Report of four cases, pathology, and classification. Pathol Res Pract 1988;184:77–85.

171a. Sarlomo-Rikala M, Kovatich A, Barusevicius A, Miettinen M. CD117: a sensitive marker for gastrointestinal stromal tumors that is more specific than CD34. Mod Pathol 1998;11:728–34.

172. Umemoto S, Makuuchi H, Amemiya T, et al. Intra-abdominal desmoid tumors in familial polyposis coli: a case report of tumor regression by prednisolone therapy. Dis Colon Rectum 1991;34:89–93.

173. Waddell WR, Gerner RE, Reich MP. Nonsteroid antiinflammatory drugs and tamoxifen for desmoid tumors and carcinoma of the stomach. J Surg Oncol 1983;22:197–211.

174. Waddell WR, Kirsch WM. Testolactone, sulindac, warfarin, and vitamin K1 for unresectable desmoid tumors. Am J Surg 1991;161:416–21.

175. Yoshida MA, Ikeuchi T, Iwama T, et al. Chromosome changes in desmoid tumors developed in patients with familial adenomatous polyposis. Jpn J Cancer Res 1991;82:916–21.

Infantile Desmoid Tumor

176. Ayala AG, Ro JY, Goepfert H, Cangir A, Khorsand J, Flake G. Desmoid fibromatosis: a clinicopathologic study of 25 children. Semin Diagn Pathol 1986;3:138–50.

177. Chung EB. Pitfalls in diagnosing benign soft tissue tumors in infancy and childhood. Pathol Annu 1985;2:323–46.

178. Enzinger FM, Weiss SW. Soft tissue tumors. 3rd ed. St Louis: Mosby, 1995:251–6.

179. Fromowitz FB, Hurst LC, Nathan J, Badalamente M. Infantile (desmoid type) fibromatosis with extensive ossification. Am J Surg Pathol 1987;11:66–75.

180. Rosenberg HS, Stenback WA, Spjut HJ. The fibromatoses of infancy and childhood. Perspect Pediatr Pathol 1978;4:269–348.

181. Schmidt D, Klinge P, Leuschner I, Harms D. Infantile desmoid–type fibromatosis. Morphological features correlate with biological behaviour. J Pathol 1991;164:315–9.

Inflammatory Myofibroblastic Tumor

182. Coffin CM, Humphrey PA, Dehner LP. Extrapulmonary inflammatory myofibroblastic tumor: a clinical and pathologic survey. Semin Diag Pathol 1998;15:85–101.

182a. Coffin CM, Watterson J, Priest JR, Dehner LP. Extrapulmonary inflammatory myofibroblastic tumor (inflammatory pseudotumor). A clinicopathologic and immunohistochemical study of 84 cases. Am J Surg Pathol 1995;19:859–72.

182b. Griffin CA, Hawkins AL, Dvorak C, Henkle C, Ellingham T, Perlman EJ. Recurrent involvement of 2p23 in inflammatory myofibroblastic tumours. Cancer Res 1999;59:2776–80.

183. Meis JM, Enzinger FM. Inflammatory fibrosarcoma of the mesentery and retroperitoneum. A tumor closely simulating inflammatory pseudotumor. Am J Surg Pathol 1991;15:1146–56.

183a. Meis-Kindblom JM, Kjellström C, Kindblom LG. Inflammatory fibrosarcoma: update, reappraisal, and perspective

on its place in the spectrum of inflammatory myofibroblastic tumors. Semin Diag Pathol 1998;15:133–43.

183b. Su LD, Atayde-Perez A, Sheldon S, Fletcher JA, Weiss SW. Inflammatory myofibroblastic tumor: cytogenetic evidence supporting clonal origin. Mod Pathol 1998;11:364–8.

Inflammatory Myxohyaline Tumor of Distal Extremities

183c. Meis-Kindblom JM, Kindblom LG. Acral myxoinflammatory fibroblastic sarcoma: a low grade tumor of the hands and feet. Am J Surg Pathol 1998;22:911–24.

183d. Montgomery EA, Devaney KO, Giordano TJ, Weiss SW. Inflammatory myxohyaline tumor of distal extremities

with virocyte or Reed-Sternberg-like cells: a distinctive lesion with features simulating inflammatory conditions, Hodgkin's disease, and various sarcomas. Mod Pathol 1998;11:384–91.

Adult Fibrosarcoma

184. Enzinger FM, Weiss SW. Soft tissue tumors. 3rd ed. St Louis: Mosby, 1995:269–81.

184a. Eyden BP, Manson C, Banerjee SS, Roberts IS, Harris M. Sclerosing epithelioid fibrosarcoma: a study of five cases emphasizing diagnostic criteria. Histopathology 1998;33:354–60.

185. Frankenthaler R, Ayala AG, Hartwick RW, Goepfert H. Fibrosarcoma of the head and neck. Laryngoscope 1990;100:799–802.

186. Mackenzie D. Fibroma: a dangerous diagnosis. Br J Surg 1964;51:607–14.

187. Mark RJ, Sercarz JA, Tran L, Selch M, Calcaterra TC. Fibrosarcoma of the head and neck. The UCLA experience. Arch Otolaryngol Head Neck Surg 1991;117:396–401.

188. Meis JM, Enzinger FM. Inflammatory fibrosarcoma of the mesentery and retroperitoneum. A tumor closely simulating inflammatory pseudotumor. Am J Surg Pathol 1991;15:1146–56.

188a. Meis-Kindblom JM, Kindblom LG, Enzinger FM. Sclerosing epithelioid fibrosarcoma. A variant of fibrosarcoma simulating carcinoma. Am J Surg Pathol 1995;19:979–93.

189. Pritchard DJ, Sim FH, Ivins JC, Soule EH, Dahlin DC. Fibrosarcoma of bone and soft tissues of the trunk and extremities. Orthop Clin North Am 1977;8:869–81.

190. Pritchard DJ, Soule EH, Taylor WF, Ivins JC. Fibrosarcoma—a clinicopathologic and statistical study of 199 tumors of the soft tissues of the extremities and trunk. Cancer 1974;33:888–97.

191. Scott SM, Reiman HM, Pritchard DJ, Ilstrup DM. Soft tissue fibrosarcoma. A clinicopathologic study of 132 cases. Cancer 1989;64:925–31.

192. Suh CH, Ordonez NG, Mackay B. Fibrosarcoma: observations on the ultrastructure. Ultrastruct Pathol 1993;17:221–9.

Infantile and Childhood Fibrosarcoma

193. Chung EB, Enzinger FM. Infantile fibrosarcoma. Cancer 1976;38:729–39.

194. Coffin CM, Jaszcz W, O'Shea PA, Dehner LP. So-called congenital-infantile fibrosarcoma: does it exist and what is it? Pediatr Pathol 1994;14:133–50.

195. Dehner LP, Askin FB. Tumors of fibrous tissue origin in childhood. A clinicopathologic study of cutaneous and soft tissue neoplasms in 66 children. Cancer 1976;38:888–900.

196. Gonzalez–Crussi F. Ultrastructure of congenital fibrosarcoma. Cancer 1970;26:1289–99.

197. Hays DM, Mirabal VQ, Karlan MS, Patel HR, Landing BH. Fibrosarcomas in infants and children. J Pediatr Surg 1970;5:176–83.

198. Salloum E, Caillaud JM, Flamant F, Landman J, Lemerle J. Poor prognosis infantile fibrosarcoma with pathologic features of malignant fibrous histiocytoma after local recurrence. Med Pediatr Oncol 1990;18:295–8.

199. Schofield DE, Fletcher JA, Grier HE, Yunis EJ. Fibrosarcoma in infants and children. Application of new techniques. Am J Surg Pathol 1994;18:14–24.

200. Soule EH, Pritchard DJ. Fibrosarcoma in infants and children: a review of 110 cases. Cancer 1977;40:1711–21.

Low–Grade Fibromyxoid Sarcoma

201. Devaney DM, Dervan P, O'Neill S, Carney D, Leader M. Low-grade fibromyxoid sarcoma. Histopathology 1990;17:463–5.

202. Evans HL. Low-grade fibromyxoid sarcoma. A report of 12 cases. Am J Surg Pathol 1993;17:595–600.

202a. Farinha P, Oliveira P, Soares J. Metastasising hyalinising spindle cell tumour with giant rosettes: report of a case with long survival. Histopathology 2000;36:92–3.

203. Goodlad JR, Mentzel T, Fletcher CD. Low grade fibromyxoid sarcoma: clinicopathological analysis of eleven

new cases in support of a distinct entity. Histopathology 1995;26:229–37.

204. Lane K, Shannon R, Weiss S. Hyalinizing spindle cell tumor with giant rosettes. Am J Surg Pathol 1997;21:1481–8.

204a. Woodruff JM, Antonescu CR, Erlandson RA, Bowland PJ. Low grade fibrosarcoma with palisaded granuloma-like bodies (giant rosettes): report of a case that metastasized. Am J Surg Pathol 1999;23:1423–8.

Myofibrosarcoma

205. Mentzel T, Dry S, Katenkamp D, Fletcher CD. Low grade myofibroblastic sarcoma. Analysis of 18 cases in the spectrum of myofibroblastic tumors. Am J Surg Pathol 1998;22:1228–38.

205a. Mentzel T, Fletcher CD. The emerging role of myofibroblasts in soft tissue neoplasia. Am J Clin Pathol 1997;107:2–5.

206. Smith DM, Mahmoud HH, Jenkins JB, Rao B, Hopkins KP, Parham DM. Myofibrosarcoma of the head and neck in children. Pediatr Pathol Lab Med 1995;15:403–18.

3
FIBROUS HISTIOCYTOMAS

INTRODUCTION

The concept of the fibrous histiocytoma was developed approximately 30 years ago to provide an organizing principle and nomenclature for a group of soft tissue neoplasms and neoplastic-like lesions that were composed of a mixture of cells with the hematoxylin and eosin (H&E) morphology of fibroblasts and histiocytes but were otherwise undifferentiated. The initial focus was on a group of sarcomas that contained large bizarre cells that either possessed foamy cytoplasm, and thus were thought by some to resemble lipoblasts, or were endowed with abundant eosinophilic cytoplasm that caused them to resemble rhabdomyoblasts. Against these interpretations was the absence of the characteristic nuclear indentation by clear lipid vacuoles that identifies lipoblasts and the absence of demonstrable cross-striations in the cells with eosinophilic cytoplasm.

Impressed with the resemblance of many of the tumor cells to fibroblasts and histiocytes, and in the absence of convincing evidence of either lipoblastic or rhabdomyoblastic differentiation, O'Brien and Stout (23) suggested the name "malignant fibrous histiocytoma" for this group of sarcomas. Studies were then undertaken to attempt to prove that these neoplastic spindled and rounded cells were indeed histiocytes and fibroblasts. In cell cultures carried out by Ozzello and associates (24), the cells of these neoplasms were reported to assume stellate shapes and to exhibit amoeboid movement and phagocytic activity. These investigators took this as evidence of histiocytic differentiation, an interpretation that was not then universally accepted and is now generally considered to be erroneous. As a result of these observations, they proposed that the malignant fibrous histiocytomas were histiocytic neoplasms in which some of the tumor cells took on the appearance and function of fibroblasts (i.e., the tumor cells were "facultative fibroblasts").

When the electron microscope became widely available, a large number of fibrous histiocytomas, particularly the malignant variants, were examined with this instrument. The main conclusion that can be drawn from the large number of published studies is that the cells of malignant fibrous histiocytomas are no more differentiated when examined with the electron microscope than they are when examined with the light microscope (1,9,10,12,14,30). Ultrastructurally, some tumor cells have the features of fibroblasts, with elongate nuclei and prominent rough endoplasmic reticulum, while other similar cells contain intermediate filaments and the other subcellular components of myofibroblasts (3,13,13a). The cells that resemble histiocytes by light microscopy have oval or round nuclei and may contain lysosomes, lipid, and phagosomes. A fourth type of cell, without any of the above ultrastructural features, was also described in many malignant fibrous histiocytomas. These have been variously interpreted as "primitive" or "intermediate" mesenchymal cells; it has been theorized that they are the long sought after "progenitor" cells that give rise to the fibroblasts, myofibroblasts, and histiocyte-like cells that populate fibrous histiocytomas (9).

Paralleling the early histogenetic studies outlined above were other studies aimed at elucidating the clinicopathology of this large undifferentiated "fibrous histiocytoma" group. These compared traditional light microscopic histopathologic features with clinical outcome in an attempt to develop clinically relevant histopathologic subgroups. Because of their relative frequency among the sarcomas, and because they cause considerable diagnostic difficulty, the pleomorphic malignant fibrous histiocytomas were among the first to be evaluated. In 1972, Kempson and Kyriakos (18a) reported 30 pleomorphic tumors composed of fibroblasts and histiocyte-like cells that they labeled fibroxanthosarcoma, a type of malignant fibrous histiocytoma. Weiss and Enzinger in 1978 (32a) reported 200 more cases and renamed the tumor pleomorphic malignant fibrous histiocytoma, the label that is now most often used to identify these sarcomas.

Almost as soon as these morphologic features were recognized and accepted as identifying a clinically useful group of neoplasms, it became apparent that some pleomorphic malignant

Table 3-1

TUMORS INCLUDED IN THE FIBROUS HISTIOCYTOMA CATEGORY

Benign
(Managerial Groups Ia, Ib, and Ic, Table 1-10)

Dermal fibrous histiocytomas
    Dermatofibroma
    Fibroxanthoma
    Dermal histiocytomas
    Hemosiderotic (sclerosing hemangioma)
    Cellular*
    Epithelioid
    Aneurysmal (angiomatoid)*
    Palisading
    Atypical

Subcutaneous and deep benign fibrous histiocytomas

Juvenile xanthogranuloma**

Reticulohistiocytoma**

Xanthoma**

Intermediate
(Managerial Groups IIa, IIb, and IIc, Table 1-10)

Atypical fibroxanthoma

Dermatofibrosarcoma protuberans

Giant cell fibroblastoma

Plexiform fibrous histiocytoma

Angiomatoid fibrous histiocytoma

Malignant
(Managerial Group III, Table 1-10)

Pleomorphic

Myxoid (myxofibrosarcoma)

Giant cell
    High-grade variant
    Low-grade variant (giant cell tumor of soft tissue)

Inflammatory

---

*Significant incidence of recurrence.
**These are discussed in the Fascicle, Non-Melanocytic Tumors of the Skin (65a).

fibrous histiocytomas contained variably sized areas of hypocellular myxoid stroma and that the morphologic patterns of some overlapped with those of the tumor that had been previously categorized as high-grade fibrosarcoma. These observations suggested the need for a sub-classification of the malignant fibrous histiocytic neoplasms. As a result, the categories of the fibrous and myxoid types of malignant fibrous histiocytoma were created (17a,32b). In 1972,

Guccion and Enzinger (11a) described a variant marked by numerous osteoclast-like giant cells and they appended the name giant cell sarcomas to these. Kyriakos and Kempson (20) reported yet another type of fibrous histiocytoma characterized by a predominance of histiocyte-like cells set in a sea of acute inflammation. They labeled this variant inflammatory fibrous histiocytoma.

Other investigators studied the superficial fibrous histiocytomas. An initial focus of attention was atypical fibroxanthoma, a dermal lesion that is histologically identical to pleomorphic malignant fibrous histiocytoma but, paradoxically, practically never metastasizes (7,18a). About the same time, it was realized that many of the common dermal lesions previously labeled dermatofibroma, sclerosing hemangioma, dermal histiocytoma, or subepidermal nodular fibrosis were composed of cells resembling fibroblasts and histiocytes. It was apparent that these benign and possibly reactive lesions could be collected under the fibrous histiocytoma umbrella and more sensibly named dermal fibrous histiocytomas while identical lesions in the subcutaneous and deep soft tissues were classified as superficial and deep benign fibrous histiocytomas. Concomitantly, juvenile xanthogranuloma, reticulohistiocytoma, and xanthoma were added to the benign fibrous histiocytoma category. Through the years, other lesions whose constituent cells were thought to resemble histiocytes and fibroblasts have been designated as fibrous histiocytomas. These include plexiform fibrous histiocytoma, angiomatoid fibrous histiocytoma, giant cell fibroblastoma, and dermatofibrosarcoma protuberans.

Within the last two decades, enzyme histochemical and immunohistochemical techniques have been employed in a search for distinctive fibrous histiocytoma antigens or cell products that would shed light on the differentiation of these tumors. Alpha-1-antitrypsin, alpha-1-antichymotrypsin, lysozyme, and cathepsin-B are produced by histiocytes and when antibodies against these antigens became available, they were found to be present in the tumor cells of most malignant fibrous histiocytomas (5,19,21, 22,26,33). Unfortunately, a large number of nonhistiocytic cells, including tumor cells of diverse differentiation, also synthesize these enzymes (25,27,28). With only rare exceptions, investigators also have failed to find antigens thought to be specific for bone marrow–derived cells such as CD14 (LeuM-3) and CD15 (LeuM-1) in the neoplastic cells of malignant fibrous histiocytomas (2,16,17,20a,26,29,34). Recently, KP1, a CD68 monoclonal antibody that recognizes a lysosomal glycoprotein present in bone marrow–derived macrophages and myeloid cells, has been reported to decorate the cells of some but not all malignant fibrous histiocytomas (1a,17,20a,25). However, CD68 expression is not limited to macrophages and has been reported in many other neoplasms including malignant melanoma and some carcinomas. The non-neoplastic foam cells often present at the margins of malignant fibrous histiocytomas do have the staining profile of bone marrow–derived monocytes/macrophages (20a,34).

The results of immunostaining the tumor cells of dermal fibrous histiocytomas depends on the histologic features of the lesion. When foam cells are present these react as histiocytes. Nonfoam cells in some lesions express actin and factor XIIIa is expressed in dermatofibroma and other benign fibrous histiocytomas. The immunohistochemical profile of fibrous histiocytomas with recurring or low metastatic potential is variable and there is no firm evidence that the constituent cells are bone marrow–derived macrophages. CD68 staining has been reported in plexiform fibrous histiocytomas, angiomatoid fibrous histiocytomas, and atypical fibroxanthomas, and one group has reported that the cells in angiomatoid fibrous histiocytoma are desmin positive (7). Over 90 percent of dermatofibrosarcoma protuberans are composed of cells that express an antigen recognized by CD34 (31).

In summary, electron microscopy and immunohistochemistry indicate that in most fibrous histiocytomas the constituent cells, other than the obvious foamy macrophages, are not histiocytes; rather they are fibroblasts, myofibroblasts, and primitive undifferentiated mesenchymal cells, some of which take on phagocytic properties and in doing so acquire epitopes shared with cells of the monocyte/macrophage system (8,11,20a,34). In fact, a subset of the sarcomas with malignant fibrous histiocytoma features such as the dedifferentiated areas in dedifferentiated liposarcoma develop as a result of dedifferentiation of a nonfibrohistiocytic differentiated mesenchymal neoplasm. It may be that a significant number of malignant fibrous histiocytomas are the result of dedifferentiation rather than originating as neoplasms that are undifferentiated except for the fibroblasts and myofibroblasts. Should the name "fibrous histiocytoma" be changed and the tumors reclassified to reflect these facts (4)? On the whole, we think not (18). Names serve many purposes in clinical medicine, only one of which is to reflect the latest scientific truth; their primary function must always be to facilitate unambiguous communication between clinicians and pathologists concerning patient management issues. Patient management considerations argue that diseases should have stable names, and unless renaming or reclassifying a group of tumors has managerial implications, familiar and accepted names, in our opinion, should stay. More important to us than changing the name to fit the latest scientific study is the assurance that pathologists are using a shared set of morphologic criteria to diagnose the fibrous histiocytomas. The clinicopathology of the many lesions encompassed by the term "fibrous histiocytoma" has been delineated by numerous studies over the last 30 years and an extensive published experience has been accumulated and organized using the classificatory structure suggested by this clinical investigation (6,32). This means that the definition of the fibrous histiocytomas is based upon H&E morphologic features and that they are tumors and tumor-like conditions in which otherwise undifferentiated tumor cells are thought to take on the light microscopic phenotype of fibroblasts and histiocytes. Tumors are included or not included in the category on this basis.

Are too many sarcomas with focal or subtle evidence of differentiation along lines other than those that define the fibrous histiocytomas placed in the malignant fibrous histiocytoma (MFH) category? Fletcher argues in the affirmative on the basis of a retrospective study of 159 tumors originally diagnosed as pleomorphic sarcomas (8a,15). One hundred and one of these had been diagnosed since MFH became a generally accepted label, 48 of which have been subclassified as pleomorphic MFH or compatible with MFH. Utilizing more H&E sections, electron microscopy, and immunohistochemistry Fletcher was able to demonstrate evidence of differentiation as he defined it in 117 of the 159 tumors (97 were interpreted as a type of sarcoma other than MFH and 20 were not sarcomas) while 42 of these pleomorphic sarcomas lacked evidence of cellular differentiation other than that expected in pleomorphic MFH. While everyone would agree with classifying tumors on the basis of reproducible and generally agreed upon evidence of cellular differentiation, what counts as evidence of differentiation in a pleomorphic sarcoma is often controversial. For example, opinion differs among investigators about whether desmin expression is specific for muscle differentiation. If it is considered to be specific in and of itself the incidence of leiomyosarcoma and rhabdomyosarcoma will increase at the expense of pleomorphic MFH because all tumors that otherwise meet the definition of MFH but contain desmin-positive cells will be classified as muscle tumors. Another example is the difference of opinion about whether small quantities of tumor bone should cause a sarcoma to be classified as osteosarcoma rather than pleomorphic MFH with focal bone formation.

What is at stake when areas of differentiation are or are not found in an otherwise pleomorphic MFH? Currently, detecting subtle or focal differentiation in an otherwise MFH or an otherwise pleomorphic undifferentiated sarcoma does not alter therapy and often requires the application of costly technology. Surely, it is of interest scientifically to determine how often apparent pleomorphic MFHs do contain differentiated cells not apparent by H&E morphology, and studies should be undertaken to determine whether detecting such differentiation has clinical implications, but it can be argued that this type of investigation should be limited to randomized clinical trials or funded research. If research uncovers specific tumors within the group now encompassed under the rubric of pleomorphic MFH that have significant differences in prognosis or response to therapy they can then be separately identified. Of course, distinguishing malignant lymphoma, metastatic carcinoma, and metastatic melanoma from a primary pleomorphic MFH is of utmost importance, and whatever procedures are needed to accomplish this should be employed.

The tumors currently included in the fibrous histiocytoma category include a group of benign lesions, some of which are reactive and most of which occur in the skin and subcutaneous tissue; a group of neoplasms with a significant incidence of recurrence but with low metastatic potential, most of which are superficial; and the MFHs, many, but not all of which develop in the deep soft tissues (Table 3-1). The latter comprises four morphologically defined variants that have as their common theme cells that take on the appearance of fibroblasts and histiocytes.

BENIGN FIBROUS HISTIOCYTOMAS (MANAGERIAL GROUPS Ia, Ib, AND Ic, TABLE 1-10)

The nomenclature commonly employed for the benign fibrohistiocytic tumors is presented in Tables 3-1 and 3-2. While the fibrous histiocytomas that arise in the skin are also discussed in the Fascicle, Non-Melanocytic Tumors of the Skin (65a), they enter into the differential diagnoses of soft tissue tumors with sufficient frequency to warrant their discussion here.

Benign Dermal Fibrous Histiocytomas

Definition. Benign dermal fibrous histiocytomas (DFH) are nodular proliferations composed of fibrocytes, fibroblasts, myofibroblasts, histiocytes, and histiocyte-like cells mixed together in variable proportions. By definition, these lesions arise in, and are centered in, the dermis but subcutaneous extension can occur.

General Considerations. The category of benign DFH includes dermatofibroma, sclerosing hemangioma, dermal histiocytoma, and fibroxanthoma (57,66,68,76). These lesions have also been grouped together under the heading of *subepidermal nodular fibrosis.* We applaud the lumping but prefer the label dermal fibrous histiocytoma because these lesions are composed of fibroblasts and histiocytic-appearing cells (Table 3-2). In addition, true histiocytes are present in some DFHs as evidenced by xanthoma cells, multinucleated foam cells, and immunohistochemical studies. Recently, several more variants of benign DFH have been described (48). These include the epithelioid, aneurysmal (angiomatoid), palisading, cellular, clear cell, and atypical (fibrous histiocytoma with "monster" cells) types (37,44,47,48, 54,55,58,63,65,70,72,75,77). For diagnosis it is preferable to use the subtype name, e.g., dermatofibroma; dermal fibrous histiocytoma,

Table 3-2

THE CLINICAL AND HISTOLOGIC FEATURES OF THE VARIANTS OF BENIGN DERMAL FIBROUS HISTIOCYTOMA

Variant	Clinical Features	Histologic Features
1) Common dermal fibrous histiocytoma (dermatofibroma, dermal histiocytoma, fibroxanthoma)	Solitary, slowly growing, red-brown nodules usually on the extremities of young adults, most often women; usually 1 to 2 cm	Usually circumscribed but not encapsulated; hyperplasia and hyperpigmentation of epidermis; proliferation of variable numbers of haphazardly arranged spindle cells, foam cells, histiocyte-like cells, and giant cells; can be mainly fibrous (dermatofibroma), contain equal amounts of fibrous tissue and foam cells (fibroxanthoma), or be mainly foam cells (dermal histiocytoma); cholesterol clefts can be present and collagen is usually prominent in the fibrous lesions
2) Cellular fibrous histiocytoma	5 percent of dermal fibrous histiocytomas; most common on extremities and head and neck of young males; usually over 2 cm; about a quarter recur	Epidermal hyperplasia less common and lesion often extends into the subcutaneous tissue; predominantly spindled cells with prominent eosinophilic cytoplasm; inflammatory cells, foam cells, and giant cells are common but may be inconspicuous; necrosis and ulceration in about 10 percent; around half contain actin-positive cells at least focally; hyalinized collagen surrounded by tumor cells common at the edge
3) Aneurysmal fibrous histiocytoma	Less than 2 percent of dermal fibrous histiocytomas; slowly growing blue to brown nodules most common in extremities of middle-aged adults; usually appear cystic and polypoid; about 20 percent recur	Blood-filled spaces not lined by endothelium that vary from clefts to cavernous channels; these are present focally or diffusely; abundant hemosiderin-filled mono- and multinucleated cells, foam cells, and inflammatory cells but inflammation much less than in angiomatoid fibrous histiocytoma; typical features of common dermal fibrous histiocytomas are present in all lesions but may be focal; epidermal hyperplasia usually present
4) Hemosiderotic fibrous histiocytoma (sclerosing hemangioma)	Same as common fibrous histiocytoma except that lesions are usually blue to black	Same as common fibrous histiocytoma except that capillary proliferation is prominent and large numbers of histiocytes contain hemosiderin; nuclei can be atypical and normal mitoses can be numerous
5) Epithelioid fibrous histiocytoma (epithelioid cell histiocytoma, adventitial cellular myxofibroblastoma)	Most commonly presents as polypoid red nodule in the lower extremities of middle-aged adults, but can occur at many sites	Epidermal hyperplasia common but the lesion often extends to the epidermis without an uninvolved layer of dermis; may have collarette; composed of round cells with abundant eosinophilic cytoplasm, round vesicular nucleus, and red nucleolus; multinucleated giant cells are unusual but bi- and trinucleated cells are not uncommon; foam cells are usually present; transition to a dermatofibroma pattern is frequently seen
6) Atypical fibrous histiocytoma (pseudosarcomatous fibrous histiocytoma with monster cells)	Same as common dermal fibrous histiocytoma except that more patients are middle-aged and involvement of the trunk is common; lesions may be polypoid	Same as common dermal fibrous histiocytoma except that huge multinucleated giant cells with bizarrely shaped nuclei with very dense chromatin are present; mononuclear foam cells may also be large and have large irregular nuclei; hemosiderin is common; mitotic figures are sparse and normal and lesion is less cellular than atypical fibroxanthoma
7) Palisading dermal fibrous histiocytoma	Same as common dermal fibrous histiocytoma except for a predilection for acral sites	Same as common dermal fibrous histiocytoma except that focal groups of spindle cells feature nuclear palisading; tumor cells are S-100 protein negative

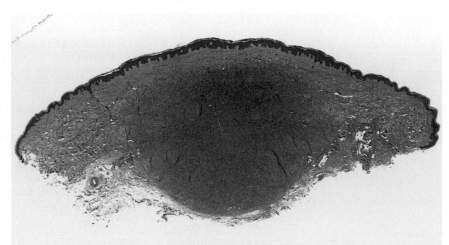

Figure 3-1
DERMAL FIBROUS
HISTIOCYTOMA

Benign fibrous histiocytomas occur most commonly in the dermis. At low magnification they often have a more basophilic appearance than the surrounding dermis as well as an uninvolved zone of dermis between the lesion and the often hyperplastic epidermis.

cellular variant; dermal fibrous histiocytoma, aneurysmal variant; etc.

Clinical Features. Patients who develop the dermatofibroma, sclerosing hemangioma (hemosiderotic), dermal histiocytoma, and fibroxanthoma types of DFH are most often adults between the ages of 20 and 60 years but these lesions have been reported to occur at all ages (57, 76). The majority of the patients are women. Dermatofibromas are slowly growing, and occur most commonly in the skin of the lower extremities, although they can develop in any part of the body. Usually, they are hard, white, or red to tan nodules, while the sclerosing hemangioma (hemosiderotic) type may be blue or black because of hemosiderin deposition. In the latter circumstance, DFH can be confused clinically with malignant melanoma. Less commonly, they are polypoid. The cellular variant is more common in males, occurs chiefly in young adults, and has a predilection for the extremities and the head and neck region (49,54,64). It is usually larger than the common dermatofibroma. The aneurysmal variant occurs most commonly on the extremities of middle-aged adults and appears as a blue-black, often cystic lesion (47,70). The epithelioid variant is also more common in middle-aged individuals and occurs in all sites although involvement of the extremities is most common; it is often polypoid (55,72,77). The atypical variant has clinical features identical to the common dermatofibroma type of DFH except that some are polypoid (48). Typically, most types of DFH are small (less than 2 cm) but they can reach 10 cm or more.

Pathologic Findings. Grossly, these dermal tumors are almost always uninodular, firm, white to yellow to bluish black nodules. Rare examples are multinodular, and blue-black nodules may be soft or cystic. The overlying skin is almost always intact and may be hyperpigmented. A noninvolved zone between the tumor and the epidermis can sometimes be appreciated macroscopically. The epithelioid, aneurysmal, and atypical variants may be polypoid.

The epidermis overlying a DFH is frequently hyperplastic and there is usually hyperpigmentation of the basal cell layer. Characteristically, an uninvolved rim of dermis lies between the epidermis and the lesion, except for the epithelioid variant which usually grows in contact with the epidermis (fig. 3-1). Inflammatory cells, if present, are usually sparse, focal, perivascular, and located at the edge of the lesion. Occasionally, they can be numerous and intralesional and rarely, germinal centers may be formed (42). By definition, DFH must be centered in the dermis but extension of part of the tumor into the superficial subcutaneous tissue is permitted and in fact is rather common. Two patterns of extension have been observed: the most common is characterized by short spikes of connective tissue that extend along septa into the fat, and the less common by a rounded blunt pushing border against the fat (fig. 3-2) (60). Intravascular growth has been reported (67).

The most common types of DFH display a spectrum of histologic patterns varying from tumors that are predominantly fibroblastic (dermatofibroma), to those that are a mixture of fibroblasts

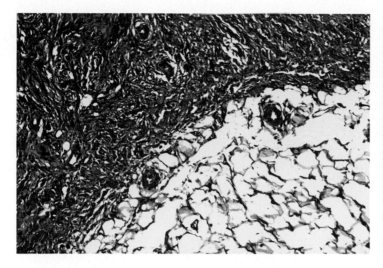

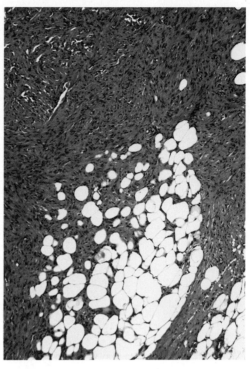

Figure 3-2
DERMAL FIBROUS HISTIOCYTOMA
The border between a dermal fibrous histiocytoma and the subcutaneous fat is usually sharp (above) but fat can be trapped at the edge (right). In the latter circumstance, care must be taken to exclude DFSP which characteristically infiltrates between fat cells.

and foam cells or histiocyte-like cells (fibroxanthoma), to those that are predominantly composed of foam cells and/or histiocyte-like cells with no or only focal evidence of fibrous differentiation (dermal histiocytoma) (figs. 3-3, 3-4). Lesions that are composed of equal numbers of fibroblasts and foamy macrophages also have been labeled as fibroxanthoma. Pure xanthomas are composed exclusively of foamy histiocytes and, for largely historical reasons, are still labeled as xanthoma rather than DFH.

The most commonly encountered tumor is the one most often designated as *dermatofibroma*, a predominantly fibrous lesion. This tumor is usually well circumscribed but not encapsulated. The constituent fibroblasts and myofibroblasts that form this very common lesion are loosely bundled and arranged in a more or less random pattern, although they may take on a tufting or storiform arrangement focally or, rarely, more diffusely (figs. 3-4, 3-5). Dermatofibroma is more cellular than the surrounding dermis and more cellular at its center than at the periphery. The constituent nuclei are larger than the nuclei of the nearby normal dermal fibrocytes and division figures are absent or sparse. Collagen is usually plentiful and more dense and refractile

at the periphery, and individual collagen bundles at the periphery are surrounded by infiltrating tumor cells. Rare lesions have heavily collagenized, paucicellular centers and have been labeled as the atrophic variant (43). The fibrous pattern blends imperceptibly into one in which histiocytes and histiocyte-like cells, including foam cells, are mixed with the fibroblasts; the number of fibrocytes and histiocyte-like cells varies from lesion to lesion. When histiocytes are the exclusive tumor cell, the term *dermal histiocytoma* is sometimes used. Cells that have phagocytized hemosiderin may be found; multinucleated giant cells, some with foamy cytoplasm, are common; and cholesterol clefts may be present (fig. 3-6). On occasion, one finds striking vascular proliferation which is associated with hemorrhage and extensive hemosiderin deposition, and for these the term *sclerosing hemangioma* (or more recently, *hemosiderotic variant*) has been devised. Phagocytosis of hemosiderin may be prominent to massive in such lesions and the pigmented phagocytic cells may have enlarged nuclei with dense chromatin that cause concern for malignancy (fig. 3-7). Sometimes the vessels in such lesions take on a staghorn (pericytic) appearance. Occasionally, the cells in

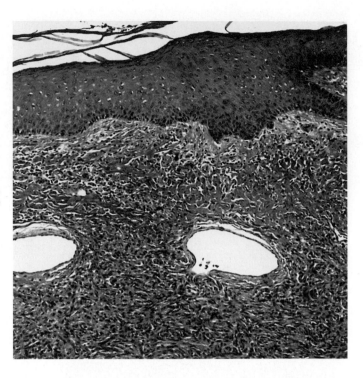

Figure 3-3
DERMAL FIBROUS HISTIOCYTOMA
The usual benign dermal fibrous histiocytoma is more cellular than the surrounding dermis and hence the basophilia.

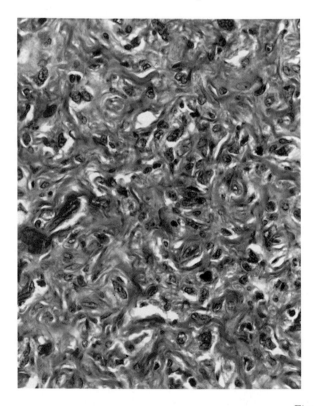 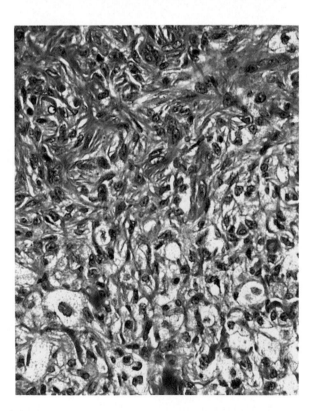

Figure 3-4
DERMAL FIBROUS HISTIOCYTOMA
Benign fibrous histiocytomas vary from those that appear mostly fibrous (dermatofibroma) with abundant collagen (left) to those that are composed of more histiocyte-like cells and foam cells (right).

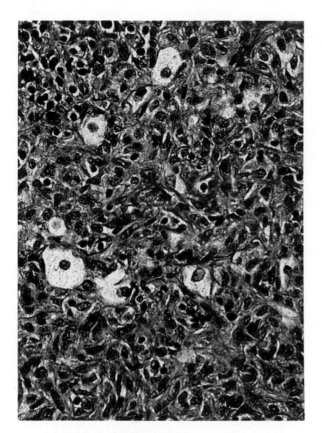

Figure 3-5
DERMAL FIBROUS HISTIOCYTOMA

A benign dermal fibrous histiocytoma (dermatofibroma) with foam cells, fibroblasts, and histiocyte-like cells. Foam cells are a useful marker for this lesion. In this example the lesional cells are randomly arranged, but they can be in fascicles or in a storiform pattern.

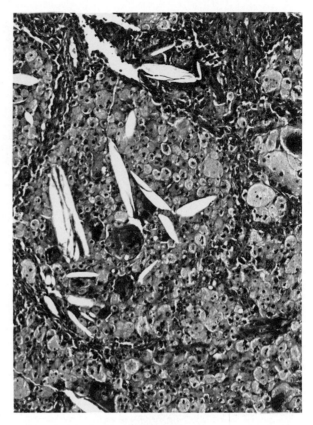

Figure 3-6
DERMAL FIBROUS HISTIOCYTOMA

Less commonly, dermal fibrous histiocytomas feature a predominance of histiocytes and even cholesterol clefts.

DFH may be palisaded in a pattern reminiscent of the Verocay bodies in schwannoma (*palisading variant*) (71). A study has suggested that in children juvenile xanthogranuloma is a part of this spectrum of lesions although it is usually classified separately (64).

Other less common histologic variants of DFH have been described and a review of these has been published (48). The *cellular variant* has also been labeled as benign fibrous histiocytoma with potential for local recurrence, and *"atypical" fibrous histiocytoma* (49,54,64). The latter term is best not used because of possible confusion with the pleomorphic variant and atypical fibroxanthoma (see below). Histologically, the cellular variant is marked by a higher degree of cellularity than the usual DFH, the usually elongated constituent cells are often arranged in fas-

cicles or a storiform pattern, and typically the eosinophilic cytoplasm is easily seen (fig. 3-8). Normal mitotic figures are common and may surpass 10 per 10 high-power fields. Collagen is usually abundant and the lesion often extends into the subcutaneous tissue (60). Necrosis is present in around 10 percent of cases, and less commonly, there is ulceration of the epidermis. Inflammation, foam cells, and giant cells are present in most lesions although they may be inconspicuous (fig. 3-9).

The *aneurysmal variant* is marked by polypoid growth and blood-filled spaces that are most prominent near the center of the lesion and vary from clefts to cavernous lakes (fig. 3-10) (47,70). Endothelial cells do not line the spaces but numerous capillaries are present in the surrounding stroma along with hemosiderin, hemosiderin macrophages, foam cells, and inflammatory cells. The spindled cells typical of DFH are always

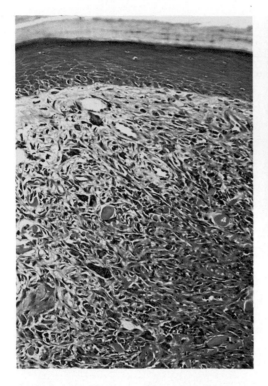

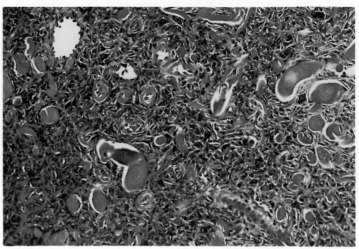

Figure 3-7
DERMAL FIBROUS HISTIOCYTOMA,
HEMOSIDEROTIC VARIANT
This variant, also known as sclerosing hemangioma variant, is marked by large amounts of hemosiderin. There may be considerable sclerosis as in the above figure.

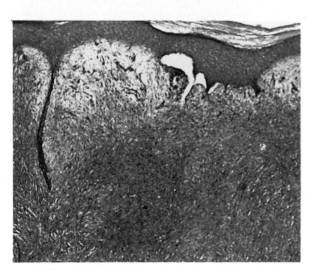

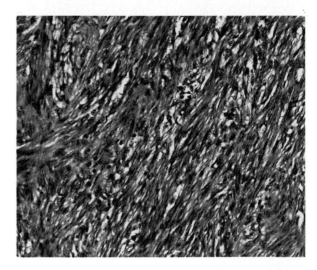

Figure 3-8
DERMAL FIBROUS HISTIOCYTOMA, CELLULAR VARIANT
This variant is more cellular than the usual dermatofibroma and the generally elongate cells may be arranged in fascicles or a storiform pattern.

present but may be inconspicuous. Cellular atypia is uncommon but up to 10 mitotic figures per 10 high-power fields have been reported. DFHs with abundant hemosiderin but without the aneurysmal blood-filled spaces are considered to be the *sclerosing hemangioma (hemosiderotic) variant.*

The *epithelioid variant* occurs most commonly on the thigh, is characteristically polypoid or nodular, and often features an epithelial collarette (37,55,65,72,77). This lesion often extends into the superficial subcutaneous tissue and may flatten the epidermis but it has a well-demarcated

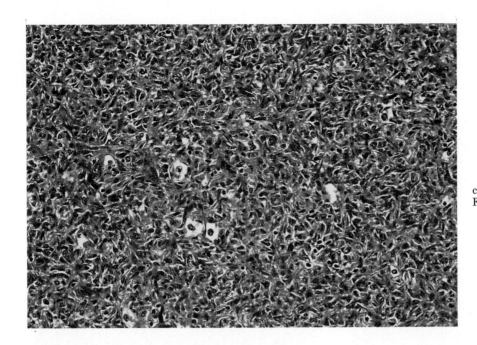

Figure 3-9
DERMAL FIBROUS
HISTIOCYTOMA,
CELLULAR VARIANT
An example in which the tumor
cells are more histiocyte-like.
Foam cells are present.

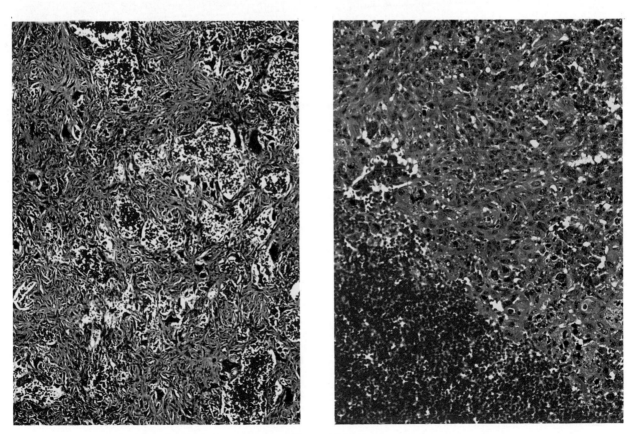

Figure 3-10
DERMAL FIBROUS HISTIOCYTOMA, ANEURYSMAL VARIANT
The aneurysmal variant features nonendothelial-lined blood-filled spaces that vary from clefts to lakes.

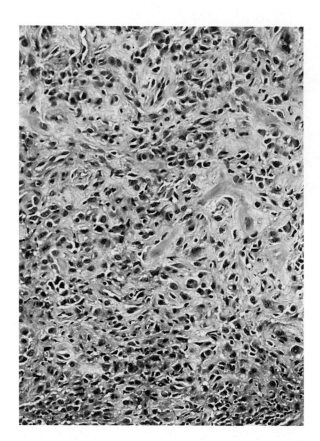 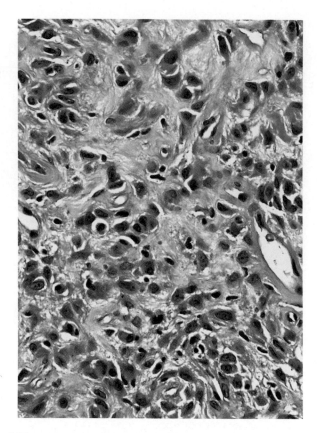

Figure 3-11
DERMAL FIBROUS HISTIOCYTOMA, EPITHELIOID VARIANT
The majority of cells in this variant take on histiocyte-like features with more abundant cytoplasm. Spindled cells are absent or sparse.

margin. The characteristic constituent cells are uniform, have abundant eosinophilic cytoplasm and a large oval vesicular nucleus with a small nucleolus, and are separated by delicate collagen fibers (figs. 3-11, 3-12). By definition, they must constitute 50 percent or more of the tumor cell population. These epithelioid cells blend into variable numbers of the more characteristic spindle cells found in all DFHs. Foam cells and binucleate or trinucleate cells are common but multinucleated giant cells are unusual. Inflammation is muted, mitotic figures are rare, and necrosis and hemorrhage are not seen.

Rare examples of DFH contain strikingly enlarged pleomorphic cells, many of which are multinucleate. These cells have irregular, hyperchromatic, sometimes multiple nuclei, prominent nucleoli, and most often foamy or hemosiderin-laden cytoplasm (fig. 3-13). Some cells have nu-

clei with intense hyperchromasia but the chromatin is smooth and dense suggesting degeneration. When numerous, they can impart an appearance that is worrisome for sarcoma, but mitotic figures are sparse or absent, cellularity is not as high as it is in most sarcomas, and necrosis is absent. Spindled cells, histiocyte-like cells, and foamy macrophages make up the rest of the cellular population. Stromal collagen fibers and usually inflammatory cells are common, and the epidermis is usually hyperplastic. DFHs containing these bizarre enlarged cells have been labeled as "atypical" or "pseudosarcomatous"; we prefer the atypical label or, more fancifully, "dermatofibroma with monster cells" (44,63,68,75). Very rarely, DFHs are composed predominantly of clear cells (78) or granular cells. In the latter circumstance, the tumor can resemble granular cell tumor.

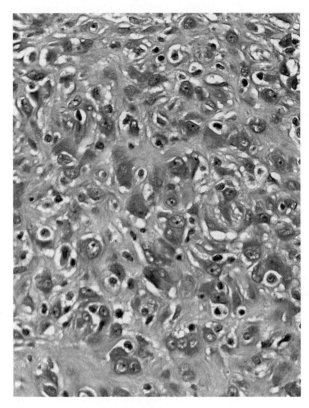

Figure 3-12
DERMAL FIBROUS HISTIOCYTOMA,
EPITHELIOID VARIANT

Another example of epithelioid benign fibrous histiocytoma. The cells have histiocytic features and are set in a hyalinized stroma.

Special Studies. Immunohistochemical reports indicate that variable numbers of the tumor cells in most DFHs, except those that are predominantly or exclusively fibrous, decorate with one or another antibody known to react against, but not be specific for, macrophages (46, 56,62,74). About 30 to 50 percent of DFHs contain spindled cells that react with muscle-specific actin or smooth muscle actin (40). This supports myofibroblastic differentiation by at least some of the tumor cells. S-100 protein and desmin are essentially not expressed by the lesional cells. Less than 5 percent of DFHs are composed of cells that contain an antigen recognized by CD34, and these are almost exclusively of the cellular variant in which staining is most often weak and focal (41,59). Nearly 90 percent of DFHs contain variable numbers of cells that express an antigen recognized by an antibody against the clotting enzyme factor XIIIa (35,38,

39,41,50,51,59,69). This antibody also recognizes dermal dendrocytes in the normal skin, and whether the reactive cells in DFHs are lesional or overrun dermal dendrocytes is controversial. Electron microscopy reveals fibroblasts, myofibroblasts, and in some lesions, cells with the ultrastructural features of histiocytes. These studies support the light microscopic observation that true histiocytes as well as histiocyte-like cells are often present within DFH.

Differential Diagnosis. The differential diagnosis of the benign DFH is large because many other lesions are composed of similar-appearing cells. The main considerations include dermatofibrosarcoma protuberans (DFSP), plexiform fibrous histiocytoma, smooth muscle tumors, neurofibroma, desmoplastic malignant melanoma, spindle cell carcinoma, hemangiopericytoma, Kaposi's sarcoma, atypical fibroxanthoma, pleomorphic fibroma, juvenile xanthogranuloma, and reticulohistiocytoma. Probably the most common problem is distinguishing DFH, particularly the cellular variant, from DFSP (36,60, 76a). A comparison of the histologic and immunohistochemical features of the two lesions is presented in Table 3-3. Thick bundles of collagen in the center of the lesion, a perivascular inflammatory infiltrate of lymphocytes and plasma cells at the periphery, foam cells, diffusely distributed multinucleated giant cells, hemosiderin deposits, and epidermal hyperplasia are characteristic features of DFH and are quite unusual in DFSP. However, rare DFSPs may contain centrally located thick collagen bundles. The pattern of extension into the subcutaneous tissue is also very useful in distinguishing these two lesions (60). Benign DFH may extend into the subcutaneous tissue, either with a blunt pushing margin or with short extensions of fibrous tissue into fat (76a). DFSP typically involves the subcutaneous tissue extensively and also has two patterns of growth. In the first, vertically oriented slender tumor cells extend between fat cells, leaving intact fat cells that then appear to be scattered throughout the lesion ("honeycomb" or "lace-like" pattern). Intralesional fat occurs very rarely in DFH, although a few trapped fat cells may be present at the periphery of the tumor. In the second pattern, the cells of DFSP lie with their nuclei predominantly parallel to the skin surface, resulting in layers of fat

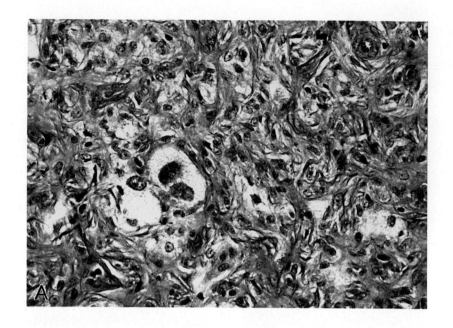

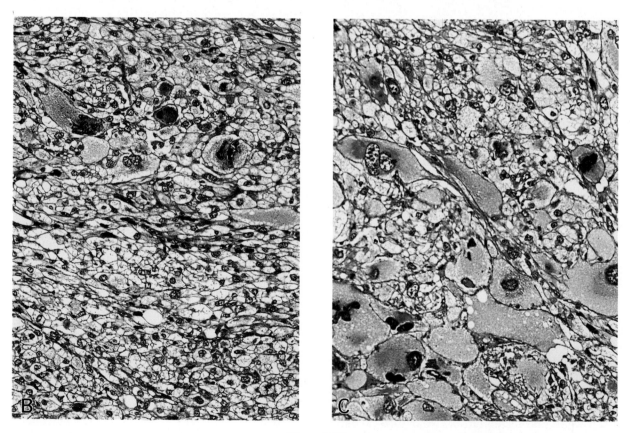

Figure 3-13
DERMAL FIBROUS HISTIOCYTOMA, ATYPICAL VARIANT
Atypical benign fibrous histiocytoma features cells with enlarged, often hyperchromatic nuclei, however, mitotic figures are sparse.

Table 3-3

THE DIFFERENTIAL DIAGNOSIS OF BENIGN FIBROUS HISTIOCYTOMA, DERMATOFIBROSARCOMA PROTUBERANS (DFSP), PLEXIFORM FIBROUS HISTIOCYTOMA, AND NODULAR FASCIITIS

		Benign Fibrous Histiocytoma	DFSP	Plexiform Fibrous Histiocytoma	Nodular Fasciitis
1)	Location	Usually dermis, may extend a short distance into the subcutaneous tissue; rare examples arise in the subcutaneous tissue (benign subcutaneous fibrous histiocytoma)	Subcutaneous and dermis	Subcutaneous, sometimes with extension into the lower dermis	Subcutaneous (or deeper)
2)	Margins	Usually circumscribed with only short extensions of tumor into subcutaneous tissue	Always infiltrating; pattern of infiltration is characteristic (see text)	Plexiform with long extensions of fibrous tissue	Infiltrating
3)	Cells	Polymorphous: fibrocytes, myofibroblasts, giant cells, histiocyte-like cells, hemosiderin laden macrophages, foam cells	Monomorphous: uniform cells with hard-to-see cytoplasm arranged in a repetitive storiform pattern; giant and foam cells are rare	Polymorphous: fibrous tissue resembling that seen in desmoids alternating with nodules of multinucleated giant cells and histiocyte-like cells	Monomorphous: cells with vesicular, uniform, often enlarged nuclei resembling fibroblasts in granulation tissue arranged in loose bundles; multinucleated giant cells may be present
4)	Stroma	Often collagenous, particularly at the periphery; thick collagen fibers may be present but are often difficult to find in the cellular variant	Usually inconspicuous; the lesion is cellular; collagen is usually absent and not ropy (except for rare collagenous variant)	Finely collagenous as in desmoid fibromatosis	Granulation tissue-like to myxoid; rarely hyalinized
5)	Immuno-histo-chemistry	Cells in most reported to express factor XIIIa; staining may be focal and questions have been raised about whether the positive cells are lesional cells; CD34 staining very rare and if present focal and weak; 30 percent have cells that express muscle actin; desmin and S-100 protein are negative	Over 90 percent have numerous cells that express CD34; rare tumors may contain a small number of cells that express factor XIIIa; actin may be positive; S-100 protein, desmin are negative	Giant cells express CD68; fibroblasts may express actin but are CD68 negative	Cells are smooth muscle actin positive

cells interposed between layers of spindle cells ("pearl necklace" pattern), a pattern not seen in DFH. Mixtures of these two patterns of infiltration may be found in the same tumor. Numerous mitotic figures are more often a feature of DFSP, as is a prominent myxoid stroma, although the latter is not uncommon in subcutaneous DFH (see below). Cellular DFH contains cells with more abundant eosinophilic cytoplasm than the cells in DFSP. DFSP is rarely less than 2 cm and more often 4 to 5 cm.

Nearly all reports indicate that CD34 is expressed by the cells of almost all DFSPs but only rarely by the cells of DFH (most reports indicate that less than 5 percent of DFHs contain CD34-positive cells and those that do are usually the cellular variant and the staining in such tumors is weak and focal) (35,38,41,59,75a). Factor XIIIa is expressed by at least some cells in about 90 percent of DFHs whereas factor XIIIa is only infrequently expressed by the cells of DFSP, and even if factor XIIIa-positive cells are present in DFSP they are focal, most frequently at the edge of the lesion and probably reactive. Whether the factor XIIIa-positive cells in DFH are lesional or overrun dendritic cells is controversial, but the presence of large numbers of such cells in a dermal tumor favors, but is not specific for, DFH (35).

Plexiform fibrous histiocytoma and DFH share some features; however, most DFHs are centered in the dermis, whereas plexiform fibrous histiocytoma most often is centered in the subcutaneous tissue, although involvement of the lower dermis is common. Most plexiform fibrous histiocytomas are characterized by areas of purely fibrous tissue alternating with nodules of histiocyte-like and giant cells, rather than a diffuse mixture of the two cell types, as is common in DFH. Although benign DFH may extend into the subcutaneous tissue with ray-like extensions of fibrous tissue, the rays are short and attached to the dermal mass, whereas the extensions of fibrous tissue in plexiform fibrous histiocytoma characteristically are long and extend for considerable distance. Nodules of histiocyte-like and giant cells may be present in these long fibrous rays.

Neural neoplasms share morphologic features with the fibrous histiocytomas, particularly those featuring palisaded cells, but for practical purposes all benign nerve sheath tumors contain cells that express S-100 protein and many nerve sheath tumors contain cells that express CD34. S-100 protein is practically never expressed by the lesional cells of DFH, although dendritic cells are present in many and these stain with S-100 protein. Less than 5 percent of DFHs contain cells that express CD34. The cells of neurofibroma have wavy nuclei, an unusual feature in DFH, and they are smaller than the nuclei in the usual DFH.

Smooth muscle tumors are composed of cells with discernible eosinophilic cytoplasm arranged in bundles. The tufting or storiform pattern often found in DFH is largely absent, as are foam cells. In addition, smooth muscle cells may express desmin and desmin is largely absent in the constituent cells of DFH.

Desmoplastic malignant melanoma can mimic a DFH. Whenever a fibrous-appearing lesion is encountered in the skin, particularly the skin of the head and neck of an adult patient, the possibility of desmoplastic malignant melanoma should be considered. There are two features that, if present, are particularly useful in identifying this lesion. First, there may be a melanocytic proliferation, usually of the lentigo maligna type, at the dermo-epidermal junction. Second, there may be infiltration of nerves by tumor cells near the base of the lesion, and this may cause the nerves to become enlarged. The fibroblastic-appearing cells in desmoplastic malignant melanoma are frequently arranged in fascicles, and mitotic figures and enlarged atypical cells with abnormal nuclei are characteristically mixed among the spindled cells. In most desmoplastic malignant melanomas, at least some of the tumor cells express S-100 protein although HMB45 is usually negative.

Benign DFH composed predominantly of fibrocytes conceivably could be confused with the desmoid type fibromatosis. However, desmoid type fibromatoses do not primarily develop in the dermis, and fibromatoses involving the subcutaneous tissue and dermis also infiltrate the underlying muscle. Fibromatoses are large lesions, lack a histiocyte-like component, and have cells arranged in a fascicular rather than a storiform pattern. Fibrosarcomas are composed of spindled cells arranged in bundles that intersect at acute angles. They almost never arise in the skin except as a component of DFSP (see DFSP below). Spindle cell carcinomas typically are more cellular, with less collagen than the fibrous histiocytomas. Keratin stains should be applied to lesions whose appearance raises the possibility of spindle cell carcinoma.

The cells composing hemangiopericytomas share many features with those of DFH, and indeed, areas indistinguishable from hemangiopericytoma can be found in several types of fibrous histiocytomas. Both hemangiopericytoma and DFH may feature cells with a tufted arrangement and staghorn vessels, but hemangiopericytomas lack a histiocyte-like component, foam cells, or giant cells, and they are rare in the dermis.

Kaposi's sarcoma contains spindled cells but does not feature epidermal hyperplasia, basal cell hyperpigmentation, multinucleated giant cells, or foam cells and lacks the blood lakes of the aneurysmal variant of DFH (45). The constituent cells of Kaposi's sarcoma are frequently CD34 and CD31 positive.

Distinguishing DFH from the other benign fibrohistiocytic lesions is usually not difficult. Juvenile xanthogranuloma is a lesion that occurs almost always in the skin of children and infants, although there may be lesions in other organs. This lesion is predominantly a histiocytic one and the histiocytes usually have vacuolated or foamy cytoplasm. Touton type giant cells featuring nuclei arranged in a ring are a hallmark of this lesion, but the number of giant cells varies considerably from area to area of the same tumor and from tumor to tumor. Reticulohistiocytoma is also a predominantly histiocytic lesion that occurs most often in adults. The histiocytes, which may be multinucleated, have glassy eosinophilic cytoplasm; mitotic figures may be quite numerous and nuclear pleomorphism may be prominent. It is these multinucleated giant cells that are most helpful in distinguishing this lesion from the epithelioid variant of DFH because the latter practically never contains multinucleated cells. Atypical fibroxanthoma has a morphologic pattern identical to that of pleomorphic MFH; it is distinguished from the latter on the basis of its location in the dermis and absence of necrosis. The high cellularity, marked pleomorphism, anaplasia of the constituent cells, and presence of abnormal division figures all serve to distinguish atypical fibroxanthoma from the usual benign fibrous histiocytoma. Atypical DFH with giant or monster cells may raise the question of atypical fibroxanthoma but the former is less cellular and does not contain numerous or abnormal division figures. The lesion known as pleomorphic fibroma can resemble dermatofibroma with atypical cells because of the enlarged cells with hyperchromatic nuclei, but it lacks foam cells and epidermal hyperplasia, and the atypical cells appear to be fibroblasts rather than histiocyte-like cells (61).

The aneurysmal variant can resemble several types of tumors. One of these is spindle cell hemangioma which features endothelial-lined, cavernous vascular spaces and a prominent rather than an inconspicuous spindle cell population. Angiosarcoma contains complex interanastomosing channels at least somewhere in the tumor and the tumor cells dissect between collagen bundles, features not found in the aneurysmal variant of DFH. The vast majority of angiosarcomas occur on the face and scalp, uncommon sites for the aneurysmal variant, and the typical patient with angiosarcoma is elderly. Angiomatoid fibrous histiocytoma and the aneurysmal variant both feature blood-filled spaces, but the former is usually subcutaneous, associated with an intense lymphoplasmacytic infiltrate that often features germinal centers (see Angiomatoid Fibrous Histiocytoma below).

Treatment and Prognosis. DFHs are benign and, except for the cellular and aneurysmal variants, both of which recur in up to 25 to 30 percent of cases, rarely ever recur unless they are very large. Multinodularity has been noted to be a marker for risk of recurrence but whether the risk from multinodularity is independent of size is unknown (54). Recurrences are almost never aggressive and almost always are cured by reexcision. Two patients with the cellular variant of DFH have developed lymph node and lung metastases following local recurrence. However, even with lung metastasis, the course seems to be indolent (52).

Benign Subcutaneous and Deep Fibrous Histiocytomas

Definition. These tumors, composed of fibrocytes, fibroblasts, myofibroblasts, and histiocyte-like cells in variable proportions are, by definition, centered in the subcutaneous tissue, or arise within the deep soft tissue or central body cavities. They are histologically identical to the DFH except that a storiform pattern is more consistently present and the tumor is usually better circumscribed (53).

Clinical Features. Subcutaneous and deep benign fibrous histiocytomas are rare in comparison to DFH. Of the cases reported, most have occurred on the extremities, usually within the subcutaneous tissue, but skeletal muscle and the abdominal cavity have been reported to be involved as well. These tumors present as asymptomatic masses with an average size of about 4 to 5 cm (range, 2 to 15 cm). Most develop in individuals between the ages of 20 and 40 years, but they have been found in patients of all ages.

Pathologic Findings. Characteristically, the subcutaneous and deep benign fibrous histiocytomas are bounded by a fibrous capsule which gives them a circumscribed appearance grossly. Most are single nodules but occasionally they may be multinodular. The tumors are usually firm, and the cut surfaces pale to light brown. Low-power microscopy confirms the gross impression of circumscription (fig. 3-14). In most tumors the constituent cells resemble fibroblasts and myofibroblasts, with bland, uniform, and elongate to oval nuclei that have dense to vesicular chromatin (fig. 3-15). The appearance of the cells is related to the cellularity of the lesion and the stroma. More cellular lesions tend to be composed of cells with vesicular nuclei; more collagenous ones by cells with the elongate, dense nuclei characteristic of mature fibrocytes. Pleomorphism is absent and if mitotic figures are present, they are sparse and normal. Even in cellular lesions, the mitotic activity is usually not greater than 5 mitotic figures per 10 high-power fields. Giant cells and foam cells are unusual (unlike in DFH) and when present are most often focal, but in some lesions they are prominent and diffuse (fig. 3-16) (73). When xanthoma cells are numerous cholesterol clefts may be noted. Rarely, giant cells are so numerous that the question of giant cell tumor of tendon sheath arises. Usually a storiform pattern is more prominent than in DFH and in many lesions it is diffuse, resulting in an appearance reminiscent of DFSP (fig. 3-17). In addition, areas indistinguishable from hemangiopericytoma, including a staghorn vascular pattern, are found within some tumors (fig. 3-18). Microscopic, often stellate, foci of necrosis may be seen. Vascular invasion by a subcutaneous benign fibrous histiocytoma has been reported (67).

The stroma in these deeper benign fibrous histiocytomas may be partially or predominantly myxoid and contain arborizing blood vessels or, alternatively, collagen may be prominent and dense. In fact, in some tumors the collagen is stellate and dense enough to meet the definition of "amianthoid" fibers. Metaplastic bone has been observed (73).

Except for the foam cells, the tumor cells have not been reported to express antigens characteristic of bone marrow–derived macrophages. The

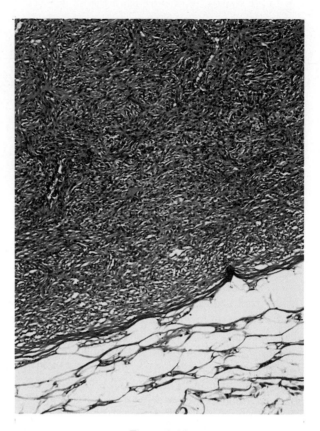

Figure 3-14
SUBCUTANEOUS BENIGN FIBROUS HISTIOCYTOMA
The circumscription and the absence of trapped fat help identify this as a benign fibrous histiocytoma rather than DFSP or other tumors.

immunohistochemical profile of the few cases studied has been identical to that of the DFH.

Differential Diagnosis. A common problem is uncertainty about whether a benign fibrous histiocytoma is dermal or subcutaneous. This distinction is important since DFHs, except for the cellular and aneurysmal variants, almost never recur, and subcutaneous ones do in approximately 15 to 30 percent of cases, apparently without regard to histologic pattern (see Treatment and Prognosis below). We restrict the definition of benign DFH to lesions involving the dermis, but some of these extend into the subcutaneous tissue; when there is doubt about the location the clinician can be informed that recurrence is possible. Most of the remainder of the differential diagnosis of the benign subcutaneous and deep fibrous histiocytomas is the same as that for DFH described above. DFSP looms particularly large

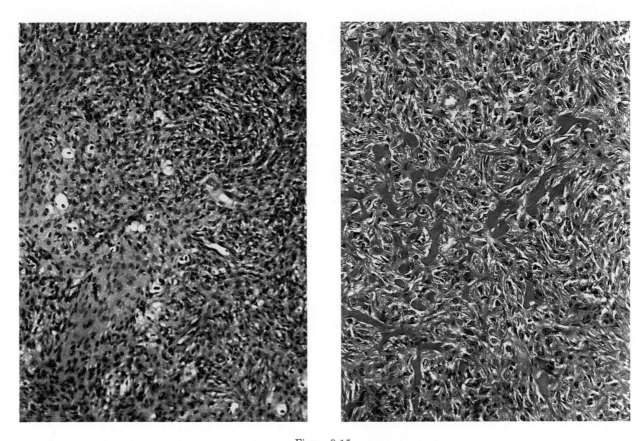

Figure 3-15
SUBCUTANEOUS BENIGN FIBROUS HISTIOCYTOMA
Subcutaneous benign fibrous histiocytomas may be cellular (left) or have a more fibrous stroma (right).

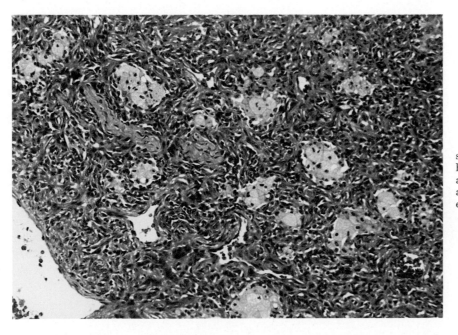

Figure 3-16
SUBCUTANEOUS BENIGN
FIBROUS HISTIOCYTOMA
Foam cells are less common in subcutaneous benign fibrous histiocytomas but when present are a useful marker because foam cells are rare in DFSP, the usual differential diagnostic consideration.

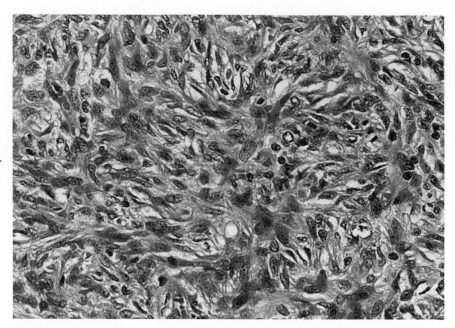

Figure 3-17
SUBCUTANEOUS BENIGN
FIBROUS HISTIOCYTOMA
A storiform pattern at least focally and cellular uniformity mark benign fibrous histiocytomas. If there is concern for DFSP, a CD34 stain should be performed.

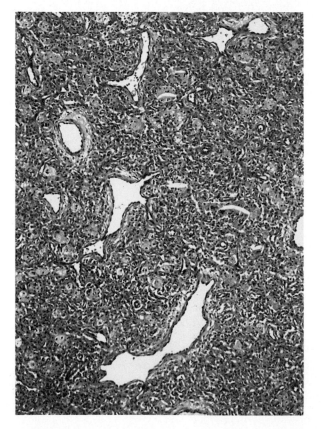

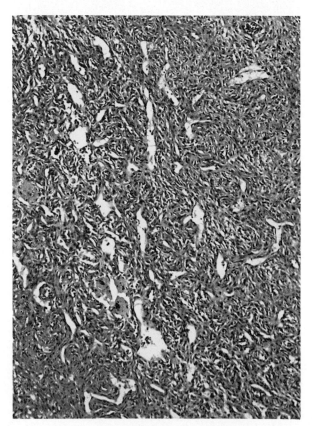

Figure 3-18
SUBCUTANEOUS BENIGN FIBROUS HISTIOCYTOMA
A pericytic vascular pattern may be found in benign fibrous histiocytomas so this possibility should be considered when such a pattern is encountered.

in this differential diagnosis. DFSP is an infiltrating lesion while benign fibrous histiocytomas are circumscribed. Moreover, DFSP is characterized by a single cell type arranged in a repetitive storiform pattern while in subcutaneous fibrous histiocytoma there is often a mixture of fibroblasts, myofibroblasts, and histiocyte-like cells. The stroma is often collagenized in fibrous histiocytoma while collagen is unusual in DFSP. Foam cells and multinucleated giant cells are practically never found in DFSP. If the cells are CD34 positive the lesion is probably best regarded as DFSP unless the morphologic features are entirely wrong for this tumor.

Atypical fibroxanthoma is replaced by pleomorphic MFH in the differential diagnosis of benign subcutaneous and deep fibrous histiocytoma because tumors with the features of atypical fibroxanthoma occurring in the subcutaneous and deep soft tissues are classified as pleomorphic MFH. The paucity of mitotic figures, the absence of abnormal division figures, an overall appearance identical or similar to DFH, and the uniformity of the constituent cells all serve to distinguish benign subcutaneous fibrous histiocytoma from pleomorphic MFH and other malignant neoplasms.

Nodular fasciitis can resemble subcutaneous and deep benign fibrous histiocytomas. The features we find most helpful in making this distinction are summarized in Table 3-3. When the cells in a benign fibrous histiocytoma are predominantly mature fibrocytes rather than the granulation type fibroblasts that compose nodular fasciitis, and when the background is collagenous rather than the loose background characteristic of nodular fasciitis, the distinction is easy. Most importantly, normal mitotic figures are almost always numerous in nodular fasciitis while they are typically difficult to find in benign fibrous histiocytomas. There are cases, however, in which the distinction between the two is difficult. When this occurs, the difficulty should be explained to the clinician and the patient warned that the lesion might recur.

Treatment and Prognosis. Benign subcutaneous and deep fibrous histiocytomas may recur but they do not metastasize. Recurrences are not destructive nor are they uncontrolled, and all patients with recurrences have been cured by reexcision. Because so few tumors have

been reported the relapse rate is largely unknown, but based on a few cases it appears to be in the range of 20 to 30 percent. Size and completeness of excision probably affect the recurrence rate and, as for DFH, multinodularity has been reported as a morphologic feature that predicts an increased risk of recurrence.

Juvenile Xanthogranuloma, Reticulohistiocytoma, and Xanthoma

These skin lesions, included in the World Health Organization (WHO) classification of benign fibrous histiocytomas, are presented in the Fascicle Non-Melanocytic Tumors of the Skin (65a) and are not discussed here other than in the differential diagnosis sections.

INTERMEDIATE FIBROUS HISTIOCYTOMAS (MANAGERIAL GROUPS IIa, IIb, AND IIc, TABLE 1-10)

The WHO classification includes five tumors in this category: atypical fibroxanthoma, dermatofibrosarcoma protuberans (including pigmented forms), giant cell fibroblastoma, plexiform fibrous histiocytoma, and angiomatoid fibrous histiocytoma. Dermatofibroma protuberans (DFSP) is composed of a monomorphic proliferation of cells that resemble fibroblasts rather than the biphasic population of fibroblasts and histiocyte-like (or histiocytes) required by the definition of fibrous histiocytomas. It is included in the fibrous histiocytoma category because of its storiform pattern (a pattern associated with fibrous histiocytomas) and because some observers have concluded that a subset of the tumor cells are "histiocyte-like." Early tissue culture studies also suggested histiocytic differentiation, an observation now largely refuted. We think the morphologic features better support a fibrous tumor and the recent observations that the tumor cells in almost all DFSPs express CD34 supports the concept that these cells are differentiating along the same lines as the CD34-positive spindle cells found in the normal dermis. For these reasons, we think it most logical to move this tumor and its close relative, giant cell fibroblastoma, to the fibrous tumor category (assuming the CD34-positive dermal spindle cells are fibrocytes). However, in the interest of classificatory uniformity, because of the uncertainty concerning the direction of differentiation of the CD34-positive spindle cells in the normal dermis, and because there are no clinical implications whether DFSP is classified as fibrous or fibrohistiocytic, we have reluctantly chosen to follow the lead of WHO and retained DFSP in the fibrous histiocytoma category (see also Introduction to this chapter).

Giant cell fibroblastoma, originally considered to be a fibrous tumor, does contain giant cells and fibroblasts and thus is biphasic; however, the giant cells appear more fibrocytic than histiocyte-like making this tumor a better candidate for a fibrous tumor category than DFSP. Giant cell fibroblastoma is linked to DFSP because areas of otherwise characteristic DFSP may contain giant cell fibroblastoma, both DFSP and giant cell fibroblastoma may recur with the other's pattern, and they share rearrangements of chromosomes 17 and 22 (122,139).

Most, but not all, plexiform fibrous histiocytomas are biphasic, being composed of fibroblasts (or myofibroblasts) and, focally, cells resembling histiocytes, including multinucleated giant cells. Thus, it seems reasonable to classify this tumor as a fibrous histiocytoma even though ultrastructural examination supports fibroblastic or myofibroblastic differentiation of both sets of cells.

The place in the pantheon of soft tissue tumors for angiomatoid fibrous histiocytoma, recently removed from the malignant fibrous histiocytoma category to the "intermediate" category on the basis of new information about patient outcome, is also controversial. The plump cells with lightly eosinophilic cytoplasm have been interpreted both as histiocyte-like and myofibroblastic. The tumor cell staining with desmin reported in some laboratories supports myofibroblastic differentiation; however, desmin expression has been reported to be "focal and weak" by other investigators and is present in less than half the tumors. Because the direction of differentiation of these tumors is unsettled we have followed custom and retained angiomatoid lesions among the fibrous histiocytomas. Among this "intermediate" group of neoplasms, only atypical fibroxanthoma seems to wear the mantle of fibrous histiocytoma comfortably, because it is histologically identical to pleomorphic MFH (this conclusion assumes one accepts pleomorphic MFH as a fibrous histiocytoma; see Introduction to this chapter).

Atypical Fibroxanthoma

Definition. Atypical fibroxanthoma (AFX) is a cellular, circumscribed, compressive neoplasm composed of spindled fibroblasts, myofibroblasts, round histiocyte-like cells, and often, giant cells (87,88,90,93,94,105). Tumors containing cells demonstrating any other line of differentiation are excluded. The tumor is centered in the dermis with no more than superficial involvement of the subcutaneous tissue. Nuclear pleomorphism is marked and mitotic figures, often abnormal, are easily found. However, tumor cell necrosis not connected to surface ulceration and vascular invasion by tumor cells definitionally excludes AFX. Recently, the definition of AFX has been expanded to include cellular, primarily monomorphic, fibroblastic spindle cell lesions located in the dermis that feature numerous mitotic figures including abnormal forms (80). Pleomorphism may be present in such tumors but is typically mild. A mixture of the two patterns in a single tumor is common.

Clinical Features. AFX occurs almost exclusively in the sun-damaged skin of the elderly, usually on the ear, nose, forehead, or cheek. A much smaller subset has been reported to occur in non–sun-damaged skin on the trunk and extremities of younger individuals, usually in burn scars or in sites of prior radiation (82). We suspect that at least most, if not all, of these are other lesions such as atypical DFH with monster cells (see above) or a sarcoma, particularly pleomorphic leiomyosarcoma or pleomorphic MFH, rather than AFX. The lesions of AFX are typically rapidly growing, most often ulcero-nodular, and frequently umbilicated centrally. The lesions vary from less than 1 cm to over 10 cm, with most measuring less than 2 cm.

Pathologic Findings. Grossly, most AFXs are exophytic nodules that frequently demonstrate a central ulcer (88,93,96). Microscopically, the morphologic features are identical to or very similar to those of pleomorphic MFH; distinction between the two is based on location (fig. 3-19). By definition, AFX is a tumor centered in and predominantly involving the dermis. Identical neoplasms with more than minimal involvement of the subcutis should be interpreted as pleomorphic MFH. AFXs grow with circumscribed compressive margins; they push aside the surrounding

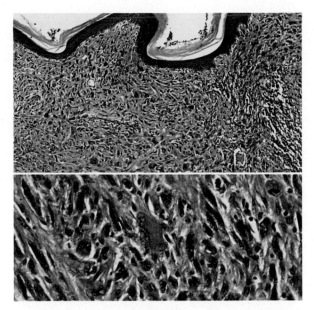

Figure 3-19
ATYPICAL FIBROXANTHOMA
The usual atypical fibroxanthoma has an appearance identical to pleomorphic MFH but it is limited to the dermis. It features high cellularity and is composed of cells with marked pleomorphism, easily found mitotic figures, and chromatin abnormalities of the type found in malignant cells. It is distinguished from atypical benign fibrous histiocytoma by the latter three characteristics.

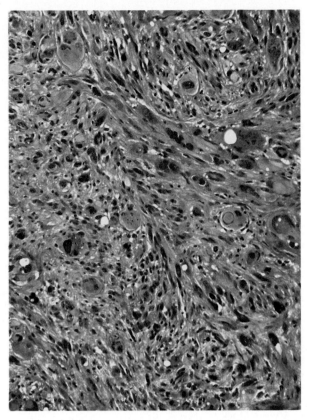

Figure 3-20
ATYPICAL FIBROXANTHOMA
The marked pleomorphism and high cellularity found in most atypical fibroxanthomas are seen in this photomicrograph.

pilosebaceous units and eccrine glands at the periphery of the advancing tumor mass. The overlying epidermis is almost always thinned and, at the center of the lesion, frequently ulcerated. This pattern of growth creates an elevated nodule with an epithelial collar. However, a few lesions grow down into the dermis rather than upward as a protruding nodule. The tumor cells frequently extend right up to the remaining epidermis and can appear to merge with it. The overlying epidermis rarely displays actinic atypia; however, solar elastosis is usually prominent in the surrounding dermis.

Two variants have been described; both are cellular (80,88,93,96). In the pleomorphic variant, spindled cells of varying sizes, sometimes arranged in poorly formed bundles, are interposed haphazardly among round histiocyte-like cells, a large number of which are enlarged and varying numbers of which are multinucleated (fig. 3-20). The round cells may have foamy cytoplasm, and not infrequently some, particularly those that are enlarged or multinucleate, have bizarre, hyperchromatic, irregular nuclei and

enlarged nucleoli (fig. 3-21). Other round cells have abundant eosinophilic cytoplasm. Mitotic figures characteristically abound and abnormal forms are the norm. A storiform pattern is unusual and if present is poorly developed. This variant is identical to pleomorphic MFH. In the primarily spindled variant the fibroblasts have pale eosinophilic cytoplasm with poorly defined cell margins, and most are arranged in bundles (fig. 3-22). However, at least mild pleomorphism is present focally in almost all tumors. The tumor cell nuclei are usually vesicular with coarse chromatin. Numerous mitotic figures are present and abnormal division forms are common. In neither variant is differentiation other than fibroblastic, histiocytic, or histiocyte-like allowed, although metaplastic (not tumor) bone and cartilage is permitted (81). AFXs with osteoclast-like giant cells have been reported (107).

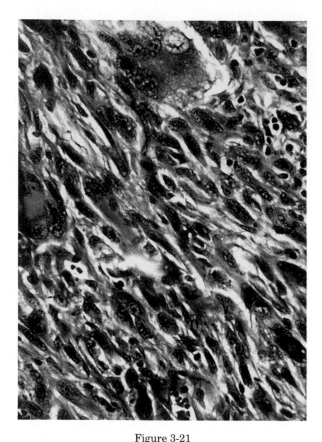

Figure 3-21
ATYPICAL FIBROXANTHOMA
High-power view of atypical fibroxanthoma shows the bizarre cells that are characteristically present.

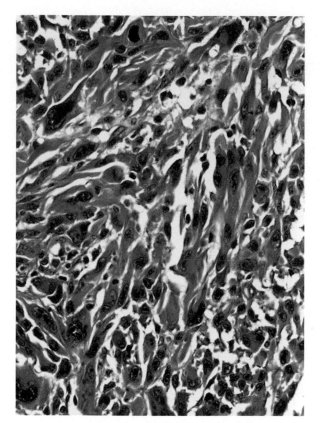

Figure 3-22
ATYPICAL FIBROXANTHOMA, SPINDLED VARIANT
In this variant the generally spindled cells have eosinophilic cytoplasm. Pleomorphism is generally less.

Vascular invasion, infiltrating margins, and tumor cell necrosis other than the acceptable surface ulceration are not allowed in the definition of AFX, and otherwise atypical fibroxanthomas with these features should be considered potentially capable of metastasizing and classified as pleomorphic MFH (80,98).

Special Studies. The definition of AFX requires that the constituent tumor cells be negative for keratin and S-100 protein. If the former is positive, carcinoma cannot be excluded; if the latter is positive, the tumor is likely to be malignant melanoma. However, S-100 protein–positive reactive dendritic cells (Langerhans cells) are commonly present within AFX and these cells should not be interpreted as tumor cells (99,102,108). Interpretation can be tricky because in a few AFXs as many as 40 to 50 percent of the cells may be reactive dendritic cells. H&E sections should be carefully compared with S-100 protein–stained sections to be sure of the identity of the S-100 protein–positive cells. The tumor cells in AFX react with smooth muscle actin or muscle-specific actin in 30 to 65 percent of cases (98,99,102). Anti-smooth muscle actin seems to be the more sensitive antibody. Desmin is practically never expressed and some investigators think that a negative reaction for desmin should be definitional for AFX (98,103); presumably, an otherwise atypical fibroxanthoma that contained desmin-positive tumor cells would be interpreted by them as a leiomyosarcoma.

AFX cells have been reported to express various antigens also expressed by, but not specific for, histiocytes (83,84,95,96,99). These include alpha-1-antitrypsin, alpha-1-antichymotrypsin, ferritin, lysozyme, and cathepsin B. The presence of each of these antigens in the tumor cells of AFX has been touted at one time or another as evidence of histiocytic differentiation but, because none of these is specific for bone marrow–derived monocytes/macrophages, this claim is not supportable. The corollary is that none of these antibodies is useful diagnostically because of their lack of specificity. Recently, KP1, a monoclonal CD68 antibody that recognizes an epitope of a lysosomal glycoprotein present in a number of different cells of the monocyte/macrophage system, has been reported to be positive in about half of AFXs (98,101). However, CD68 may be expressed by the constituent cells of other neoplasms including malignant melanoma and some carcinomas (86,104). A recent report describes the four staining profiles found in a large series of AFXs: CD68 positive and actin negative, CD68 negative and actin positive, both antibodies positive, and both antibodies negative (98). In the setting of an equivocal S-100 protein result we think a positive actin stain helps exclude melanoma since we are unaware of such tumors being actin positive.

Investigators examining AFX with the electron microscope generally have come to the same conclusion as those who have performed ultrastructural examination of pleomorphic MFH, namely, that the constituent cells are fibroblasts, myofibroblasts, and primitive mesenchymal cells, sometimes with evidence of phagocytosis (79,106). Electron microscopy has extremely limited use as a diagnostic tool for AFX. A flow cytometry study reported that 93 percent of the tumors were diploid, a very surprising result that has been contradicted recently by other investigators who report that 8 out of 10 AFXs were aneuploid (100,109). Almost all pleomorphic MFHs, the morphologically identical tumor, are aneuploid.

Differential Diagnosis. Because many other neoplasms have histologic patterns that mimic AFX, the differential diagnosis is lengthy. In fact, we think a diagnosis of AFX should only be made when other possibilities have been excluded, and this exercise, in all likelihood, will require the use of a panel of immunohistochemical reagents. The initial immunohistochemical panel we commonly use is composed of antibodies against S-100 protein, keratin, actin, desmin, and leukocyte common antigen (98). The main differential diagnostic considerations are malignant melanoma (desmoplastic and spindle cell), spindle cell squamous carcinoma, leiomyosarcoma, neu-

ral tumor, pleomorphic MFH, DFH with giant cells, and metastasis. A careful search for evidence of atypical melanocytes or the changes of lentigo maligna melanoma as well as enlarged nerves surrounded by spindled tumor cells at the base of the lesion, a feature of desmoplastic melanoma, is always indicated when thinking about a diagnosis of AFX (97). Over 95 percent of malignant melanomas (including spindled and desmoplastic melanomas) express S-100 protein, a marker not expressed by the lesional cells of AFX. S-100 protein–positive dendritic cells often scattered throughout AFX should not be interpreted as lesional cells. AFX is also negative for HMB45. Actin expression by melanoma cells has not been reported so the presence of actin-positive but S-100 protein-, keratin-, and leukocyte common antigen-negative cells in a lesion that otherwise meets the criteria for AFX provides support for that diagnosis. The cells in about half of AFXs express antigens recognized by the CD68 antibody but this antigen also can be present in melanoma cells. Intercellular bridges between tumor cells or keratinization is evidence of squamous cell carcinoma (85). Many well-differentiated squamous cell carcinomas of the skin contain cells that express keratin but the percentage of spindle cell carcinomas in the skin that do so is largely unknown.

The cells in AFX lack the bundle arrangement of spindle cells that marks the usual leiomyosarcoma, and dermal leiomyosarcomas are seldom as pleomorphic as most AFXs. About half of AFXs contain cells that express one or another muscle actin but desmin expression is unusual. The rare dermal tumor with the morphologic features of AFX in which the tumor cells express desmin can either be interpreted as a desmin-positive AFX or a leiomyosarcoma, depending on whether or not the observer considers desmin expression specific for muscle differentiation. Clinically, it does not make a difference because it is very rare for either tumor limited to the dermis to metastasize, although both may recur. Essentially all neurofibromas, including those with enlarged cells ("ancient" or "atypical" neurofibroma), contain cells that express S-100 protein. Pleomorphic MFH is distinguished from AFX by location. Any tumor with the histologic and immunohistologic features of AFX that extends more than a short distance into the subcutaneous tissue should be classified as pleomorphic MFH because significant involvement of the subcutaneous tissues is a predictor of metastatic potential. This also applies to lesions that originally met the criteria for AFX but recur within the subcutaneous tissue and to dermal tumors that meet the histologic and immunologic criteria for AFX but also feature vascular invasion or tumor cell necrosis away from surface ulceration. DFH with "monster" or "pseudosarcomatous" cells lacks the cellularity, mitotic activity, and abnormal division figures found in AFX.

Treatment and Prognosis. The combined recurrence rate in three early series of AFX was 7 percent, and no metastases were reported (88, 93,94). Subsequently, rare cases with spread to regional lymph nodes and distant metastases were reported (89,91,92). Factors reported to predispose to metastasis include tumor cell necrosis, vascular invasion, and significant involvement of the subcutaneous or deeper tissue. By current definition, AFX is a circumscribed dermal tumor with no more than minor involvement of the subcutaneous tissue. When there is a greater extent of subcutaneous involvement, whether by the initial tumor or by a recurrence, the lesion should be interpreted as a pleomorphic MFH. Excluding such lesions as well as those with vascular invasion and more than minimal focal tumor cell necrosis, the recurrence and metastasis rates for AFX are nearly, if not, zero.

Dermatofibrosarcoma Protuberans

Definition. DFSP is a nodular or plaque-like infiltrating tumor that involves the skin and subcutaneous tissue. It is composed of a bland, monomorphic, uniform population of cells with scant cytoplasm, resembling fibroblasts and fibrocytes, arranged in a repetitive storiform pattern. Pigmented melanocytes, sometimes numerous, are present in 5 to 10 percent of DFSPs (*pigmented DFSP, Bednar tumor*).

General Considerations. The cells that constitute DFSP morphologically resemble fibrocytes and fibroblasts; there is not a population of histiocytes or histiocyte-like cells as required by the definition of fibrous histiocytomas, although some of the fibroblasts in DFSP do have open vesicular nuclei similar to those of histiocytes (136). The cells that form DFSP are arranged in a repetitive

storiform pattern as are focal groups of cells in some of the other fibrous histiocytomas and this, plus the interpretation of some of the cells as histiocyte-like, have provided the impetus to classify this tumor as a fibrohistiocytic tumor rather than a fibrous neoplasm. It has been observed that the cells in nearly all DFSPs express CD34, an antigen also expressed by a population of perivascular, perifollicular, periappendageal, and interstitial cells in the normal dermis (110,111,114, 131,135,152). Whether these cells are fibroblasts or a subpopulation of dendrocytes is uncertain but it does appear that DFSP is a neoplasm whose constituent cells are differentiating along the same lines as these dermal spindle cells.

DFSP and giant cell fibroblastoma are closely related, at least to the extent that the patterns of both tumors can be found in the same neoplasm and each tumor can recur as the other (116,130a). Moreover, both have supernumerary ring chromosomes containing sequences from chromosomes 17 and 22 and both possess the same (t17:22) translocation (122,139,140,146). On this basis, we think the conclusion about the proper classificatory niche for DFSP also applies to giant cell fibroblastoma and wherever DFSP goes, so should giant cell fibroblastoma (see Giant Cell Fibroblastoma below).

DFSP is defined as a cutaneous and subcutaneous tumor. Rarely, however, identical neoplasms can be encountered in the deep soft tissues and the central body cavities, particularly the retroperitoneum. In the latter location, a tumor with the histologic features of DFSP may be the dedifferentiated portion of a dedifferentiated liposarcoma. Our experience indicates deep infiltrative lesions with the histologic pattern of DFSP behave in the same way as the superficial DFSPs.

The sarcoma part of the label dermatofibrosarcoma protuberans implies metastatic potential, something the tumor possesses only on occasions so rare as to be anecdotal unless there is evidence of dedifferentiation to morphologic sarcoma. Clinicians may not be aware of this and pathologists might consider an explanation about potential behavior in the pathology report if the clinician has little experience with DFSP. This is further discussed in the Treatment and Prognosis section below.

Clinical Features. DFSP is most often diagnosed in individuals between the ages of 20 and 40 years, although the tumor may arise in infants and children as well as teenagers and middle-aged persons (119,121,127,137,138,151). It is distinctly unusual in the elderly. The tumors are most common on the trunk (about half the cases); the remainder are almost evenly divided between the head and neck area and the proximal upper and lower extremities. The distal extremities are seldom involved and the hands and feet are almost never involved. Some lesions develop in sites of previous trauma, particularly scars.

Most patients present with lesions over 2 cm; in fact the average size at the time of excision is 4 to 5 cm. Early DFSP grows as a plaque and only later develops the nodular or protuberant configuration that gives the tumor its name. Multinodular growth is almost universal among larger tumors. The tumors are characteristically slowly growing, at least initially, and because of this it is not uncommon for patients to have ignored them for considerable periods of time, even as long as 10 to 15 years. Following a prolonged initial phase, a period of rapid growth may ensue and this usually causes the patient to seek treatment. Growth of the tumor, even if slow, is continuous and DFSP can reach enormous size.

Gross Findings. Grossly, the tumor, whether a plaque or a nodule(s), is gray-white unless large numbers of melanocytes are present, in which case it is brown to black. If nodular, the tumor usually stretches, thins, and sometimes ulcerates the overlying skin. As noted, the average size is 4 to 5 cm and very few resected DFSPs are less than 2 cm. The dermis and subcutaneous tissue are both involved in almost all cases although only subcutaneous tumors have been recorded. Many DFSPs appear deceptively circumscribed grossly but all are infiltrative microscopically. Involvement of underlying skeletal muscle is rare except for tumors arising in the head and neck. Some tumors may have a gelatinous consistency corresponding to a myxoid stroma and cysts are noted in some. Hemorrhage is uncommon and tumor cell necrosis is rare.

Microscopic Findings. At low magnification the required repetitive storiform pattern, characterized by innumerable whorls of tumor cells radiating out from centers that usually contain a vessel(s), is apparent in many areas of most

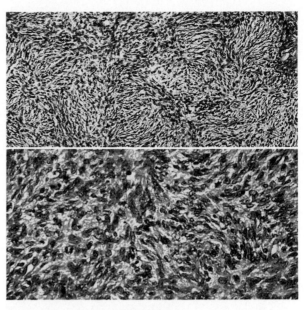

Figure 3-23
DERMATOFIBROSARCOMA PROTUBERANS
A repetitive pattern of uniform, small cells radiating like pinwheels from centers that often contain a vessel is the hallmark of DFSP.

DFSPs but may be difficult to find, particularly in the plaque stage (fig. 3-23) (119,121,127,151). The tumor is usually highly and uniformly cellular but may be less so in areas. At the edges, the universally infiltrating margins are almost always marked by fat cells entrapped by proliferating tumor cells. The tumor frequently grows immediately beneath the epidermis, although a thin rim of uninvolved dermis is sometimes seen. The overlying epidermis is thinned and sometimes ulcerated, not hyperplastic as it characteristically is in the dermal fibrous histiocytomas. With higher magnification, the tumor cells are bland, uniform, and monomorphic (fig. 3-24). Their nuclei vary from elongate and small, with mildly dense chromatin indistinguishable from fibrocyte nuclei, to nuclei that are larger, round, and vesicular. Whatever the nuclear configuration cytoplasm is faintly eosinophilic, sparse, and hard to discern and cytoplasmic margins are indistinct.

The morphologic definition of DFSP specifically disallows significant anaplasia or pleomorphism and multinucleated giant cells are rare, and if present, focal. We allow otherwise characteristic DFSPs to demonstrate mild pleomorphism and atypia in one or two microscopic fields and still be classified as true DFSP. Finding

139

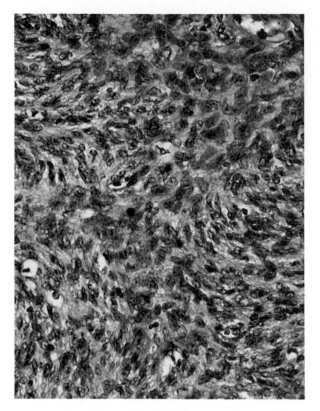

Figure 3-24
DERMATOFIBROSARCOMA PROTUBERANS
DFSP typically contains little intercellular collagen, the cells are uniform, and significant pleomorphism is not allowed. Foam cells and giant cells are rare and their presence should cause the observer to think about the possibility of benign fibrous histiocytoma.

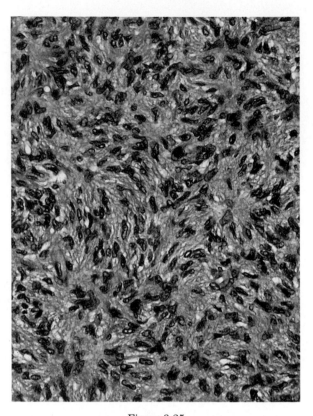

Figure 3-25
DERMATOFIBROSARCOMA PROTUBERANS
In this example fine strands of collagen are present.

mitotic figures is not unusual but in most tumors they do not exceed 5 per 10 high-power fields; however, tumors with 10 to 15 or more normal mitotic figures per 10 high-power fields have been reported. Abnormal division figures are almost never found.

Typically, collagen fibers in the center of the tumor are nonpolarizable, discrete, and thin; broad sheets of keloid-like collagen are not a feature of the usual DFSP except at the edges (fig. 3-25). However, rare examples contain central thick collagen bundles and have been dubbed the *collagenous variant* (133). Foam cells are rare and if present are usually at the edge of the tumor. Hemosiderin is rare and inflammatory cells are sparse, if present at all. Adnexal structures are frequently preserved and surrounded by tumor cells. Thin-walled, often capillary-sized vessels are randomly distributed throughout the tumor

and are often present in the center of the spirals of radiating tumor cells. In the plaque stage a storiform pattern may be muted or absent, and the thin tumor cells lie parallel to the surface of the skin and infiltrate wavy collagen (fig. 3-26).

All DFSPs are infiltrative and the pattern of infiltration of the subcutaneous fat is distinctive enough to be helpful in identifying this tumor (133). The better known pattern is often designated as "honeycomb" and is characterized by tumor cells extending between and surrounding groups of preexisting fat cells, which remain viable. The result is fat present within the tumor (fig. 3-27A,B). The less well known pattern is one in which multiple layers of tumor cells, usually with their nuclei parallel to the surface, isolate and trap small, often linear, groups of fat cells. This can result in a line of one or more layers of fat cells that has been likened to a string of pearls (fig. 3-27C). Both patterns of infiltration may be present in the same tumor (fig. 3-28).

Ordinarily, DFSP is a cellular neoplasm so stroma is sparse. However, in some tumors cellularity is decreased focally or diffusely to such a degree that stroma, frequently myxoid but also on occasion hyalinized collagen, becomes more abundant (134). A myxoid stroma is particularly a feature of recurrent tumors. When the stroma is myxoid the histologic pattern is one of sparse cellularity, small uniform cells with scant cytoplasm, and often an arborizing vascular pattern. When myxoid areas are extensive or predominant rather than focal, the term *myxoid variant* has been applied (129). Rarely, the entire tumor is myxoid and in this circumstance, definitive diagnosis is possible only if a recurrent tumor demonstrates histologic patterns characteristic of DFSP or, in the case of a recurrence, if the original tumor had such areas, although a CD34-positive myxoid tumor in the dermis or subcutaneous tissue is most likely DFSP.

About 5 to 10 percent of DFSPs feature melanin-containing cells that appear to be melanocytes ultrastructurally (fig. 3-29). Such tumors are commonly labeled as *pigmented DFSP* or, less commonly, as *Bednar tumors* (124,125,128, 142). They occur in the same age range as DFSP but the majority of patients are black. The melanocytes have elongate, often bipolar, heavily pigmented cytoplasm; they are most numerous deep in the tumor and they are S-100 protein positive, and HMB45 and epithelial membrane antigen negative. The remainder of the tumor has the characteristic cellular features of DFSP and the nonpigmented tumor cells are S-100 protein negative.

The origin of melanocytes within DFSP, which is clearly not a melanocytic tumor, is uncertain, but a plausible theory suggests colonization of the tumor by melanocytes from the overlying epidermis or skin adnexae (128). Two cases of DFSP have been reported to contain granular cells similar to those found in granular cell tumor (115). Unlike usual granular cell tumors, the granular cells in DFSP do not contain S-100 protein.

Rarely, DFSP may contain areas of fibrosarcoma, heralded by sweeping bundles of spindled cells intersecting at acute angles instead of tumor cells arranged in a storiform pattern (figs. 3-30, 3-31). Mitotic activity is usually increased and nuclear chromatin is often coarser than that found in cells composing the usual DFSP. These

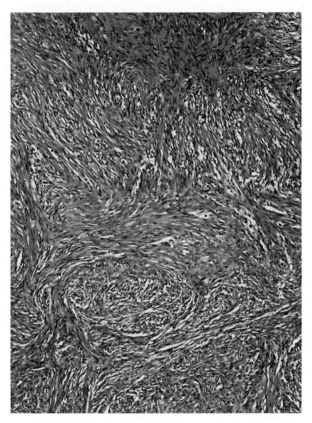

Figure 3-26
DERMATOFIBROSARCOMA PROTUBERANS
In some DFSPs the storiform pattern is muted or absent. A CD34 stain is usually helpful if characteristic storiform areas cannot be found.

features should prompt a diagnosis of "DFSP with areas of fibrosarcoma" (121,123,126,138a, 153). Such areas usually form a nodule but may be focal, so thorough sectioning is important. Most fibrosarcomatous areas are found in the subcutaneous part of the tumor but occasionally the dermis is involved. The interface between the DFSP and fibrosarcoma may be sharp or indistinct. Trapped fat cells, a prominent feature of most DFSPs, are lost or muted in fibrosarcoma but myxoid change may be present in fibrosarcomatous areas. Fibrosarcoma is more common in recurrences of DFSP but may be found in the original resection specimen. The extent of the fibrosarcomatous change, the grade of the nuclei, and the level of mitotic activity have all been reported to affect the metastatic potential, so recording these in the pathology report is worthwhile (153). Rarely, actin-positive myoid cells are

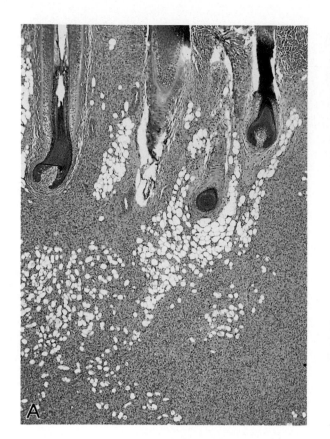

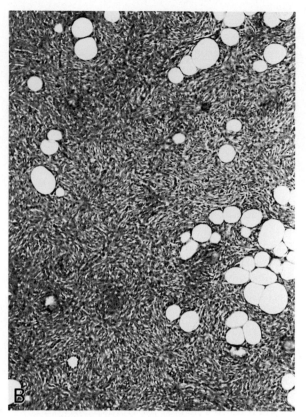

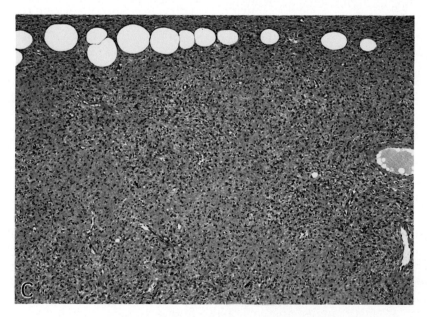

Figure 3-27

DERMATOFIBROSARCOMA PROTUBERANS

Most DFSPs infiltrate fat, leaving residual fat cells surrounded by tumor cells. This pattern is so characteristic of DFSP that it is a useful diagnostic feature. In C, the residual fat cells are in a linear arrangement which has been likened to a string of pearls, a feature very characteristic of DFSP and rare in benign fibrous histiocytoma.

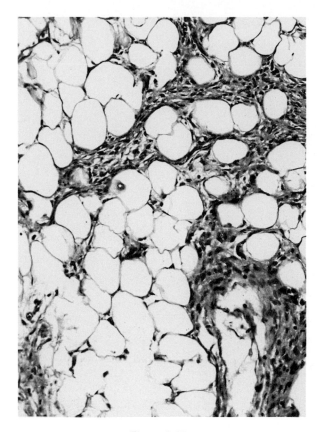

Figure 3-28
DERMATOFIBROSARCOMA PROTUBERANS
Higher magnification shows how tumor cells infiltrate in and among fat cells.

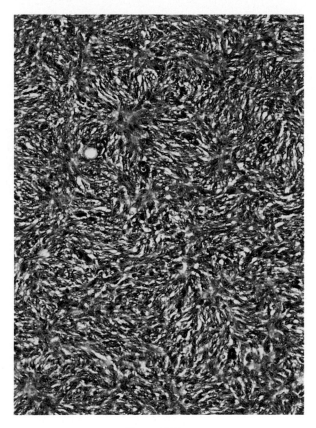

Figure 3-29
DERMATOFIBROSARCOMA PROTUBERANS
Pigmented cells are found in some DFSPs.

found in fibrosarcomatous areas or even in DFSP itself (fig. 3-32).

Very rarely, DFSP contains areas in which the cells are large and pleomorphic (fig. 3-33). In these areas, giant cells, some multinucleated, are common, mitotic activity is usually elevated, and abnormal division figures are not unusual. The definition of DFSP requires cellular uniformity and insignificant chromatin abnormalities. Therefore, significant cellular pleomorphism, as defined in the Microscopic Findings section above, excludes a diagnosis of pure DFSP and when pleomorphic areas are focal we label the tumor "DFSP with areas of malignant fibrous histiocytoma" (141). We do this because significant pleomorphism confers metastatic capability. A diffusely pleomorphic tumor with a storiform pattern is considered to be pleomorphic MFH. Areas indistinguishable from hemangiopericytoma may occur in DFSP.

Although unusual, DFSP may contain areas of giant cell fibroblastoma, DFSP may recur as giant cell fibroblastoma, and giant cell fibroblastoma may recur as DFSP (see Giant Cell Fibroblastoma below). When both are present in the same tumor the two patterns usually merge imperceptibly into one another. When multinucleated giant cells are seen in DFSP the observer should search for more typical areas of giant cell fibroblastoma (121). The giant cells in the latter lack the chromatin abnormalities and pleomorphism of the giant cells in MFH.

Special Studies. The monoclonal antibody that has been raised against the human hematopoietic progenitor cell antigen CD34 has been shown to react with the tumor cells of DFSP in nearly 100 percent of cases, including areas of giant cell fibroblastoma if they are present, although fibrosarcomatous areas are not always positive (110,111,114,130,131,135,138a,152). Unfortunately, this antibody also reacts with an

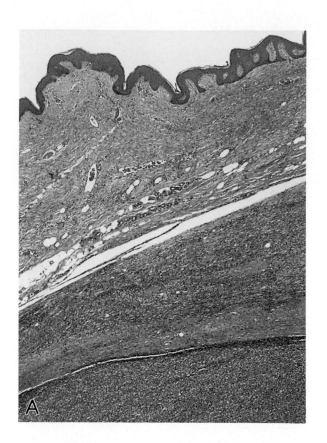

Figure 3-30
DERMATOFIBROSARCOMA
PROTUBERANS WITH FIBROSARCOMA
DFSP with a nodule of fibrosarcoma. The areas of DFSP demonstrate characteristic trapping of fat cells while the fibrosarcoma is more cellular.

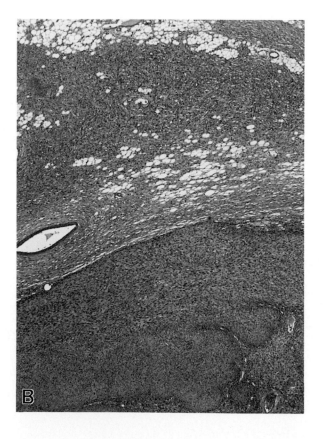

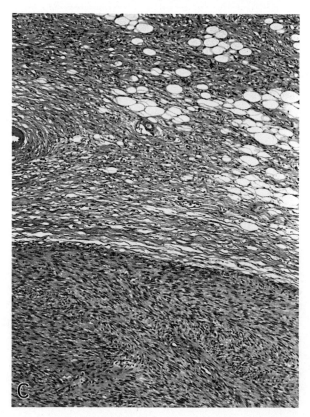

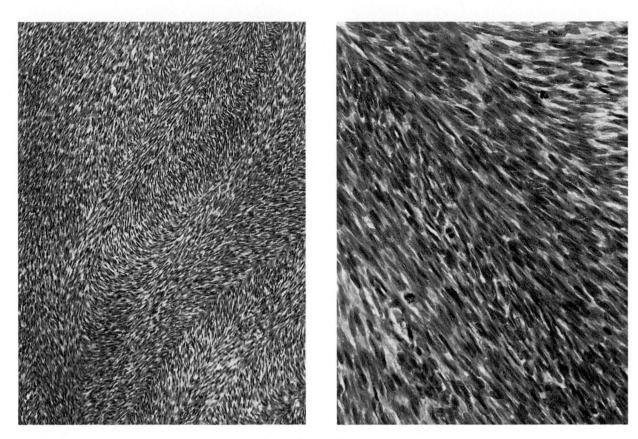

Figure 3-31
FIBROSARCOMA ARISING IN DERMATOFIBROSARCOMA PROTUBERANS
The cells in areas of fibrosarcoma are spindled and uniform but hyperchromatic and arranged in a "herring bone" rather than a storiform pattern.

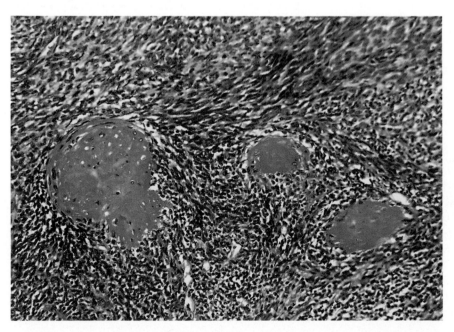

Figure 3-32
FIBROSARCOMA ARISING
IN DERMATOFIBROSARCOMA
PROTUBERANS
Rarely, myoid nodules composed of CD34 and desmin-negative but actin-positive cells with eosinophilic cytoplasm are encountered in fibrosarcomatous areas of DFSP. They also occur in ordinary DFSP and are of no known significance.

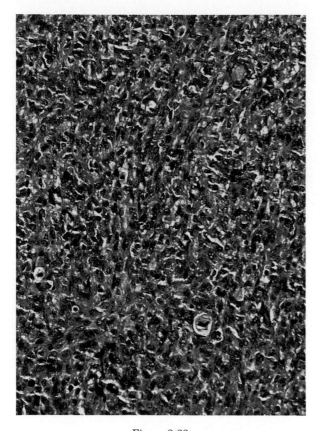

Figure 3-33
PLEOMORPHIC SARCOMA ARISING IN
DERMATOFIBROSARCOMA PROTUBERANS
Some sarcomas that develop in DFSP are pleomorphic
and contain cells whose nuclear chromatin is granular.

Electron microscopy is of limited value in the diagnosis of DFSP and is seldom used for that purpose. Ultrastructural examination has led to conflicting conclusions. Some investigators report that the tumor cells are fibroblasts, others find histiocytes or histiocyte-like cells in addition to the fibroblasts, while yet others have suggested perineural differentiation (112,127). Ultrastructurally, the pigmented cells in pigmented DFSP contain melanosomes (125,128).

Investigators have reported supernumerary ring chromosomes composed of sequences from chromosomes 17 and 22 in DFSP as well as random trisomies (118,122,139,140,144,150). Additional work revealed that the ring chromosomes were amplicons of sequences of chromosomes 17 and 22, specifically 17q23-24 and 22q11-12 (146). Interestingly, giant cell fibroblastoma has an essentially identical translocation. The translocation breakpoints have been cloned and reveal that these rearrangements fuse the COL1A1 gene on chromosome 17 with the PGGFB gene on chromosome 22 (148).

Differential Diagnosis. Differential diagnostic considerations for DFSP are much the same as for dermal fibrous histiocytoma (see above). In fact, the most frequent differential diagnostic consideration when a lesion has features suggesting it may be DFSP is dermal fibrous histiocytoma, particularly when the specimen is small. The parameters we have found useful in making a distinction between these two tumors are described in the Differential Diagnosis section of dermal fibrous histiocytomas above.

Occasionally, benign subcutaneous fibrous histiocytomas can have a repetitive storiform pattern but these tumors are circumscribed, not infiltrative as is DFSP. Specifically, the extensive trapping of fat cells by infiltrating tumor cells, almost a signature feature of DFSP, is nonexistent in benign subcutaneous fibrous histiocytomas. Moreover, current evidence indicates that the latter are CD34 negative. Tumors in the deep soft tissues and central body cavities with the pattern of DFSP and with infiltrating margins are usually categorized as fibrous histiocytomas with recurring potential. Neural neoplasms may contain cells that resemble those in DFSP but a repetitive storiform pattern is absent except in perineurioma which is epithelial membrane antigen positive. Moreover, benign

ever-increasing number of other cells including endothelial cells, smooth muscle cells, nerve sheath cells, the cells of hemangiopericytoma, and the cells composing solitary fibrous tumors. However, importantly, it seldom reacts with the cells of the other types of fibrous histiocytomas (see Dermal Fibrous Histiocytomas above). The tumor cells composing DFSP are S-100 protein, desmin, and epithelial membrane antigen negative but may be muscle actin positive (113,120, 136). Some reports indicate that DFSPs essentially do not contain cells that react to antibodies against factor XIIIa while other investigators report factor XIIIa–positive cells in a small subset of DFSPs (110,114,131). Such cells are focal and the staining is generally reputed to be weak. The melanocytes in pigmented DFSP are S-100 protein positive, and HMB45 and epithelial membrane antigen negative (128).

neural neoplasms practically always contain cells that express S-100 protein while the lesional cells of DFSP are S-100 protein negative. Malignant peripheral nerve sheath tumors (MPNST) arise from a nerve, arise in a neurofibroma, or develop in a patient with neurofibromatosis. About half the reported cases of MPNST contain S-100 protein–positive cells. CD34 is expressed by the cells composing most benign and many malignant nerve sheath tumors; consequently, this antibody, which is expressed by nearly 100 percent of DFSPs, is of no value in distinguishing the two (152).

Plexiform fibrous histiocytoma lacks the repetitive storiform pattern of DFSP, the stroma is more collagenous, and giant cells and histiocyte-like cells, often in nodular aggregates, are present, a feature usually absent and never arranged in nodules in DFSP. Moreover, DFSP lacks a plexiform growth pattern. Smooth muscle tumors lack a storiform pattern and the constituent cells have more abundant cytoplasm than the cells of DFSP. The cells of spindle cell and desmoplastic malignant melanoma almost always express S-100 protein and they are not arranged in a storiform pattern. The tumor cells of DFSP are S-100 protein negative although melanocytes in pigmented DFSPs do express S-100 protein. The storiform arrangement of the nonpigmented cells helps exclude melanoma. An atypical melanocytic proliferation at the dermal-epidermal junction is not a feature of DFSP.

Areas indistinguishable from hemangiopericytoma can, on rare occasion, be found in DFSP; as long as areas characteristic of DFSP are found elsewhere in the tumor it is considered to be DFSP. Likewise, tumors with the patterns of DFSP and fibrosarcoma are considered to be DFSP with fibrosarcoma. Pure fibrosarcoma limited to the skin and subcutis is extremely rare so thorough sectioning of any apparent superficial fibrosarcoma, searching for areas of DFSP, is warranted.

DFSPs with paucicellular myxoid stroma can cause diagnostic difficulty because these myxoid areas may be indistinguishable from the bland myxoid areas found in several other types of soft tissue neoplasms, including the bland areas in myxoid MFH. Identification of the tumor depends not on the myxoid areas but on finding distinctive patterns elsewhere in the tumor or in recurrence, e.g., a storiform pattern for DFSP, lipoblasts for myxoid liposarcoma, pleomorphism for myxoid MFH, etc. A CD34 stain is also useful.

Tumors with a repetitive storiform pattern, diffuse significant cellular pleomorphism, and nuclear atypia are definitively relegated to the pleomorphic MFH category if they involve the subcutis or to the atypical fibroxanthoma category if they are limited to the dermis. Tumors otherwise resembling DFSP with focal pleomorphism and atypia are designated as DFSP with pleomorphic MFH. Such tumors are very rare. Unfortunately, the number of atypical and pleomorphic cells and the degree of atypia required to distinguish DFSP from pleomorphic MFH has never been quantified; we allow tumor cells to demonstrate mild pleomorphism and atypia in one or two microscopic fields and still be classified as DFSP. If pleomorphism and atypia are more severe or more extensive, we place the tumor in the pleomorphic MFH category or DFSP with MFH if such areas are focal because the limited evidence available suggests this degree of pleomorphism and atypia are associated with metastatic potential. On the other hand, giant cells with uniform nuclei, particularly giant cells of the type found in giant cell fibroblastoma, can be found in tumors that behave as does the usual DFSP (121).

Giant cell fibroblastoma and DFSP can be mixed together and when this occurs the usual designation is DFSP with giant cell fibroblastoma (116) (see Giant Cell Fibroblastoma below).

Treatment and Prognosis. Recurrence is a common occurrence for patients with DFSP and the literature suggests an incidence of around 20 to 50 percent (121,123,127,145,147,151). There seems to be poor correlation between size of tumor and recurrence but the completeness of excision and the distance of margins from tumor have been reported to affect the recurrence rate (121, 145,147,149). Several reports suggest that excision with at least 2 cm of free margin will reduce the relapse rate significantly (145,147). Because the cells of DFSP are typically uniform and bland, and because only small numbers of tumor cells may be present among numerous fat cells at the edge of a DFSP, frozen section diagnosis of margins can be difficult. We take a conservative approach because the superficial location of DFSP allows ready access for reexcision. Recurrences may be multiple, they may be destructive with tumor infiltrating underlying muscle and, rarely, bone, and they may be uncontrolled. The literature suggests the recurrence rate for the pigmented variety of DFSP is less than that for ordinary DFSP but fewer than 75 cases of pigmented DFSP have been reported (124).

Whether DFSP without areas of fibrosarcoma or pleomorphic MFH ("pure" DFSP) ever metastasizes is not clear (117,132,138,143). Many reports of metastasizing DFSP contain pathologic descriptions indicating fibrosarcomatous areas or giant cells suggesting pleomorphic MFH. Other reports provide incomplete histologic descriptions. When these are excluded, metastasis from pure DFSP is very rare and in our opinion nearer to 0.5 percent than the 4 percent figure given in some reports. Most of the handful of acceptable cases of pure metastasizing DFSP have had mitotic counts in excess of 5 mitotic figures per 10 high-power fields and most have been composed of cells with coarser chromatin than is found in the usual DFSP. On the other hand, DFSPs with fibrosarcomatous areas have about a 20 percent incidence of metastasis and a recurrence rate of about 75 percent, although this appears to be affected by the presence of necrosis, the level of mitotic activity, and the degree of chromatin abnormalities and cellular pleomorphism (123,138a,153). DFSPs with focal pleomorphic MFH are probably capable of metastasizing but the metastatic rate is largely unknown because so few cases have been reported. If there is doubt about whether focal pleomorphism or chromatin abnormalities in an otherwise DFSP are sufficient to indicate a significant risk of metastasis, this uncertainty should be expressed in the pathology report.

DFSPs with areas of giant cell fibroblastoma behave as pure DFSPs.

Giant Cell Fibroblastoma

Definition. Giant cell fibroblastoma (GCF) is characterized by spindled fibrocytes, stellate cells, and multinucleated giant cells set in a solid fibromyxoid to hyalinized stroma. This stroma is dissected by vascular-like spaces (angiectoid spaces), often gaping and of varying size, lined by the stromal cells including the giant cells.

General Considerations. The light and electron microscopic features of the constituent cells of GCF indicate they are fibroblasts; histiocytes and histiocyte-like cells are not a part of this tumor. This supports classifying GCF as a fibrous tumor. However, areas of GCF may develop in DFSP, and DFSP may recur as GCF; GCF may contain foci of DFSP or recur as DFSP; and DFSP and GCF share the same cytogenetic abnormalities (155,156,158–159,164–166). These observations suggest that both are closely related and should be placed within the same category of soft tissue tumors. Indeed, there is evidence to support classifying DFSP as a fibrous tumor (or a tumor of dermal spindled dendritic cells; see the introductory paragraph under Intermediate Tumors above). Unfortunately, custom and the revised WHO classification of soft tissue tumors places DFSP among the fibrous histiocytomas. We object to this classificatory maneuver but in the spirit of nomenclatural uniformity and because nothing of clinical importance hinges on whether the tumors are classified as fibrous or as fibrous histiocytomas, we follow the WHO mandate. This forces classification of GCF as a fibrous histiocytoma as well. As is noted throughout this chapter, DFSP and GCF are not the only neoplasms upon which the mantle of "fibrous histiocytoma" sits uneasily.

Clinical Features. GCF is most often discovered during the first 4 years of life and about 90 percent are diagnosed by age 10; however, sporadic cases are found in adults up to the seventh decade (154,157,160–162). Most develop on the trunk but at least 20 percent occur in the extremities, and any subcutaneous site except the hands and feet can be involved. The dermis is seldom involved and deep soft tissues are not known to be affected. Most patients are males, and the tumor is almost always less than 5 cm in diameter and usually painless.

Pathologic Findings. Grossly, GCF is an unencapsulated, gray-white and most often gelatinous mass. White fibrous streaks may cross the tumor. Microscopically, the most striking features that greet the observer at low magnification are the giant cells and the irregular, vascular-like (angiectoid) spaces that frequently dominate the landscape of this tumor (fig. 3-34) (154,157,160,161). The giant cells not only are scattered throughout the more solid areas, they also line the angiectoid spaces. At higher magnification, the solid areas contain elongate to stellate cells set within a stroma that varies from myxoid to collagenous

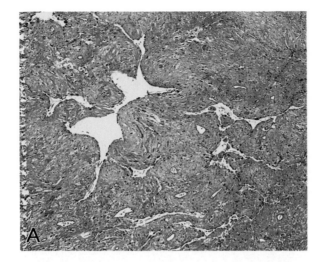

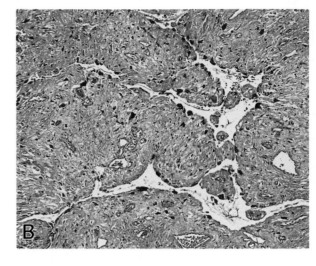

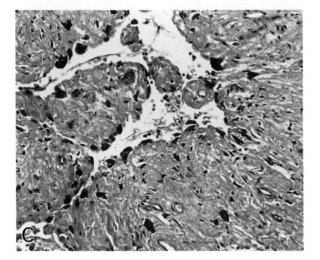

Figure 3-34
GIANT CELL FIBROBLASTOMA
The eye-catching feature of this tumor is the angiectoid spaces which are often lined by giant cells as seen in these three photomicrographs.

(fig. 3-35). Areas of hyalinization are not uncommon. The elongate cells sometimes have wavy nuclei, their cytoplasm is indistinct, and most frequently they are arranged in ill-defined, randomly placed fascicles. The spindled and stellate cells have small, bland, uniform nuclei with inconspicuous nucleoli. In contrast, the multinucleate cells have large, often vesicular nuclei with prominent nucleoli (fig. 3-36). Even though enlarged these nuclei are generally uniformly sized within a given cell and are sometimes arranged around the periphery of the cell in a floret pattern. The cytoplasm of the giant cells is usually angulated and eosinophilic. Mononuclear giant cells also may be found. Mitotic figures are almost never identified.

Many of the angiectoid spaces are elongate and feature irregular branching side channels. They vary from small slit-like spaces to gaping channels that resemble the vascular spaces of a cavernous lymphangioma (fig. 3-34). They are lined by the multinucleated giant cells, mononucleated round to spindled cells, and collagen fibers. Angiectoid spaces are randomly placed throughout the tumor and may be more numerous in some areas than in others. The spaces are usually empty but some contain amorphous, lightly eosinophilic material or sometimes a few red blood cells.

The solid areas vary in cellularity from hypocellular with abundant myxoid stroma to moderately cellular with less myxoid material.

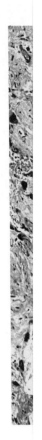

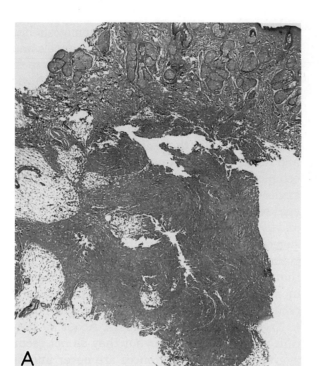

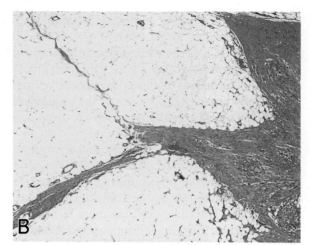

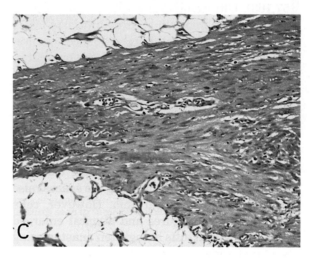

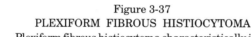

Figure 3-37
PLEXIFORM FIBROUS HISTIOCYTOMA
Plexiform fibrous histiocytoma characteristically is a subcutaneous proliferation composed in part of bland fibrous tissue which radiates outward from the center of the lesion.

the upper extremity, while the remainder are more or less equally distributed in the lower extremities, trunk, and the head and neck area.

Pathologic Findings. PFHs develop in the superficial subcutaneous tissue and lower dermis, but they can extend from their primary site into the upper dermis above or occasionally into skeletal muscle below. They are reported to range from 0.3 to 6.0 cm but most are 1 to 3 cm in diameter. They are gray-white and firm on cut section.

Low-power microscopy is distinctive because of the ray-like extensions of fibrous tissue into the surrounding fat (fig. 3-37) (168,170). There is almost always a considerable rim of normal dermis above the lesion, and the overlying epidermis is usually of normal thickness. The proportion of the tumor's two major components, bundles of fibrocytes/fibroblasts and clusters of

histiocyte-like/giant cells, varies from lesion to lesion. At one end of this spectrum are tumors composed predominantly of histiocyte-like cells and giant cells arranged in nodules, both within the fibrous tissue in the main tumor mass and within the arms of fibrous tissue radiating out from the main mass. When fully developed, this arrangement results in numerous round collections of histiocyte-like cells and giant cells (figs. 3-38, 3-39). Sometimes the nodules are composed partially or completely of plump spindle cells instead of round cells and sometimes the nodules are confluent (fig. 3-40). At the other end of the spectrum are the lesions that are exclusively, or almost exclusively, formed of fibrocytes in which the bland, thin spindle cells form a central fibrous mass with long radiating arms of fibrous tissue that extend into the surrounding

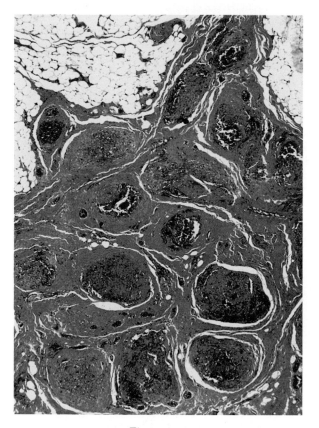

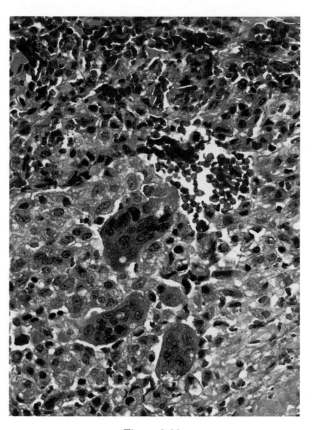

Figure 3-38
PLEXIFORM FIBROUS HISTIOCYTOMA
Within the fibrous tissue of most but not all plexiform fibrous histiocytomas are variable numbers of nodules composed of histiocyte-like cells and giant cells. Hemorrhage is also frequently present. In this example, the nodules of histiocyte-like cells predominate over fibrous tissue. This pattern is so characteristic that it should cause the observer to think of this tumor.

Figure 3-39
PLEXIFORM FIBROUS HISTIOCYTOMA
The histiocyte-like cells have pale-staining cytoplasm. Giant cells are present.

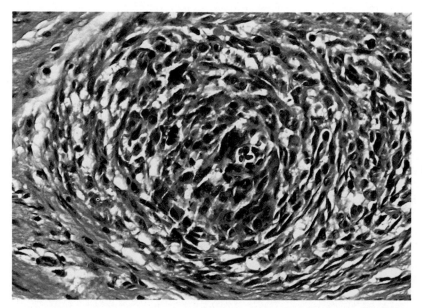

Figure 3-40
PLEXIFORM FIBROUS
HISTIOCYTOMA
Sometimes the nodules are composed of cells with elongate nuclei.

153

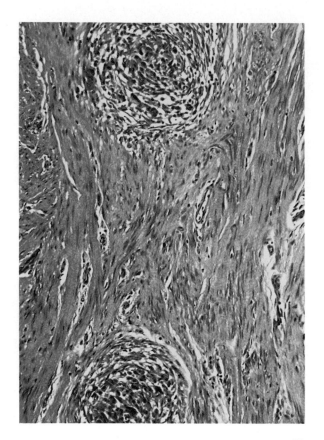 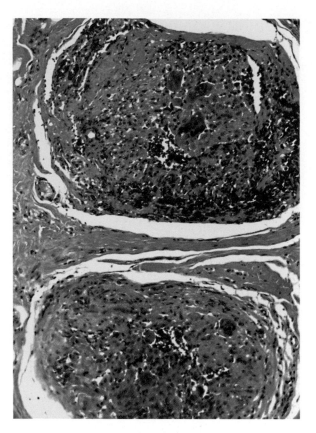

Figure 3-41
PLEXIFORM FIBROUS HISTIOCYTOMA
A more or less equal mixture of fibrous tissue and nodules is present in this tumor.

subcutaneous tissue. Lesions with a more or less equal mixture of fibrocytes and histiocyte-like cells are seen about as frequently as those with a predominance of histiocyte-like cells (fig. 3-41).

At higher magnification, the histiocyte-like cells and the multinucleated giant cells have rather abundant, pale-staining, granular cytoplasm and central nuclei. Hemorrhage is common within the nodules and serves as an aid in identifying this lesion. Not surprisingly, hemosiderin deposits can result from the hemorrhage. An infiltrate of lymphocytes and plasma cells may be seen around some nodules. The fibrous tissue component, whether abundant or sparse, resembles that seen in desmoid fibromatosis, i.e., spindled fibrocytes partially arranged in fascicles and set within dense collagen (fig. 3-42). When cut transversely, the rays of fibrous tissue also take on the appearance of nodules of fibrous tissue within the subcutaneous fat. Hyalinization may be prominent and rarely osseous metaplasia may be observed.

Mitotic figures are unusual and if present sparse; they are more common in recurrences. Pleomorphism is not a feature of this lesion in either the fibrous or histiocyte-like areas. Intravascular growth has been noted in some tumors and xanthoma cells form in rare cases.

Special Studies. In the studies published thus far, the tumor cells of PFH have been negative for S-100 protein, keratin, CD45, HLA-DR, factor VIII, desmin, and lysozyme (169,170). The giant cells stain strongly with CD68 as do a proportion of the histiocyte-like cells and the plump spindled cells within the nodules, but the fibroblasts outside the nodules are CD68 negative. These fibroblasts express smooth muscle actin; occasionally, the histiocyte-like cells are weakly smooth muscle actin positive. Electron microscopy reveals undifferentiated cells, myofibroblasts, and fibroblasts (168,170). The neoplastic cells do not have the ultrastructural features of histiocytes. Based on the ultrastructural and

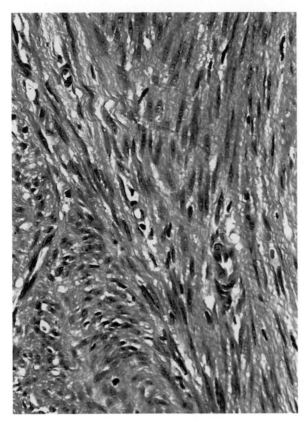

Figure 3-42
PLEXIFORM FIBROUS HISTIOCYTOMA
The fibrous tissue resembles that found in desmoid fibromatosis.

immunohistochemical results thus far reported, there is no good evidence that any of the cells that form PFH are bone marrow–derived macrophages; rather they appear to be myofibroblasts and undifferentiated mesenchymal cells that have taken on an epitope that recognizes anti-CD68. Clonal chromosomal abnormalities have been reported in one tumor (173).

Differential Diagnosis. The lesion most likely to be confused with PFH is a benign dermal or subcutaneous fibrous histiocytoma. Unlike PFH, neither of these lesions features long plexiform extensions of fibrous tissue and neither is characterized by nodules of histiocyte-like cells and multinucleated giant cells within the subcutaneous tissue and dermis. Benign dermal and subcutaneous fibrous histiocytomas rather commonly contain foam cells, a rare feature of PFH, and if there are fibrous extensions from the central mass of a benign fibrous histiocytoma into the subcu-

taneous tissue, they are short. In addition, benign fibrous histiocytomas usually arise in older individuals and the lesions are circumscribed.

The absence of pleomorphism and the sparse mitotic activity in PFH exclude atypical fibroxanthoma, pleomorphic MFH, and giant cell sarcoma of soft parts. Nodular fasciitis is usually composed of fibroblasts with more open, larger nuclei than are found in PFH and the fibroblasts are arranged in large bundles that grow as gently undulating S- and C-shaped structures instead of the linear bundles that characterize PFH. Giant cells may be present in nodular fasciitis but they are not arranged in nodules, and mitotic figures are usually easy to find. A plexiform pattern is rare.

Because of the patient age at which PFH is found and because of the rays of fibrous tissue extending from the lesion, fibrous hamartoma of infancy enters into the differential diagnosis. However, fibrous hamartoma has a myxoid stroma and contains immature cells in addition to the strands of mature fibrous tissue, and it never features multinucleated giant cells. Plexiform neurofibromas are always S-100 protein positive; PFH is S-100 protein negative except for entrapped dendritic cells. Histologically, PFH may remind the observer of desmoid fibromatosis but the plexiform architecture, superficial location, small size, and nodules of giant and histiocyte-like cells all serve as markers of PFH, not desmoid tumor. Myofibromatosis is generally circumscribed, lacks giant cells, and often there are small blue cells and staghorn vessels in a part of the tumor, usually the center.

Most angiomatoid fibrous histiocytomas are marked by a chronic inflammatory infiltrate so prominent it makes one think of a lymph node. Moreover, the red blood cells are in large lakes rather than the small foci of hemorrhage characteristic of PFH. Smooth muscle tumors often are desmin positive in contrast to PFH, and lack its nodular and plexiform pattern.

DFSP is characterized by a repetitive storiform pattern not present in PFH and nodules of giant cells are absent in DFSP.

Treatment and Prognosis. About a third of the reported cases of PFH are known to have recurred, but recurrences are not destructive or uncontrolled (165,167). A few tumors have recurred more than once. A few patients have had metastases to the regional lymph nodes and less than a dozen have had metastases to the lungs (171,172,179). The metastatic rate of the cases reported in the literature seems to be around 10 to 15 percent so PFH is properly placed among the intermediate tumors in managerial category IIc, Table 1-10.

Angiomatoid Fibrous Histiocytoma

Definition. Angiomatoid fibrous histiocytoma (AFH) is a neoplasm composed of spindled and round plump ("histiocyte-like") cells associated with cystic areas of hemorrhage and intense marked chronic inflammation.

General Considerations. On the basis of recent outcome data (175), WHO has sensibly moved AFH from the malignant fibrous histiocytomas to the intermediate (managerial group IIc, Table 1-10) category of fibrous histiocytomas and the term malignant has been dropped from the name. However, there is ongoing controversy whether AFH should be classified as a fibrous histiocytoma at all or whether it is a myoid tumor (178,179,182,183). By light microscopy, the tumor is composed of cells resembling fibroblasts and round cells with rather abundant cytoplasm that have been likened to histiocytes. Ultrastructurally, the tumor cells have the features of myofibroblasts, phagocytic cells, and undifferentiated cells, i.e., the ultrastructural features are those of most of the other tumors included in the fibrous histiocytoma category. Utilizing immunohistochemical techniques, one group of investigators found that the tumor cells were CD68 positive in approximately 50 percent of the cases they studied while desmin was weakly and focally expressed in half of the cases (3 of 6) (182). In our experience, 40 percent of tumors contain desmin-positive cells. Currently, the direction of differentiation of AFH must be considered inconclusive, but based on the light microscopic appearance and the increasing evidence of desmin expression by tumor cells, it will probably be confirmed as a myofibroblastic tumor.

Clinical Features. AFH is a slowly growing, pink to blue, cystic tumor that occurs predominantly in children and young adults (median age, 15 years) (174,175,177,180). Nearly 90 percent are discovered before age 30 while the remaining 10 percent occur at all other ages up to 70 years. The

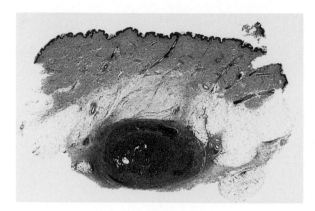

Figure 3-43
ANGIOMATOID FIBROUS HISTIOCYTOMA
The heavy chronic inflammatory infiltrate characteristic of angiomatoid fibrous histiocytoma causes it to resemble a lymph node. Consequently, when an out-of-place apparent lymph node is found in the soft tissue, the possibility of angiomatoid fibrous histiocytoma should be considered.

extremities are most often affected (65 to 85 percent), but these tumors may also develop in the trunk and the head and neck area. About 80 percent develop in the subcutaneous tissue, less than 20 percent involve skeletal muscle or periosteum, and rare examples are centered in the dermis. Most patients complain of a mass. Some have had the following systemic findings: anemia, fever, weight loss, generalized lymphadenopathy, and protein abnormalities (175,177,181). Excision of the lesion may relieve these symptoms and signs.

Pathologic Findings. Grossly, AFH is usually small (median, about 2.5 cm) but the size varies from less than 1 cm to (rarely) over 10 cm. Most often, the lesion is cystic and filled with blood or bloody fluid. Microscopically, the low-power view of the usual lesion is distinctive because the almost inevitable intense chronic inflammatory infiltrate causes it to resemble a lymph node out of place in the soft tissue (fig. 3-43) (175, 177,179,180). At higher magnification, spindled cells and round cells with eosinophilic cytoplasm are most prominent in the center of the lesion, where they form nodules or sheets of cells that are separated by cystic spaces. The latter are almost always filled with red blood cells and are lined by lesional cells (fig. 3-44). In fact, cystic spaces filled with blood are so prominent in some examples of AFH the observer may be concerned about a hemangioma or a vascular malformation.

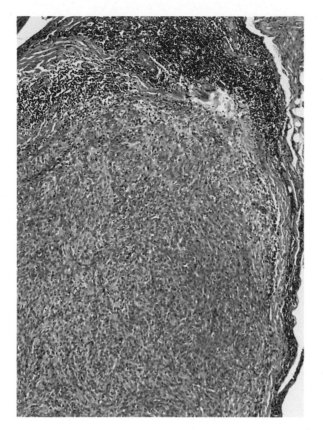 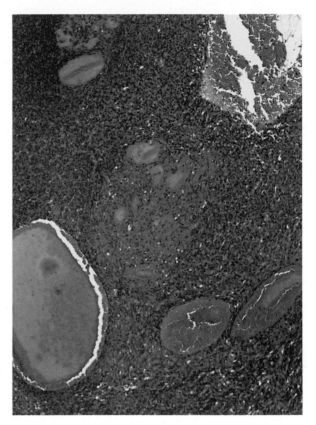

Figure 3-44
ANGIOMATOID FIBROUS HISTIOCYTOMA
In addition to chronic inflammation, angiomatoid fibrous histiocytoma is characterized by nodules of cells with round to elongate nuclei. These surround cystic spaces filled with red blood cells.

Thrombosis may also be a prominent feature. The chronic inflammatory infiltrate is most intense at the periphery and is composed mainly of plasma cells and lymphocytes. Follicular centers develop in some lesions. The edge of the lesion is marked by a delimiting fibrous capsule containing chronic inflammation and histiocyte-like cells. Hemosiderin is often present here as well as in other parts of the mass. The margin is circumscribed in about 75 percent of cases.

The constituent fibroblasts and round cells typically have vesicular nuclei with no to mild pleomorphism, resulting in an overall "bland" appearance, but occasional tumors contain moderately pleomorphic cells (fig. 3-45). Mitotic figures are usually difficult to find. Tumor cells line the cystic spaces but dilated, endothelial-lined vascular spaces are also a prominent feature of most of these tumors. A few lesions contain foam cells, and in a handful the constituent cells are arranged in a storiform pattern. Multinucleated giant cells are rare, as is stromal calcification.

This usual histologic pattern varies. In about a fifth of the cases, pleomorphism is moderate or rarely, marked; in a few, the mitotic index is greater than 5 mitotic figures per 10 high-power fields; and in about 10 percent of cases, inflammation is so subdued that the resemblance to a lymph node is lost. Rarely, the stroma may be myxoid.

Special Studies. Ultrastructural examination reveals the expected for a fibrous histiocytoma: histiocyte-like cells, fibroblasts, and myofibroblasts, along with undifferentiated cells (174,180). Desmin-positive cells have been reported in some lesions as noted in the General Considerations section above (179,182). Smooth muscle actin apparently is not expressed by the tumor cells and muscle-specific antigen is positive in only a minority of cases. Staining for CD68 has been reported in some tumor cells in about half the

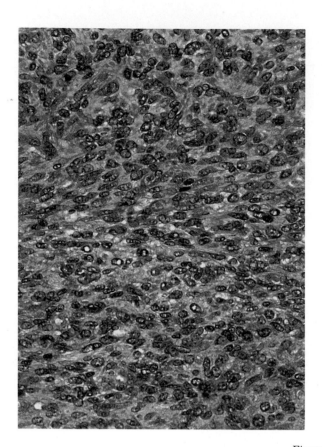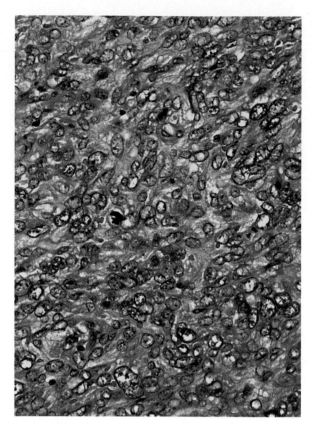

Figure 3-45
ANGIOMATOID FIBROUS HISTIOCYTOMA
Left: The cells surrounding the spaces are typically uniform and elongate to round.
Right: However, moderate nuclear pleomorphism is found in some lesions.

cases. The tumor cells are negative for keratin, S-100 protein, CD45, factor VIII–associated antigen, CD31, myoglobin, and muramidase (179,182). The few cases subjected to DNA analysis have revealed the cells to be diploid (176).

Differential Diagnosis. The initial impression when viewing an AFH is a lymph node within the soft tissue or an inflamed hemangioma. Against a lymph node, in addition to the unusual location, is the lack of a capsular sinus or other architectural features of a normal lymph node. Higher power magnification reveals cystic spaces lined by lesional cells that do not have the features of endothelium and do not express endothelial antigens. Thus, immunohistochemistry can aid in excluding hemangioma and angiosarcoma. Moreover, the tumor lacks the interconnecting, anastomosing channels and papillae of angiosarcoma. The spindle cells and the areas of hemorrhage may raise the question of Kaposi's sar-

coma, but the slit-like spaces that characterize the latter are absent. Moreover, almost all AFHs are in the subcutis, not in the dermis, and the cells are CD31 negative. The staghorn vessels that mark hemangiopericytomas are lacking in AFH and histiocyte-like cells are more prominent than they are in hemangiopericytoma.

Another differential diagnostic concern is distinguishing a benign dermal fibrous histiocytoma (DFH) with areas of cystic hemorrhage (aneurysmal variant of DFH) from AFH. In both the hemorrhagic spaces are lined by nonendothelial tumor cells, but a larger number of histiocyte-like or myoid-like round cells are found in AFH than in the aneurysmal variant. Numerous foam cells and prominent multinucleated giant cells, common features of DFH, are present, at least focally, in most examples of the aneurysmal variant, but are rare in AFH. AFH usually occurs in the subcutaneous tissue rather than the dermis.

In about half the cases, the round cells in AFH are desmin positive while such positivity has not been reported to date in the cells in the aneurysmal variant of DFH. The inflammatory infiltrate associated with DFH is usually focal and peripheral, and not diffuse and intense, sometimes with follicular centers, as is the case for most AFHs. Extensive hemosiderin may be found in both. Patients with AFH are usually younger than those with the aneurysmal variant of DFH and they may have the symptoms listed in the Clinical Features section above.

Because it is composed of histiocyte-like cells, because chronic inflammation may be prominent, and because it often contains cystic spaces, the diffuse form of tenosynovial giant cell tumor (diffuse form of giant cell tumor of tendon sheath) can resemble AFH. However, the spaces in diffuse tenosynovial giant cell tumors are not filled with blood, usually the giant cells are more numerous than those in AFH, and the cells are not desmin positive.

AFH lacks the pleomorphism and anaplasia of the malignant fibrous histiocytomas and it usually occurs in young rather than in older individuals. Smooth muscle tumors enter into the differential diagnosis; indeed, as noted above, some tumor cells express desmin. AFH rather than a smooth muscle tumor is diagnosed when hemorrhagic cysts lined by spindle cells with sparse cytoplasm and round cells with more abundant eosinophilic cytoplasm are associated with diffuse intense chronic inflammation.

Treatment and Prognosis. Although initially thought to be more often aggressive, a recent study of a large number of angiomatoid fibrous histiocytomas reports that nearly 85 percent of patients with AFH are cured by the initial excision while about 15 percent experience local recurrence or local metastasis to the nearby soft tissue (177, 182). Recurrences may be multiple. Metastasis to regional lymph nodes and distant metastases are rare (approximately 1 to 2 percent). Patients whose tumors recur or metastasize locally are almost always cured by reexcision, even if more than one recurrence or local metastasis develops. Morphologic features significantly related to an increased risk of recurrence are infiltrating margins, incomplete excision, and tumor below the subcutis. Features that have not been shown to predict outcome are the degree of pleomorphism,

the level of mitotic activity, the severity of the inflammatory response, the size of the tumor, and the age of the patient (182).

MALIGNANT FIBROUS HISTIOCYTOMAS (MANAGERIAL GROUP III, TABLE 1-10)

The lesions usually accepted as types of malignant fibrous histiocytoma (MFH) are presented in Table 3-1. Concepts concerning these tumors and the current status of our knowledge about the direction of differentiation of their constituent cells are discussed in the Introduction at the beginning of this chapter. The myxoid variant sits uneasily among these tumors because to many pathologists the proper label is *myxofibrosarcoma*, a name that implies a fibrous tumor. However, other pathologists, impressed that the myxoid areas are frequently interspersed among areas indistinguishable from pleomorphic MFH, prefer to classify the myxoid variant as a type of fibrous histiocytoma. Because the latter view is still held in the WHO Classification and to avoid clinical confusion, we have retained the label myxoid MFH but have placed myxofibrosarcoma in parenthesis.

Pleomorphic Variant Malignant Fibrous Histiocytoma (Storiform and Pleomorphic Malignant Fibrous Histiocytoma, Fibroxanthosarcoma)

Definition. Pleomorphic MFH is a pleomorphic anaplastic sarcoma composed of varying proportions of fibroblasts, myofibroblasts, histiocyte-like cells including multinucleated giant cells, and undifferentiated cells. Tumors formed by cells with any other recognizable line of differentiation, e.g., rhabdomyoblastic, smooth muscle, bony, or fatty differentiation, are definitionally excluded from the category.

Clinical Features. Pleomorphic MFH is almost always discovered in individuals over the age of 50; it is very rare in children (187,213,218). In fact, the diagnosis should be made with great caution in individuals under the age of 30. The most commonly affected site is the deep soft tissues of the extremities but examples may be encountered in the subcutaneous tissue of the extremities, soft tissues of the trunk, and rarely, almost any other site, including organs (190–193,199,200,214,215). Deep pleomorphic MFHs

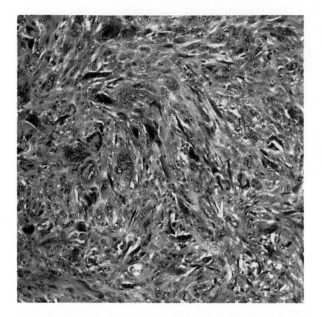 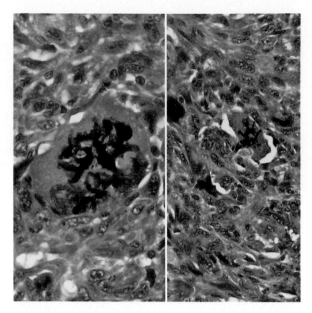

Figure 3-46
PLEOMORPHIC MALIGNANT FIBROUS HISTIOCYTOMA
Left: The low-power appearance of pleomorphic MFH is striking because of the cellularity, the marked pleomorphism, and the bizarre nuclei as well as the whirled arrangement of the cells.
Right: Enlarged cells with bizarre chromatin patterns are common in pleomorphic MFH.

are usually large while superficial examples are smaller at the time of diagnosis. A few patients present with malaise, fever, and weight loss, and in the case of retroperitoneal lesions, abdominal pain. Rare patients have hypoglycemia. Pleomorphic MFH almost never presents as a metastasis without a very large mass in the primary site, an attribute that is helpful to know about when evaluating patients with metastatic pleomorphic neoplasms and an occult primary.

Pleomorphic MFH is the most common sarcoma to develop in sites of prior radiation in adults (196). A long interval (average, 10 to 12 years) has been noted between the radiation and the diagnosis of almost all postradiation sarcomas including pleomorphic MFH. Pleomorphic MFH may also arise in chronic ulcers and scars (186,195).

Gross Findings. Grossly, pleomorphic MFH is a fleshy, often multilobulated mass that typically features areas of hemorrhage and necrosis. Deep tumors in the extremities are usually between 5 and 10 cm while the average tumor in the retroperitoneum is even larger. Infiltration may be macroscopically evident although the

tumors all too often appear grossly circumscribed. On cut section, the non-necrotic tumor is usually gray-tan, but if xanthoma cells are present they may impart a yellowish hue. Hemorrhage and necrosis are so common as to be almost universal and can be extensive enough to almost destroy the tumor. In this latter circumstance, numerous sections from the edges of the mass may be needed to find viable tumor cells.

Microscopic Findings. At low-power magnification, the first impression of the usual pleomorphic MFH is one of a bizarre malignant neoplasm (fig. 3-46, left); many contain some of the most outlandish cells found in any human neoplasm (fig. 3-46, right). The basic requirement for diagnosis is a malignant neoplasm composed of spindled fibroblasts, myofibroblasts, round histiocyte-like cells, and undifferentiated cells; definitionally, the tumor cells cannot display other lines of differentiation (fig. 3-47) (192,199–201,205,214,215). Most often the spindled cells and myofibroblasts are randomly arranged, although focally they may grow in small fascicles and bundles. However, the intersecting, organized,

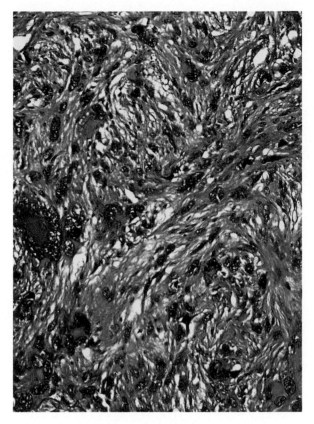

Figure 3-47
PLEOMORPHIC MALIGNANT
FIBROUS HISTIOCYTOMA
This view of pleomorphic MFH reveals the required admixture of fibroblasts and histiocyte-like cells including multinucleated forms.

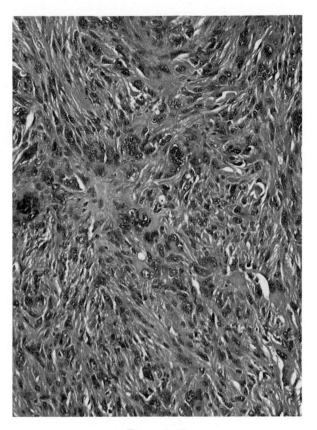

Figure 3-48
PLEOMORPHIC MALIGNANT
FIBROUS HISTIOCYTOMA
A vague storiform pattern, often focal, is common in pleomorphic MFH.

long fascicular arrangement typical of the spindled cells composing fibrosarcoma and leiomyosarcoma is largely absent. It is also common for the spindled cells to arrange themselves in a vague storiform pattern, at least focally, but this pattern is not present in all tumors and thus is not required for the diagnosis (fig. 3-48). Even when present it is often poorly developed. The histiocyte-like cells tend to be round, typically have more abundant cytoplasm than the spindled cells, and vary from cells that are small and relatively uniform to those that are large to huge and pleomorphic (fig. 3-49). Some of the latter may be multinucleated. Sometimes the tumor cells, particularly the larger examples, have strikingly abundant or elongated eosinophilic cytoplasm that causes them to resemble rhabdo-

myoblasts, or they may have vacuolated cytoplasm that suggests lipoblasts (fig. 3-50). Phagocytosis by these cells is common.

The nuclei of the tumor cells vary from relatively small and regular to enormous, jagged, and irregular. Mitotic figures should be easy to find and abnormal forms are almost universal. The latter may develop some of the most bizarre arrangements of chromosomes seen in any type of tumor (fig. 3-51). Reactive histiocytes including xanthoma cells are common and tend to be concentrated at the periphery of the tumor. The stroma is almost always collagenous but there is variation from tumors so cellular that it is difficult or impossible to identify the collagen to those in which the tumor cells are trapped in dense sheets of it. Myxoid areas may be present but by

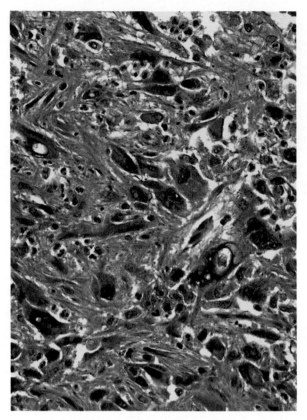

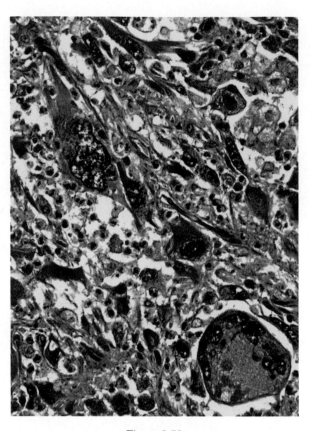

Figure 3-49
PLEOMORPHIC MALIGNANT
FIBROUS HISTIOCYTOMA

The cells with bizarre nuclei and abundant eosinophilic cytoplasm raise the question of a muscle tumor. There is little or no difference in the management of patients with soft tissue leiomyosarcoma and those with pleomorphic MFH.

Figure 3-50
PLEOMORPHIC MALIGNANT
FIBROUS HISTIOCYTOMA

Pleomorphic MFH with strap-like cells mimicking rhabdomyosarcoma. This is discussed in the Differential Diagnosis portion of the text.

Figure 3-51
PLEOMORPHIC MALIGNANT
FIBROUS HISTIOCYTOMA

Numerous mitotic figures, including bizarre abnormal forms, are the rule in pleomorphic MFH.

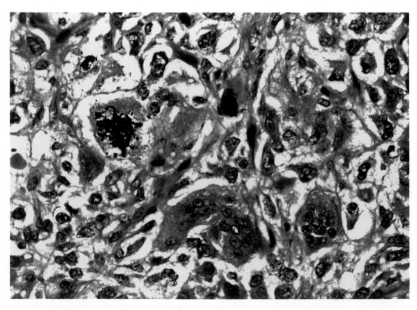

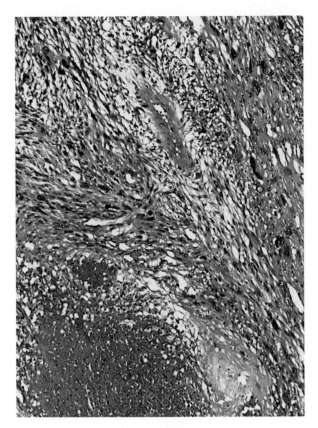

Figure 3-52
PLEOMORPHIC MALIGNANT
FIBROUS HISTIOCYTOMA
Tumor cell necrosis is so frequent in pleomorphic MFH
that it is a useful feature in distinguishing this tumor from
benign and recurring fibrous histiocytomas.

our definition (see below) hypocellular myxoid areas cannot exceed 10 percent of the area of the tumor (if hypocellular myxoid stroma is in excess of 10 percent of the volume of the tumor, the proper classification is myxoid MFH [myxofibrosarcoma]).

Focal chronic inflammation is ubiquitous in pleomorphic MFH, and a diffuse infiltration of lymphocytes and plasma cells is common. Acute inflammation is also common, either as the sole inflammatory element or mixed with chronic inflammatory cells. However, a massive infiltrate of acute inflammatory cells without significant chronic inflammation in a tumor with a predominant histiocyte-like population of cells should prompt consideration of inflammatory MFH (see below). Necrosis is common in pleomorphic MFH and is often associated with hemorrhage (fig. 3-52).

The basic morphologic pattern described above may vary considerably and the range of histologic patterns permitted by most investigators for this tumor is fairly wide. At the spindled cell end of the spectrum are neoplasms indistinguishable from dermatofibrosarcoma protuberans except that round to oval, enlarged, pleomorphic, often multinucleated cells with abnormal nuclei are present within the tumor. Mitotic activity is usually high. Also considered to be pleomorphic MFHs are tumors indistinguishable from fibrosarcoma except for the presence of enlarged pleomorphic cells, at least focally. Areas identical to hemangiopericytoma may be encountered focally, and staghorn vessels may also be found in areas more characteristic of MFH. However, the degree of pleomorphism required for pleomorphic MFH is not allowed in pure hemangiopericytoma. At the histiocytic end of the spectrum are tumors composed predominantly of pleomorphic histiocyte-like cells and in some of these, only careful search turns up the required fibroblasts or myofibroblasts.

Many pleomorphic MFHs contain otherwise undifferentiated cells that cannot be easily recognized as fibroblastic, myofibroblastic, or histiocyte-like. The available evidence indicates that these undifferentiated cells are primitive mesenchymal cells that have acquired phagocytic capacity. What is not allowed in pleomorphic MFH are cells that exhibit recognizable differentiation along known cell lines other than fibroblastic and myofibroblastic (194,205). Consequently, neoplastic lipoblasts, lipocytes, and neoplastic smooth or skeletal muscle cells are not allowed, and if present even focally are sufficient evidence to place the tumor in the fatty or muscle tumor category. Whether any bone or cartilage formed by neoplastic cells (tumor bone or cartilage) should be allowed in a tumor certified as a pleomorphic MFH is controversial. Focal neoplastic bone, osteoid, or cartilage was allowed by at least one group of investigators (215). We think pleomorphic sarcomas in which the tumor cells form bone or cartilage, however focal, fit the definition of soft tissue osteosarcoma or chondrosarcoma and should be classified as such.

Metaplastic bone or cartilage is present in about 1 percent of pleomorphic MFHs and should be distinguished from bone or cartilage laid down by tumor cells because the latter qualifies the

163

tumor as osteosarcoma or chondrosarcoma (188). The cells in the metaplastic osteocartilaginous areas do not display the anaplasia and pleomorphism of the tumor cells in osteosarcoma or chondrosarcoma, and metaplastic osteocartilaginous tissue tends to be focal, small in amount, and located mainly at the periphery near or within the fibrous capsule of the tumor.

Also separated from the pleomorphic MFH category are MFHs with large numbers of osteoclast-like giant cells (giant cell sarcoma) or large numbers of acute inflammatory cells (inflammatory MFH) (214). If the stroma is greater than 10 percent myxoid and the myxoid stroma is hypocellular, an otherwise pleomorphic MFH is classified as myxoid MFH (a tumor that is also classified as myxofibrosarcoma) (214).

Special Studies. The results of numerous ultrastructural studies of the MFHs have been summarized in the General Considerations section at the beginning of this chapter. Briefly, most of these reports conclude that the cells in pleomorphic MFH are fibroblasts, myofibroblasts, and primitive mesenchymal cells, some of which take on phagocytic capacity. The role of electron microscopy in diagnosis is very limited; its most common use is to search for evidence of Z bands or thick and thin filaments that would indicate the tumor is a pleomorphic rhabdomyosarcoma rather than pleomorphic MFH, or to search for evidence of neural differentiation. Electron microscopy has little or no advantage over hematoxylin and eosin (H&E)-stained sections or immunohistochemistry in proving fatty, vascular, or smooth muscle differentiation, and neural tumors can almost always be identified without resorting to electron microscopy.

A large number of pleomorphic MFHs have been subjected to immunohistochemical staining. CD68, a glycoprotein associated with myeloid cells and histiocytes and recognized by the antibody KP1, is expressed by the cells of some but not all MFHs, but this antigen (or an epitope of it) may be expressed by nonhistiocytic tumors as diverse as lymphoma, malignant melanoma, and some carcinomas (189,198,202). To our knowledge, LeuM-3 (CD14) and LeuM-1 (CD15), markers of bone marrow–derived histiocytes, are not expressed by the tumor cells of MFH (216). Antibodies against factor XIIIa, a fibrin stabilizing factor, react with dendritic cells in

organs and the soft tissue including the skin. Factor XIIIa–positive cells are present in many MFHs but unfortunately they are also present in many other types of mesenchymal tumors and inflammatory processes so this antibody has little diagnostic utility (208). Muscle actins are reported to be expressed by the tumor cells in as many as one third of pleomorphic MFHs (189, 197). The incidence of desmin expression depends on how tumors are defined; if all desmin-positive sarcomas are classified as muscle tumors then desmin expression in MFH is zero. If otherwise pleomorphic MFHs are classified as such even if tumor cells express desmin, then less than a third of pleomorphic MFHs contain desmin-positive cells (197,202). We think there should be evidence other than just desmin expression before a tumor is categorized as demonstrating muscle differentiation, e.g., fasciculation of tumor cells for leiomyosarcoma and other immunologic or ultrastructural evidence of skeletal muscle differentiation for rhabdomyosarcoma. Desmin expression in otherwise pleomorphic MFHs is often focal and weak. A few MFHs contain tumor cells that express keratin; this is usually focal and weak (202,206). CD45 (leukocyte common antigen), S-100 protein, and CD34 stains are negative.

What is the status of immunohistochemistry as a tool for diagnosing MFH? Unfortunately, the constituent cells of pleomorphic MFH have not yet been found to express antigens that are unique enough to this tumor to provide strong support for the diagnosis; however, immunohistochemistry is extremely useful and sometimes vital in excluding other neoplasms, particularly lymphoma, carcinoma, melanoma, and other nonmesenchymal and mesenchymal tumors that at times can mimic MFH. If immunohistochemistry is used, the basic panel of antibodies usually includes CD45, one or more keratins, and S-100 protein. Other antibodies are used as indicated and often include muscle actin, desmin, T- and B-cell markers, HMB45, epithelial membrane antigen, and CD68.

Flow cytometry and morphometry have been utilized to predict the course of patients with MFH. Preliminary data suggest that S-phase fraction and morphometry provide some prognostic information beyond that provided by tumor grade, but further studies are needed to prove this is a cost-effective approach (185,212). Ki-67 staining has been reported to correlate with nuclear grade, number of mitoses, and the extent of necrosis, but not with outcome (217). Chromosomal analysis of most pleomorphic MFHs has revealed complex aberrations that vary from tumor to tumor (204,207,209).

Differential Diagnosis. The most important consideration when contemplating a diagnosis of pleomorphic MFH, or any primary sarcoma for that matter, is to exclude metastatic carcinoma, melanoma, and lymphoma. Whether this requires the routine use of immunohistochemical stains, i.e., should a diagnosis of pleomorphic MFH ever be made without performing immunohistochemical stains to help rule out these three possibilities?, has not been settled to all pathologists' satisfaction, but certainly if the clinical and histologic features are not absolutely characteristic of pleomorphic MFH we suggest using a panel of immunohistochemical stains as noted in the section immediately above. The cells in high-grade pleomorphic T-cell lymphoma do not always express leukocyte common antigen (CD45), so there may be consideration for T- and B-cell markers, and Hodgkin's disease sometimes enters the differential diagnosis. Only about 1 percent of melanomas are S-100 protein negative but if suspicion for melanoma is high and the S-100 protein is negative, HMB45 staining may be useful (203). Obtaining historical information, encouraging imaging studies to search for tumor elsewhere, and cutting large numbers of sections are maneuvers that also help exclude metastasis and lymphoma. Glycogen and mucin stains are sometimes useful.

Other major considerations in the differential diagnosis are the other high-grade pleomorphic sarcomas, particularly pleomorphic liposarcoma, pleomorphic rhabdomyosarcoma, leiomyosarcoma, malignant peripheral nerve sheath tumor, osteosarcoma, and chondrosarcoma. The lengths a pathologist should go to prove focal or inconspicuous differentiation in a pleomorphic sarcoma is the subject of considerable debate but the observation that current clinical patient management is the same for all the pleomorphic sarcomas is worth considering (see the Introduction at the beginning of this chapter) (194). Certainly, taking one section for each 1 to 2 cm of tumor up to 10 to 12 sections and carefully

searching for lipoblasts and evidence of origin from a nerve or a neurofibroma is reasonable. Electron microscopy can identify Z bands and thick and thin filaments in skeletal muscle cells as well as provide evidence of neural differentiation but it is expensive. If electron microscopy is used, care must be taken not to mistake normal cells for tumor cells. Desmin and actin stains identify muscle cells but actin is not specific for muscle cells since it decorates myofibroblasts and fibroblasts, and there is accumulating evidence that cells other than those demonstrating smooth muscle or skeletal muscle differentiation can contain antigens that react with the desmin antibody. About half of the tumors reported to be malignant peripheral nerve sheath tumors have been composed, at least focally, of S-100 protein–positive cells.

Metaplastic bone and cartilage can be present in pleomorphic MFH and should not be construed as evidence of chondrosarcoma or osteosarcoma (188). Metaplastic bone is formed by cells with small bland nuclei and it lacks the irregular random pattern of neoplastic bone; rather it resembles the bone in healing fractures or myositis ossificans. It is most often limited to the fibrous capsule of the tumor and is distinctly focal. On the other hand, neoplastic bone and cartilage is laid down by tumor cells.

Pleomorphic liposarcoma has histologic features identical to pleomorphic MFH except that some tumor cells are differentiated as lipoblasts. These may be focal and sparse. Dedifferentiated liposarcoma, a particular concern in the retroperitoneum, can be distinguished from pleomorphic MFH only by finding its atypical lipomatous tumor component. A diagnosis of pleomorphic rhabdomyosarcoma requires a pleomorphic sarcoma pattern plus tumor cells, most often with abundant eosinophilic cytoplasm, differentiating as skeletal muscle, i.e., cross-striations by light microscopy (rarely ever found) or the ultrastructural features of skeletal muscle cells. Desmin, muscle-specific actin, and MyoD1 or myogenin expression by tumor cells that are "strap-like" or have abundant eosinophilic cytoplasm is generally considered specific for skeletal muscle differentiation in an otherwise pleomorphic MFH.

Leiomyosarcoma requires tumor cells that have the light or electron microscopic features of smooth muscle cells. This means that spindled

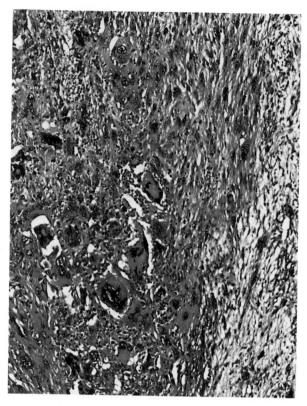

Figure 3-53
MYXOID VARIANT OF MALIGNANT FIBROUS
HISTIOCYTOMA (MYXOFIBROSARCOMA)

The usual myxoid MFH (myxofibrosarcoma) has myxoid areas (at right) as well as areas more characteristic of pleomorphic MFH. The myxoid portion usually contains pleomorphic cells but the cells may be uniform as long as pleomorphic MFH is present somewhere in the tumor.

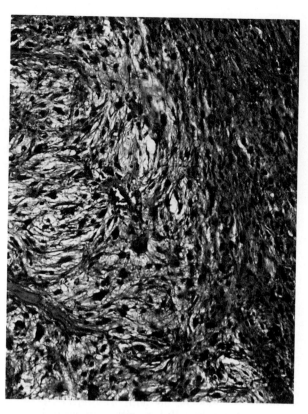

Figure 3-54
MYXOID VARIANT OF MALIGNANT FIBROUS
HISTIOCYTOMA (MYXOFIBROSARCOMA)

Some myxoid MFHs feature myxoid areas alternating with solid tumor that is not as pleomorphic as the usual pleomorphic MFH.

under discussion. Myxofibrosarcoma is just as, and in the minds of some, more, acceptable.

Clinical Features. The clinical features of myxoid MFH are identical to those of pleomorphic MFH except that a higher percentage of cases develop in the subcutaneous tissue and a retroperitoneal location is rare (219,226,229).

Gross Findings. Myxoid MFH, as its name would suggest, is gelatinous or frankly mucinous, either diffusely or focally, and when the myxoid areas are diffuse these tumors are grossly indistinguishable from other myxoid neoplasms such as myxoid liposarcoma. Myxoid MFHs tend to form multiple, macroscopically visible nodules of tumor.

Microscopic Findings. The classic myxoid MFH is composed of variable proportions of paucicellular to moderately cellular myxoid

tumor mixed with cellular tumor often identical to that found in pure pleomorphic MFH (figs. 3-53, 3-54) (219,225,226,229). The myxoid areas that count toward classification of the tumor as the myxoid variant may be diffuse or focal but in aggregate make up greater than 10 percent or greater than 50 percent of the tumor volume depending on whether one uses the definition of Mentzel et al. (225) or Weiss and Enzinger (229). The cells in the myxoid areas vary from small and bland to enlarged bizarre and pleomorphic (figs. 3-55–3-57). Either type of cell may predominate but in most tumors there is a mixture. The small bland cells have elongate to round regular nuclei and scant cytoplasm. These blend imperceptibly into cells with larger, often irregular nuclei and more abundant eosinophilic or vacuolated cytoplasm. Finally, bizarre, enlarged, often huge cells with round to jagged irregular nuclear outlines, abundant cytoplasm, and

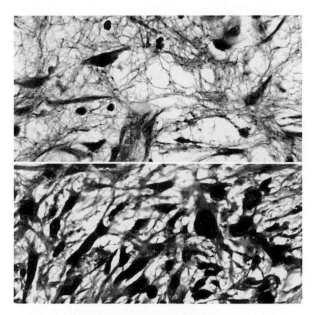

Figure 3-55
MYXOID VARIANT OF MALIGNANT FIBROUS
HISTIOCYTOMA (MYXOFIBROSARCOMA)

Myxoid MFH may be purely myxoid and not contain areas of pleomorphic MFH. To qualify as a myxoid MFH, at least some of the constituent cells of the purely myxoid neoplasm must be pleomorphic, as seen here. Such tumors vary from paucicellular (top) to moderately cellular (bottom). Tumors more cellular than the one illustrated in the bottom panel are usually not diagnosed as myxoid.

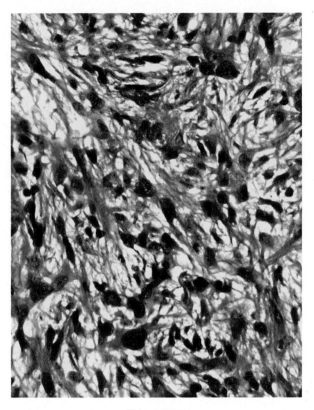

Figure 3-56
MYXOID VARIANT OF MALIGNANT FIBROUS
HISTIOCYTOMA (MYXOFIBROSARCOMA)

Characteristic myxoid area in a myxoid MFH (myxofibrosarcoma), demonstrating moderate cellularity.

marked hyperchromasia round out the roster of cells that can be found in the myxoid areas (figs. 3-55, 3-56). Any of these cells may have vacuolated or bubbly cytoplasm and thus resemble lipoblasts; however, their nuclei are characteristically central, the strands or spikes of chromatin that extend from the indented nucleus of a lipoblast are absent, and the vacuoles are not usually sharply circumscribed and clear as are fat vacuoles (see definition of lipoblasts in the Introduction to chapter 4). The cytoplasmic vacuolar material often stains with Alcian blue. Mitotic figures are usually easy to find and abnormal forms are the rule in pleomorphic areas. Blood vessels are prominent and may take on an arborizing pattern of the type found in myxoid liposarcoma or, more often, form arcs or curves. Acute and chronic inflammation are found in some tumors, particularly those that have areas of pleomorphic MFH. Necrosis is generally limited to tumors with areas of pleomorphic MFH.

Although classic myxoid MFHs have solid areas indistinguishable from pleomorphic MFH, tumors within this category may be purely myxoid (219, 225,226). The minimum requirement for inclusion is an otherwise undifferentiated tumor with a myxoid stroma throughout in which the constituent cells demonstrate at least mild pleomorphism (fig. 3-57), that is, at least some tumor cell nuclei are enlarged and hyperchromatic, and have irregular outlines. Mitotic figures, including abnormal forms, are often present. Blood vessels may be numerous and prominent, and arranged in gently curvilinear arches or in a plexiform pattern reminiscent of the vessels found in myxoid liposarcoma (225). Rarely, a pericytic vascular pattern is present. The tumor cells tend to condense around the vessels. Pure myxoid MFHs vary from hypocellular to modestly cellular and there is a continuum of nuclear atypia, pleomorphism, abnormal mitotic figures, and increasing cellularity that blends into the solid pattern of pleomorphic MFH. Myxoid lesions composed of

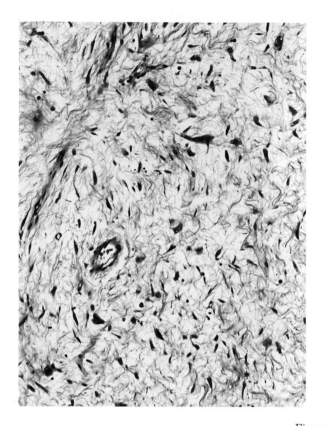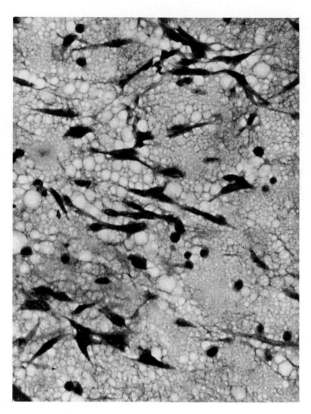

Figure 3-57
MYXOID VARIANT OF MALIGNANT FIBROUS HISTIOCYTOMA (MYXOFIBROSARCOMA)
Myxoid MFH should be graded. The cells composing this tumor exhibit the minimal degree of pleomorphism required for a diagnosis of grade I MFH. Figures 3-54 and 3-59 represent grade II MFH while figure 3-53 is grade III because of the areas of pleomorphic MFH present in the tumor.

cells that do not meet these requirements should not be placed in the myxoid MFH (myxofibrosarcoma) category (fig. 3-58).

Because of significant differences in patient outcome between purely hypocellular myxoid MFHs and those that are more cellular and pleomorphic, myxoid MFH should be graded. The grading criteria provided by Mentzel and associates (225) utilize a three-tier scheme and are easy to apply. Low-grade myxoid MFHs are hypocellular throughout and their matrix is entirely myxoid (fig. 3-57). High-grade tumors have solid pleomorphic areas indistinguishable from pleomorphic MFH in addition to myxoid areas (fig. 3-53). Intermediate-grade lesions are myxoid throughout but are more cellular than the low-grade ones and pleomorphism is more obvious. Giant cells and abnormal division figures are often present. Tiny areas of solid tumor are acceptable in intermediate tumors (figs. 3-54, 3-59).

In summary, in order for a tumor to qualify as myxoid MFH the neoplastic cells must not be differentiated except as fibroblasts, myofibroblasts, or histiocyte-like cells; the myxoid areas used to make the diagnosis must account for over 10 percent of the volume of the tumor; and at least focally significant pleomorphism with enlarged cells must be present in the myxoid areas, the cellular areas, or both. Whenever myxoid MFH (myxofibrosarcoma) is diagnosed a grade should be specified; we use the terms low, intermediate, and high grade.

Special Studies. Electron microscopy reveals the expected: fibroblasts and primitive cells. Thus, this procedure is not useful diagnostically except on rare occasions when it is needed to exclude another neoplasm (221,223). Rarely, CD68 and factor XIIIa may be focally positive and some tumors contain actin-positive cells. As is the case for pleomorphic MFH, the main value

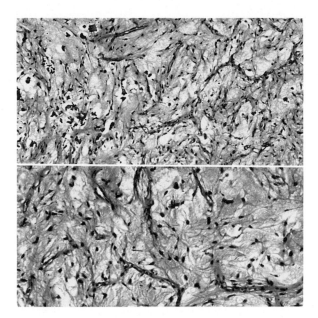
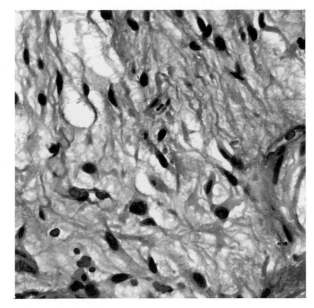

Figure 3-58
BLAND SOFT TISSUE MYXOID LESION

Purely myxoid lesions without pleomorphism as shown here should not be placed in the myxoid MFH category. Contrast this with figure 3-57. Such lesions recur but have no metastatic potential. Most fit into the juxta-articular myxoma or cellular intramuscular myxoma category but sometimes "myxoid lesion with recurrent potential" must be used as a diagnostic label.

of immunohistochemistry is to exclude other neoplasms. In more than 50 percent of myxoid MFHs, ring chromosomes have been identified but the constituents of these chromosomes remain unknown (228).

Differential Diagnosis. The prime entities in the differential diagnosis are myxoid liposarcoma, myxoid chondrosarcoma, neural neoplasms, pleomorphic MFH, leiomyosarcoma with myxoid stroma, metastatic mucinous carcinoma, myxoid melanoma, and bland myxoid tumors composed of uniform cells (224). A diagnosis of pleomorphic MFH versus myxoid MFH is based on the amount of myxoid stroma in the neoplasm (less or more than 10 percent). The stromal cells, particularly those in the hypocellular areas of myxoid MFH may be indistinguishable from the undifferentiated stromal cells in myxoid liposarcoma, but myxoid liposarcoma also contains lipidic cells and does not contain the pleomorphic cells required, at least focally, for a diagnosis of myxoid MFH. Myxoid liposarcoma only rarely arises in the subcutaneous tissue whereas myxoid MFH not infrequently develops in this site. S-100 protein stains can help exclude neural neoplasms as can electron microscopy and knowledge about the

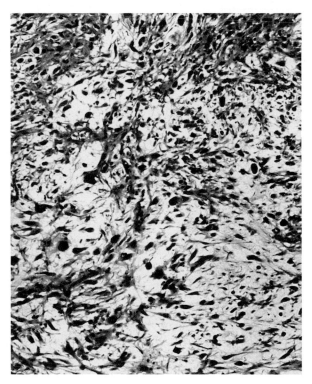

Figure 3-59
MYXOID VARIANT OF MALIGNANT
FIBROUS HISTIOCYTOMA (MYXOFIBROSARCOMA)
Grade II myxoid MFH.

relationship of the tumor to a nerve (malignant peripheral nerve sheath tumors arise from a nerve or a neurofibroma, or develop in a patient with neurofibromatosis). S-100 protein will also identify almost all myxoid melanomas. Keratin, epithelial membrane antigen, and mucin stains are adjuncts that often help identify metastatic carcinoma. Myxoid chondrosarcoma has a microscopic lobular architecture and the chain-like arrangement of uniform cells extending from the periphery of the lobules to the center is unlike the cellular pattern in myxoid MFH. Moreover, the cells in myxoid chondrosarcoma are usually small and uniform and do not demonstrate the degree of pleomorphism and anaplasia found at least focally in myxoid MFH.

Aggressive angiomyxoma, juxta-articular myxoma, intramuscular myxoma including cellular forms, and superficial angiomyxoma lack the pleomorphism and nuclear atypia required for low-grade myxoid MFH. Recently, Evans (220a) has reported a type of bland fibromyxoid tumor that has metastatic potential even without significant cellular pleomorphism. This he has labeled low-grade fibromyxoid sarcoma, and it is characterized by not only paucicellular myxoid stroma, bland cells, and a low mitotic count but also by abundant fibrous tissue and a whorled or storiform arrangement of the constituent cells (see Fibrous Tumors). Almost all are deep and large, and they are slow growing even when metastatic. Nodular fasciitis may have a myxoid stroma but it lacks the pleomorphism required for even low-grade myxoid MFH.

Treatment and Prognosis. The reason for distinguishing myxoid MFH (myxofibrosarcoma) from pleomorphic MFH is the supposedly better prognosis for patients with the former as compared to the latter. As it turns out the prognosis for patients with high-grade myxoid MFH is for practical purposes the same as for pleomorphic MFH (approximately 50 to 60 percent recurrence rate, 20 to 30 percent metastasis rate) (219,225–227, 229). However, low-grade myxoid MFH almost never metastasizes, although it has a recurrence rate in the same range as high-grade myxoid MFH and pleomorphic MFH, and it may become more pleomorphic and cellular (and hence higher grade) in recurrence. Intermediate-grade myxoid MFH appears to behave as does the high-grade variety, although the number of cases with follow-up is small. As is the case for pleo-morphic MFH, the prognosis of those with high-grade lesions depends on size and location, whether superficial or deep: patients with large, deep, lesions do significantly worse than those with superficial tumors, but of course most superficial tumors are small when discovered.

Giant Cell Variant Malignant Fibrous Histiocytoma (Giant Cell Sarcoma; Giant Cell Tumor of Soft Tissue)

Definition. Some giant cell variants are otherwise pleomorphic MFHs containing large numbers of osteoclast-like giant cells, while others have histologic features very similar to giant cell tumor of bone.

General Considerations. This category of tumor is defined by the presence of large numbers of giant cells with uniform nuclei that resemble osteoclasts. It is undoubtedly heterogeneous and includes tumors that are otherwise pleomorphic MFHs as well as tumors indistinguishable from giant cell tumor of bone (230,230a,231,233,233a). In addition, about half of the very small number of the tumors reported have contained bone or cartilage, some at least apparently formed by neoplastic cells, although some such foci are metaplastic. As long as the neoplastic bone or cartilage is focal and inconspicuous, Guccion and Enzinger (231) elected to use the label giant cell MFH rather than soft tissue osteosarcoma or chondrosarcoma. If the neoplastic bone or cartilage is "prominent," these investigators suggest classifying the histologically identical tumor as a soft tissue osteosarcoma or chondrosarcoma. We disagree with this approach and instead classify soft tissue sarcomas in which the tumor cells form bone or cartilage, even if it is small in amount and focal, as osteosarcoma or chondrosarcoma. If such tumors contain large numbers of osteoclast-like giant cells we refer to them as giant cell–rich osteosarcoma as is done for identical tumors of bone. Our policy is to label tumors that are histologically otherwise pleomorphic MFHs containing large numbers of osteoclastic-like giant cells but not tumor bone or cartilage as the high-grade giant cell variant of MFH, while tumors that resemble giant cell tumors of bone with uniform mononuclear cells as giant cell tumor of soft tissue.

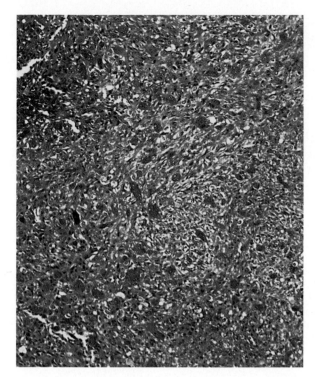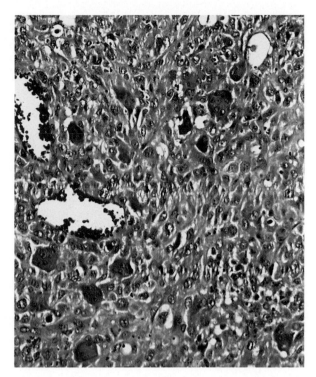

Figure 3-60
GIANT CELL MALIGNANT FIBROUS HISTIOCYTOMA
Giant cell MFH takes two forms. The high-grade variant, illustrated here, is an otherwise pleomorphic MFH which contains osteoclast-like giant cells with uniform nuclei.

Clinical Features. The clinical features are essentially the same as those for pleomorphic MFH except that a higher percentage of tumors arise in the subcutaneous tissue and skin (230,231). The majority of the less than 100 cases of giant cell sarcoma reported have occurred in the extremities, although the trunk is a common site for these neoplasms.

Pathologic Findings. Grossly, the giant cell variants of MFH that resemble pleomorphic MFH are often necrotic and hemorrhagic. As would be expected, superficial tumors are usually smaller than deep ones.

Microscopically, at low power, nodularity is a distinctive feature of many of the high-grade tumors; the nodules are composed of neoplastic cells surrounded by dense fibrous tissue that contains numerous blood vessels, some of which are dilated. At higher magnification, the histologic pattern of the high-grade tumors is identical to that found in pleomorphic MFH except for the many multinucleated cells that resemble osteoclasts (fig. 3-60). In addition to the osteo-clast-like giant cells, fibroblasts, and myofibroblasts, randomly arranged or in small irregular bundles, alternate with histiocyte-like cells including nonosteoclast-like giant cells with one or more bizarre, irregular, hyperchromatic nuclei. The elongated cells tend to aggregate around the periphery of the tumor nodules. The degree of nuclear anaplasia of the histiocyte-like cells and fibroblasts varies from tumor to tumor but it is at least moderate and can be marked. Superficial tumors tend to be composed of cells with fewer chromatin abnormalities. In about three fourths of the tumors histiocyte-like cells predominate. Mitotic figures are easy to find and abnormal forms are common. However, the feature that distinguishes this tumor from pleomorphic MFH is the large number of osteoclast-like giant cells (fig. 3-60). These differ from the tumor giant cells by the greater number of nuclei that tend to be regular with evenly distributed chromatin. Nucleoli are usually prominent. Studies in our laboratory indicate the osteoclast-like cells in giant cell sarcoma have a histiocytic phenotype,

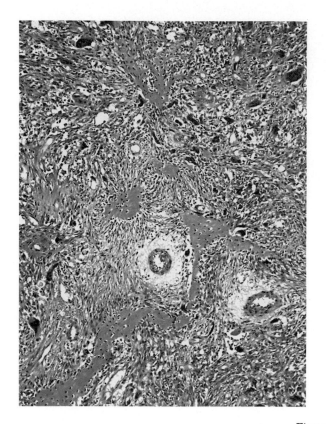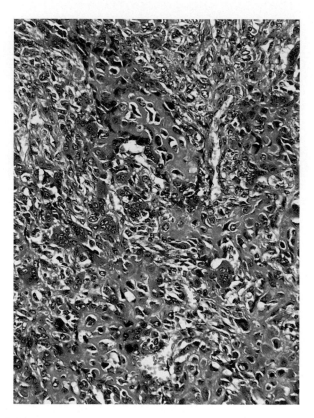

Figure 3-61
GIANT CELL–RICH OSTEOSARCOMA

Focally, the cells of tumors indistinguishable from high-grade giant cell MFH may form tumor bone and osteoid. We classify such tumors as giant cell–rich osteosarcoma.

as determined by immunohistochemical techniques, suggesting they are reactive histiocytes and not neoplastic cells. The stroma is generally collagenous, and hemorrhage and necrosis are present in most tumors. As noted, if neoplastic bone or cartilage (i.e., bone laid down by tumor cells) is present, we classify the tumor as giant cell–rich osteosarcoma or chondrosarcoma (fig. 3-61). On the other hand, metaplastic bone or cartilage is acceptable in a giant cell variant.

The low-grade giant cell variant, now often known as giant cell tumor of soft tissue, is usually multinodular, and the mononuclear cells are small and uniform with scant cytoplasm, i.e., they resemble the stromal cells in giant cell tumor of bone (fig. 3-62) (230a,233a). The osteoclast-like giant cells are distributed throughout the tumor and have histologic features identical to those in the high-grade tumors described above. Mitotic figures are usually easy to find and often exceed 5 per 10 high-power fields. Vascular invasion is common. Metaplastic

bone formation is often present and bone may form a shell around the tumor. Both the mononuclear and the giant cells are reported to express CD68 (KP1) (233).

Differential Diagnosis. The high-grade giant cell variant differs from pleomorphic MFH only by the presence of easily found, multinucleated giant cells with numerous, uniform, relatively bland but sometimes large nuclei. Multinucleated giant cells with irregular pleomorphic and hyperchromatic nuclei don't count and tumors with giant cells with bizarre nuclei, no matter how numerous, should be classified as pleomorphic MFH rather than giant cell sarcoma unless large numbers of osteoclast-like cells with uniform nuclei are also present. Otherwise pleomorphic MFHs with only rare or scattered osteoclast-like giant cells are also relegated to the pleomorphic MFH category. The low-grade giant cell variant of MFH is identical to giant cell tumor of bone. Bone radiographs are

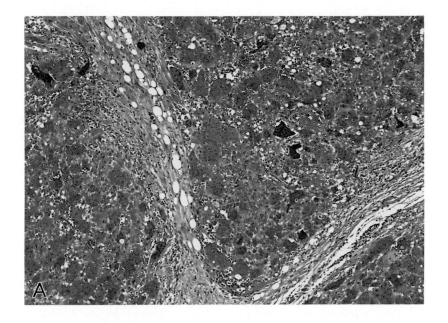

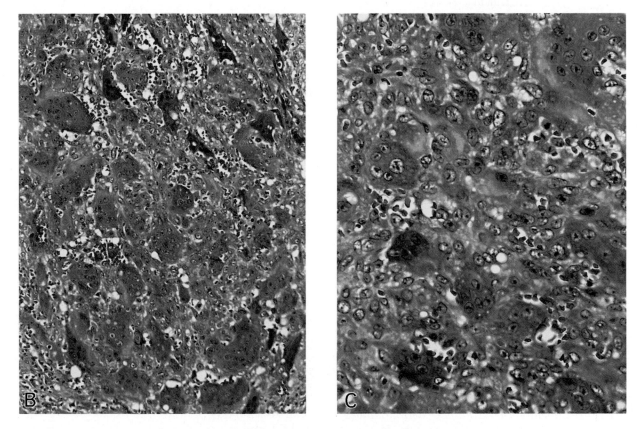

Figure 3-62
GIANT CELL TUMOR OF SOFT TISSUE

The other form of giant cell MFH is low grade and closely resembles giant cell tumor of bone. The giant cells resemble osteoclasts and the constituent cells are not pleomorphic.

always in order when a diagnosis of either high- or low-grade giant cell MFH is contemplated in order to rule out a bone primary. Distinction of the low-grade giant cell variant from localized tenosynovial giant cell tumor (giant cell tumor of tendon sheath) is based on location of the latter near a joint, particularly the joints of the hands, feet and knee, and its usually small size. Histologically, the two may be indistinguishable. Diffuse tenosynovial giant cell tumors (extra-articular villonodular synovitis) contain fewer giant cells and lack the nodularity and high mitotic index that characterize the giant cell variant of MFH. Metastasis from giant cell carcinoma is a consideration but the giant cells are pleomorphic and do not contain the uniform nuclei of the osteoclast-like giant cells found in the giant cell variant. Keratin stains may be useful when giant cell carcinoma is a consideration. Leiomyosarcomas may also have prominent osteoclast-like giant cells so they should be considered in the differential diagnosis (232).

Treatment and Prognosis. The behavior of the high-grade giant cell variant is similar to that of pleomorphic MFH (see above). Deep tumors, as would be expected, are larger at discovery and tend to have a higher frequency of metastasis; however, superficial tumors have a high rate of recurrence (231). The low-grade variant resembling giant cell tumor of bone has a low metastatic rate but recurrences are common (230a,233,233a).

Inflammatory Malignant Fibrous Histiocytoma

Definition. Inflammatory MFH is composed predominantly or exclusively of histiocyte-like cells, including giant cell forms associated with massive acute inflammation, in the absence of necrosis. Foam cells are often present and may be prominent.

General Considerations. This variant of MFH was thought important enough to be classified separately because it can easily be mistaken for an inflammatory process, lymphoma, carcinoma, or melanoma. Areas of pleomorphic MFH are present in some but not all inflammatory variants, but if present, they are almost always inconspicuous. The inflammatory variant has been reported in the older literature under the title of xanthogranuloma and xanthosarcoma (234–239). This is a rare neoplasm and only a handful of cases have been reported. In fact, some examples in the older literature might be classified differently after immunohistologic evaluation.

Clinical Features. Inflammatory MFH usually occurs in middle-aged adults (mean age, approximately 50 years) although it has been reported in children as well as the elderly (234–237). Most of the tumors occur in the retroperitoneum but a number have been found in the pleura and other sites (235,236,238). Some patients present with symptoms that result from the presence of a large mass while others report fever and symptoms suggesting an infectious process (236). Some of the latter have leukocytosis which characteristically disappears along with the fever when the tumor is removed.

Pathologic Findings. The average size of these tumors is 8 to 10 cm as befits their often deep sites of origin, and they are usually firm, lobulated, and yellow to yellow-white. Areas of hemorrhage and necrosis are unusual. Microscopically, the characteristic low-power impression is one of histiocyte-like and xanthoma cells floating in a sea of acute inflammatory cells, but paradoxically, necrosis is absent (fig. 3-63) (235,236). The histiocyte-like cells vary from those with enlarged but bland vesicular nuclei to huge cells with bizarre, irregular, hyperchromatic and sometimes multiple nuclei (fig. 3-64). The cytoplasm of the tumor cells varies from foamy to eosinophilic. In addition, foamy histiocytes with small central often pyknotic nuclei inhabit most tumors and in some cases are predominant. The proportion of bland histiocytes and bland histiocyte-like cells to enlarged cells with bizarre nuclei varies from situations in which the latter cells are rare and difficult to find to those in which such cells are numerous in every section. Because large abnormal cells are required to identify the inflammatory variant, they should be sought (fig. 3-65). Not infrequently, such cells are in division, sometimes abnormal division. Consequently, searching for large and abnormal mitotic figures is often rewarding. Thus, the usual inflammatory MFH is composed of a spectrum of cells that vary from classic xanthoma cells with pyknotic nuclei, to histiocyte-like cells with bland vesicular nuclei, to histiocyte-like cells with atypical enlarged nuclei, to bizarre giant cells. In addition to the prominent acute inflammatory infiltrate, lymphocytes, plasma cells, and

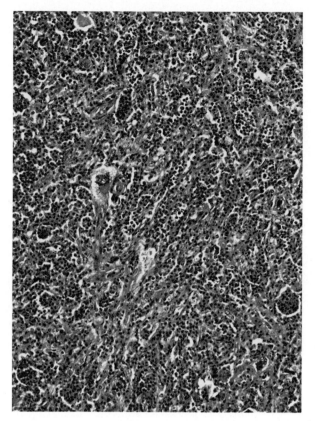

Figure 3-63
INFLAMMATORY MALIGNANT
FIBROUS HISTIOCYTOMA
Sheets of acute inflammatory cells punctuated by large histiocyte-like cells characterize inflammatory MFH.

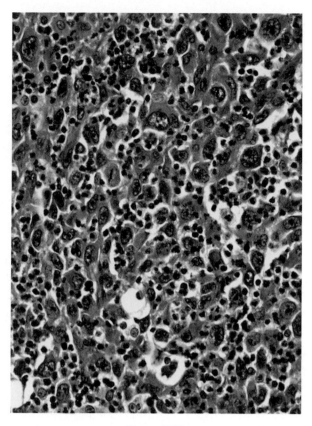

Figure 3-64
INFLAMMATORY MALIGNANT
FIBROUS HISTIOCYTOMA
Large histiocyte-like cells with prominent nucleoli sometimes accompanied by fibroblasts are the neoplastic cells of inflammatory MFH. Lymphoma and carcinoma must be excluded by appropriate immunohistochemical stains.

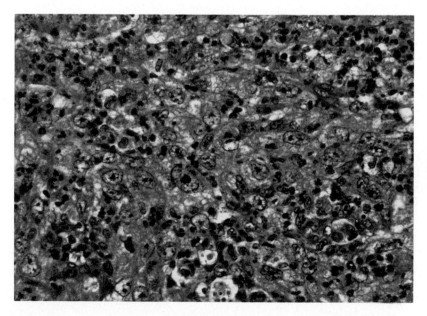

Figure 3-65
INFLAMMATORY MALIGNANT
FIBROUS HISTIOCYTOMA
Inflammatory MFH with large numbers of histiocyte-like cells. The resemblance to lymphoma is striking.

eosinophils are commonly observed. Sometimes these are numerous and rarely the acute inflammation is subdued in comparison to the large number of other inflammatory cells. Finally, a fibrous or myofibroblastic spindled component, with or without admixed histiocyte-like cells, is found in some but not all inflammatory MFHs. In many instances these areas resemble ordinary pleomorphic MFH, a very helpful finding.

At present, too few of these tumors have been subjected to immunohistochemical staining to accurately determine their immunologic profile but in some of the cases we have examined the tumor cells do not differ significantly from those in pleomorphic MFH. However, it is also plausible that tumors that would have been classified as inflammatory MFH in the past are now classified as another type of tumor after immunohistologic evaluation.

Differential Diagnosis. Many other types of neoplasms share histologic features with inflammatory MFH; as a result, the diagnosis is an exercise in exclusion. The mimics can be placed into five categories: 1) inflammatory processes; 2) lymphomas, both Hodgkin's and non-Hodgkin's types; 3) metastatic carcinoma and melanoma; 4) other sarcomas, particularly liposarcoma; and 5) other fibrous histiocytomas. Because of the magnitude and importance of this differential diagnosis, resort to a panel of immunohistochemical stains is almost always required. When the enlarged atypical cells required for inflammatory MFH are focal or minimally deviated from reactive histiocytes, xanthogranulomatous inflammatory processes such as malacoplakia, Whipple's disease, and xanthogranulomatous pyelonephritis extending out of the kidney into the retroperitoneum are considerations. The cells in malacoplakia and Whipple's disease contain PAS-positive intracytoplasmic material that is diastase resistant. Such material is sparse, if present at all, in the cells of inflammatory MFH. A careful search for enlarged cells with atypical nuclei, enlarged cells in division, and areas more characteristic of MFH is often required to distinguish inflammatory MFH from inflammation. Careful and thorough sectioning is required because many inflammatory MFHs contain large areas of banal foam cells indistinguishable from those found in inflammatory processes. Cultures also may be helpful.

Immunohistochemical stains using a panel approach are often helpful when the question of lymphoma, carcinoma, or melanoma arises. Some anaplastic lymphomas are histologically identical to inflammatory MFH and may not express CD45 common leukocyte antigen, so we suggest utilizing T- and B-cell markers to exclude lymphoma if a CD45 stain is negative. However, most lymphomas are not accompanied by the intense, acute inflammatory response that is characteristic of inflammatory MFH. Lipoblasts are required for a diagnosis of liposarcoma; these are defined in the Introduction to chapter 4. The foamy histiocytes and the histiocyte-like tumor cells in inflammatory MFH have mainly central nuclei that are not deformed by clear vacuoles as is required for lipoblasts. Atypical lipomatous tumors (well-differentiated liposarcoma) may dedifferentiate to MFH, including the inflammatory variant, although the dedifferentiated pattern is usually that of pleomorphic MFH. The key to the correct diagnosis is identifying the atypical lipomatous portion of the tumor. To accomplish this it is sometimes necessary to go back to the gross specimen and submit sections of what grossly appears to be normal fat or repeat the imaging studies to be sure all of the tumor has been removed.

Distinguishing other types of fibrous histiocytoma from the inflammatory variant is accomplished by recognizing the presence of the large numbers of acute inflammatory cells and the absence of necrosis in the latter. Other types of MFH may contain acute and chronic inflammation but necrosis is common in any high-grade MFH. It is the sheet-like arrangement of the acute and sometimes chronic, inflammatory cells with interspersed histiocyte-like cells and the absence of necrosis that is the hallmark of the inflammatory variant of MFH. Two observations have been helpful to us when faced with a lesion that may be an inflammatory MFH. First, this is an uncommon neoplasm and all of the other possibilities in the differential diagnosis should be carefully excluded before making this diagnosis. Second, both neoplastic and inflammatory processes in the retroperitoneum are notoriously treacherous and difficult to diagnose correctly; consequently many sections and liberal use of histochemical and immunohistochemical stains are often rewarding maneuvers.

Treatment and Prognosis. About two thirds of inflammatory MFHs recur and about a third metastasize (234,236). As is the case for the other MFHs, deep location and large size are adverse prognostic variables.

THE QUESTION OF A FIBROUS VARIANT

It has become customary for most pathologists to classify sarcomas that meet the criteria of fibrosarcoma, except that they contain easily identified, enlarged, pleomorphic round cells, including multinucleated giant cells, as MFH rather than labeling them "pleomorphic fibrosarcoma" as was often done in the past. While such tumors are usually included within the pleomorphic MFH group, some investigators have suggested a category of "fibrous variant" of MFH (199). Because the clinical features and the outcome are identical to pleomorphic MFH, we do not think adding yet another morphologic variant to the MFH category is advantageous. What is important to understand is that fibrosarcoma as now defined must be composed of uniform spindled cells arranged in bundles that intersect at acute angles, and that round cells and significantly pleomorphic cells are not allowed.

REFERENCES

Introduction

1. Alguacil-Garcia A, Unni KK, Goellner JR. Malignant fibrous histiocytoma: an ultrastructural study of six cases. Am J Clin Pathol 1978;69:121–9.
1a. Binder SW, Said JW, Shintaku IP, Pinkus GS. A histiocyte-specific marker in the diagnosis of malignant fibrous histiocytoma. Use of monoclonal antibody KP-1 (CD68). Am J Clin Pathol 1992;97:759–63.
2. Brecher ME, Franklin WA. Absence of mononuclear phagocyte antigens in malignant fibrous histiocytoma. Am J Clin Pathol 1986;86:344–8.
2a. Calonje E, Fletcher CD. Myoid differentiation in dermatofibrosarcoma protuberans and its fibrosarcomatous variant: clinicopathologic analysis of 5 cases. J Cutan Pathol 1996;23:30–6.
3. Churg AM, Kahn LB. Myofibroblasts and related cells in malignant fibrous and fibrohistiocytic tumours. Hum Pathol 1977;8:205–18.
4. Dehner LP. Malignant fibrous histiocytoma. Nonspecific morphologic pattern, specific pathologic entity, or both? [Editorial] Arch Pathol Lab Med 1988;112:236–7.
5. du Boulay CE. Demonstration of alpha-I-antitrypsin and alpha-I-antichymotrypsin in fibrous histiocytomas using the immunoperoxidase technique. Am J Surg Pathol 1982;6:559–64.
6. Fisher C. Fibrohistiocytic tumors. In: Weiss SW, Brooks JJ, eds. Soft tissue tumors. Baltimore: Williams & Wilkins, 1996:162–80.
7. Fletcher CD. Angiomatoid "malignant fibrous histiocytoma": an immunohistochemical study indicative of myoid differentiation. Hum Pathol 1991;22:563–8.
8. Fletcher CD. Commentary. Histopathology 1987;11:433–7.
8a. Fletcher CD. Pleomorphic malignant fibrous histiocytoma: fact or fiction? A critical reappraisal based on 159 tumors diagnosed as pleomorphic sarcoma. Am J Surg Pathol 1992;16:213–28.
8b. Fretzin DF, Helwig EB. Atypical fibroxanthoma of the skin. A clinicopathologic study of 140 cases. Cancer 1973;31:1541–52.
9. Fu YS, Gabbiani G, Kaye GI, Lattes R. Malignant soft tissue tumours of probable histiocytic origin (malignant fibrous histiocytomas): general considerations and electron microscopic and tissue culture studies. Cancer 1975;35:176–98.
10. Fukuda T, Tsuneyoshi M, Enjoji M. Malignant fibrous histiocytoma of soft parts: an ultrastructural quantitative study. Ultrastruct Pathol 1988;12:117–29.
11. Genberg M, Mark J, Hakelius L, Ericsson J, Nistér M. Origin and relationship between different cell types in malignant fibrous histiocytoma. Am J Pathol 1989;135:1185–96.
11a. Guccion JG, Enzinger FM. Malignant giant cell tumor of soft parts. An analysis of 32 cases. Cancer 1972;29:1518–29.
12. Harris M. The ultrastructure of benign and malignant fibrous histiocytomas. Histopathology 1980;4:29–44.
13. Hayashi Y, Kikuchi-Tada A, Jitsukawa K, Sato S, Anzai T, Kawashima M. Myofibroblasts in malignant fibrous histiocytoma—histochemical, immunohistochemical, ultrastructural and tissue culture studies. Clin Exper Dermatol 1988;13:402–5.
13a. Hirose T, Kudo E, Hasegawa T, Abe J, Hizawa K. Expression of intermediate filaments in malignant fibrous histiocytomas. Hum Pathol 1989;20:871–7.
14. Hoffman MA, Dickersin GR. Malignant fibrous histiocytoma: an ultrastructural study of eleven cases. Hum Pathol 1983;14:913–22.

15. Hollowood K, Fletcher CD. Malignant fibrous histiocytoma: morphologic pattern or pathologic entity? Semin Diagn Pathol 1995;12:210–20.
16. Iwasaki H, Isayama T, Ohjimi Y, et al. Malignant fibrous histiocytoma. A tumor of facultative histiocytes showing mesenchymal differentiation in cultured cell lines. Cancer 1992;69:437–47.
17. Iwasaki H, Yoshitake K, Ohjimi Y, et al. Malignant fibrous histiocytoma. Proliferative compartment and heterogeneity of "histiocytic" cells. Am J Surg Pathol 1992;16:735–45.
17a. Kearney MM, Soule EH, Ivins JC. Malignant fibrous histiocytoma: a retrospective study of 167 cases. Cancer 1980;45:167–78.
18. Kempson RL, Hendrickson MR. What is a fibrohistiocytic tumor? In: Fletcher CD, McKee PH, eds. Pathobiology of soft tissue tumors. Edinburgh: Churchill Livingstone, 1990:105–40.
18a. Kempson RL, McGavran MH. Atypical fibroxanthomas of the skin. Cancer 1964;17:1463–71.
19. Kindblom LG, Jacobsen GK, Jacobsen M. Immunohistochemical investigations of tumors of supposed fibroblastic-histiocytic origin. Hum Pathol 1982;13:834–40.
20. Kyriakos M, Kempson RL. Inflammatory fibrous histiocytoma: an aggressive and lethal lesion. Cancer 1976;37:1584–606.
20a. Lawson CW, Fisher C, Gatter KC. An immunohistochemical study of differentiation in malignant fibrous histiocytoma. Histopathology 1987;11:375–83.
21. Meister P, Nathrath W. Immunohistochemical markers of histiocytic type [Letter]. Hum Pathol 1980;11:300–1.
22. Nakanishi S, Hizawa K. Enzyme histochemical observation of fibrohistiocytic tumors. Acta Pathol Jpn 1984;34:1003–16.
23. O'Brien JE, Stout AP. Malignant fibrous xanthomas. Cancer 1964;17:1445–55.
24. Ozzello L, Stout AP, Murray MR. Cultural characteristics of malignant histiocytomas and fibrous xanthomas. Cancer 1963;16:331–44.
25. Pulford KA, Rigney EM, Micklem KJ, et al. KP1: a new monoclonal antibody that detects a monocyte/macrophage associated antigen in routinely processed tissue sections. J Clin Pathol 1989;42:414–21.
26. Roholl PJ, Kleijne J, van Basten CD, van der Putte SC, van Unnik J. A study to analyze the origin of tumor cells in malignant fibrous histiocytomas. A multiparametric characterization. Cancer 1985;56:2809–15.
27. Soini Y, Miettinen M. Alpha-1-antitrypsin and lysozome. Their limited significance in fibrohistiocytic tumors. Am J Clin Pathol 1989;91:515–21.
28. Soini Y, Miettinen M. Widespread immunoreactivity for alpha-1-antichymotrypsin in different types of tumors. Am J Clin Pathol 1988;89:131–6.
29. Strauchen JA, Dimitriu-Bona A. Malignant fibrous histiocytoma. Expression of monocyte/macrophage differentiation antigens detected with monoclonal antibodies. Am J Pathol 1986;124:303–9.
30. Taxy JB, Battifora H. Malignant fibrous histiocytoma: an electron microscopic study. Cancer 1977;40:254–67.
31. van de Rijn M, Rouse RV. CD34: a review. Appl Immunohistochem 1994;2:71–80.
32. Weiss SW. Malignant fibrous histiocytoma. A reaffirmation. Am J Surg Pathol 1982;6:773–84.
32a. Weiss SW, Enzinger FM. Malignant fibrous histiocytoma: an analysis of 200 cases. Cancer 1978;41:2250–66.
32b. Weiss SW, Enzinger FM. Myxoid variant of malignant fibrous histiocytoma. Cancer 1977;39:1672–85.
33. Wolfe HJ, Palmer PE. Alpha-I-antitrypsin: its immunohistochemical localization and significance in diagnostic pathology. In: DeLellis RA, ed. Diagnostic immunohistochemistry. New York: Masson, 1981:227–38.
34. Wood GS, Beckstead JH, Turner RR, Hendrickson MR, Kempson RL, Warnke RA. Malignant fibrous histiocytoma tumor cells resemble fibroblasts. Am J Surg Pathol 1986;10:323–35.

Benign Fibrous Histiocytomas

35. Abenoza P, Lillemoe T. CD34 and factor XIIIa in the differential diagnosis of dermatofibroma and dermatofibrosarcoma protuberans. Am J Surg Pathol 1993;17:429–34.
36. Ackerman AB, Mendonca AM, Guo Y. Dermatofibroma vs. dermatofibrosarcoma protuberans. In: Differential diagnosis in dermatopathology, 2nd ed. Philadelphia: Lea & Febiger, 1992:170–3.
37. Addington SL, Pulitzer DR, Hoda SA, Reed RJ. Adventitial cellular myxofibroblastoma of the skin [Abstract]. Mod Pathol 1994;7:43A.
38. Altman DA, Nickoloff BJ, Fivenson DP. Differential expression of factor XIIIa and CD34 in cutaneous mesenchymal tumors. J Cutan Pathol 1993;20:154–8.
39. Arrese-Estrada J, Pierard GE. Factor XIIIa-positive dendrocytes and the dermal microvascular unit. Dermatology 1990;180:51–3.
40. Azumi N, Rubin MA, Boyle L, Hartmann DP. Desmin, muscle-specific actin and alpha-smooth muscle actin expression in non-muscular sarcomas and sarcoma-like lesions [Abstract]. Mod Pathol 1994;7:4A.
41. Baer SC, Raymond AK, Ordonez NG. CD34 and factor XIIIa expression in dermatofibrosarcoma protuberans: specificity, sensitivity, and pattern of immunostaining [Abstract]. Mod Pathol 1994;7:44A.
42. Barker SM, Winkelmann RK. Inflammatory lymphadenoid reactions with dermatofibroma/histiocytoma. J Cutan Pathol 1986;13:222–6.
43. Beer M, Eckert F, Schmoeckel C. The atrophic dermatofibroma. J Am Acad Dermatol 1991;25:1081–2.
44. Beham A, Fletcher CD. Atypical "pseudosarcomatous" variant of cutaneous benign fibrous histiocytoma: report of eight cases. Histopathology 1990;17:167–9.
45. Blumenfeld W, Egbert BM, Sagebiel RW. Differential diagnosis of Kaposi's sarcoma. Arch Pathol Lab Med 1985;109:123–7.
46. Burgdorf WH, Duray P, Rosai J. Immunohistochemical identification of lysozyme in cutaneous lesions of alleged histiocytic nature. Am J Clin Pathol 1981;75:162–7.
47. Calonje E, Fletcher CD. Aneurysmal benign cutaneous fibrous histiocytoma: clinicopathologic analysis of a tumor frequently misdiagnosed as a vascular lesion. Histopathology 1995;26:323–31.
48. Calonje E, Fletcher CD. Cutaneous fibrohistiocytic tumors: an update. Adv Anat Pathol 1994;1:2–15.

49. Calonje E, Mentzel T, Fletcher CD. Cellular benign fibrous histiocytoma. Clinicopathologic analysis of 74 cases of a distinctive variant of cutaneous fibrous histiocytoma with frequent recurrence. Am J Surg Pathol 1994;18:668–76.

50. Cerio R, Griffiths CE, Cooper KD, Nickoloff BJ, Headington JT. Characterization of factor XIIIa positive dermal dendritic cells in normal and inflamed skin. Br J Dermatol 1989;121:421–31.

51. Cerio R, Spaull J, Oliver GF, Wilson-Jones E. A study of factor XIIIa and MAC 387 immunolabeling in normal and pathological skin. Am J Dermatopathol 1990;12:221–33.

52. Colome-Grimmer MI, Evans HL. Metastasizing cellular dermatofibroma: a report of two cases. Am J Surg Pathol 1996;20:1361–7.

53. Fletcher CD. Benign fibrous histiocytoma of subcutaneous and deep soft tissue: a clinicopathologic analysis of 21 cases. Am J Surg Pathol 1990;14:801–9.

54. Franquemont DW, Cooper PH, Shmookler BM, Wick MR. Benign fibrous histiocytoma of the skin with potential for local recurrence: a tumor to be distinguished from dermatofibroma. Mod Pathol 1990;3:158–63.

55. Glusac EJ, Barr RJ, Everett MA, Pitha J, Santa Cruz DJ. Epithelioid cell histiocytoma: a report of 10 cases including a new cellular variant. Am J Surg Pathol 1994;18:583–90.

56. Gonzalez SB. Benign fibrous histiocytoma of the skin. An immunohistochemical analysis of 30 cases. Pathol Res Pract 1985;180:486–9.

57. Gonzalez SB, Duarte I. Benign fibrous histiocytoma of the skin. A morphologic study of 290 cases. Pathol Res Pract 1982;174:379–91.

58. Helm KF, Helm T, Helm F. Palisading cutaneous fibrous histiocytoma. An immunohistochemical study demonstrating differentiation from dermal dendrocytes. Am J Dermatopathol 1993;15:559–61.

59. Hsi ED, Nickoloff BJ. Dermatofibroma (DF) and dermatofibrosarcoma protuberans (DFSP): an immunohistochemical study reveals distinctive antigenic profiles [Abstract]. Mod Pathol 1994;7:46A.

60. Kamino H, Jacobson M. Dermatofibroma extending into the subcutaneous tissue. Differential diagnosis from dermatofibrosarcoma protuberans. Am J Surg Pathol 1990;14:1156–64.

61. Kamino H, Lee JY, Berke A. Pleomorphic fibroma of the skin: a benign neoplasm with cytologic atypia. A clinicopathologic study of eight cases. Am J Surg Pathol 1989;13:107–13.

62. Kanitakis J, Schmitt D, Thivolet J. Immunohistologic study of cellular populations of histiocytofibromas ("dermatofibromas"). J Cutan Pathol 1984;11:88–94.

63. Leyva WH, Santa Cruz DJ. Atypical cutaneous fibrous histiocytoma. Am J Dermatopathol 1986;8:467–71.

64. Marrogi AJ, Dehner LP, Coffin CM, Wick MR. Benign cutaneous histiocytic tumors in childhood and adolescence, excluding Langerhans' cell proliferations. A clinicopathologic and immunohistochemical analysis. Am J Dermatopathol 1992;14:8–18.

65. Mehregan AH, Mehregan DR, Broecker A. Epithelioid cell histiocytoma. A clinicopathologic and immunohistochemical study of eight cases. J Am Acad Dermatol 1992;26:243–6.

65a. Murphy GF, Elder DE. Non-melanocytic tumors of the skin. Atlas of Tumor Pathology, 3rd Series, Fascicle 1. Washington, D.C.: Armed Forces Institute of Pathology, 1991.

66. Niemi KM. The benign fibrohistiocytic tumours of the skin. Acta Dermatol Venereol (Suppl) 1970;50:1–66.

67. Nguyen GK, Johnson ES. Invasive benign histiocytoma [Letter]. Am J Surg Pathol 1987;11:487–8.

68. Reed RJ. New concepts in surgical pathology of the skin. New York: Wiley, 1976.

69. Reid MB, Gray C, Fear JD, Bird CC. Immunohistological demonstration of factors XIIIa and XIIIs in reactive and neoplastic fibroblastic and fibro-histiocytic lesions. Histopathology 1986;10:1171–8.

70. Santa Cruz DJ, Kyriakos M. Aneurysmal ("angiomatoid") fibrous histiocytoma of the skin. Cancer 1981;47:2053–61.

71. Schwob VS, Santa Cruz DJ. Palisading cutaneous fibrous histiocytoma. J Cutan Pathol 1986;13:403–7.

72. Singh Gomez C, Calonje E, Fletcher CD. Epithelioid benign fibrous histiocytoma of skin: clinicopathologic analysis of 20 cases of a poorly known variant. Histopathology 1994;24:123–9.

73. Smith NM, Davies JB, Shrimankar JS, Malcolm AJ. Deep fibrous histiocytoma with giant cells and bone metaplasia. Histopathology 1990;17:365–7.

74. Soini Y. Cell differentiation in benign cutaneous fibrous histiocytomas. An immunohistochemical study with antibodies to histiomonocytic cells and intermediate filament proteins. Am J Dermatopathol 1990;12:134–40.

75. Tamada S, Ackerman AB. Dermatofibroma with monster cells. Am J Dermatopathol 1987;9:380–7.

75a. van de Rijn M, Rouse RV. CD34: a review. Appl Immunohistochem 1994;2:71–80.

76. Vilanova JR, Flint A. The morphological variants of fibrous histiocytoma. J Cutan Pathol 1974;1:155–64.

76a. Wick MR, Ritter JH, Lind AC, Swanson PE. The pathological distinction between "deep penetrating" dermatofibroma and dermatofibrosarcoma protuberans. Semin Cutan Med Surg 1999;18:91–8.

77. Wilson Jones E, Cerio R, Smith NP. Epithelioid cell histiocytoma: a new entity. Br J Dermatol 1989;120:185–95.

78. Zelger BW, Steiner H, Kutzner H. Clear cell dermatofibroma. Case report of an unusual fibrohistiocytic lesion. Am J Surg Pathol 1996;20:483–91.

Atypical Fibroxanthoma

79. Abdelatif OM, Khankhanian NK, Crosby JH, Chamberlain CR, Seigler MM, Tom GD. Malignant fibrous histiocytoma and malignant melanoma: the role of immunohistochemistry and electron microscopy in the differential diagnosis. Mod Pathol 1989;2:477–85.

80. Calonje E, Wadden C, Wilson-Jones E, Fletcher CD. Spindle-cell non-pleomorphic atypical fibroxanthoma: analysis of a series and delineation of a distinctive variant. Histopathology 1993;22:247–54.

81. Chen KT. Atypical fibroxanthoma of the skin with osteoid production. Arch Dermatol 1980;116:113–4.

82. Dahl I. Atypical fibroxanthoma of the skin. A clinicopathological study of 57 cases. Acta Pathol Microbiol Scand [A] 1976;84:183–97.

83. Eckert F, Burg G, Braun-Falco O, Schmid U, Gloor F. Immunostaining in atypical fibroxanthoma of the skin. Pathol Res Pract 1989;184:27–34.

84. Eusebi V, Ceccarelli C, Piscioli F, Cristofolini M, Azzopardi JG. Spindle cell tumours of the skin of debatable origin. An immunocytochemical study. J Pathol 1984;144:189–99.

85. Evans HL, Smith JL. Spindle cell squamous carcinomas and sarcoma-like tumors of the skin. A comparative study of 38 cases. Cancer 1980;45:2687–97.

86. Facchetti F, Bertalot G, Grigolato PG. KP1 (CD68) staining of malignant melanomas. Histopathology 1991;19:141–5.

87. Finlay-Jones LR, Nicoll P, Ten Seldam RE. Pseudosarcoma of the skin. Pathology 1971;3:215–22.

88. Fretzin DF, Helwig EB. Atypical fibroxanthoma of the skin. A clinicopathologic study of 140 cases. Cancer 1973;31:1541–52.

89. Glavin FL, Cornwell ML. Atypical fibroxanthoma of the skin metastatic to a lung. Report of a case, features by conventional and electron microscopy, and a review of relevant literature. Am J Dermatopathol 1985;7:57–63.

90. Helwig EB. Tumor seminar. In: Proceedings of the 18th Annual Tumor Seminar presented by the San Antonio Society of Pathologists. Texas State J Med 1963;59:652–89.

91. Helwig EB, May D. Atypical fibroxanthoma of the skin with metastasis. Cancer 1986;57:368–76.

92. Jacobs DS, Edwards WD, Ye RC. Metastatic atypical fibroxanthoma of skin. Cancer 1975;35:457–63.

93. Kempson RL, McGavran MH. Atypical fibroxanthomas of the skin. Cancer 1964;17:1463–71.

94. Kroe DJ, Pitcock JA. Atypical fibroxanthoma of the skin. Report of ten cases. Am J Clin Pathol 1969;51:487–92.

95. Kuwano H, Hashimoto H, Enjoji M. Atypical fibroxanthoma distinguishable from spindle cell carcinoma in sarcoma-like skin lesions. A clinicopathologic and immunohistochemical study of 21 cases. Cancer 1985;55:172–80.

96. Leong AS, Milios J. Atypical fibroxanthoma of the skin: a clinicopathological and immunohistochemical study and a discussion of its histogenesis. Histopathology 1987;11:463–75.

97. Lodding P, Kindblom LG, Angervall L. Metastases of malignant melanoma simulating soft tissue sarcoma. A clinicopathological, light, and electron microscopic and immunohistochemical study of 21 cases. Virchows Arch [A] 1990;417:377–88.

98. Longacre TA, Smoller BR, Rouse RV. Atypical fibroxanthoma. Multiple immunologic profiles. Am J Surg Pathol 1993;17:1199–209.

99. Ma CK, Zarbo RJ, Gown AM. Immunohistochemical characterization of atypical fibroxanthoma and dermatofibrosarcoma protuberans. Am J Clin Pathol 1992;97:478–83.

100. McCalmont TH, Thompson CT. Ploidy analysis of atypical fibroxanthoma using thick section fluorescent in-situ hybridization (FISH) [Abstract]. Mod Pathol 1994;7:47A.

101. Pulford KA, Rigney EM, Micklem KJ, et al. KP1: a new monoclonal antibody that detects a monocyte/macrophage associated antigen in routinely processed tissue sections. J Clin Pathol 1989;42:414–21.

102. Ricci A, Cartun RW, Zakowski MF. Atypical fibroxanthoma. A study of 14 cases emphasizing the presence of Langerhans' histiocytes with implications for differential diagnosis by antibody panels. Am J Surg Pathol 1988;12:591–8.

103. Silvis NG, Swanson PE, Manivel JC, Kaye VN, Wick MR. Spindle-cell and pleomorphic neoplasms of the skin. A clinicopathologic and immunohistochemical study of 30 cases, with emphasis on "atypical fibroxanthoma." Am J Dermatopathol 1988;10:9–19.

104. Tsang WY, Chan JK. KP1 (CD68) staining of granular cell neoplasms: is KP1 a marker for lysosomes rather than the histiocytic lineage? Histopathology 1992;21:84–6.

105. Vargas-Cortes F, Winkelmann RK, Soule EH. Atypical fibroxanthomas of the skin. Further observations with 19 additional cases. Mayo Clin Proc 1973;48:211–8.

106. Weedon D, Kerr JF. Atypical fibroxanthoma of skin: an electron microscope study. Pathology 1975;7:173–7.

107. Wilson PR, Strutton GM, Stewart MR. Atypical fibroxanthoma: two unusual variants. J Cutan Pathol 1989;16:93–8.

108. Winkelmann RK, Peters MS. Atypical fibroxanthoma. A study with antibody to S-100 protein. Arch Dermatol 1985;121:753–5.

109. Worrell JT, Ansari MQ, Ansari SJ, Cockerell CJ. Atypical fibroxanthoma: DNA ploidy analysis of 14 cases with possible histogenetic implications. J Cutan Pathol 1993;20:211–5.

Dermatofibrosarcoma Protuberans

110. Abenoza P, Lillemoe T. CD34 and factor XIIIa in the differential diagnosis of dermatofibroma and dermatofibrosarcoma protuberans. Am J Surg Pathol 1993;17:429–34.

111. Aiba S, Tabata N, Ishii H, Ootani H, Tagami H. Dermatofibrosarcoma protuberans is a unique fibrohistiocytic tumour expressing CD34. Br J Dermatol 1992;127:79–84.

112. Alguacil-Garcia A, Unni KK, Goellner JR. Histogenesis of dermatofibrosarcoma protuberans. An ultrastructural study. Am J Clin Pathol 1978;69:427–34.

113. Azumi N, Rubin MA, Boyle L, Hartmann DP. Desmin, muscle-specific actin and alpha-smooth muscle actin expression in non-muscular sarcomas and sarcoma-like lesions [Abstract]. Mod Pathol 1994;7:4A.

114. Baer SC, Raymond AK, Ordonez NG. CD34 and factor XIIIa expression in dermatofibrosarcoma protuberans: specificity, sensitivity, and pattern of immunostaining [Abstract]. Mod Pathol 1994;7:44A.

115. Banerjee SS, Harris M, Eyden BP, Hamid BN. Granular cell variant of dermatofibrosarcoma protuberans. Histopathology 1990;17:375–8.

116. Beham A, Fletcher CD. Dermatofibrosarcoma protuberans with areas resembling giant cell fibroblastoma: report of two cases. Histopathology 1990;17:165–7.

117. Brenner W, Schaefler K, Chhabra H, Postel A. Dermatofibrosarcoma protuberans metastatic to a regional lymph node: report of a case and review. Cancer 1975;36:1897–902.

118. Bridge JA, Neff JR, Sandberg AA. Cytogenetic analysis of dermatofibrosarcoma protuberans. Cancer Genet Cytogenet 1990;49:199–202.

119. Burkhardt BR, Soule EH, Winkelmann RK, Ivins JC. Dermatofibrosarcoma protuberans: study of fifty-six cases. Am J Surg 1966;111:638–44.
120. Calonje E, Fletcher CD. Myoid differentiation in dermatofibrosarcoma protuberans and its fibrosarcomatous variant: clinicopathologic analysis of 5 cases. J Cutan Pathol 1996;23:30–6.
121. Connelly JH, Evans HL. Dermatofibrosarcoma protuberans: a clinicopathologic review with emphasis on fibrosarcomatous areas. Am J Surg Pathol 1992;16:921–5.
122. Dal Cin P, Sciot R, de Wever I, et al. Cytogenetic and immunohistochemical evidence that giant cell fibroblastoma is related to dermatofibrosarcoma protuberans. Genes Chrom Cancer 1996;15:73–5.
123. Ding J, Hashimoto H, Enjoji M. Dermatofibrosarcoma protuberans with fibrosarcomatous areas. A clinicopathologic study of nine cases and a comparison with allied tumors. Cancer 1989;64:721–9.
124. Ding J, Hashimoto H, Sugimoto T, Tsuneyoshi M, Enjoji M. Bednar tumor (pigmented dermatofibrosarcoma protuberans): an analysis of six cases. Acta Pathol Jpn 1990;40:744–54.
125. Dupree WB, Langloss JM, Weiss SW. Pigmented dermatofibrosarcoma protuberans (Bednar tumor): a pathologic, ultrastructural, and immunohistochemical study. Am J Surg Pathol 1985;9:630–9.
126. Eisen RN, Tallini G. Metastatic dermatofibrosarcoma protuberans with fibrosarcomatous change in the absence of local recurrence. A case report of simultaneous occurrence with a malignant giant cell tumor of soft parts. Cancer 1993;72:462–8.
127. Fletcher CD, Evans BJ, Macartney JC, Smith N, Wilson Jones E, McKee PH. Dermatofibrosarcoma protuberans: a clinicopathological and immunohistochemical study with a review of the literature. Histopathology 1985;9:921–38.
128. Fletcher CD, Theaker JM, Flanagan A, Krausz T. Pigmented dermatofibrosarcoma protuberans (Bednar tumor): melanocytic colonization or neuroectodermal differentiation? A clinicopathological and immunohistochemical study. Histopathology 1988;13:631–43.
129. Frierson HF, Cooper PH. Myxoid variant of dermatofibrosarcoma protuberans. Am J Surg Pathol 1983;7:445–50.
130. Goldblum JR. CD34 positivity in fibrosarcomas which arise in dermatofibrosarcoma protuberans. Arch Pathol Lab Med 1995;119:238–41.
130a. Harvell JD, Kilpatrick SE, White WL. Histogenetic relations between giant cell fibroblastoma and dermatofibrosarcoma protuberans. Am J Dermatopathol 1998;20:339–45.
131. Hsi ED, Nickoloff BJ. Dermatofibroma (DF) and dermatofibrosarcoma protuberans (DFSP): an immunohistochemical study reveals distinctive antigenic profiles [Abstract]. Mod Pathol 1994;7:46A.
132. Kahn LB, Saxe N, Gordon W. Dermatofibrosarcoma protuberans with lymph node and pulmonary metastases. Arch Dermatol 1978;114:599–601.
133. Kamino H, Jacobson M. Dermatofibroma extending into the subcutaneous tissue: differential diagnosis from dermatofibrosarcoma protuberans. Am J Surg Pathol 1990;14:1156–64.
134. Kamino H, McDonagh D, Burchette JL, Tam ST. Collagenous variant of dermatofibrosarcoma protuberans [Abstract]. Mod Pathol 1994;7:46A.
135. Kutzner H. Expression of the human progenitor cell antigen CD34 (HPCA-1) distinguishes dermatofibrosarcoma protuberans from fibrous histiocytoma in formalin-fixed, paraffin-embedded tissue. J Am Acad Dermatol 1993;28:613–7.
136. Lautier R, Wolff HH, Jones RE. An immunohistochemical study of dermatofibrosarcoma protuberans supports its fibroblastic character and contradicts neuroectodermal or histiocytic components. Am J Dermatopathol 1990;12:25–30.
137. McKee PH, Fletcher CD. Dermatofibrosarcoma protuberans presenting in infancy and childhood. J Cutan Pathol 1991;18:241–6.
138. McPeak CJ, Cruz T, Nicastri AD. Dermatofibrosarcoma protuberans: an analysis of 86 cases–five with metastases. Ann Surg 1967;166:803–16.
138a. Mentzel T, Beham A, Katenkamp D, Dei Tos AP, Fletcher CD. Fibrosarcomatous ("high-grade") dermatofibrosarcoma protuberans: clinicopathologic and immunohistochemical study of a series of 41 cases with emphasis on prognostic significance. Am J Surg Pathol 1998;22:576–87.
139. Minoletti F, Miozzo M, Pedeutour F, et al. Involvement of chromosomes 17 and 22 in dermatofibrosarcoma protuberans. Genes Chromo Cancer 1995;13:62–5.
140. Naeem R, Lux ML, Huang SF, Naber SP, Corson JM, Fletcher JA. Ring chromosomes in dermatofibrosarcoma protuberans are composed of interspersed sequences from chromosomes 17 and 22. Am J Pathol 1995;147:1553–8.
141. O'Dowd J, Laidler P. Progression of dermatofibrosarcoma protuberans to malignant fibrous histiocytoma: report of a case with implications for tumor histogenesis. Hum Pathol 1988;19:368–70.
142. Onoda N, Tsutsumi Y, Kakudo K, et al. Pigmented dermatofibrosarcoma protuberans (Bednar tumor): an autopsy case with systemic metastasis. Acta Pathol Jpn 1990;40:935–40.
143. Patil PK, Patel SG, Krishnamurthy S, Mistry RC, Deshpande RK, Desai PB. Dermatofibrosarcoma protuberans metastatic to the lung. A case report. Tumori 1992;78:49–51.
144. Pedeutour F, Coindre JM, Nicolo G, Bouchot C, Ayraud N, Turc Carel C. Ring chromosomes in dermatofibrosarcoma protuberans contain chromosome 17 sequences: fluorescence in situ hybridization. Cancer Genet Cytogenet 1993;67:149.
145. Roses DF, Valensi Q, LaTrenta G, Harris MN. Surgical treatment of dermatofibrosarcoma protuberans. Surg Gynecol Obstet 1986;162:449–52.
146. Rubin B, Fletcher J, Fletcher C. The histologic, genetic, and biological relationships between dermatofibrosarcoma protuberans and giant cell fibroblastoma: an unexpected story. Advances in Anatomic Pathology 1997;4:336–41.
147. Rutgers EJ, Kroon BB, Albus-Lutter CE, Gortzak E. Dermatofibrosarcoma protuberans: treatment and prognosis. Eur J Surg Oncol 1992;18:241–8.
148. Simon MP, Pedeutour F, Sirvent N, Grosgeorge J, et al. Deregulation of the platelet-derived growth factor B-chain gene via fusion with collagen gene COL1A1 in dermatofibrosarcoma protuberans and giant-cell fibroblastoma. Nat Genet 1997;15:95–8.
149. Smola MG, Soyer HP, Scharnagl E. Surgical treatment of dermatofibrosarcoma protuberans: a retrospective study of 20 cases with review of literature. Eur J Surg Oncol 1991;17:447–53.

150. Stephenson CF, Berger CS, Leong SP, Davis JR, Sandberg AA. Ring chromosome in a dermatofibrosarcoma protuberans. Cancer Genet Cytogenet 1992;58:52–4.
151. Taylor HB, Helwig EB. Dermatofibrosarcoma protuberans: a study of 115 cases. Cancer 1962;15:717–25.
152. van de Rijn M, Rouse RV. CD34: a review. Appl Immunohistochem 1994;2:71–80.
153. Wrotnowski U, Cooper PH, Shmookler BM. Fibrosarcomatous change in dermatofibrosarcoma protuberans. Am J Surg Pathol 1988;12:287–93.

Giant Cell Fibroblastoma

154. Abdul-Karim FW, Evans HL, Silva EG. Giant cell fibroblastoma: a report of three cases. Am J Clin Pathol 1985;83:165–70.
155. Alguacil-Garcia A. Giant cell fibroblastoma recurring as dermatofibrosarcoma protuberans. Am J Surg Pathol 1991;15:798–801.
156. Beham A, Fletcher CD. Dermatofibrosarcoma protuberans with areas resembling giant cell fibroblastoma: report of two cases. Histopathology 1990;17:165–7.
157. Chou P, Gonzalez-Crussi G, Mangkornikanok M. Giant cell fibroblastoma. Cancer 1989;63:756 62.
158. Coyne J, Kaftan SM, Craig RD. Dermatofibrosarcoma protuberans recurring as a giant cell fibroblastoma. Histopathology 1992;21:184–7.
158a. Dal Cin P, Sciot R, de Wever I, et al. Cytogenetic and immunohistochemical evidence that giant cell fibroblastoma is related to dermatofibrosarcoma protuberans. Genes Chrom Cancer 1996;15:73–5.
159. De Chadarévian J, Coppola D, Billmire DF. Bednar tumor pattern in recurring giant cell fibroblastoma. Am J Clin Pathol 1993;100:164–6.
160. Dymock RB, Allen PW, Stirling JW, Gilbert EF, Thornbery JM. Giant cell fibroblastoma. A distinctive, recurrent tumor of childhood. Am J Surg Pathol 1987;11:263–71.
161. Fletcher CD. Giant cell fibroblastoma of soft tissue: a clinicopathological and immunohistochemical study. Histopathology 1988;13:499–508.
161a. Harvell JD, Kilpatrick SE, White WL. Histogenetic relations between giant cell fibroblastoma and dermatofibrosarcoma protuberans. Am J Dermatopathol 1998;20:339–45.
162. Hirose T, Sasaki M, Shintaku M, et al. Giant cell fibroblastoma: a case report. Acta Pathol Jpn 1990;40:540–4.
163. Kanai Y, Mukai M, Sugiura H, et al. Giant cell fibroblastoma: a case report and immunohistochemical comparison with ten cases of dermatofibrosarcoma protuberans. Acta Pathol Jpn 1991;41:552–60.
164. Michal M, Zamecnik M. Giant cell fibroblastoma with a dermatofibrosarcoma protuberans component. Am J Dermatol 1992;14:549–52.
164a. Minoletti F, Miozzo M, Pedeutour F, et al. Involvement of chromosomes 17 and 22 in dermatofibrosarcoma protuberans. Genes Chromo Cancer 1995;13:62–5.
164b. Rubin B, Fletcher J, Fletcher C. The histologic, genetic, and biological relationships between dermatofibrosarcoma protuberans and giant cell fibroblastoma: an unexpected story. Advances in Anatomic Pathology 1997;4:336–41.
165. Shmookler BM, Enzinger FM. Giant cell fibroblastoma. A juvenile form of dermatofibrosarcoma protuberans. Cancer 1989;64:2154–61.
166. Simon MP, Pedeutour F, Sirvent N, et al. Deregulation of the platelet-derived growth factor B-chain gene via fusion with collagen gene COL1A1 in dermatofibrosarcoma protuberans and giant-cell fibroblastoma. Nat Genet 1997;15:95–8.
167. Suster S, Rosai J. Hamartoma of the scalp with ectopic meningothelial elements: a distinctive benign soft tissue lesion that may simulate angiosarcoma. Am J Surg Pathol 1990;14:1–11.

Plexiform Fibrous Histiocytoma

168. Enzinger FM, Zhang R. Plexiform fibrohistiocytic tumor presenting in children and young adults. An analysis of 65 cases. Am J Surg Pathol 1988;12:818–26.
169. Giard F, Bonneau R, Raymond GP. Plexiform fibrohistiocytic tumor. Dermatologica 1991;183:290–3.
170. Hollowood K, Holley MP, Fletcher CD. Plexiform fibrohistiocytic tumour: clinicopathological, immunohistochemical and ultrastructural analysis in favour of a myofibroblastic lesion. Histopathology 1991;19:503–13.
171. Remstein ED, Arndt CA, Nascimento AG. Plexiform fibrohistiocytic tumor: clinicopathologic analysis of 22 cases. Am J Surg Pathol 1999;23:662–70.
172. Salomao D, Nascimento A. Plexiform fibrohistiocytic tumor with systemic metasases—a case report. Am J Surg Pathol 1997;21:469–76.
173. Smith S, Fletcher CD, Smith MA, Gusterson BA. Cytogenetic analysis of a plexiform fibrohistiocytic tumor. Cancer Genet Cytogenet 1990;48:31–4.

Angiomatoid Fibrous Histiocytoma

174. Argenyi ZB, Van Rybroek JJ, Kemp JD, Soper RT. Congenital angiomatoid malignant fibrous histiocytoma. A light-microscopic, immunopathologic, and electron-microscopic study. Pediatr Dermatopathol 1988;10:59–67.
175. Costa MJ, Weiss SW. Angiomatoid malignant fibrous histiocytoma: a follow-up study of 108 cases with evaluation of possible histologic predictors of outcome. Am J Surg Pathol 1990;14:1126–32.
176. El-Naggar AK, Ro JY, Ayala AG, Hinchey WW, Abdul-Karim FW, Batsakis JG. Angiomatoid malignant fibrous histiocytoma: flow cytometric DNA analysis of six cases. J Surg Oncol 1989;40:201–4.
177. Enzinger FM. Angiomatoid malignant fibrous histiocytoma: a distinct fibrohistiocytic tumor of children and young adults simulating a vascular neoplasm. Cancer 1979;44:2147–57.
178. Fletcher CD. Angiomatoid fibrous histiocytoma [Letter]. Am J Surg Pathol 1992;16:426–7.

179. Fletcher CD. Angiomatoid "malignant fibrous histiocytoma": an immunohistochemical study indicative of myoid differentiation. Hum Pathol 1991;22:563–8.

180. Pettinato G, Manivel JC, De Rosa G, Petrella G, Jaszcz W. Angiomatoid malignant fibrous histiocytoma: cytologic, immunohistochemical, ultrastructural, and flow cytometric study of 20 cases. Mod Pathol 1990;3:479–87.

181. Seo IS, Frizzera G, Coates TD, Mirkin LD, Cohen MD. Angiomatoid malignant fibrous histiocytoma with extensive lymphadenopathy simulating Castleman's disease. Pediatr Pathol 1986;6:233–47.

182. Smith ME, Costa MJ, Weiss SW. Evaluation of CD68 and other histiocytic antigens in angiomatoid malignant fibrous histiocytoma. Am J Surg Pathol 1991;15:757–63.

183. Wegmann W, Heitz PU. Angiomatoid malignant fibrous histiocytoma: evidence for the histiocytic origin of tumor cells. Virchows Arch [A] 1985;406:59–66.

Pleomorphic Malignant Fibrous Histiocytoma

184. Ariel IM. Incidence of metastases to lymph nodes from soft-tissue sarcomas. Semin Surg Oncol 1988;4:27–9.

185. Becker RL, Venzon D, Lack EE, Mikel UV, Weiss SW, O'Leary TJ. Cytometry and morphometry of malignant fibrous histiocytoma of the extremities. Prediction of metastasis and mortality. Am J Surg Pathol 1991;15:957–64.

186. Berth-Jones J, Fletcher A, Graham-Brown R. Cutaneous malignant fibrous histiocytoma. A rare but serious malignancy. Acta Derm Venereol 1990;70:254–6.

187. Bertoni F, Capanna R, Biagini R, et al. Malignant fibrous histiocytoma of soft tissue. An analysis of 78 cases located and deeply seated in the extremities. Cancer 1985;56:356–67.

188. Bhagavan BS, Dorfman HD. The significance of bone and cartilage formation in malignant fibrous histiocytoma of soft tissue. Cancer 1982;49:480–8.

189. Binder SW, Said JW, Shintaku IP, Pinkus GS. A histiocyte-specific marker in the diagnosis of malignant fibrous histiocytoma. Use of monoclonal antibody KP-1 (CD68). Am J Clin Pathol 1992;97:759–63.

190. De Bruin MJ, Pelger RC, Meijer WS, Giard RW. Malignant fibrous histiocytoma of the spermatic cord. J Urol 1989;142:131–3.

191. Ekfors TO, Rantakokko V. An analysis of 38 malignant fibrous histiocytomas in the extremities. Acta Pathol Microbiol Scand [A] 1978;86:25–35.

192. Enjoji M, Hashimoto H, Tsuneyoshi M, Iwasaki H. Malignant fibrous histiocytoma. A clinicopathologic study of 130 cases. Acta Pathol Jpn 1980;30:727–41.

193. Enzinger FM. Malignant fibrous histiocytoma 20 years after Stout. Am J Surg Pathol 1986;10:43–53.

194. Fletcher CD. Pleomorphic malignant fibrous histiocytoma: fact or fiction? A critical reappraisal based on 159 tumors diagnosed as pleomorphic sarcoma. Am J Surg Pathol 1992;16:213–28.

195. Fletcher CD. Soft tissue sarcomas apparently arising in chronic tropical ulcers. Histopathology 1987;11:501–10.

196. Goette DK, Deffer TA. Postirradiation malignant fibrous histiocytoma. Arch Dermatol 1985;121:535–8.

197. Hirose T, Kudo E, Hasegawa T, Abe J, Hizawa K. Expression of intermediate filaments in malignant fibrous histiocytomas. Hum Pathol 1989;20:871–7.

198. Iwasaki H, Yoshitake K, Ohjimi Y, et al. Malignant fibrous histiocytoma. Proliferative compartment and heterogeneity of "histiocytic" cells. Am J Surg Pathol 1992;16:735–45.

199. Kearney MM, Soule EH, Ivins JC. Malignant fibrous histiocytoma: a retrospective study of 167 cases. Cancer 1980;45:167–78.

200. Kempson RL, Kyriakos M. Fibroxanthosarcoma of the soft tissues. A type of malignant fibrous histiocytoma. Cancer 1972;29:961–76.

201. Lattes R. Malignant fibrous histiocytoma. A review article. Am J Surg Pathol 1982;6:761–71.

202. Lawson CW, Fisher C, Gatter KC. An immunohistochemical study of differentiation in malignant fibrous histiocytoma. Histopathology 1987;11:375–83.

203. Lodding P, Kindblom LG, Angervall L. Metastases of malignant melanoma simulating soft tissue sarcoma: a clinicopathological, light and electron microscopic and immunohistochemical study of 21 cases. Virchows Arch [A] 1990;417:377–88.

204. Mandahl N, Heim S, Arheden K, Rydholm A, Willén H, Mitelman F. Rings, dicentrics, and telomeric association in histiocytomas. Cancer Genet Cytogenet 1988;30:23–33.

205. Meister P. Malignant fibrous histiocytoma. History, histology, histogenesis. Pathol Res Pract 1988;183:1–7.

206. Miettinen M, Soini Y. Malignant fibrous histiocytoma. Heterogeneous patterns of intermediate filament proteins by immunohistochemistry. Arch Pathol Lab Med 1989;113:1363–6.

207. Molenaar WM, DeJong B, Buist J, et al. Chromosomal analysis and the classification of soft tissue sarcomas. Lab Invest 1989;60:266–74.

208. Nemes Z, Thomazy V. Factor XIIIa and the classic histiocytic markers in malignant fibrous histiocytoma: a comparative immunohistochemical study. Hum Pathol 1988;19:822–9.

209. Örndal C, Mandahl N, Carlén B, et al. Near-haploid clones in a malignant fibrous histiocytoma. Cancer Genet Cytogenet 1992;60:147–51.

210. Pezzi CM, Rawlings MS, Esgro JJ, Pollock RE, Romsdahl MM. Prognostic factors in 227 patients with malignant fibrous histiocytoma. Cancer 1992;69:2098–103.

211. Rydholm A, Syk I. Malignant fibrous histiocytoma of soft tissue: correlation between clinical variables and histologic malignancy grade. Cancer 1986;57:2323–4.

212. Stenfert Kroese MC, Rutgers DH, Wils IS, van Unnik JA, Rohol PJ. The relevance of the DNA index and proliferation rate in the grading of benign and malignant soft tissue tumors. Cancer 1990;65:1782–8.

213. Tracy T, Neifeld JP, DeMay RM, Salzberg AM. Malignant fibrous histiocytomas in children. J Pediatr Surg 1984;19:81–3.

214. Weiss SW. Malignant fibrous histiocytoma. A reaffirmation. Am J Surg Pathol 1982;6:773–84.

215. Weiss SW, Enzinger FM. Malignant fibrous histiocytoma: an analysis of 200 cases. Cancer 1978;41:2250–66.

216. Wood GS, Beckstead JH, Turner RR, Hendrickson MR, Kempson RL, Warnke RA. Malignant fibrous histiocytoma tumor cells resemble fibroblasts. Am J Surg Pathol 1986;10:323–35.

217. Zehr RJ, Bauer TW, Marks KE, Weltevreden A. Ki-67 and grading of malignant fibrous histiocytomas. Cancer 1990;66:1984–90.

218. Zuppan CW, Mierau GW, Wilson HL. Malignant fibrous histiocytoma in childhood: a report of two cases and review of the literature. Pediatr Pathol 1987;7:303–18.

Myxoid Variant, Malignant Fibrous Histiocytoma (Myxofibrosarcoma)

219. Angervall L, Kindblom LG, Merck C. Myxofibrosarcoma. A study of 30 cases. Acta Pathol Microbiol Scand 1977;85:127–40.

220. Enzinger RM, Weiss SW. Soft tissue tumors. 3rd edition. St. Louis: Mosby, 1995.

220a.Evans HL. Low-grade fibromyxoid sarcoma. A report of 12 cases. Am J Surg Pathol 1993;17:595–600.

221. Kindblom LG, Merck C, Angervall L. The ultrastructure of myxofibrosarcoma. A study of 11 cases. Virchows Arch [A] 1979;381:121–39.

222. Kindblom LG, Merck C, Svendsen P. Myxofibrosarcoma: a pathologico-anatomical, microangiographic and angiographic correlative study of eight cases. Br J Radiol 1977;50:876–87.

223. Lagacé R, Delage C, Seemayer TA. Myxoid variant of malignant fibrous histiocytoma: ultrastructural observations. Cancer 1979;43:526–34.

224. Mackenzie DH. The myxoid tumors of somatic soft tissues. Am J Surg Pathol 1981;5:443–58.

225. Mentzel T, Calonje E, Wadden C, et al. Myxofibrosarcoma. Clinicopathologic analysis of 75 cases with emphasis on the low-grade variant. Am J Surg Pathol 1996;20:391–405.

226. Merck C, Angervall L, Kindblom LG, Odén A. Myxofibrosarcoma. A malignant soft tissue tumor of fibroblastic-histiocytic origin. A clinicopathologic and prognostic study of 110 cases using multivariate analysis. Acta Pathol Microbiol Immunol Scand 1983;91:3–40.

227. Montgomery EA, Laskin WB, Ayala GE, Aaron AD, Azumi N. Myxoid malignant fibrous histiocytoma: an aggressive neoplasm [Abstract]. Mod Pathol 1994;7:9A.

228. Orndal C, Mandahl N, Rydholm A, et al. Supernumerary ring chromosomes in five bone and soft tissue tumors of low or borderline malignancy. Cancer Genet Cytogenet 1992;60:170–5.

229. Weiss SW, Enzinger FM. Myxoid variant of malignant fibrous histiocytoma. Cancer 1977;39:1672–85.

Giant Cell Variant, Malignant Fibrous Histiocytoma

230. Angervall L, Hagmar B, Kindblom LG, Merck C. Malignant giant cell tumor of soft tissues. A clinicopathologic, cytologic, ultrastructural, angiographic, and microangiographic study. Cancer 1981;47:736–47.

230a.Folpe A, Morris RJ, Weiss SW. Soft tissue giant cell tumour of low malignant potential: a proposal for the reclassification of malignant giant cell tumour of soft parts. Mod Pathol 1999;12:894–902.

231. Guccion JG, Enzinger FM. Malignant giant cell tumor of soft parts. An analysis of 32 cases. Cancer 1972;29:1518–29.

232. Mentzel T, Calonje E, Fletcher CD. Leiomyosarcoma with prominent osteoclast-like giant cells. Analysis of eight cases closely mimicking the so-called giant cell variant of malignant fibrous histiocytoma. Am J Surg Pathol 1994;18:258–65.

233. Nascimento AG. Giant cell tumors of soft parts [Abstract]. Mod Pathol 1993;6:9A.

233a.Oliveira AM, Dei Tos AP, Fletcher CD, Nascimento AG. Primary giant cell tumor of soft tissues: a study of 22 cases. Am J Surg Pathol 2000;24:248–56.

Inflammatory Variant, Malignant Fibrous Histiocytoma

234. Kahn LB. Retroperitoneal xanthogranuloma and xanthosarcoma (malignant fibrous xanthoma). Cancer 1973;31:411–22.

235. Kay S. Inflammatory fibrous histiocytoma (? xanthogranuloma). Report of two cases with ultrastructural observations in one. Am J Surg Pathol 1978;2:313–9.

236. Kyriakos M, Kempson RL. Inflammatory fibrous histiocytoma. An aggressive and lethal lesion. Cancer 1976;37:1584–606.

237. Merino MJ, LiVolsi VA. Inflammatory malignant fibrous histiocytoma. Am J Clin Pathol 1980;73:276–81.

238. Nistal M, Regadera J, Jareño E, Paniagua R. Inflammatory malignant fibrous histiocytoma of the spermatic cord. Urol Int 1988;43:188–92.

239. Papadimitriou JA, Matz LR. Retroperitoneal xanthogranuloma. A case report with electron microscopic observations. Arch Pathol 1967;83:535–42.

❖❖❖

4
LIPOMATOUS TUMORS

INTRODUCTION

In order for a tumor to be classified as being of adipose tissue type, at least some of the constituent neoplastic cells must demonstrate fatty differentiation manifested by vacuolated clear cytoplasm resulting from lipid accumulation. The cytoplasmic vacuoles, which may be single or multiple, must be clear and sharply delimited and bulge against or distort the nucleus in order to be recognized as lipidic (5). In mature adipocytes, as in non-neoplastic fat, lipomas, and some other types of fatty tumors, the cytoplasmic lipid, in a large single vacuole, pushes the nucleus to the edge of the cell and deforms it into a thin crescent. Adipocytes in lipogenic neoplasms (both malignant and benign) other than lipoma may have a larger central or peripheral nucleus, which characteristically is indented by one or more fat vacuoles in such a way that spikes of chromatin project between the fatty vacuoles. These cells, most often termed "lipoblasts," usually are smaller than mature lipocytes and their lipid vacuoles tend to be smaller. It is unusual for non-neoplastic fat to contain lipoblasts, so they are useful markers of tumorous fatty differentiation; however, lipoblasts can be found in some non-neoplastic lesions such as fat necrosis and lipogranulomas. Because many different types of cells in the soft tissues have vacuolated cytoplasm, nuclear deformation by one or more sharply marginated clear vacuoles is required before a cell is deemed to demonstrate lipidic differentiation. We have found fat stains to be technically unreliable and we do not use them; rather, lipidic cells are recognized by their clear cytoplasmic vacuoles as described above.

Mimics of lipogenic cells include histiocytes (the nucleus is usually central and not deformed and vacuoles are characteristically small; fig. 4-1), metastatic signet ring carcinoma cells (mucin and keratin stains are most often helpful), the cells of clear cell melanoma (S-100 protein and HMB45 stains are positive; be careful, fat cells are also S-100 protein positive), and mesenchymal cells producing cytoplasmic acid mucopolysaccharide (the nucleus is usually not deformed, the vacu-oles are not completely clear and empty; rather they may have the tinctorial qualities of the surrounding stroma and Alcian blue stains may be positive). If any of these cells are interpreted as lipogenic, the lesion of which they are a part may well be misdiagnosed as a fatty tumor. Another trap also awaits the diagnostic pathologist: normal fat infiltrated by a nonfatty neoplasm. When this occurs, the non-neoplastic fat cells can appear to be a part of the neoplasm at first glance. In most instances, non-neoplastic fat cells are found at the periphery, not the center, of nonfatty tumors and usually the fat cells in fatty tumors are smaller than normal fat cells. Attention to the location of the adipocytes and awareness of the morphologic features of fatty tumors almost always allow correct interpretation.

The classification and nomenclature of adipose tissue tumors are in a state of flux because of controversy concerning the status of the terms "well-differentiated liposarcoma" and "round cell liposarcoma" (1,6,8,16,17,24). We suggest the

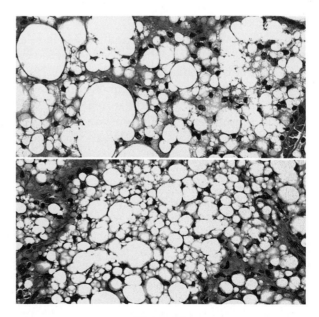

Figure 4-1
SILICONE GRANULOMA
Fat necrosis and foreign material can cause histiocytes to closely resemble neoplastic lipoblasts.

Table 4-1

COMPARISON OF WHO AND THE AUTHORS' CLASSIFICATION OF LIPOMATOUS TUMORS

WHO	Classification Used in this Fascicle
Benign	**Benign (Managerial Groups Ia and Ib, Table 1-10)**
Lipoma	Lipoma
Lipoblastoma	Lipoblastoma
Lipomatosis	Lipomatosis
Angiolipoma	Angiolipoma
Spindle cell/pleomorphic lipoma	Spindle cell/pleomorphic lipoma
Angiomyolipoma	Angiomyolipoma
Myelolipoma	Myelolipoma
Hibernoma	Hibernoma
Atypical lipoma	Chondroid lipoma
	Myolipoma
	Subcutaneous atypical lipomatous tumor
Intermediate	**Intermediate (Managerial Groups IIa, IIb, and IIc, Table 1-10)**
None	Atypical lipomatous tumors located in sites other than the subcutaneous tissue
Malignant	**Malignant (Managerial Group III, Table 1-10)**
Well-differentiated liposarcoma	Dedifferentiated liposarcoma
Lipoma-like	Myxoid liposarcoma
Sclerosing	Paucicellular
Inflammatory	Cellular
Myxoid liposarcoma	Pleomorphic liposarcoma
Round cell (poorly differentiated myxoid) liposarcoma	Unclassified liposarcoma
Pleomorphic liposarcoma	
Dedifferentiated liposarcoma	

term "atypical lipomatous tumor" (7) for neoplasms that in the past have been classified as well-differentiated liposarcoma (Table 4-1). Our reasons for this are presented more fully in the sections of this chapter devoted to atypical lipomatous tumors and dedifferentiated liposarcomas. Briefly, we think the atypical lipomatous tumor terminology is more appropriate because these neoplasms do not metastasize and because they cause death very rarely if at all unless located in the retroperitoneum or another central body site in close proximity to vital structures. Atypical lipomatous tumors can become dedifferentiated, i.e., develop a component of cellular, nonlipogenic sarcoma with metastatic capability, and we recognize this occurrence with the term "dedifferentiated liposarcoma" (this happens most often in the retroperitoneum). We think it best not to use the term sarcoma until dedifferentiation has occurred and the tumor develops metastatic capability.

A second area of controversy concerns the category of round cell liposarcoma. We think there is compelling histologic and cytogenetic evidence that most of the tumors that have been labeled as such are in fact cellular myxoid liposarcomas (1,6,7,9). For this reason, we do not think round cell liposarcoma should be considered a separate neoplasm (Table 4-1).

Immunohistochemistry has some use in the diagnosis of adipose tissue tumors. Normal fat cells and the lipidic cells in many fatty tumors express S-100 protein. Generally, S-100 protein is only positive in those cells having obvious (cytoplasmic) adipocytic differentiation, and not "prelipoblastic" or undifferentiated/pleomorphic cells in an adipocytic neoplasm, although it may stain some cells without fat vacuoles in myxoid liposarcoma (3,4,11). CD34 strongly stains the spindle cells in spindle cell lipoma and marks a network of spindle cells in ordinary lipomas, myxoid liposarcomas, and atypical lipomatous tumors (21). It also stains the atypical and floret cells in atypical lipomatous tumors and pleomorphic lipomas. Of course, immunohistochemistry may be useful in excluding other neoplasms that mimic lipomatous tumors such as metastatic carcinoma, balloon cell melanoma, and signet ring cell lymphoma. Electron microscopy practically never has a role in the diagnosis of fatty tumors. Most investigators report ultrastructural evidence of lipomatous differentiation when fatty tumors are examined with the electron microscope (2,10,12,13,18,20,22,23), but the lipid vacuoles that identify these tumors can almost always be discerned by light microscopy. Even if fatty differentiation is questionable by light microscopy, alternative diagnoses rarely have sufficient effect on therapy or prognosis to justify the cost of electron microscopy (this is especially true of pleomorphic liposarcoma, where the problem usually arises). Imaging studies provide helpful clues that a mass may be composed, at least partially, of fat cells, but histologic diagnosis is still required (14,15). Nonrandom cytogenetic alterations have been reported in some fatty tumors and may prove to be of diagnostic importance in the future (9,19). These are summarized in the descriptions of the individual tumor types.

The following discussion of the fatty tumors is organized according to the classification presented in Table 4-1.

BENIGN LIPOMATOUS TUMORS (MANAGERIAL GROUPS Ia AND Ib, TABLE 1-10)

Lipoma

Definition. A lipoma is a tumor mass composed of mature adipocytes with uniform nuclei identical to the cells that form normal adult fat.

General Considerations. Whether lipoma is a benign neoplasm, a local hyperplasia of fat cells, or both, is uncertain. Published reports indicate that clonal chromosomal abnormalities are present in about half of the over 250 lipomas studied, suggesting that at least some lipomas are neoplasms. The majority of these rearrangements have involved regions 13–15 on the long arm of chromosome 12, while a minority of the lipomas with chromosomal abnormalities have rearrangements involving chromosomes other than 12 (39,

48,58). If fibrous tissue or a myxoid stroma is focally present within a lipoma the terms fibrolipoma or myxolipoma are sometimes applied but the tumor is still considered to be a form of lipoma. If other types of tissue are present within a lipoma they are not only named along with lipoma but many such lesions are classified as separate tumors, e.g., angiolipoma, chondroid lipoma.

Clinical Features. Lipoma is by far the most common soft tissue tumor, and most occur in older adults, without any clear sex or race predilection (50). The usual lipoma is subcutaneous and most commonly located on the back, shoulder, neck, abdomen, or proximal extremities (50, 55). Lipomas are uncommon on the hands, distal extremities, and feet (52). Lipomas usually present as slowly growing, soft, asymptomatic masses, and demonstrate fat density on computerized tomography (CT) scans. They rarely contain bone (49, 52). Local recurrence or regrowth occurs occasionally after excision but is uncommon. Some patients have multiple lipomas, which may be familial. The occurrence of multiple lipomas, macrocephaly, and hemangiomas is known as the *Bannayan syndrome* (26).

Less commonly, lipomas occur in nonsubcutaneous locations, and some of these are identified by adding the site or the growth pattern to the term lipoma. These are summarized in Table 4-2. Among the more common of these is *intramuscular lipoma,* which develops within skeletal muscles (25,27,31,35,44). Intramuscular lipoma is usually found in adults but occasionally is discovered in children. It is more common in males than females, and most often develops in the large muscles of the extremities, especially the thigh, shoulder, and upper arm, although it does occur on the trunk and rarely in other muscles (30,36). Intramuscular lipomas range from small to large, are usually slow growing, and may become more prominent when the muscle is contracted. CT scans reveal an intramuscular mass with the density of fat. Most larger series report a local recurrence rate that varies from 0 to 20 percent (34,35,44). One of the lowest reported recurrence rates, 3 percent, was in a series where special attention was given to wide excision (44). Fletcher and Martin-Bates (35) have reported a higher recurrence rate for infiltrating tumors than circumscribed ones (19 percent versus 0 percent).

Table 4-2

LIPOMAS WITH UNUSUAL CLINICAL FEATURES

Tumor	Clinical Features
Intramuscular lipoma	Location within muscle; when vessels are prominent, tumor is classified as intramuscular hemangioma even though a fatty component is present
Intermuscular lipoma	In deep soft tissues between muscle
Fibrolipomatous hamartoma of nerve (neural fibrolipoma)	Fibrolipomatous mass infiltrating large nerve, usually the median nerve; often associated with macrodactyly
Nerve sheath lipoma	Circumscribed; does not infiltrate nerve bundles
Diffuse lipomatosis	Diffuse nonlocalized overgrowth of fatty tissue affecting a portion of trunk or limb; involves subcutaneous tissue and muscle but not nerves; diffuse growth distinguishes it from intramuscular lipoma
Nevus lipomatosus superficialis	Overgrowth of fat in the dermis; when confluent and linear can result in "Michelin tire man" syndrome
"Lipoma arborescens"	Overgrowth of fat in subsynovial tissue of a joint, almost always a large joint; results in villous projections of fatty tissue
Lipoma of tendon sheath	Discrete fatty mass attached to tendon sheath
Lumbosacral lipoma	Diffuse overgrowth of fat over lumbosacral spine; always associated with spina bifida or laminar defect and may be connected to spinal cord
Pelvic lipomatosis	Overgrowth of fat in perirectal and perivesical region; may involve retroperitoneum and mesentery; must be distinguished from atypical lipomatous tumor (well-differentiated liposarcoma) (see text)
Symmetrical lipomatosis (Madelung's disease)	Large symmetrical masses of fatty tissue usually in neck or upper trunk; usually affects middle-aged men, often with alcoholism or metabolic disorders
Adiposis dolorosa (Dercum's disease)	Tender or painful fatty masses in subcutaneous tissue of pelvic region and thigh; most frequent in peri- and postmenopausal women
Multiple lipomas	May be familial
Bannayan syndrome	Multiple lipomas, macrocephaly, and hemangiomas

Intermuscular lipoma is less common than intramuscular lipoma. By definition, the tumor does not involve skeletal muscle, rather it lies between muscles (35,44). The recurrence rate is essentially zero if the lesion is completely excised.

Fibrolipomatous hamartoma of nerve (*neural fibrolipoma, intraneural lipoma, perineural lipoma*) is a fibrolipomatous mass surrounding, infiltrating, and extending along a portion of a major nerve (51,57). It almost always occurs in persons under 30 years of age and is sometimes found at birth. By far the most common site of involvement is the median nerve, typically in the area of the hand, wrist, and forearm. The ulnar nerve and other nerves, including those of the feet, are occasionally affected. Neural fibrolipoma characteristically presents as a slowly growing mass, usually causing pain, tenderness, decreased sensation, paresthesia, or loss of strength. In approximately one third of cases it is accompanied by bone overgrowth that results in macrodactyly. The lesion is benign, but complete excision may be unsatisfactory because it entails removal of the involved nerve segment, resulting in loss of sensation or function.

Diffuse lipomatosis, a rare condition, is defined as a diffuse overgrowth of mature fat affecting a large portion of an extremity or portions of the trunk (45). It usually occurs in infants under 2 years of age, but it may become apparent in adults. It typically involves both subcutaneous tissue and muscle, and may be associated with bone involvement and osseous hypertrophy. It differs from neural fibrolipoma in that nerves are not affected, from intramuscular lipoma in that it is not confined to muscle, and from intermuscular lipoma in that it is not a delineated mass. Diffuse lipomatosis frequently recurs after attempted excision, often repeatedly over many years. It may become quite large and occasionally causes such distortion and loss of function of an extremity that amputation becomes necessary.

Nevus lipomatosus superficialis ("Michelin tire man" syndrome) is a hamartoma found either at birth or in the first two decades of life and is manifest by dermal nodules of fat that usually develop in the buttocks or upper thighs (28,32,41, 43). These often become confluent, and when they coalesce sufficiently they tend to form linear masses along skin folds. When this occurs, the condition has been dubbed the "Michelin tire man" syndrome because patients supposedly resemble the symbol of the French tire manufacturer, a man with tires around his body. Histologically, one finds large numbers of mature adipocytes in the dermis. Using the term "nevus lipomatosus superficialis" for localized simple intradermal lipomas, i.e., fatty skin tags, is inappropriate.

Villous lipomatous proliferation of the synovial membrane ("lipoma arborescens") is an overgrowth of fat in the subsynovial tissue, most often of a large joint, resulting in villous projections of fat lined by synovial cells. It occurs mainly in older people and is associated with joint trauma and chronic arthritis (38,60). *Lipoma of tendon sheath* is characterized by a mass of mature adipose attached to a tendon (59). It is very rare, occurs mainly in adults under the age of 40, and usually affects the tendons of the hands and wrists; less commonly, the ankle and foot are involved.

Lumbosacral lipoma is a diffuse overgrowth of mature fat overlying the lumbosacral spine. By definition, it is always associated with spina bifida or a laminar defect and is usually connected to the spinal cord or cauda equina through the defect (47,53). It may contain a meningocele or myelocele. As might be expected, lumbosacral lipoma is encountered most commonly in infants and children, although it occasionally presents in adults. It is usually asymptomatic initially, although myelopathy or radiculopathy, resulting in disturbed function in the legs, bowel, or bladder, frequently develops later. There may be an overlying sinus, skin tag, or hemangioma, or overgrowth of hair. Imaging studies demonstrate a mass with the density of fat associated with spina bifida or sacral dysgenesis.

Pelvic lipomatosis is a diffuse overproduction of fat in the perirectal and perivesical region. It chiefly affects black males, who have ranged from 9 to 80 years of age, with a median age of 48 (37,42,46). Rarely, excess fat can be found in the perianal tissues, retroperitoneum, and mesentery. Approximately 150 cases have been reported. The patients usually have urinary frequency and mild perineal pain at first but often develop constipation and more severe abdominal and back pain later. The process may eventually cause large bowel obstruction, hydronephrosis, and uremia. Imaging studies are characteristic because of the fat-density tissue (in the pelvis) that distorts the bladder and rectal contours, and separates the prostate from the seminal vesicles (29). There may also be lateral displacement and dilatation of one or both ureters, sometimes accompanied by hydronephrosis. Distinction from retroperitoneal atypical lipomatous tumor (well-differentiated liposarcoma) rests on the pelvic location, the absence of a discrete mass, and the absence of the atypical cells and fibrous or myxoid tissue found in most atypical lipomatous tumors.

Of syndromes involving lipomas, the two most important probably are *symmetrical lipomatosis (Madelung's disease)* and *adiposis dolorosa (Dercum's disease)*. Symmetrical lipomatosis almost always affects middle-aged men (33,54,56). There are large, symmetrical fatty masses, primarily in the neck and shoulder area, although the cheeks, breasts, upper arms, axillae, trunk, and mediastinum also may be involved. The deposits of bland fatty tissue involve both subcutaneous and deeper soft tissues, and may extend between muscles of the neck and upper chest, resulting at times in partial obstruction of the esophagus or trachea. Peripheral and autonomic neuropathies have been reported, and most patients have metabolic abnormalities (33). Adiposis dolorosa consists of a tender or painful accumulation of subcutaneous fat, typically in the pelvic region and lower extremities in postmenopausal women (40). It is associated with weakness, fatigability, and depression. No hormonal abnormalities have been documented.

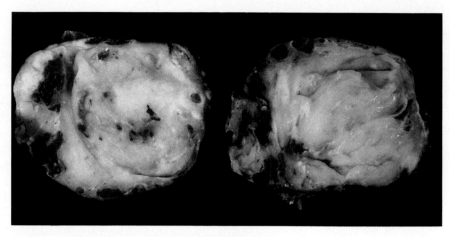

Figure 4-2
LIPOMA
Grossly, lipomas most often are indistinguishable from normal fat except that the constituent cells form a mass. The hemorrhage in this specimen is a result of surgery.

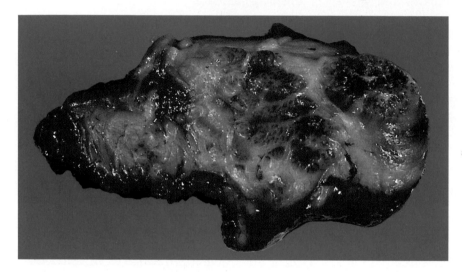

Figure 4-3
INTRAMUSCULAR LIPOMA
Yellow adipose tissue can be seen within skeletal muscle.

Pathologic Findings. Grossly, most lipomas are composed of soft, yellow fat indistinguishable from normal fat except that a mass is present (fig. 4-2). Some have a significant fibrous component reflected grossly as white tissue. Intramuscular lipomas characteristically interdigitate between muscle fibers, and this may give the muscle a striated gross appearance and make delineation of the tumor margin very difficult (fig. 4-3). Microscopically, lipomas, whether subcutaneous, located elsewhere, or part of a syndrome, are formed of mature fat cells with small, uniform, eccentric nuclei that are morphologically indistinguishable from normal adult fat cells (fig. 4-4). Because of this, a diagnosis of lipoma cannot be made unless a mass has been identified. Mitotic figures are nonexistent in lipomas unless fat necrosis is present.

Occasionally, there is a component of innocuous-appearing fibrous tissue (*fibrolipoma*), especially in neural fibrolipoma and symmetrical lipomatosis (fig. 4-5). A myxoid stroma is present in rare instances, in which case the term *myxolipoma* may be used. Cartilaginous and osseous metaplasia rarely occur in lipomas (49,52). Neural fibrolipomas extend along, surround, and infiltrate the involved nerve and typically are confined by the epineurium. Lumbosacral lipomas sometimes contain areas with large numbers of blood vessels, smooth muscle cells, or both, and occasionally, the fatty tissue near the spinal defect also contains foci of glia or ependymal structures (53). Intramuscular lipomas feature residual skeletal muscle fibers interspersed among the mature adipocytes composing the intramuscular mass (fig. 4-6).

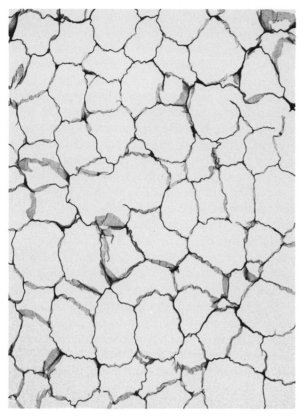

Figure 4-4
LIPOMA

The usual lipoma is composed of adult fat cells indistinguishable from normal fat cells. A diagnosis of lipoma is made because a mass was removed, not because of the histologic pattern.

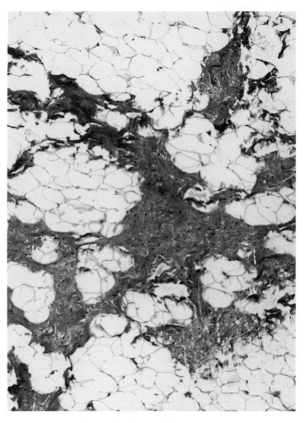

Figure 4-5
LIPOMA

Sometimes fibrous tissue is present within a lipoma and if desired such tumors can be classified as fibrolipomas. Care should be taken to examine the fibrous tissue carefully to be sure it does not contain atypical cells because the only atypical cells in an atypical lipomatous tumor may be in fibrous tissue.

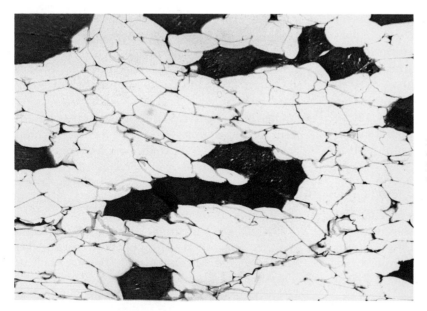

Figure 4-6
INTRAMUSCULAR LIPOMA

Intramuscular lipoma features adult fat cells between and among skeletal muscle fibers. If vessels are numerous and prominent the lesion is definitionally classified as an intramuscular hemangioma.

Special Studies. Chromosomal abnormalities, as described in the General Considerations section above, have been reported in about 50 percent of the patients studied. Fat cells are S-100 protein positive and slender spindle cells in many types of lipoma are CD34 positive (59a). Overall, immunohistochemistry plays little role in the diagnosis of lipoma.

Differential Diagnosis. A common diagnostic concern about lipoma is its distinction from non-neoplastic fat. As noted, a diagnosis of lipoma requires the presence of a mass, because histologically the usual lipoma is indistinguishable from adult fat. If a fatty mass contains abundant fibrous or myxoid tissue, these can be used to help identify the lesion as tumorous because such tissue is not usually present within normal fat.

The most troublesome diagnostic difficulty is the distinction of lipoma from atypical lipomatous tumor (well-differentiated liposarcoma). Occasional cells in lipomas may have slightly enlarged nuclei, but nuclear enlargement sufficient to be appreciated at low-power (40X) microscopy points to atypical lipomatous tumor. Care should be taken not to confuse histiocytes in fat necrosis with atypical fat cells. If there is considerable variation in fat cell size, atypical lipomatous tumor should be suspected and sufficiently enlarged nuclei carefully sought. This differential diagnostic problem is discussed further in the section concerning atypical lipomatous tumors below.

Lipomas essentially do not occur in the retroperitoneum. Retroperitoneal fatty neoplasms (there must be a mass to distinguish a neoplasm from pelvic lipomatosis and excessive fat in obesity) are capable of recurring and dedifferentiating even if they are histologically bland. In order to highlight this potential, we use the term atypical lipomatous tumor for such neoplasms in this location even though atypical cells may not be present. Retroperitoneal atypical lipomatous tumors must be distinguished from pelvic lipomatosis (see above).

Lipomas with a myxoid stroma should be distinguished from myxoid liposarcoma. The latter usually does not arise in the subcutaneous tissue, the site where lipoma is most common, and has an arborizing vascular pattern that is absent in almost all lipomas. Moreover, the microcysts found in some myxoid liposarcomas are absent in lipomas.

Intramuscular lipomas may have a prominent component of blood vessels. By convention, intramuscular tumors composed of adult fat cells and numerous prominent vessels, or a vascular pattern characteristic of capillary or cavernous hemangioma, are considered to be intramuscular hemangiomas rather than intramuscular lipomas, regardless of the amount of adipose tissue present. Distinguishing between intramuscular lipoma and intramuscular hemangioma is not critical because both have some risk of recurrence although recurrences are not destructive and neither lesion has metastatic capacity. Most of the time the distinction between the two is straightforward and problems usually arise only when the number of vessels is marginally increased. The vessels in the usual intramuscular lipoma are identical to those in ordinary lipoma.

Treatment and Prognosis. Lipomas may recur (or regrow) but they do not metastasize and recurrences are not uncontrolled. The frequency of recurrence depends on the site of the lipoma. Those lipomas with a significant incidence of recurrence are noted in the Clinical Features section above.

Lipomatosis

These rare proliferations of mature adipose tissue are presented in Table 4-2 and discussed in the Clinical Features section of Lipoma above.

Angiolipoma

Definition. An angiolipoma is a subcutaneous tumor made up of mature fat and prominent, easily found blood vessels. The term angiolipoma is only used to describe subcutaneous lesions composed of fat and a large number of small blood vessels.

Clinical Features. Angiolipomas usually occur in young adults and older teenagers (61,62). They are rarely larger than 2 cm, frequently multiple, and characteristically tender or painful. The most common locations are the forearm, trunk, and upper arm. Angiolipomas are familial in approximately 5 percent of instances.

Pathologic Findings. Grossly, angiolipomas are circumscribed and yellow with varying amounts of red. Microscopically, they are made up of mature fat cells admixed with small vessels (fig. 4-7). The proportion of vessels to fat varies from example to example; lesions composed almost entirely of vessels may be confused with a vascular neoplasm (62,63). A characteristic feature of angiolipoma is fibrin thrombi within the vessels, so this is useful diagnostically (fig. 4-8). Longstanding examples may demonstrate perivascular and interstitial fibrosis. The angiolipomas thus far studied have had a normal karyotype (61a,63a).

Differential Diagnosis. The term "intramuscular angiolipoma" has been used by some authors for intramuscular tumors that feature prominent vessels as well as a fatty component. Such tumors should be classified as intramuscular hemangiomas rather than angiolipomas and hence they are discussed in the chapter that concerns vascular tumors. When the vascular component of an angiolipoma becomes predominant or cellular, confusion with Kaposi's sarcoma and spindle cell hemangioendothelioma is possible. The circumscription of angiolipoma, the prominent thrombi within the vessels, the presence of some fat, and the association with other more characteristic angiolipomas should allow correct interpretation.

Treatment and Prognosis. Recurrence after excision is rare and the tumor is never aggressive.

Angiomyolipoma

This lesion, which occurs almost exclusively in the kidney, is discussed in the Fascicle, Tumors of the Kidney, Bladder, and Related Urinary Structures (58a) (see also Differential Diagnosis in the Atypical Lipomatous Tumor section below).

Myelolipoma

This lesion is discussed in the Fascicle devoted to tumors of the adrenal gland (65a). It is sufficient here to note that myelolipomas do occur, rarely, outside the adrenal gland, usually in the pelvis but also in other sites (64,65). Extra-adrenal myelolipomas are composed of varying proportions of fat and bone marrow elements, and thus are indistinguishable from adrenal myelolipomas. It is important to exclude extramedullary hematopoiesis secondary to myeloproliferative disorders, anemia, and skeletal disorders. Myelolipoma is well circumscribed and lymphocytic infiltration is often conspicu-

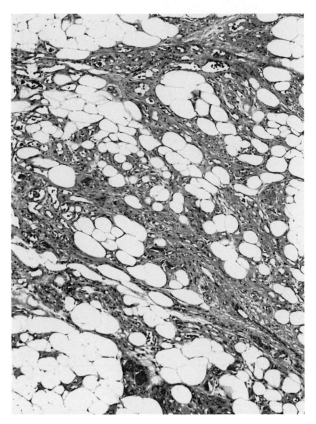

Figure 4-7
ANGIOLIPOMA
This lesion is characterized by mature fat cells mixed with variable numbers of blood vessels.

ous. Extramedullary hematopoiesis is not circumscribed, fat is not an integral part of the lesion, and disproportionate erythroid hyperplasia is common.

Hibernoma

Definition. Hibernoma is a benign neoplasm composed of multivacuolated fat cells of the type found in brown fat (66,68a).

Clinical Features. Hibernoma occurs predominantly in young adults. The most common location is the scapular and interscapular region, followed by the thigh; other sites of involvement that have been reported include the chest wall, back, axilla, and groin. Hibernomas are typically slowly growing and painless, and usually measure between 5 and 10 cm in diameter when they are diagnosed.

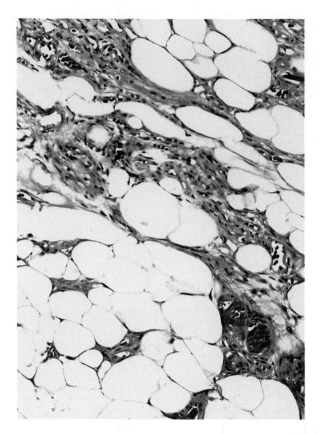 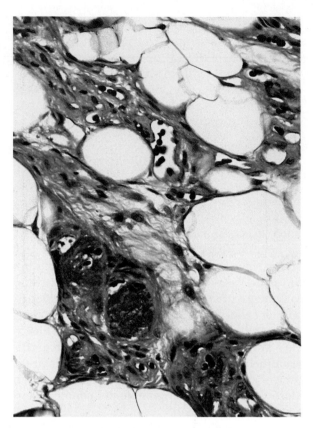

Figure 4-8
ANGIOLIPOMA
A hallmark of angiolipoma is the vascular thrombi seen here.

Pathologic Findings. Grossly, hibernomas are soft, well circumscribed, and tan to red-brown on cut section. Microscopically, they exhibit a well-defined lobular pattern and are composed of uniform round to oval cells with small central nuclei and granular to multivacuolated eosinophilic cytoplasm (figs. 4-9, 4-10) (68,68a). Univacuolated fat cells are often admixed, sometimes in sufficient number to produce an appearance intermediate between that of hibernoma and ordinary lipoma (fig. 4-11). Cytogenetic evaluation of two hibernomas showed abnormalities of chromosome 11 (67).

Differential Diagnosis. Hibernomas are distinctive and seldom is there difficulty in recognizing them. It is possible that the brown fat cells of a hibernoma could be confused with the cells of a granular cell tumor; however, the cytoplasm in the latter is not vacuolated. Occasional atypical lipomatous tumors (well-differentiated liposarcomas)

have a proportion of multivacuolated cells, but they also demonstrate enlargement and atypia of at least some nuclei, they may have a fibrous or myxoid component, and they lack a well-defined lobular pattern. Myxoid and pleomorphic liposarcomas may also contain multivacuolated cells but otherwise bear little resemblance to hibernoma. Myxoid liposarcomas feature signet ring lipoblasts and arborizing vessels not found in hibernoma and pleomorphic liposarcomas resemble pleomorphic malignant fibrous histiocytoma (MFH) except that they also contain lipoblasts. If the question of rhabdomyoma arises, a desmin stain should allow correct classification.

Treatment and Prognosis. Hibernomas have shown no tendency to recur after excision. We do not think there is a malignant hibernoma; the rare cases that have been reported as such are probably examples of pleomorphic liposarcoma or cellular myxoid liposarcoma.

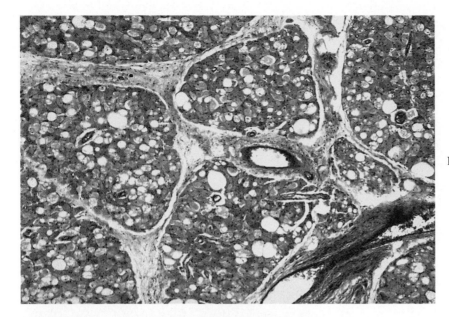

Figure 4-9
HIBERNOMA
Hibernoma is characteristically lobulated.

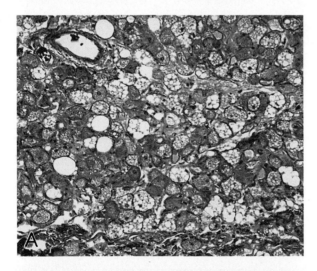

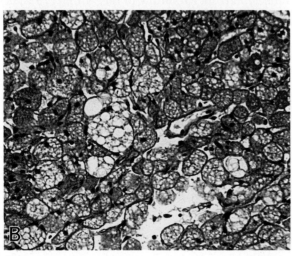

Figure 4-10
HIBERNOMA
The cells composing hibernoma have abundant cytoplasm that varies from granular to multivacuolated.

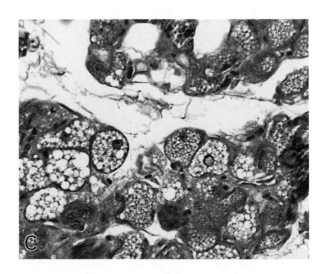

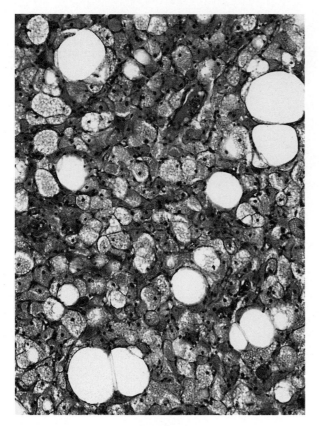

Figure 4-11
HIBERNOMA
Variable numbers of adult fat cells may be found in hibernomas. As long as granular or multivacuolated brown fat cells are present anywhere in the lesion it is considered to be a hibernoma.

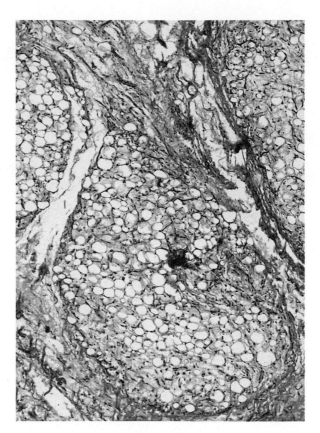

Figure 4-12
LIPOBLASTOMA
The lobular architecture of lipoblastoma is illustrated.

Lipoblastoma and Lipoblastomatosis

Definition. Lipoblastoma is a tumor that occurs exclusively or almost exclusively in infants, children, and, less often, teenagers. It is composed of small, immature fat cells separated by a myxoid matrix and admixed with a variable number of adult fat cells. Chung and Enzinger (72) recommend the term lipoblastoma for circumscribed subcutaneous examples and lipoblastomatosis for deep lesions and for all diffuse or infiltrative lesions whether superficial or deep.

Clinical Features. Lipoblastoma and lipoblastomatosis usually occur during the first 3 years of life, and are twice as frequent in boys than girls (72,73,77,78,83,84). These lesions develop very rarely, if at all, after age 20. They are usually painless. The upper and lower extremities are the most common locations, although many other soft tissue sites have been involved (69,72, 73,78,81). The majority of lipoblastomatous tumors are subcutaneous and circumscribed i.e., they are lipoblastomas, while the minority are situated in deeper locations such as skeletal muscle, retroperitoneum, or mesentery (79). The latter are almost always diffuse and infiltrating although diffuse lesions may be superficial (72).

Pathologic Findings. The cut surface of a lipoblastomatous lesion is paler than an ordinary lipoma and has a myxoid quality. The typical microscopic picture of lipoblastoma (tosis) is that of multiple, well-defined, paucicellular lobules formed by small signet ring fat cells and uniform stellate and spindled cells with scant cytoplasm, set within myxoid intercellular material that contains a plexiform vascular network (figs. 4-12, 4-13). Scattered mature fat cells are commonly present (84). The lobular architecture can usually be appreciated on magnetic resonance images (MRI), CT scans, and ultrasonograms

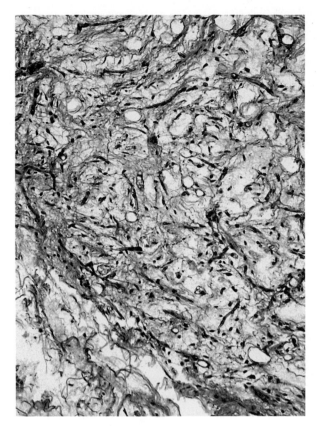

Figure 4-13
LIPOBLASTOMA
This higher power view of lipoblastoma demonstrates a plexiform vascular pattern, myxoid matrix, and small fat cells, features indistinguishable from myxoid liposarcoma. Distinction is based on the age of the patient, the lobular architecture, the lack of areas with increased cellularity, and the superficial location of many lipoblastomas as described in the text.

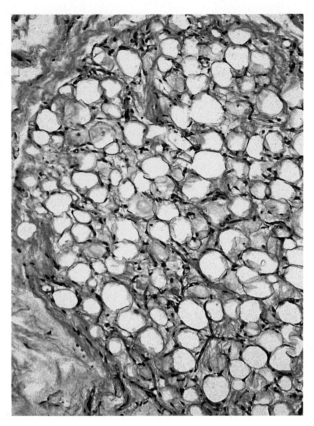

Figure 4-14
LIPOBLASTOMA
In this area, fat cells are larger, have come to predominate, and have almost crowded out the myxoid stroma. When this occurs, lipoblastomas can resemble lipomas.

(76,78,81). The lobules are separated by connective tissue septa that are usually narrow but may be quite wide. In the latter circumstance, the tumor may appear to be of fibrous type at first glance. The degree of fat cell maturation varies from tumor to tumor and within individual tumors; in some lobules the cells are small, stellate and round or spindled, and lack fat vacuoles; in others they have a "signet ring" appearance; and in yet others the two cell types are mixed together, with or without mature fat cells. Occasionally, the cells are sufficiently multivacuolated to resemble brown fat cells. The amount of myxoid matrix is inversely proportional to the degree of fatty maturation, and capillaries are typically numerous and plexiform

when the myxoid stroma is abundant. Rarely, nearly all the cells approach the appearance of adult fat cells and then only focally will the characteristic myxoid matrix be found (fig. 4-14). Nonsubcutaneous, more diffuse examples have identical morphologic features except for a less well-defined lobular pattern; sometimes the lobular pattern is lost altogether in the diffuse lesions. Deep lesions also frequently contain entrapped muscle fibers. Extramedullary hematopoiesis is occasionally present.

Sequential biopsies of recurrent lipoblastomatoses may demonstrate extensive to complete maturation to mature fat, although this is not invariable. Recent reports on a few cases indicate that the chromosomes in the cells composing lipoblastomas usually demonstrate rearrangements affecting 8q (74,75,80).

Differential Diagnosis. The histologic features of lipoblastoma and lipoblastomatosis are usually indistinguishable from those of paucicellular myxoid liposarcoma except for the prominent lobulation seen in many examples of lipoblastoma. Ultrastructural studies also demonstrate the similarities between these lesions (70). However, as noted above, rearrangements involving chromosome 8q are characteristic of lipoblastomas (74,75, 80), while almost all myxoid liposarcomas have a reciprocal 12;16 translocation t(12;16)(q13;p11) (see Myxoid Liposarcoma). More cases need to be studied before these chromosomal abnormalities can be depended on to distinguish these two lesions but the preliminary data are encouraging. Fortunately, myxoid liposarcoma rarely occurs below the age of 20, and lipoblastoma and lipoblastomatosis occur mostly in infants and children under the age of 10. Shmookler and Enzinger (82) have reported myxoid liposarcomas in individuals under the age of 21; however, all except one of the patients were over the age of 10. We think the accuracy of the diagnosis of myxoid liposarcoma in infants and children in some reports must be questioned (71); however, in infants and children myxoid fatty tumors with areas of significant cellularity should raise the question of myxoid or other liposarcomas because lipoblastoma is characterized by low cellularity. In addition to cellularity, location is also helpful because myxoid liposarcoma practically never arises in the subcutaneous tissue where most but not all lipoblastomas develop. Microcystic spaces can be found in both tumors (78). Because lipoblastomatosis can be composed almost entirely of adult fat cells, particularly in recurrence, this possibility should be considered when an infiltrating lipoma-like lesion is found in an infant or child.

Lipoblastomatosis containing prominent fibrous tissue and adult type fat cells can resemble infantile fibromatosis. Usually infantile fibromatosis is composed only of fibrous tissue and mature entrapped fat cells while most often lipoblastomatosis features myxoid stroma and plexiform capillaries as described above, at least focally.

Treatment and Prognosis. The superficial, circumscribed form rarely recurs after excision, but recurrence is frequent with the diffuse variant and multiple recurrences are not uncommon. Lipoblastomatous lesions, whether circumscribed or diffuse, do not metastasize.

Chondroid Lipoma

Definition. Chondroid lipoma is a rare, benign, fatty neoplasm characterized histologically by nests, strands, and sheets of generally uniform, small to medium-sized cells with variable fatty vacuolation set within a myxoid to hyalinized (chondroid) matrix. Mature fat cells may be present but mature cartilage is not.

Clinical Features. The 20 patients reported by Meis and Enzinger (86) (in the only sizable series of chondroid lipomas so far published) ranged in age from 14 to 70 years, with a median of 36 years. Sixteen patients were female. The tumors were most commonly located in the proximal extremities and limb girdles, although they also occurred in a variety of other soft tissue sites. Some examples were subcutaneous and others intramuscular. Tumor size varied from 1.5 to 11 cm, with a median of 4 cm.

Pathologic Findings. Chondroid lipomas are characteristically well circumscribed, and range from yellow to white to tan on cut section (fig. 4-15). Microscopically, they demonstrate small to medium-sized cells with variable fatty cytoplasmic vacuolation, often arranged in clusters or rows in a basophilic or eosinophilic homogenous matrix that resembles but is not cartilage (fig. 4-16). Mature fat cells are also typically present and may predominate (fig. 4-17). Nuclear pleomorphism and mitotic figures are generally absent, being seen in only one of Meis and Enzinger's cases (86). Mature cartilage is not present.

Special Studies. Immunohistochemically, there is consistent staining for S-100 protein and vimentin, and focal staining for keratin in a minority of cases (85,87). Ultrastructurally, the tumor cells have the features of white adipocytes without evidence of cartilaginous differentiation (87).

Differential Diagnosis. The major differential diagnostic considerations are myxoid liposarcoma and extraskeletal myxoid chondrosarcoma. Myxoid liposarcoma may have cell cords and clusters, although these are relatively uncommon and are less extensive and elaborate than those in chondroid lipoma. However, its characteristic plexiform vascular network is not a feature of chondroid lipoma. The cell arrangements in extraskeletal myxoid chondrosarcoma are more like those of chondroid lipoma, and the intercellular matrix is similar as well (hence the name,

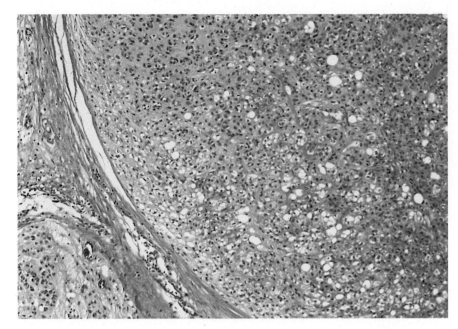

Figure 4-15
CHONDROID LIPOMA
Chondroid lipomas are characteristically sharply demarcated
from the surrounding tissue and
grow in lobules.

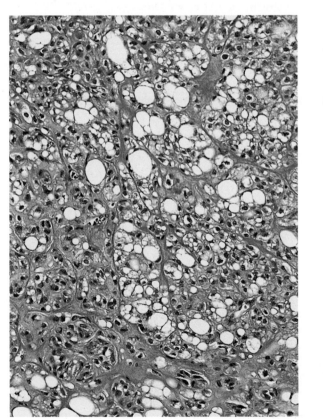 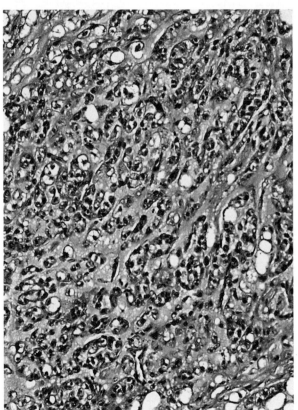

Figure 4-16
CHONDROID LIPOMA
Left: Small to medium-sized cells with variably vacuolated cytoplasm often arranged in clusters or rows mark chondroid lipoma.
Right: When these are set in a basophilic matrix the resulting appearance can mimic cartilage.

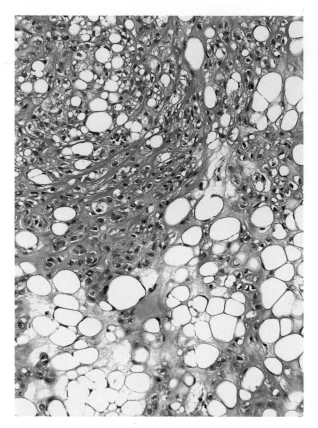

Figure 4-17
CHONDROID LIPOMA
Mature fat cells are almost always present, at least focally.

chondroid lipoma), but extraskeletal myxoid chondrosarcoma typically displays prominent lobulation, the cells lack fatty vacuoles, mature fat is not present, and the matrix is myxoid rather than hyaline-like or chondroid. Soft tissue chondroma might be a consideration; however, it usually occurs on the hands and feet, does not demonstrate fat, and features at least focally mature hyaline cartilage which is not found in chondroid lipoma.

Treatment and Prognosis. The tumor is benign; recurrence and metastases have not been reported.

Myolipoma

Definition. Myolipoma is a tumor composed of bland smooth muscle and adult fat.

General Considerations. Tumors that combine mature adipocytes with bland smooth muscle cells are well known in the uterus where they

are considered to be leiomyomas with fatty metaplasia because fat cells are not normally present in the myometrium (and hence such tumors are labeled lipoleiomyomas). Meis and Enzinger (87a) reported nine similar lesions in the soft tissues under the rubric of myolipoma.

Clinical Features. Six of the nine patients were women and all had lesions in the pelvis, retroperitoneum, suprapubic region, or inguinal canal, so it is possible their myolipomas might be related to smooth muscle tumors of the genital tract. The three males had myolipomas of the inguinal canal, anterior abdominal wall, and subcutaneous tissue of the back. As far as we know, these are the only nine soft tissue myolipomas that have been reported, although similar lesions occur in the breast.

Pathologic Findings. All nine tumors were composed of variable amounts of bland, uniform smooth muscle cells and mature fat cells. Mitotic figures were absent. They varied in size from 3 to 26 cm; seven were over 12 cm.

Differential Diagnosis. The lesion that is most easily mistaken for myolipoma is low-grade leiomyosarcoma infiltrating fat. Low-grade leiomyosarcomas may be composed of bland, uniform smooth muscle cells, so a large number of sections should be taken to be sure that the adipose tissue mixed with the smooth muscle cells is an integral part of the tumor rather than normal fat infiltrated by neoplastic smooth muscle cells, and that mitotic figures are absent. In fact, if an apparent myolipoma is encountered in the retroperitoneum it might be prudent to obtain consultation. Of great importance is the observation that the smooth muscle cells in myolipoma are uniform and cytologically bland and mitoses are absent. Histologically bland smooth muscle tumors in the soft tissues outside the retroperitoneum can also recur, so the same care in diagnostic interpretation should be taken as for retroperitoneal myolipoma. A pelvic myolipoma in a woman could be associated with the genitalia and if it is, criteria for uterine smooth muscle tumors may be applicable.

Angiomyolipoma contains abnormal blood vessels in addition to smooth muscle and fat, at least some of the constituent cells are HMB45 positive, and most involve the kidney. Atypical lipomatous tumors may demonstrate smooth muscle metaplasia but the presence of fatty tissue mixed with fibrous tissue and atypical cells points to the correct diagnosis.

Treatment and Prognosis. None of the nine tumors recurred, but follow-up information was available for only four patients and two of these had been followed for less than a year (87a). Well-differentiated leiomyosarcoma may take years to recur.

Spindle Cell and Pleomorphic Lipomas

Definition. Spindle cell lipoma has three components: 1) adult fat cells; 2) small, uniform spindle cells with indistinct, often wispy cytoplasm; and 3) brightly eosinophilic, dense collagen. These are mixed in varying proportions. Pleomorphic lipomas contain cells with enlarged, hyperchromatic nuclei, often multiple and arranged in a ring or semicircle (floret cells), in addition to adult fat and dense collagen bundles. Pleomorphic lipoma may be combined with spindle cell lipoma in the same neoplasm. Because of its morphologic overlap with atypical lipomatous tumor (see below), we restrict the category of pleomorphic lipoma to tumors located in the subcutaneous tissue of the neck, back, or shoulder.

General Considerations. Currently, there is disagreement among soft tissue pathologists, including the authors of this Fascicle, about pleomorphic lipoma. This term has been used for tumors that contain adult fat, dense mature collagen, and cells with large atypical hyperchromatic nuclei, some of which feature multiple nuclei arranged in a ring or semicircle (floret cells) (89,104). Some investigators consider such tumors to be part of the spectrum of spindle cell lipoma because elements of spindle cell lipoma may be present; most occur in the subcutaneous tissue of the back, neck, and shoulders where spindle cell lipoma is most common; and like spindle cell lipoma they rarely recur, at least when in those sites. This position is further strengthened by cytogenetic studies. Over 60 percent of atypical lipomatous tumors arising elsewhere than the subcutis of the shoulder, back, and neck have supernumerary ring chromosomes, a rare occurrence for pleomorphic lipomas in those locations (94b,103a). Furthermore, 16q alterations are common in spindle cell and pleomorphic lipomas and rare in atypical lipomatous tumors (103a). Other investigators would classify pleomorphic lipoma as a variant of atypical lipomatous tumor (see below) because floret cells, thick collagen bundles, and even areas resembling spindle cell lipoma may be found in atypical lipomatous tumors elsewhere than the subcutis of the neck, back, and shoulder, including nonsubcutaneous locations where these histologic features do not indicate a nearly zero chance of recurrence.

As is the case with many nomenclatural controversies, little is at stake clinically because the behavior of pleomorphic lipomas, spindle cell lipomas, and atypical lipomatous tumors is determined by location, not histologic differences. None of these recur except rarely as long as they are in the subcutaneous tissue of the neck, back, and shoulders, but identical tumors in the deep soft tissues may recur. We think the nomenclatural stance taken in the definition above is reasonable from a clinical management point of view because it labels tumors with a significant chance of recurrence as atypical lipomatous tumor.

Clinical Features. Spindle cell lipomas usually occur in the subcutaneous tissue of the posterior neck, shoulder area, or upper back (88,94, 95,98), although examples do develop at other sites (90,93,97,99,101–103,105). They are almost always subcutaneous, but a few tumors with essentially identical histologic features have been reported within muscle and in other deep locations. Some of the authors of this Fascicle classify deep-seated tumors with the features of spindle cell lipoma as atypical lipomatous tumor with spindle cell features. Almost all patients with spindle cell lipoma are middle-aged or older men, but the tumor occasionally occurs in women and younger males. Spindle cell lipoma can rarely be multiple or familial (94a). By definition, tumors classified as pleomorphic lipoma (see General Considerations above) are in the subcutaneous tissue of the posterior neck, shoulder, or back. Identical tumors elsewhere are classified as atypical lipomatous tumor. Pleomorphic lipoma overwhelmingly occurs in middle-aged and older males.

Pathologic Findings. Spindle cell lipoma is characteristically well-circumscribed and ranges from fatty to myxoid on cut section (fig. 4-18). Microscopically, there is a mixture of mature fat cells and uniform, small spindle cells with scant wispy and often elongated cytoplasm; the latter may be set within a myxoid matrix (88,94,95).

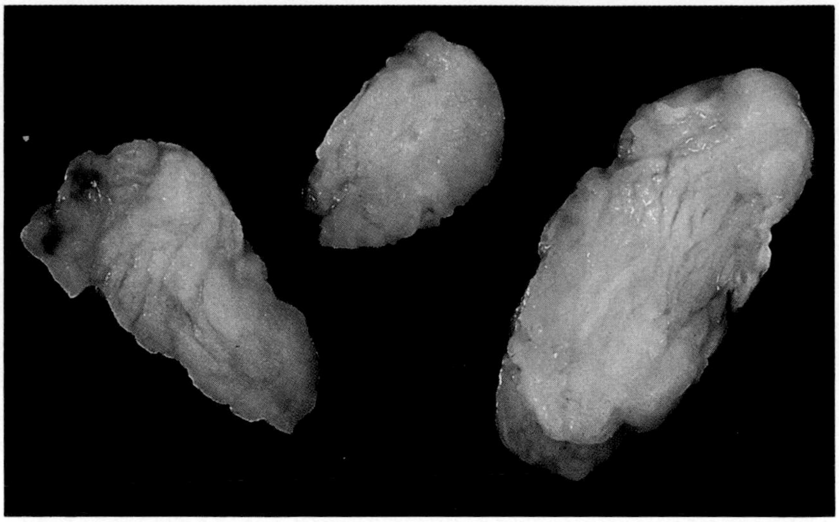

Figure 4-18
SPINDLE CELL LIPOMA
When large numbers of fat cells are present spindle cell lipoma is yellow, a feature that can be helpful diagnostically.

The spindle cells occasionally contain small cytoplasmic vacuoles. Prominent thick collagen bundles are a feature of almost all spindle cell lipomas (figs. 4-19). The proportion of fat to spindle cells varies considerably, and one or the other may be predominant. Not infrequently, the adult fat cells are smaller than the usual mature adipocyte. The spindle cells may be closely packed or more widely spaced, and may demonstrate nuclear palisading (figs. 4-20, 4-21). Vascularity is usually not prominent. Rarely, the vessels are arborizing and come to resemble those in myxoid liposarcoma, particularly if the stroma is myxoid; in other instances, the tumor vessels may be round and thickened (95,106). Occasionally there are prominent cleft-like or vascular-like spaces that may merge and even result in a pseudovillous pattern (fig. 4-22); these have been interpreted both as vessels and as a result of interstitial matrix breakdown (96). However, endothelial markers such as CD31 and factor VIII are negative, indicating that these spaces are not blood vessels. Mitotic figures are rare.

Pleomorphic lipomas contain variable numbers of cells with enlarged, atypical nuclei, both in fatty and nonfatty (fibrous or myxoid) areas, including floret cells (figs. 4-23, 4-24) (89,104). The latter are cells with multiple, enlarged, hyperchromatic nuclei arranged in a circle or semicircle (fig. 4-25). Adult fat and mature collagen bundles of the type seen in spindle cell lipoma are also present, and frequently there is a component of spindle cell lipoma. As explained above, the term "pleomor-

phic lipoma" should only be used for subcutaneous tumors located in the back, neck, or shoulders. We think neoplasms with the same histologic features located elsewhere should be classified as atypical lipomatous tumors.

Special Studies. The spindle cells in spindle cell lipoma are CD34 positive (105a) and the fat cells react with S-100 protein (91). The cells lining the spaces in the pseudoangiomatous variant do not react with endothelial markers.

Ultrastructural studies support the conclusion reached by light microscopy that spindle cell lipoma is composed of a biphasic cellular population of adipocytes and undifferentiated mesenchymal cells (92). Chromosomal analysis of spindle cell and pleomorphic lipomas has demonstrated variable abnormal karyotypes (94b,100). Most show an unbalanced aberration involving 16q resulting in monosomy or partial loss of 16q, but others have demonstrated abnormalities of 13q and 6p. A few have had ring chromosomes. Interestingly, 6p, 13q, and 12q may be abnormal in atypical lipomatous tumors but supernumerary ring chromosomes are frequently present in this tumor while they are rare in spindle cell and pleomorphic lipomas.

Differential Diagnosis. Most spindle cell lipomas contain all three elements: spindle cells, adult fat, and thick eosinophilic collagen fibers. When these are present in equal or nearly equal proportions, the appearance is distinctive and not easily confused with other entities. Spindle cell lipomas with few fat cells have a predominance of

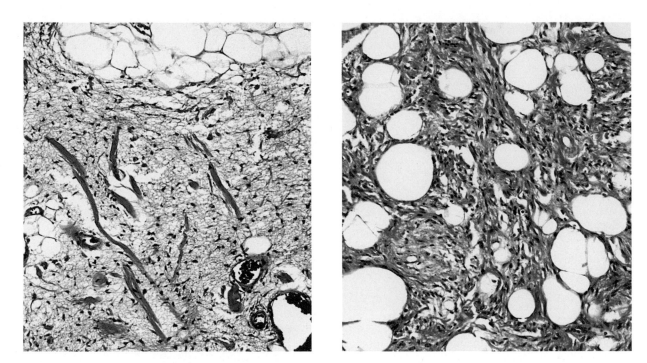

Figure 4-19
SPINDLE CELL LIPOMA
The three components of spindle cell lipoma, namely, fat cells, spindle cells, and ropy collagen, can be seen in these two low-power photomicrographs.

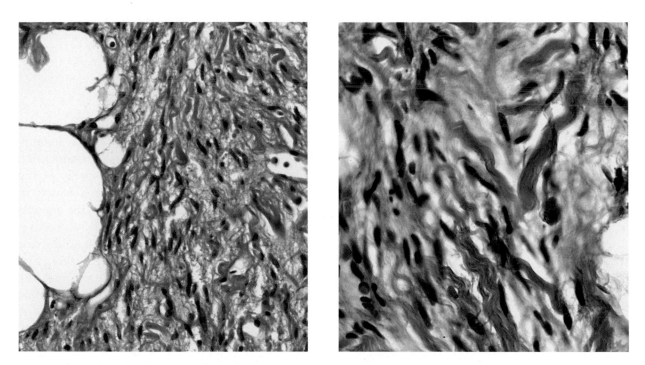

Figure 4-20
SPINDLE CELL LIPOMA
The spindle cells have small, slender, uniform nuclei and inconspicuous cytoplasm. Note the thick collagen fibers typically found in spindle cell lipoma.

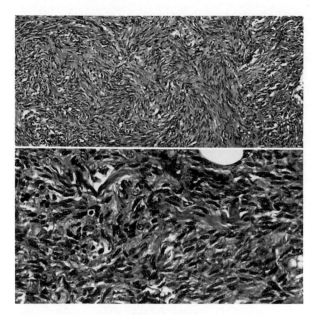

Figure 4-21
SPINDLE CELL LIPOMA
In some tumors spindle cells are the predominant element. In this circumstance a search for fat cells is indicated.

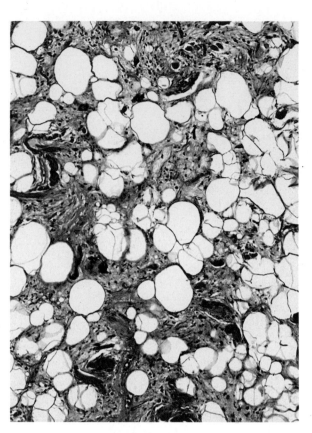

Figure 4-23
PLEOMORPHIC LIPOMA
Large atypical cells with dense chromatin, mature fat, and thick collagen bundles are the low-power features that characterize pleomorphic lipomas. Distinction from atypical lipomatous tumor is based on location.

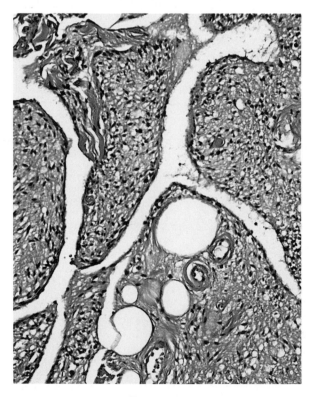

Figure 4-22
SPINDLE CELL LIPOMA
Occasionally, clefts or vascular-like spaces may be found in spindle cell lipoma.

spindle cells and thus resemble nonfatty spindle cell neoplasms such as neurofibroma, leiomyoma, or schwannoma, but these classification errors can be avoided by careful study of the spindle cells, which lack well-defined neural or smooth muscle features. Moreover, the spindle cells in spindle cell lipoma are CD34 positive, S-100 protein negative (although the adipocytes may be positive for this marker) (91,105a), and do not express desmin. The collagen and the spindle cells in spindle cell lipoma resemble those in solitary fibrous tumor and indeed the spindle cells in both are CD34 positive. However, solitary fibrous tumor does not contain fat cells (see also General Considerations above). It is unlikely that a spindle cell lipoma would be confused with sarcoma because the cells of the former are uniform and bland. The rare spindle cell lipoma-like

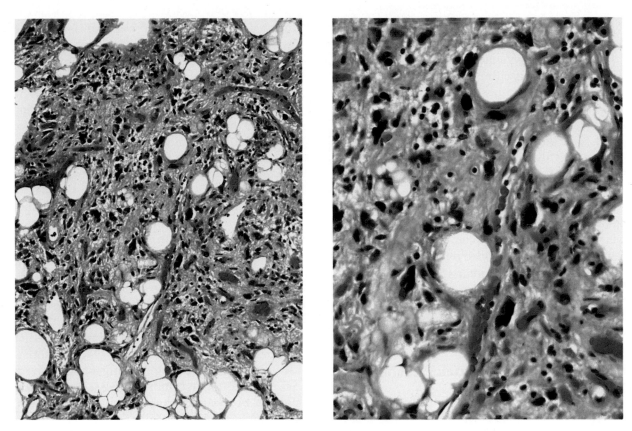

Figure 4-24
PLEOMORPHIC LIPOMA
Often the pleomorphic cells are numerous, at least focally, in pleomorphic lipomas.

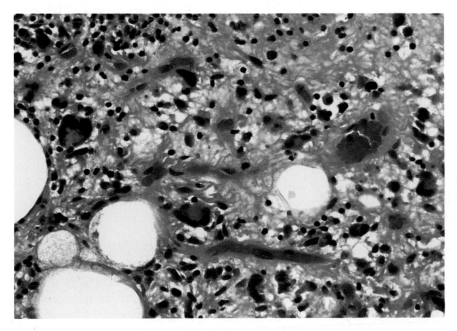

Figure 4-25
PLEOMORPHIC LIPOMA
Multinucleated cells with the hyperchromatic nuclei arranged in a semicircle (floret cells) are characteristic of pleomorphic lipoma but also may be seen in atypical lipomatous tumors.

tumor with myxoid stroma that is deep-seated would be more cellular than intramuscular and juxta-articular myxomas and would usually lack the arborizing vascular pattern of myxoid liposarcoma. Myxoid liposarcomas rarely arise in the subcutaneous tissue, do not contain thick, mature collagen bundles, and usually do not have a large proportion of spindled cells. The differential diagnosis of pleomorphic lipoma is essentially the same as that of atypical lipomatous tumor (see below).

Treatment and Prognosis. It is uncommon for a spindle cell or pleomorphic lipoma, as defined above, to recur after excision, and if it does, recurrences are easily controlled by reexcision. Spindle cell and pleomorphic lipomas do not metastasize.

INTERMEDIATE LIPOMATOUS TUMORS (MANAGERIAL GROUP IIb, TABLE 1-10)

Atypical Lipomatous Tumor

This term includes well-differentiated liposarcoma, atypical lipoma, and pleomorphic lipomas located outside the subcutaneous tissue of the neck, shoulder, and back.

Definition. Atypical lipomatous tumor is a neoplasm composed of mature fat cells and almost always fibrous or myxoid tissue. A variable number of the tumor cells, whether in the fat or the fibrous or myxoid tissue, have enlarged, irregular, hyperchromatic nuclei.

General Considerations. Except for pleomorphic lipoma, the neoplasms we include under the heading of atypical lipomatous tumor have traditionally been designated "well-differentiated liposarcoma" (117c,120,124,127,133a,142a). In the past, some investigators have suggested that atypical lipomatous tumors located in the subcutis and intramuscular (or intermuscular) sites be designated "atypical lipoma" and "atypical intramuscular lipoma," respectively, because they do not metastasize or cause patient death, but that those in the retroperitoneum and other central body sites continue to be classified as "well-differentiated liposarcoma" because they can cause patient death by uncontrolled local growth (117, 117a). However, these tumors are the same histologically whatever their site of origin, and they do not metastasize regardless of location unless they undergo dedifferentiation (see Dedifferentiated Liposarcoma below). Because of these observations, we think it more logical and more conceptually correct to group them under one term, atypical lipomatous tumor (Table 4-1) (118). Weiss and Rao (142a) have argued for retention of the term well-differentiated liposarcoma for intramuscular atypical lipomatous tumors as well as those in central body sites because of the risk of transformation into dedifferentiated liposarcoma. We certainly acknowledge the risk of dedifferentiation but nevertheless maintain that terminology should be determined by the potential reflected in the current morphology of the tumor rather than what the tumor may become (after all, colonic adenomas, salivary mixed tumors, and neurofibromas are not considered malignant). When the tumor dedifferentiates, then it can be labeled as sarcoma, i.e., dedifferentiated liposarcoma. Whatever term is used for atypical lipomatous tumors, what is most important is that the physicians caring for the patient have a clear understanding of the tumor's potential and be aware of the relationship of location to behavior (see Clinical Features below and Table 4-3). We realize that some pathologists will continue to classify central body atypical lipomatous tumors as well-differentiated liposarcoma, and there is little harm in this. However, use of this term for subcutaneous and intramuscular lesions carries with it a significant risk of overtreatment. Our views concerning pleomorphic lipoma have been presented in the Spindle Cell Lipoma section above.

The WHO classification divides well-differentiated liposarcoma into three subtypes, lipoma-like, sclerosing, and inflammatory, without defining how much fibrous tissue is required to place the tumor in the sclerosing category rather than the lipoma-like category or how much inflammation is required for the inflammatory type (143). Because these subcategories have no clinical significance, we do not use them with the atypical lipomatous tumor terminology. Mixtures of the three histologic patterns in the same tumor are common.

Clinical Features. Atypical lipomatous tumors occur mainly in middle-aged or older persons (108a,115–116,124,127,142a). They arise in a wide variety of soft tissue locations, which may be usefully grouped as subcutaneous, intramuscular

Table 4-3

BEHAVIOR OF ATYPICAL LIPOMATOUS TUMORS IN RELATION TO LOCATION

Behavior	Subcutaneous	Location Intramuscular or Intermuscular	Central Body Sites (Including Spermatic Cord and Groin)
Potential for recurrence	Yes (low)	Yes	Yes
Uncontrolled recurrence	No	No	Yes
Metastasis without a dedifferentiated component	No	No	No
Metastasis when a dedifferentiated component is present	Possible (dedifferentiation very rare and reliable data not available)	Yes (but apparently uncommon; only a few cases have been reported)	Yes

(including intermuscular), and central body sites including the groin and spermatic cord. The most common intramuscular site for atypical lipomatous tumors is the thigh, followed by the arm and buttock (108a,117,127,142a). The principal central body site is the retroperitoneum, although a lesser but significant number develop in the inguinal area along the spermatic cord and less commonly in the mediastinum (109,110,112,127,130). The only visceral site of predilection (albeit an uncommon one) appears to be the larynx (107,133,144). Whatever their location, atypical lipomatous tumors typically present as a painless mass that varies from soft to firm depending on the amount of fibrous tissue within it. Retroperitoneal examples often produce abdominal swelling and distension, and spermatic cord lesions may mimic a hernia. Atypical lipomatous tumors can grow to be quite large, and those in the retroperitoneum are among the largest neoplasms that occur in humans. On CT scan, the tumors contain tissue with the density of fat mixed with denser tissue; the extent of the latter depends on the amount of fibrous or myxoid tissue in the neoplasm. Calcific densities due to ossification are an unusual finding.

Pathologic Findings. Grossly, atypical lipomatous tumors usually consist of masses of yellow, mature-appearing fat that most often contain variable amounts of fibrous or myxoid tissue. In some cases, the fibrous and myxoid components constitute the majority of the neoplasm. In intramuscular and central body sites, some atypical lipomatous tumors are obviously infiltrative whereas others are seemingly circumscribed,

but there is no clear evidence that the latter are less likely to recur. Subcutaneous tumors are characteristically well circumscribed. When an atypical lipomatous tumor (especially one in the retroperitoneum) contains relatively discrete fibrous or myxoid areas, the surgeon may not realize that the fatty portions of the neoplasm are neoplastic and may fail to remove them (thus complicating pathologic diagnosis).

Microscopically, atypical lipomatous tumors are made up at least partially of adult type fat cells. Some of these may be smaller than the usual adult adipocyte, or the size may range from smaller to larger. Scattered among the fat cells are variable numbers of cells with enlarged, irregular, dense nuclei (fig. 4-26). Almost always there is a component of myxoid or fibrous tissue (or both) which varies from slight to extensive, and not infrequently this component also contains some of the cells with enlarged, atypical nuclei (fig. 4-27). Occasionally, all the atypical cells are in the fibrous or myxoid component. Whether in the fat or in the fibrous or myxoid stroma, these enlarged cells are required for the diagnosis, and their distinguishing feature is their large irregular nucleus which is composed of dense, often smooth chromatin (figs. 4-28, 4-29). The cytoplasm of the atypical cells, whether in the fat or fibrous tissue, may contain single or multiple clear vacuoles that distort the nucleus. Such cells meet the definition of lipoblasts but not all the atypical cells contain these vacuoles (fig. 4-30). Clear nuclear pseudo-inclusions are commonly present (figs. 4-26B, 4-30, left) and floret cells may be found (fig. 4-31). The

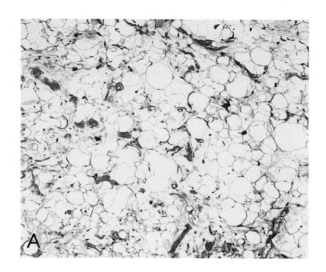

Figure 4-26
ATYPICAL LIPOMATOUS TUMOR

Atypical lipomatous tumor (well-differentiated liposarcoma) is a tumor composed at least in part of adult fat. The key feature that identifies a tumor as an atypical lipomatous tumor is a population of cells with enlarged, dense, irregularly shaped nuclei. These cells are large enough to be seen at low magnification (A) and should be searched for when examining apparent lipomas, particularly if a fatty tumor is deep-seated.

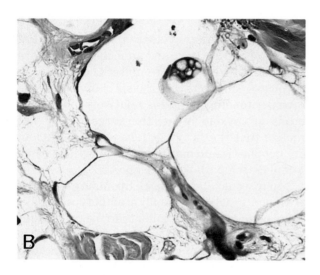

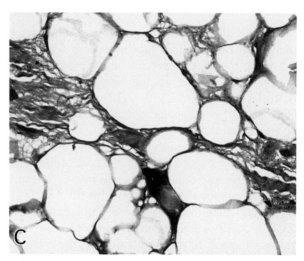

stromal collagen fibers may be coarse and mature or (more often) fine (fig. 4-32). In some instances, atypical lipomatous tumors may contain extensive sheets of paucicellular fibrous tissue which may contain atypical cells; these tumors have been given the name *sclerosing variant* (*sclerosing liposarcoma*). Rarely, central body atypical lipomatous tumors may appear exclusively myxoid, fibrous, or sclerotic in the initial mass and only in recurrence is fatty differentiation clearly demonstrable. Obviously, in this circumstance, one cannot make a diagnosis of fatty tumor until there is evidence of fatty differentiation, and such tumors are best interpreted as unclassified myxoid or fibrous neoplasms containing atypical cells with a comment that they could represent atypical lipomatous tumor.

In general, cellularity is low both in the myxoid-fibrous areas of atypical lipomatous tumor and in the fatty areas, and mitotic figures are uncommon (they may be enlarged and atypical, however). Moderately cellular fibrous or myxoid areas having a somewhat increased number of mitotic figures may be present (fig. 4-33), and have led to differences in interpretation. In a recent study reported by Henricks and associates (121), atypical lipomatous tumors with areas demonstrating cellularity in the range found in desmoid fibromatosis or slightly greater and low mitotic activity were associated with metastasis and considered to be low-grade dedifferentiated liposarcoma. However, we have not observed metastasis in this situation, and thus prefer to reserve the term "dedifferentiated

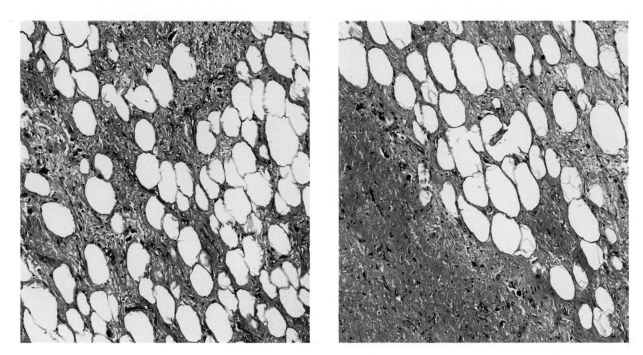

Figure 4-27
ATYPICAL LIPOMATOUS TUMOR
Low-power views of a characteristic atypical lipomatous tumor in which diagnostic large cells with irregular hyperchromatic nuclei are present mainly within fibrous tissue, a frequent feature.

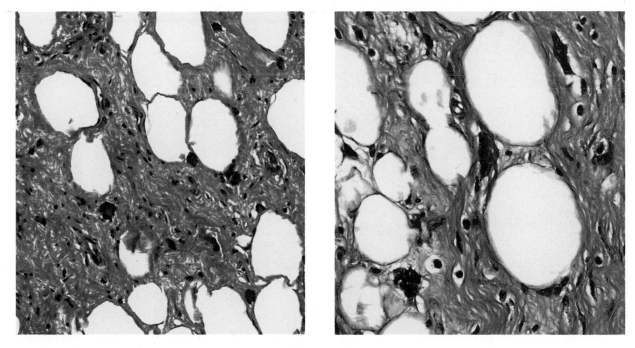

Figure 4-28
ATYPICAL LIPOMATOUS TUMOR
Another example in which the large hyperchromatic cells required for a diagnosis of atypical lipomatous tumor are in fibrous tissue. Fibrous tissue is almost always present in these tumors.

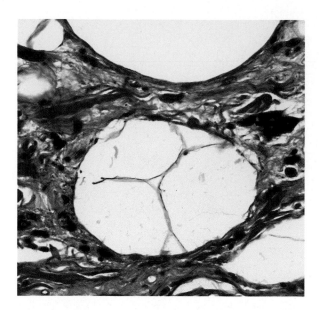
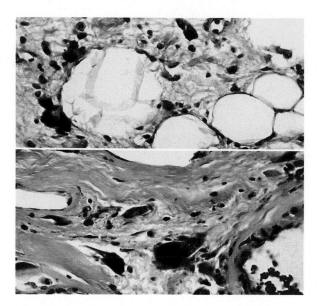

Figure 4-29
ATYPICAL LIPOMATOUS TUMOR
The large hyperchromatic nuclei often have bizarre shapes.

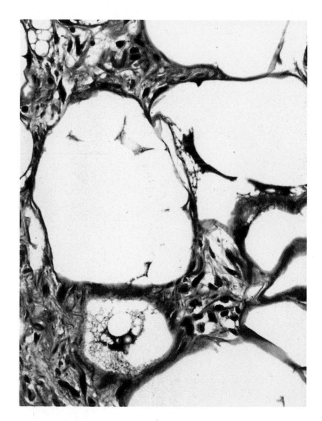
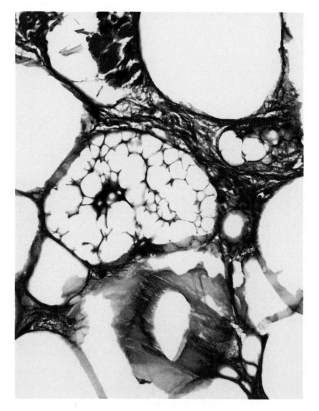

Figure 4-30
ATYPICAL LIPOMATOUS TUMOR
Sometimes the large cells in atypical lipomatous tumor have the features of lipoblasts, with vacuoles distorting the nucleus as seen here. Clear nuclear pseudoinclusions are common.

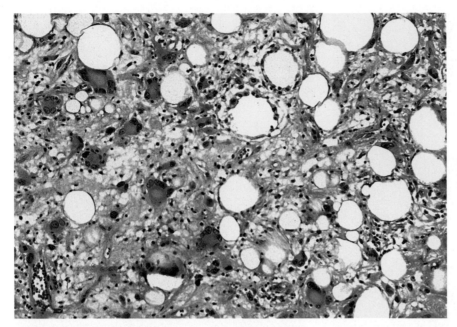

Figure 4-31
ATYPICAL
LIPOMATOUS TUMOR
Floret cells in an atypical lipomatous tumor. These may be found in deep as well as subcutaneous tumors.

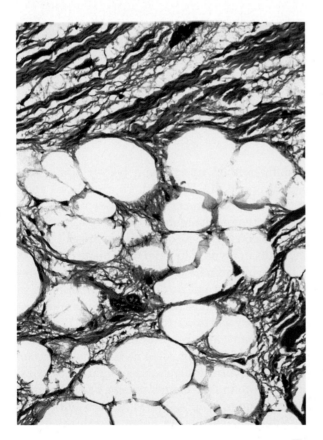

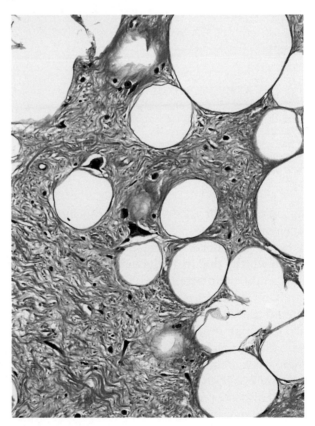

Figure 4-32
ATYPICAL LIPOMATOUS TUMOR
The collagen fibers may be thick (left) or fine (right). Note the variation in the size of the fat cells, a feature that is common in atypical lipomatous tumor.

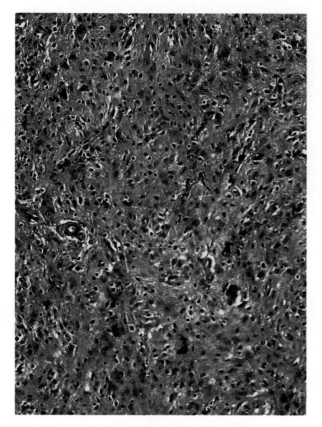

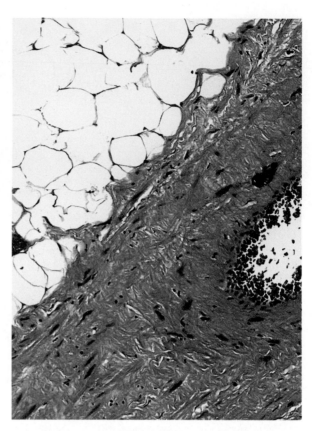

Figure 4-33
ATYPICAL LIPOMATOUS TUMOR

This fibrous area is moderately cellular in contrast to the usually paucicellular fibrous and myxoid zones found in atypical lipomatous tumors. We do not consider such areas of increased cellularity evidence of dedifferentiated liposarcoma when the maximum mitotic rate is less than 5 mitotic figures per 10 high-power fields (see text).

Figure 4-34
ATYPICAL LIPOMATOUS TUMOR

Sometimes the large atypical cells are present within the walls of blood vessels.

liposarcoma" for cases in which there are non-lipogenic areas with high-grade features (117a, 118) (see Dedifferentiated Liposarcoma below). It is noteworthy that in all the cases considered to be low-grade dedifferentiated liposarcoma in the study of Henricks et al. in which metastasis occurred there was first a local recurrence demonstrating high-grade dedifferentiated liposarcoma or an incomplete excision that could have left high-grade elements behind. The tumors reported as spindle cell liposarcoma by Dei Tos and associates (113) featured cellular areas composed of relatively bland-appearing spindle cells with few mitotic figures as well as areas characteristic of atypical lipomatous tumor; metastasis was not observed in their cases except when dedifferentiation (as defined in the section concerning dedifferentiated liposarcoma below) had supervened previously. The authors considered spindle cell liposarcoma a nondedifferentiated variant of atypical lipomatous tumor.

Occasionally, atypical nuclei are present in vessel walls in atypical lipomatous tumors (fig. 4-34). Chronic inflammation (lymphoplasmacytic) is frequently notable and rarely may be prominent, to the point of demonstrating germinal centers (*inflammatory variant*) (fig. 4-35) (108,126). Fat necrosis may also be present. An unusual and interesting finding in some cases is heterologous mesenchymal metaplasia; cartilaginous, osseous, and smooth muscle elements have been observed in such tumors (fig. 4-36) (117a,117b,139).

Special Studies. In about two thirds of the cases fat cells are S-100 protein positive and some of the spindle cells, including the atypical cells, may be CD34 positive (113a,138a). However, immunohistochemistry is seldom needed to make

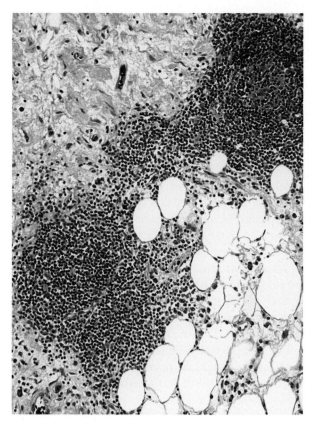

Figure 4-35
ATYPICAL LIPOMATOUS TUMOR
Atypical lipomatous tumors sometimes display prominent chronic inflammation. When this occurs there is potential for misinterpretation as an inflammatory process.

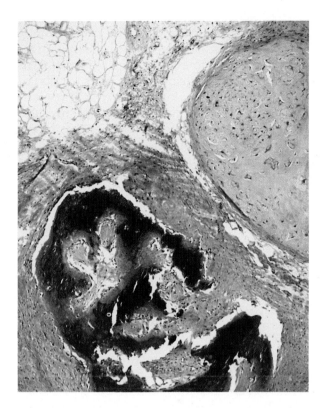

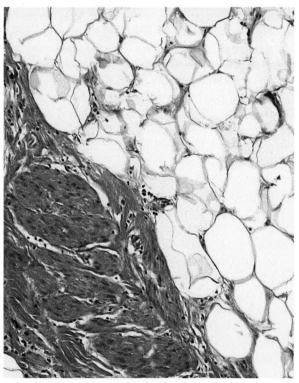

Figure 4-36
ATYPICAL LIPOMATOUS TUMOR
Metaplastic bone and cartilage (top) or smooth muscle (bottom) may occasionally be found in atypical lipomatous tumors.

the diagnosis because atypical lipomatous tumor is almost always recognizable by light microscopy, and immunohistochemistry is of little value in distinguishing among the usual differential diagnostic considerations. Recent studies have shown that over 90 percent of patients with atypical lipomatous tumors have variable clonal chromosomal abnormalities. The only consistent abnormality, found in over 60 percent of cases in a recent study, is the presence of supernumerary ring chromosomes derived from the 13–15 region of chromosome 12 (131,131a). Other alterations involve 12q, 6p, 8q, and 13q. Interestingly, 12q13–15 is the same region that is altered in lipomas, but ring chromosomes are very rare in lipomas. Of note is the rarity of aberrations of 16q13 in atypical lipomatous tumors, whereas alterations of this chromosome are common in spindle cell and pleomorphic lipomas (131).

Differential Diagnosis. The most common differential diagnostic problem involving atypical lipomatous tumors is their distinction from lipomas. Atypical lipomatous tumors are distinguished by their population of cells with atypical nuclei. How large and numerous the required atypical nuclei should be before one makes a diagnosis of atypical lipomatous tumor rather than lipoma has never been defined officially, but in nonretroperitoneal sites we require that they be large enough to be discerned at scanning magnification (40X) and regard a single such nucleus as sufficient. In the retroperitoneum, any tumor mass composed in part or totally of mature fat cells must be considered to be atypical lipomatous tumor for management purposes, even if atypical cells are not found. Atypical lipomatous tumors may have large areas that are indistinguishable from lipoma because the atypical nuclei may be present in only a few areas of the tumor. It is thus necessary to examine an adequate number of sections of any lipomatous tumor, especially when the neoplasm is removed from an intramuscular or central body site. We suggest a minimum of one section per centimeter of diameter of tumor up to 10 sections routinely be taken from lipomatous tumors removed from sites other than the subcutaneous tissue. Often, some of the fat cells in atypical lipomatous tumor are smaller than adult adipocytes or vary from smaller to larger and either of these findings should intensify the search for atypical cells. As indicated previously, enlarged, atypical nuclei may be more plentiful in fibrous or myxoid areas in atypical lipomatous tumors, so these areas (which may be small) should be sought. Atypical lipomatous tumors in the retroperitoneum may be composed of cells that are indistinguishable from those found in lipomas in other sites and atypical cells may be sparse or, rarely, absent.

Distinction of atypical lipomatous tumor from the usual spindle cell lipoma is based on the dense ropy collagen; uniform spindle cells; usual subcutaneous location in the back, neck, or shoulders; and lack of enlarged atypical cells which characterize the latter. Pleomorphic lipoma, with or without a component of spindle cell lipoma, is distinguished from atypical lipomatous tumor by location: examples that arise in the subcutis of the neck, back, and shoulder are classified as pleomorphic lipoma while those that occur elsewhere are classified as atypical lipomatous tumor.

Another diagnostic difficulty occurs in relation to nonlipogenic malignant mesenchymal neoplasms that contain enlarged atypical cells, especially the myxoid and pleomorphic variants of malignant fibrous histiocytoma (MFH). Atypical lipomatous tumors that are principally composed of myxoid or fibrous tissue may be confused with these MFH variants if it is not realized that a portion of the tumor demonstrates fatty differentiation; this is of course especially likely to occur if the surgeon does not realize this either and does not remove the fatty component. In general, atypical lipomatous tumor should be suspected, particularly in the retroperitoneum, if a myxoid or fibrous neoplasm features nuclear enlargement and pleomorphism but is distinctly less cellular and less mitotically active than the usual MFH; in such cases, a fatty component should be carefully sought and CT scans should be reviewed for evidence that the mass was composed partially of fat. Conversely, MFH infiltrating fat, especially myxoid MFH in the subcutis, may be mistakenly interpreted as an atypical lipomatous tumor. This error can be avoided if one pays attention to the overall contour of the lesion (most often circumscribed in subcutaneous atypical lipomatous tumor and usually infiltrative in MFH) and the cellularity and mitotic activity, which are almost always greater in MFH.

Features used to distinguish atypical lipomatous tumor from dedifferentiated liposarcoma (atypical lipomatous tumor with areas of nonlipidic sarcoma) are discussed in the Dedifferentiated Liposarcoma section. For differences between atypical lipomatous tumor and pleomorphic liposarcoma see the section on the latter.

Some atypical lipomatous tumors contain a large number of chronic inflammatory cells. Distinguishing this from an inflammatory process involving fat is based on the presence or absence of a mass. This is particularly important in the retroperitoneum because atypical lipomatous tumors in this area may be composed of adult fat with few atypical cells but with a large component of inflammation. Great care should be taken when contemplating a diagnosis of an inflammatory process in the retroperitoneum when there is a mass lesion present. Fat necrosis can also be confused with atypical lipomatous tumor because lipid-filled macrophages can superficially resemble atypical fat cells, and the multinucleated cells and fibrosis found in some instances of fat necrosis can further the mimicry of atypical lipomatous tumor. However, macrophages typically have small, central, nonpleomorphic nuclei that are not deformed by lipid vacuoles. Ingested foreign material such as silicone can cause the cytoplasm of macrophages to become so vacuolated that the nuclei are indented, but nuclear enlargement and pleomorphism are still lacking and there is typically more variation in vacuole size in these reactive cells than in the cells that compose atypical lipomatous tumors.

Angiomyolipoma has a component of adipocytes in which fat cell nuclei may be enlarged. Because of this, there may be concern about atypical lipomatous tumor; however, angiomyolipomas also feature prominent collections of convoluted blood vessels with little or no elastic tissue and collections of smooth muscle cells, many of which are perivascular. Large abnormal vessels are not a feature of atypical lipomatous tumor, and while metaplastic smooth muscle may be found in an atypical lipomatous tumor it is not perivascular and most often it is focal and inconspicuous. Moreover, angiomyolipoma occurs almost exclusively in the kidney, with only rare cases reported in the retroperitoneum, liver, and mediastinum. The spindle cells in angiomyolipoma are HMB45 positive and the cells in atypical lipomatous tumor are HMB45 negative.

The histologic appearances of massive localized lymphedema could bring atypical lipomatous tumor to mind because of the presence of fat intersected by fibrous septa, but enlarged atypical nuclei are lacking in that lesion and it characteristically occurs in the subcutaneous tissue of the medial proximal extremities of morbidly obese persons (118a).

Treatment and Prognosis. The behavior of atypical lipomatous tumors is distinctly related to their location (Table 4-3) (108a,117,117a,118, 127,142a). Subcutaneous examples usually do not recur after complete excision; the relatively frequent incidence of recurrence observed in one series was probably a result of incomplete excision (123). Even if they recur, subcutaneous tumors do not do so aggressively. On the other hand, atypical lipomatous tumors in central body sites, including the groin and spermatic cord, typically recur frequently and repeatedly, and can cause patient death as a result of uncon-

trolled growth and destructive local infiltration. The interval to recurrence is often quite long, the median interval being 42 months in one study (118). While intramuscular atypical lipomatous tumors also recur frequently, they rarely if ever cause patient death (108a,117,127,142a). Atypical lipomatous tumors do not metastasize. They may, however, become dedifferentiated, i.e., develop a component of cellular, nonlipogenic sarcoma, most commonly MFH-like (see Dedifferentiated Liposarcoma below), and the dedifferentiated component not only recurs more quickly and aggressively than atypical lipomatous tumor but can metastasize (108a,117a,118,121,142a). Dedifferentiation is most common in atypical lipomatous tumors involving central body sites, especially the retroperitoneum, but occurs at times in intramuscular examples and very rarely in the subcutis. Much less common than dedifferentiation to nonlipogenic sarcoma is the development of an area of unclassifiable liposarcoma (see Unclassified Liposarcoma below) in a recurrent atypical lipomatous tumor. In our experience, this occurs almost entirely in the retroperitoneum, and we have not observed metastasis associated with it (118).

MALIGNANT LIPOMATOUS TUMORS (MANAGERIAL GROUP III, TABLE 1-10)

Dedifferentiated Liposarcoma

Definition. Dedifferentiated liposarcoma is a biphasic neoplasm in which one component is atypical lipomatous tumor while the other is cellular, nonlipogenic sarcoma (the dedifferentiated component).

Clinical Features. Dedifferentiated liposarcoma, like atypical lipomatous tumor, usually occurs in middle-aged or older persons (111,117a, 118,121,128). It develops most frequently in central body sites, especially the retroperitoneum and the spermatic cord, and is considerably less common in intramuscular locations (subcutaneous dedifferentiated liposarcoma [145] is very rare). Dedifferentiated liposarcoma may occur either *ab initio,* i.e., as a biphasic neoplasm in the initial excision specimen, or as a recurrence of an erstwhile atypical lipomatous tumor; in either event, the locational preference for central body sites is similar. On CT scans, fatty and nonfatty areas are seen, but nonfatty areas may simply represent fibrous or myxoid zones in an atypical lipomatous tumor and not a dedifferentiated component.

Pathologic Findings. Grossly, the dedifferentiated component may manifest as a discrete nonfatty area within an otherwise predominantly fatty mass, or it may blend more gradually with the fibrous or myxoid zones in the atypical lipomatous tumor component and thus not be sharply outlined. A softer, "fish-flesh" consistency is especially suggestive of a dedifferentiated component rather than simply a fibrous area in an atypical lipomatous tumor.

Microscopically, dedifferentiated liposarcoma is composed of both atypical lipomatous tumor and nonlipogenic high-grade sarcoma (fig. 4-37) (117a, 118,120,121,128,133a,137). The dedifferentiated areas are cellular, usually pleomorphic, and mitotically active; for the diagnosis we require that there be at least 5 mitotic figures per 10 high-power fields in some area of the tumor (117a). Our concerns about the concept of low-grade dedifferentiated liposarcoma are expressed in the pathology section of Atypical Lipomatous Tumors above. The interface between the two components may be abrupt, the two may merge, or they may be mingled. Uncommonly, the dedifferentiated sarcoma grows as nodules throughout areas of the atypical lipomatous tumor. A recent study has proposed a size requirement of at least one 10X objective field for dedifferentiation (121). Most often, dedifferentiated areas resemble pleomorphic MFH, with nuclear hyperchromatism, pleomorphism, and numerous mitotic figures making diagnosis easy (fig. 4-38).

Other patterns that might be encountered include those resembling myxoid MFH (high-grade myxofibrosarcoma), high-grade fibrosarcoma (fig. 4-39), or inflammatory MFH. A storiform pattern may be prominent (fig. 4-40). Sheets of round cells with eosinophilic cytoplasm resembling carcinoma, melanoma, or lymphoma have also been reported. Unusual features that may be present in the dedifferentiated component include nuclear palisading, a rich, hemangiopericytoma-like vascular pattern (fig. 4-41), and whorled foci (118a,129b). Another uncommon but interesting finding is nonfatty, specialized mesenchymal elements, including skeletal muscle that can have the features of rhabdomyosarcoma, smooth muscle which may come to resemble leiomyosarcoma, malignant osteoid or tumor bone, and

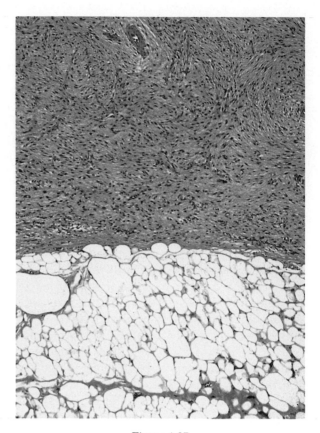

Figure 4-37
DEDIFFERENTIATED LIPOSARCOMA
So called dedifferentiation in atypical lipomatous tumor is heralded by hypercellular fibrous or myxoid areas. Here the junction between atypical lipomatous tumor and the dedifferentiated component is sharp.

angiosarcoma-like vessels (figs. 4-42, 4-43) (117c, 132,141). Metastases of dedifferentiated liposarcoma contain only the dedifferentiated component, not the atypical lipomatous tumor.

Special Studies. Immunohistochemistry is seldom needed to make a diagnosis, and when it is, it is usually to exclude another tumor type. It can also be used to confirm nonfatty differentiated mesenchymal elements, e.g., muscle, in those rare dedifferentiated liposarcomas that contain them. Ring chromosomes are very often present in the cells of dedifferentiated liposarcoma as they are in the cells of atypical lipomatous tumors (131).

Differential Diagnosis. The major differential diagnostic consideration is recognizing areas of dedifferentiation within an atypical lipomatous tumor. This is not difficult in the usual case because the dedifferentiated areas look like high-grade pleomorphic sarcoma. When there is

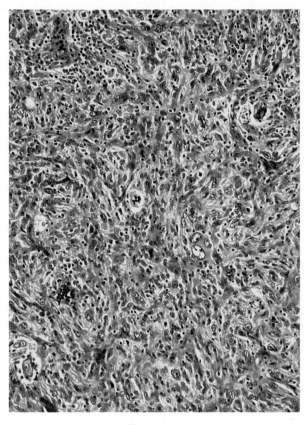

Figure 4-38
DEDIFFERENTIATED LIPOSARCOMA

This dedifferentiated component is nonlipogenic sarcoma indistinguishable from pleomorphic MFH. This is the most common pattern of dedifferentiation in dedifferentiated liposarcoma. (Correct classification requires identification of the atypical lipomatous tumor portion.)

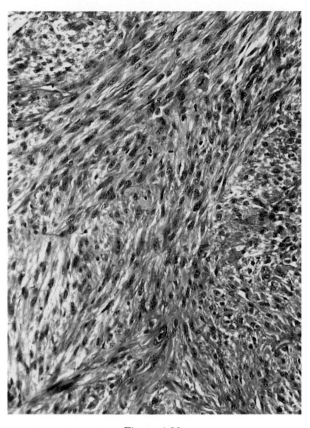

Figure 4-39
DEDIFFERENTIATED LIPOSARCOMA

A fibrosarcoma-like pattern of dedifferentiation, with less pleomorphism, is seen.

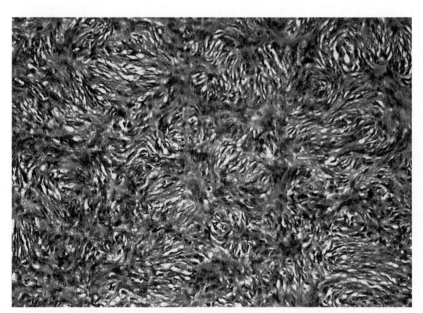

Figure 4-40
DEDIFFERENTIATED
LIPOSARCOMA

A storiform pattern is not uncommon in the dedifferentiated component.

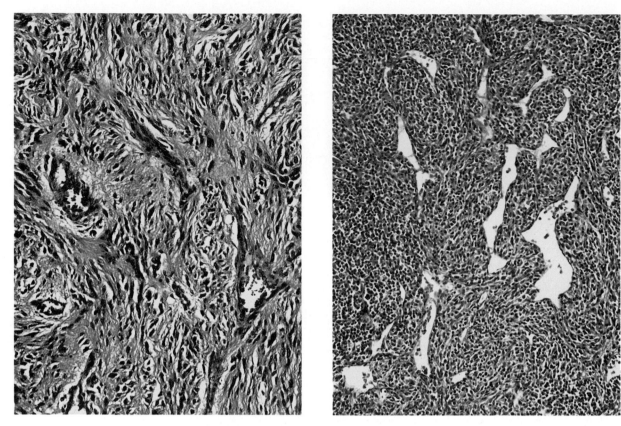

Figure 4-41
DEDIFFERENTIATED LIPOSARCOMA
Other patterns seen in dedifferentiated liposarcoma include nuclear palisading, giving the tumor a neural appearance (left), and a hemangiopericytoma-like vascular pattern (right).

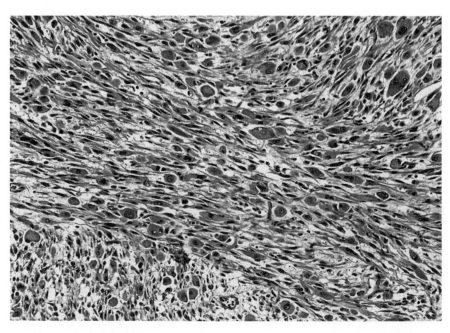

Figure 4-42
DEDIFFERENTIATED
LIPOSARCOMA
Rarely, rhadomyosarcomatous elements may be found in dedifferentiated liposarcoma.

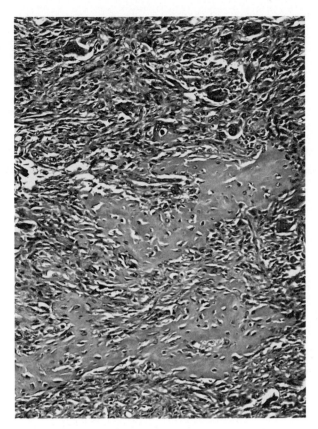

Figure 4-43
DEDIFFERENTIATED LIPOSARCOMA
This example demonstrates osteoid in the dedifferentiated component.

difficulty deciding whether the nonlipogenic component of an atypical lipomatous tumor is dedifferentiated, the mitotic index as described above in the pathology section is utilized.

Differential diagnostic problems concerning dedifferentiated liposarcoma can occur when the atypical lipomatous tumor component is inconspicuous and the dedifferentiated component greatly predominates, thus resulting in confusion with another type of (nonlipogenic) sarcoma, usually MFH. This difficulty can be obviated only by identification of the atypical lipomatous tumor component, since the dedifferentiated component has no distinguishing features. There may be some importance in this distinction because there is evidence to suggest that patients with dedifferentiated liposarcomas have a better prognosis than do those with pure pleomorphic MFH, particularly if the tumor is located outside the retroperitoneum or groin (121,128).

A much less common source of confusion is the rare angiomyolipoma in which the smooth muscle component becomes mitotically active and atypical, and thus comes to resemble the dedifferentiated component of dedifferentiated liposarcoma. The latter, however, lacks smooth muscle characteristics in all but rare cases, and if attention is paid to whether the tumor involves the kidney or the adjacent retroperitoneum diagnostic difficulties should be easily resolved because dedifferentiated liposarcoma is practically never centered in the kidney and almost all angiomyolipomas arise there. Moreover, dedifferentiated liposarcomas do not contain abnormal blood vessels of the type found in angiomyolipoma and the spindle cells in angiomyolipoma are HMB45 positive, a stain that is negative in liposarcoma.

Pleomorphic liposarcoma often has areas indistinguishable from pleomorphic MFH, a feature it shares with dedifferentiated liposarcoma, but pleomorphic liposarcoma lacks an atypical lipomatous component, i.e., it is a cellular sarcoma throughout with at least some neoplastic lipoblasts but it does not contain mature fat cells (see below). We have observed a few retroperitoneal tumors in which pleomorphic liposarcoma was combined with atypical lipomatous tumor in separate areas. Such tumors do not meet the definition of dedifferentiated liposarcoma because the sarcomatous element contains lipogenic cells, and we think the proper label is mixed atypical lipomatous tumor and pleomorphic liposarcoma. These few patients died as a result of uncontrolled local tumor growth.

Treatment and Prognosis. Dedifferentiated liposarcomas recur more quickly than atypical lipomatous tumors, and the dedifferentiated component can metastasize, most often to the lungs, liver, and bone, especially if the tumor is primary in a central body site. Although the survival of patients with dedifferentiated liposarcoma is usually longer (median, approximately 5 years) than that of patients with certain other types of high-grade or dedifferentiated sarcoma (such as dedifferentiated chondrosarcoma) and the metastasis rate may be lower, the outcome is generally unfavorable. In central body sites survival is significantly shorter for patients with dedifferentiated liposarcoma than for those with atypical lipomatous tumor alone (118,121). When a central body atypical lipomatous tumor becomes dedifferentiated in recurrence, survival from that point is similar to what is observed with dedifferentiated liposarcomas that present *ab initio* (118). The dedifferentiated component of dedifferentiated liposarcoma usually tends to progressively dominate the tumor, but occasionally this component does not reappear in subsequent recurrences, which are then composed only of atypical lipomatous tumor. As might be expected, longer survivals occur in such circumstances.

Recognizing dedifferentiation in an atypical lipomatous tumor (i.e., recognizing dedifferentiated liposarcoma) is very important because this change announces that the tumor now has metastatic capability. The features used to make this distinction are presented above. However, the risk of metastasis and death from tumor is significantly higher for tumors in central body sites than for those in intramuscular locations (121); in fact, only a few intramuscular dedifferentiated liposarcomas with metastasis have ever been reported. Dedifferentiation in subcutaneous atypical lipomatous tumors is so rare that there is no reliable information about behavior. The extent of dedifferentiation does not appear to affect outcome; location of the tumor is the only significant variable for survival (121).

Myxoid Liposarcoma: Paucicellular and Cellular

Definition. Myxoid liposarcoma is a variably cellular, fatty tumor that classically contains small, uniform, "signet ring" lipogenic tumor cells set in a myxoid matrix; numerous arborizing arched capillaries; and small, uniform, nonlipogenic cells with scant cytoplasm. Significant areas of mature fat also may be present.

General Considerations. Classifications of liposarcoma often contain a category of "round cell" liposarcoma (116,120,124,133a,143). However, we think almost all putative examples are myxoid liposarcomas with cellular areas, and we consider round cell liposarcoma as a part of the spectrum of myxoid liposarcoma (108a,117a,118). This position is strengthened by the observation that the same clonal chromosomal translocation, t(12;16)(q13;p11), is found in the cells composing both myxoid liposarcoma and round cell liposarcoma (118c,125). The stated utility of a round cell category is to call attention to a tumor that has significant metastatic potential (in contrast to the

low metastatic capacity of paucicellular myxoid liposarcoma). We suggest the metastatic potential can just as well be expressed by the term cellular myxoid liposarcoma when 25 percent or more of the tumor is cellular rather than maintaining another category of liposarcoma (108a, 117a,118). The rare, totally cellular myxoid liposarcoma (pure "round cell" liposarcoma) can be recognized by its cellular uniformity, the relatively small size of its cells, the presence of lipoblasts, usually signet ring lipoblasts, and, frequently, the presence of periarterial/perivenous hypocellular zones.

Clinical Features. Myxoid liposarcoma usually occurs in mid-adulthood, and has an incidence peak in the fifth decade (118); it rarely develops in individuals under the age of 20. Shmookler and Enzinger (134) did report a few examples in children and teenagers but all their patients except one were over the age of 10; a 7-month-old infant was reported to have "round cell" liposarcoma. By far, the most common location for myxoid liposarcoma is the thigh, although the popliteal area, groin, and buttock are also frequent sites. Myxoid liposarcoma is distinctly unusual elsewhere, including the retroperitoneum. Almost all examples arise within muscle or other deeper soft tissues and involvement of the subcutis is extraordinarily rare. Presentation is usually that of a painless mass, which is often quite large by the time it is detected. CT scans may show partial fat density or nonfat density, depending on the amount of fat in the neoplasm.

Pathologic Findings. Myxoid liposarcoma typically appears well circumscribed grossly and most often has a slimy cut surface with a variable yellow tinge (fig. 4-44). It is often lobulated. Cellular areas may have a fleshy sarcoma-like aspect, whereas areas with pronounced fatty maturation may resemble ordinary adipose tissue.

The well-known and characteristic histologic pattern of paucicellular myxoid liposarcoma is that of small uniform cells with scant cytoplasm set some distance apart within a myxoid matrix that contains numerous capillaries arranged in a plexiform pattern (fig. 4-45) (117a,118,120,122,124, 130a,136). Scattered among these cells are variable numbers of cells with a clear vacuole or vacuoles that often distort and push the frequently thin nucleus to the side of the cell (fig. 4-46). These signet ring lipoblasts are distinguished

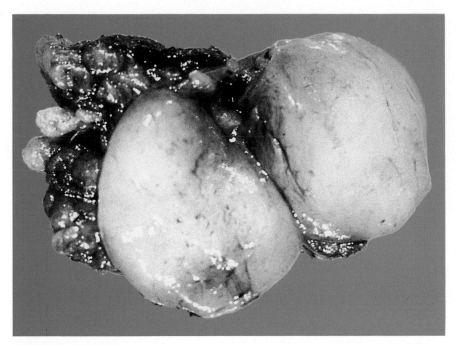

Figure 4-44
MYXOID LIPOSARCOMA
The cut surface of the usual
myxoid liposarcoma is gelatinous.

from adult fat cells by their small size. Sometimes the lipoblasts have central nuclei distorted and deformed by the fat vacuole(s). Mitotic figures are generally uncommon.

The degree of cellularity varies from this classic pattern. Some myxoid liposarcomas are more cellular and sometimes the cellularity is so high that there is little or no interstitial material; tumors this cellular have been labeled round cell liposarcomas in some classification schemes, but we think such tumors should be classified as cellular myxoid liposarcomas because they are clearly part of the spectrum of myxoid liposarcoma and not a separate entity (fig. 4-47). The rate of metastasis is related to the proportion of tumor that is cellular (117a,118,122,136) and is especially high when that proportion is 25 percent or greater, so we use this figure to define cellular myxoid liposarcoma (117a,118). Areas of high cellularity may be focal, therefore, thorough sectioning is important, and when cellular areas are present but comprise less than 25 percent of the tumor this should be noted in the pathology report along with a statement that metastatic potential may be increased (136). As the tumor becomes more cellular, the nuclei may become larger and have coarser chromatin but they remain uniform (fig. 4-48). Signet ring lipoblasts identify a largely or completely cellular tumor as myxoid liposar-

coma. Mitotic figures are often more plentiful in cellular tumors, and the plexiform vascular pattern tends to become obscured in cellular areas.

The fat cells in myxoid liposarcoma are usually small and often univacuolated, but they may be multivacuolated (fig. 4-49). When a single vacuole pushes the nucleus to the side and deforms it into a crescent, the term *signet ring lipoblast* has been used. Such cells closely resemble smaller versions of mature fat cells. An appearance so distinctive it is virtually diagnostic of myxoid liposarcoma is produced when small fat cells become numerous enough to lie back-to-back (fig. 4-50). In some myxoid liposarcomas, maturation to large mature fat cells occurs and this can progress to the point that areas of the tumor resemble lipoma (fig. 4-51). Sometimes, myxoid liposarcomas have few cells with identifiable fat vacuoles and extensive sectioning will be needed to find them since they are the key to the diagnosis. In very rare instances, lipidic cells are not found even after extensive sectioning. In this circumstance, we think the diagnosis of myxoid liposarcoma can still be made if the clinical presentation and the other histologic features are characteristic, but one should be especially careful to exclude alternatives such as low-grade myxoid MFH (low-grade myxofibrosarcoma). Of course, this maneuver constitutes a violation of the rule

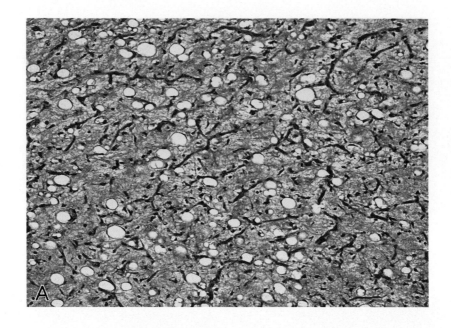

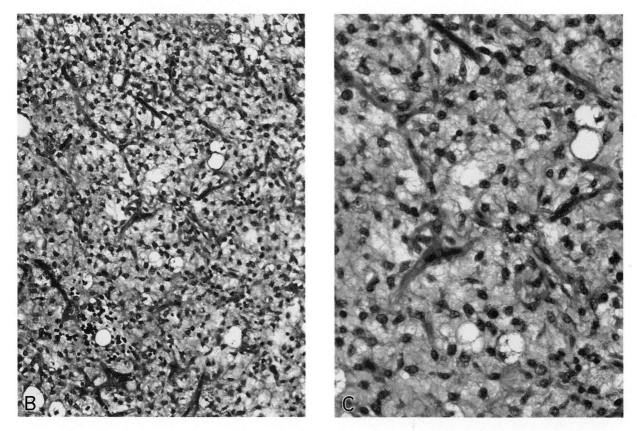

Figure 4-45
PAUCICELLULAR MYXOID LIPOSARCOMA

This is the characteristic low-power appearance of paucicellular myxoid liposarcoma composed of the required small uniform cells set in a myxoid stroma. The features that define myxoid liposarcoma are illustrated: the fine arborizing vascular pattern, signet ring lipoblasts, and nonlipidic cells with small uniform nuclei.

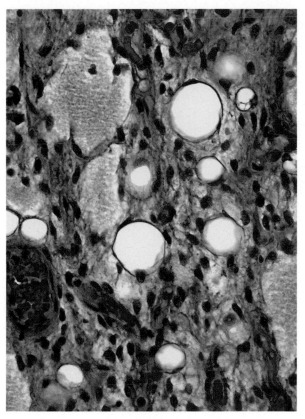

Figure 4-46
PAUCICELLULAR MYXOID LIPOSARCOMA
High-power view of signet ring lipoblasts. These differ from adult fat cells by their small size.

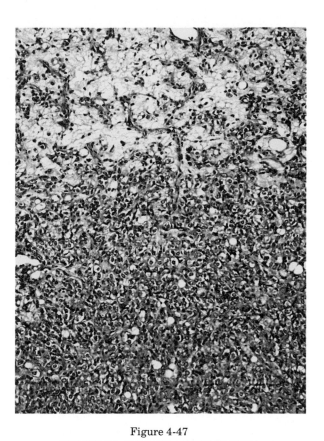

Figure 4-47
CELLULAR MYXOID LIPOSARCOMA
In most tumors cellular areas are focal if present, but when 25 percent of the tumor is cellular it is recognized as cellular myxoid liposarcoma. Careful search for cellular areas is always warranted because they herald increased metastatic potential.

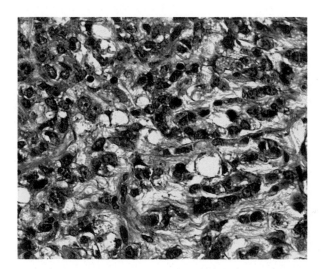

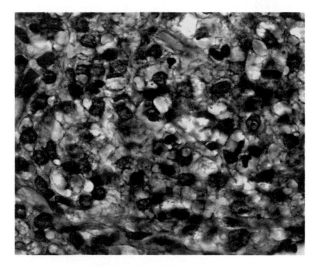

Figure 4-48
CELLULAR MYXOID LIPOSARCOMA
Even when cellular, myxoid liposarcoma is composed of cells with uniform nuclei. Significant pleomorphism is not allowed although nuclei are often more irregular and have more granular chromatin in cellular than noncellular areas.

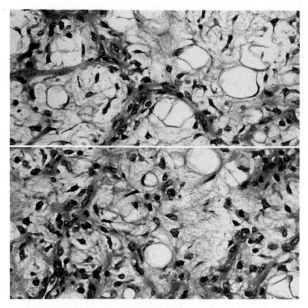

Figure 4-49
PAUCICELLULAR MYXOID LIPOSARCOMA
Signet ring lipoblasts are smaller than adult fat cells and usually have a single clear vacuole that pushes the nucleus into a crescent at the side of the cell.

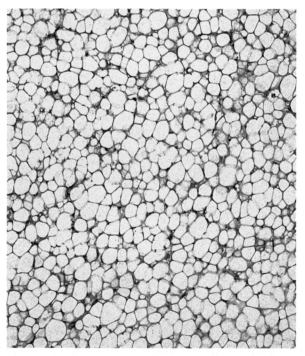

Figure 4-50
MYXOID LIPOSARCOMA
Numerous small back-to-back fat cells are characteristic of some myxoid liposarcomas and produce a distinctive appearance. Distinction from lipoma is based on the small size of the fat cells.

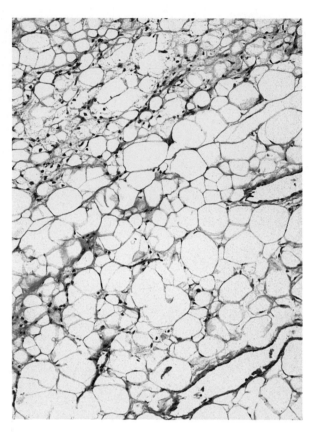

Figure 4-51
MYXOID LIPOSARCOMA
This area of a myxoid liposarcoma contains a large number of fat cells, some of which are mature and some of which, on the top left, are smaller. Such areas can lead to an erroneous diagnosis of atypical lipomatous tumor or lipoma. Thorough sectioning of deep-seated fatty tumors and those in central body sites is essential to avoid classificatory errors.

that lipidic tumors must contain lipidic cells but the behavior of tumors that have all the other features of myxoid liposarcoma except lipidic cells is the same as those that do contain such cells, so in this circumstance an exception is made.

In examples of myxoid liposarcoma with abundant myxoid interstitial material, cystic spaces, often filled with granular material, may be present within the matrix (fig. 4-52). These have been termed microcysts and on occasion they are large and bizarrely shaped (fig. 4-53). Microcysts are easily seen at low magnification and they are so distinctive that they should always cause the observer to think of myxoid liposarcoma. When larger microcysts are plentiful the pattern has been labeled *pulmonary edema-like* (fig. 4-54). A distinctive vessel-related finding

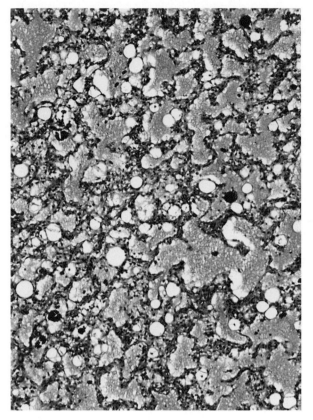

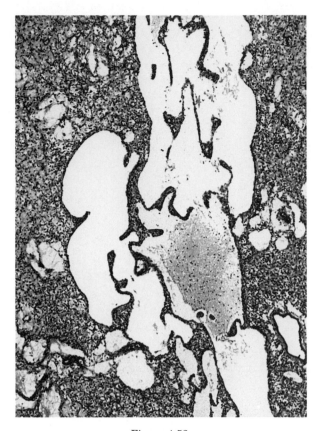

Figure 4-52
MYXOID LIPOSARCOMA
Cystic spaces (microcysts) filled with granular eosinophilic material are common in myxoid liposarcoma and serve as a useful marker of this tumor.

Figure 4-53
MYXOID LIPOSARCOMA
WITH LARGE CYSTIC SPACES
Sometimes the microcystic spaces are larger and irregularly shaped, as in this example.

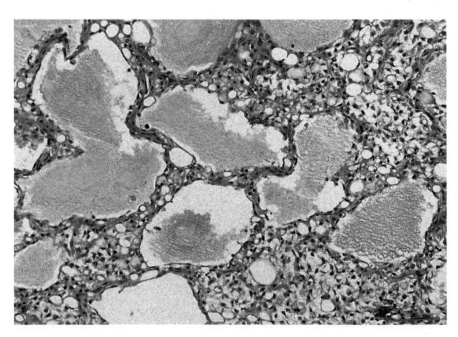

Figure 4-54
MYXOID LIPOSARCOMA
When microcysts become numerous the resulting pattern has been likened to that seen in pulmonary edema.

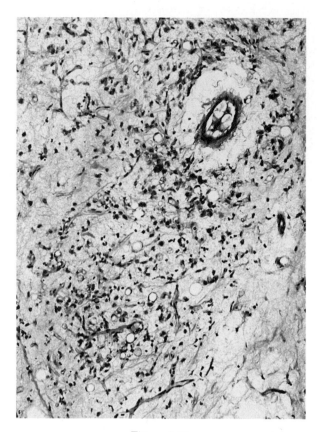

Figure 4-55
PAUCICELLULAR MYXOID LIPOSARCOMA
The hypocellular zone around a small artery is a characteristic feature of myxoid liposarcoma.

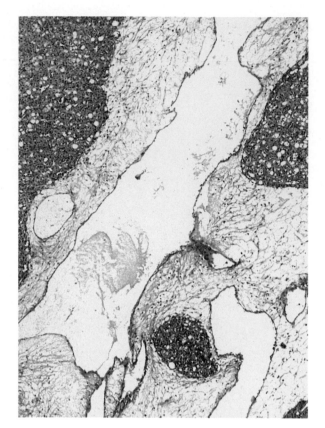

Figure 4-56
CELLULAR MYXOID LIPOSARCOMA
This tumor features large hypocellular zones around veins.

in myxoid liposarcoma, in addition to the plexiform capillary network, is the presence of hypocellular zones around small arteries and veins (figs. 4-55, 4-56).

As mentioned previously, the nuclei in myxoid liposarcoma are characteristically uniform. Although there may be an increase in nuclear size in cellular areas, significant nuclear pleomorphism is not a feature; however, rare recurrent or metastatic tumors may demonstrate this to some degree. A finding that can be confused with pleomorphism at low-power magnification is cell clusters or cords, which are occasionally seen in myxoid liposarcoma (fig. 4-57). Another uncommon finding is cell rows separated by hyalinized collagen bundles (fig. 4-58). Rarely, there is cartilaginous metaplasia (135).

Special Studies. Most reported myxoid liposarcomas subjected to cytogenetic analysis have had a translocation involving the long arm of

chromosome 12 and the short arm of chromosome 16, t(12;16)(q13;p11) (118c,114,125,129, 138,140,142). Tumors without this specific chromosomal aberration usually have had some other type of translocation that involved chromosomes 12 and 16. In addition to the 12;16 translocation, trisomy 8 was found in several tumors (138) and some have had a t(12;22) translocation with EWS/CHOP fusion. It has not been possible to identify any clinical or pathologic differences between these molecular genetic subsets (112a). The lipoblasts are often S-100 protein positive, and occasionally cells without fat vacuoles are also S-100 protein positive (113a).

Differential Diagnosis. The differential diagnosis of myxoid liposarcoma involves other neoplasms with a myxoid stroma. The cells composing myxoid MFH (myxofibrosarcoma) demonstrate greater nuclear pleomorphism, at least focally, than do the cells in myxoid liposarcoma,

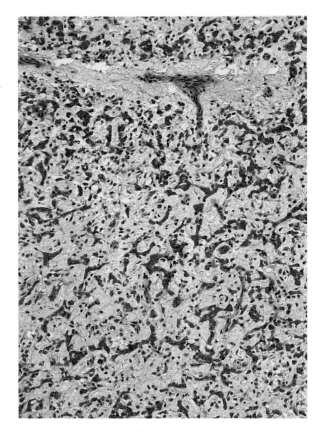

Figure 4-57
MYXOID LIPOSARCOMA
On occasion, the cells in myxoid liposarcoma line up in cords. Myxoid chondrosarcoma almost always has a similar cellular arrangement (typically more pronounced); however, lipogenesis is absent in myxoid chondrosarcoma and it also has a distinctive lobulated pattern.

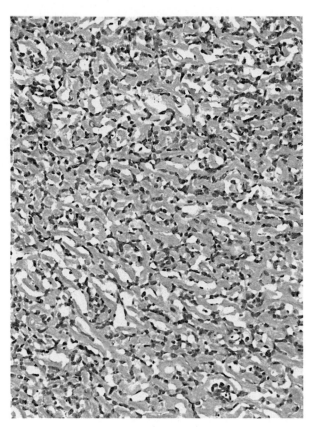

Figure 4-58
MYXOID LIPOSARCOMA
Rarely, myxoid liposarcomas feature cell rows separated by hyalinized collagen bundles.

and lack cytoplasmic fat vacuoles, although some may contain intracytoplasmic vacuoles of mucopolysaccharide which can resemble lipid. To be recognized, intracytoplasmic lipid vacuoles must appear empty, push the nucleus to the side of the cell, and distort it into a crescent (signet ring configuration), or they must scallop the nucleus. Cells containing acid mucopolysaccharide usually do not have deformed nuclei (although they may with pronounced accumulation), and the mucopolysaccharide material typically has the same tinctorial quality as the stroma and does not appear clear. Myxoid MFH often has a rich, arborizing capillary network similar to that in myxoid liposarcoma; however, hypocellular periarterial and perivenous zones and microcysts are usually lacking. Many sections may be needed to prove there are no in-tracytoplasmic lipid vacuoles within the tumor and to demonstrate the areas of significant pleomorphism which characterize myxoid MFHs. A helpful differential diagnostic feature is the observation that myxoid MFH often arises in the subcutaneous tissue, a site that is rarely involved by myxoid liposarcoma.

Myxoid chondrosarcoma is a lobulated tumor in which the uniform tumor cells are predominantly located at the periphery of the lobules and more centrally are arranged in small clusters or chains. Fat vacuoles and an arborizing vascular pattern are absent. Intramuscular myxoma contains uniform cells but is extremely paucicellular, much more so than even the least cellular myxoid liposarcoma, and it lacks fat cells and prominent vascularity.

Diagnostic difficulties involving myxoid liposarcoma sometimes occur in relation to other types of liposarcomas and lipomatous neoplasms.

Myxoid areas in atypical lipomatous tumors occasionally have plentiful capillaries, but the diagnostic problem can be resolved by identifying nuclear enlargement and pleomorphism, a feature generally not found in myxoid liposarcoma. Pleomorphic liposarcomas may have a myxoid background, but the nuclei vary more in size than those of myxoid liposarcoma (see below).

Distinction from lipoblastoma and lipoblastomatosis is discussed in the section devoted to those lesions. Spindle cell lipoma may have a myxoid stroma and contain fat cells that resemble signet ring cells, but the coarse collagen; spindle cells with elongated nuclei; usual superficial location in the back, neck, or shoulder; and absence of a plexiform vascular pattern serve to distinguish this tumor from myxoid liposarcoma. Dermatofibrosarcoma protuberans (DFSP) may have myxoid areas, and sometimes these are extensive, but cutaneous involvement and the repetitive storiform pattern that identifies DFSP exclude myxoid liposarcoma (119). Aggressive angiomyxoma occurs almost exclusively in the genital and perineal areas, and lacks fat vacuoles and an arborizing vascular pattern; rather, the vessels are large and disorganized. Signet ring lymphomas (distinguished by the immunohistochemical panel), metastatic carcinoma (PAS and keratin stains), balloon cell melanoma and clear cell sarcoma (S-100 protein and HMB45 stains—be careful, fat cells may express S-100 protein) all may enter the differential diagnosis of myxoid liposarcoma because of the presence of cytoplasmic vacuoles or cytoplasmic clearing.

Pure cellular myxoid liposarcoma (round cell liposarcoma) is composed of cells with no more than mild pleomorphism. It is distinguished from other round cell tumors by a variable number of signet ring lipoblasts.

Treatment and Prognosis. Myxoid liposarcoma has a high rate of local recurrence when treated by excision alone, but this rate is significantly reduced if postoperative radiation is used or if excision is wide. The rate of metastasis is related to the proportion of the tumor that is highly cellular (117a,118,122,136); because of this, we designate neoplasms in which 25 percent or more of the tumor is highly cellular as *cellular myxoid liposarcoma*, a term that signifies significant metastatic potential (117a,118). However, even myxoid liposarcomas that are

uniformly of low cellularity can metastasize, although this is uncommon. The time interval to metastasis may be long (median, 68 months in one of our studies), and this is true even when substantial highly cellular areas are present (118). Patients who eventually die of tumor often live for many years. One of the most distinctive clinical features of myxoid liposarcoma is its pattern of metastatic spread: the most common site of metastasis is distant soft tissue (particularly the retroperitoneum and mediastinum), followed by the spine and only then the lungs. Soft tissue metastasis has been interpreted by some in the past as multicentric origin, but we believe that the almost constant initial appearance of the tumor in the thigh in these cases and the location of the later lesions in areas unusual for primary myxoid liposarcoma speak strongly for metastasis (117a,118).

Pleomorphic Liposarcoma

Definition. Pleomorphic liposarcoma is a cellular, pleomorphic sarcoma in which at least some of the tumor cells are differentiated as lipoblasts.

Clinical Features. A rare type of liposarcoma, pleomorphic liposarcoma occurs mostly in older persons. It does not have a strong locational predilection, although it is probably most frequent in the thigh. Most examples are intramuscular or in other deep sites, although rare cases occur in the subcutis. Most pleomorphic liposarcomas are large at presentation, and CT scans usually do not demonstrate fat density.

Pathologic Findings. Pleomorphic liposarcoma usually has a sarcomatous "fish-flesh" appearance grossly and some examples are wholly or partly myxoid. A degree of yellow coloration may or may not be recognizable. Microscopically, pleomorphic liposarcoma is cellular and, as the name implies, moderately to markedly pleomorphic (fig. 4-59) (115a,117a,118). Myxoid areas are less cellular but retain the pleomorphism (fig. 4-60). Some purported "round cell" liposarcomas have actually been pleomorphic liposarcomas with rounded cells (fig. 4-61). Characteristically, the tumor cells are enlarged and cytologically malignant, with nuclei that are elongate to round to bizarre. Multinucleated giant cells are common. For the diagnosis of pleomorphic liposarcoma to be made, at least some of the tumor cells must contain clearly

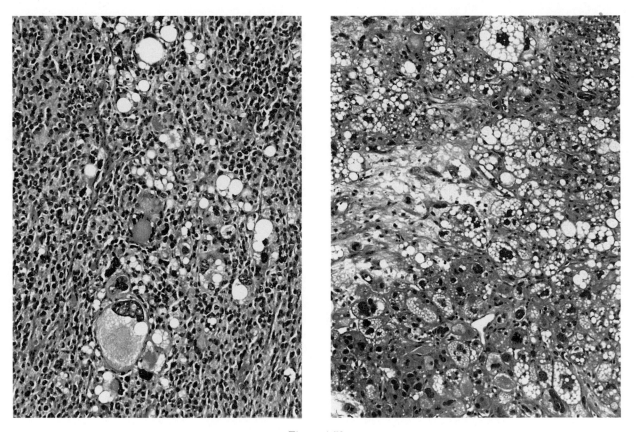

Figure 4-59
PLEOMORPHIC LIPOSARCOMA
Left: Pleomorphic liposarcoma is a pleomorphic sarcoma in which some of the cells are differentiated as lipoblasts.
Right: The lipoblasts may be multivacuolated.

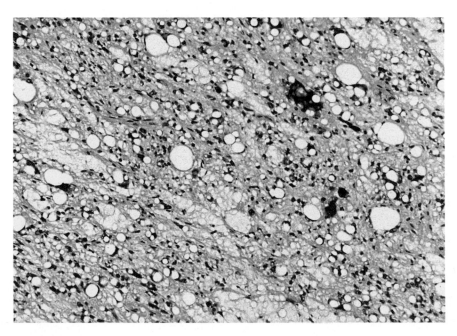

Figure 4-60
PLEOMORPHIC
LIPOSARCOMA WITH
A MYXOID STROMA
This degree of pleomorphism is not a feature of myxoid liposarcoma, not even cellular "round cell" tumors. Therefore, this tumor is placed in the pleomorphic liposarcoma category.

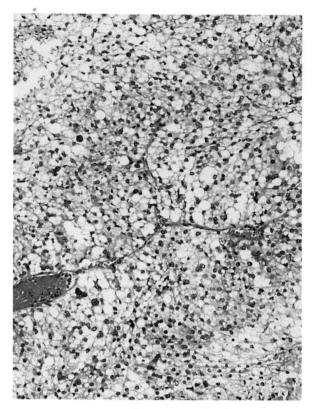

Figure 4-61
PLEOMORPHIC LIPOSARCOMA
WITH ROUNDED CELLS

Some purported examples of "round cell" liposarcoma are actually pleomorphic liposarcomas with rounded cells. The nuclear pleomorphism in this case points to the correct classification.

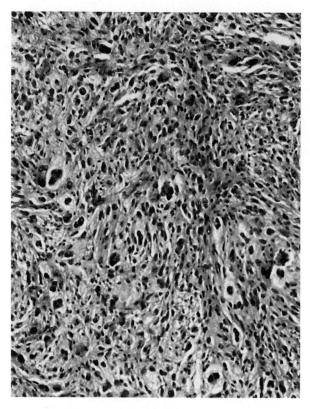

Figure 4-62
PLEOMORPHIC LIPOSARCOMA: AREA
RESEMBLING PLEOMORPHIC MALIGNANT
FIBROUS HISTIOCYTOMA

Pleomorphic liposarcoma and pleomorphic MFH have identical histologic features except that the former contains at least some lipoblasts. This photomicrograph is from an area of a pleomorphic liposarcoma that did not contain the lipidic cells found elsewhere in the tumor and thus is identical to pleomorphic MFH. Fatty differentiation may be focal in pleomorphic liposarcomas so numerous sections may be needed to find it.

identifiable cytoplasmic lipid vacuoles that are sharply outlined, appear empty, and indent the nucleus. Such cells often have enlarged irregular nuclei. Mature fat cells are not present. Pleomorphic liposarcomas often contain significant areas that do not demonstrate fatty differentiation and are indistinguishable from pleomorphic or myxoid MFH (fig. 4-62) (117a,133a). An epithelioid variant in which the tumor cells may be keratin positive has been reported (129a).

Differential Diagnosis. In the past, pleomorphic sarcomas without definite fat-containing cells (most often MFH) were sometimes misclassified as pleomorphic liposarcoma because they contained cells with vacuolated or foamy cytoplasm. The characteristics of fat vacuoles as described in the Introduction to this chapter should be kept in mind, and vacuoles that lack these features, such as those that are not crisply delimited, those that are not clear, and those that do not compress and deform the nucleus, should not be accepted as evidence of fatty differentiation. If fat vacuoles are not clearly identified and the tumor otherwise meets the requirements for pleomorphic MFH, it should be interpreted as such. There is no difference in treatment between those two tumors. There is occasional confusion between pleomorphic liposarcoma and atypical lipomatous tumor engendered by the presence of enlarged, pleomorphic nuclei in both neoplasms, but difficulties should be easily avoidable in view of the much greater cellularity and mitotic activity in pleomorphic liposarcoma and its lack of mature fat cells.

Treatment and Prognosis. Pleomorphic liposarcoma has a high propensity for both local recurrence and distant metastasis, often to widespread sites, and patient survival is typically short. We have observed a few cases in which pleomorphic liposarcoma was combined with atypical lipomatous tumor in a retroperitoneal neoplasm; the patients all died with locally recurrent tumor in which pleomorphic liposarcoma was increasingly predominant (see also Differential Diagnosis section for Dedifferentiated Liposarcoma).

Unclassified Liposarcoma

Occasional sarcomas that clearly contain lipid-forming cells do not demonstrate the characteristic features of any of the specific types of liposarcoma outlined above. Some of these tumors occur de novo, whereas others (as previously mentioned) develop in a recurrent atypical lipomatous tumor; we have seen metastasis occur in the former situation but not in the latter. In our experience, the majority of these unclassifiable liposarcomas have had a myxoid background but have demonstrated neither the typical cellular and vascular pattern required for a diagnosis of myxoid liposarcoma nor the degree of pleomorphism appropriate for pleomorphic liposarcoma; in addition, they have not formed a homogeneous group themselves. It is important to recognize these neoplasms as unclassifiable and not "force" them into an inappropriate category, a point applicable to tumors in general.

REFERENCES

Introduction

1. Azumi N, Curtis J, Kempson RL, Hendrickson MR. Atypical and malignant neoplasms showing lipomatous differentiation. A study of 111 cases. Am J Surg Pathol 1987;11:161–83.
2. Battifora H, Nunez-Alonso C. Myxoid liposarcoma: study of ten cases. Ultrastruct Pathol 1980;1:157–69.
3. Cocchia D, Lauriola L, Stolfi VM, Tallini G, Michetti F. S-100 antigen labels neoplastic cells in liposarcoma and cartilaginous tumours. Virchows Arch [A] 1983;402:139–45.
4. Dei Tos AP, Wadden C, Fletcher CD. S-100 protein staining in liposarcoma. Appl Immunohistochem 1996;4:95–101.
5. Enzinger FM, Weiss SW. Soft tissue tumors. St. Louis: Mosby, 1988.
6. Evans HL. Liposarcoma: a study of 55 cases with a reassessment of its classification. Am J Surg Pathol 1979;3:507–23.
7. Evans HL. Liposarcomas and atypical lipomatous tumors. A study of 66 cases followed for a minimum of 10 years. Surg Pathol 1988;1:41–54.
8. Evans HL, Soule EH, Winkelmann RK. Atypical lipoma, atypical intramuscular lipoma, and well-differentiated retroperitoneal liposarcoma: a reappraisal of 30 cases formerly classified as well-differentiated liposarcoma. Cancer 1979;43:574–84.
9. Fletcher CD, Akerman M, Dal Cin P, de Wever I, et al. Correlation between clinicopathologic features and karyotype in lipomatous tumors. Am J Pathol 1996;148:623–30.
10. Fu YS, Parker FG, Kaye GI, Lattes R. Ultrastructure of benign and malignant adipose tissue tumors. Pathol Ann 1980;15.67–89.
11. Hashimoto H, Daimaru Y, Enjoji M. S-100 protein distribution in liposarcoma. An immunoperoxidase study with special reference to the distinction of liposarcoma from myxoid malignant fibrous histiocytoma. Virchows Arch [A] 1984;405:1–10.
12. Kindblom LG, Säve-Söderbergh J. The ultrastructure of liposarcoma. Acta Pathol Microbiol Scand 1979;87:109–21.
13. Lagacé R, Jacob S, Seemayer TA. Myxoid liposarcoma. An electron microscopic study: biological and histogenetic considerations. Virchows Arch [A] 1979;384:159–72.
14. Lindahl S, Markhede G, Berlin Ö. Computed tomography of lipomatous and myxoid tumors. Acta Radiol Diagn 1985;26:709–13.
15. Merton DA, Needleman L, Alexander AA, Wolfson PJ, Goldberg BB. Lipoblastoma: diagnosis with computed tomography, ultrasonography, and color Doppler imaging. J Ultrasound Med 1992;11:549–52.
16. O'Connor M, Snover DC. Liposarcoma. A review of factors influencing prognosis. Am Surg 1983;49:379–84.
17. Reszel PA, Soule EH, Coventry MB. Liposarcoma of the extremities and limb girdles. A study of two hundred twenty-two cases. J Bone Joint Surg 1966;48:229–44.
18. Rossouw DJ, Cinti S, Dickersin GR. Liposarcoma. An ultrastructural study of 15 cases. Am J Clin Pathol 1986;85(6):649–67.
19. Rubin BP, Fletcher CD. The cytogenetics of lipomatous tumours. Histopathology 1997;30:507–11.

20. Shimoda T, Yamashita H, Furusato M, et al. Liposarcoma. A light and electron microscopic study with comments on their relation to malignant fibrous histiocytoma and angiosarcoma. Acta Pathol Jap 1980;30(5):779–97.

21. Suster S, Fisher C. Immunoreactivity for the human hematopoietic progenitor cell antigen (CD34) in lipomatous tumors. Am J Surg Pathol 1997;21:195–200.

22. Tsuneyoshi M, Hashimoto H, Enjoji M. Myxoid malignant fibrous histiocytoma versus myxoid liposarcoma. A comparative ultrastructural study. Virchows Arch [A] 1983;400:187–99.

23. Weiss LM, Warhol MJ. Ultrastructural distinctions between adult pleomorphic rhabdomyosarcomas, pleomorphic liposarcomas, and pleomorphic malignant fibrous histiocytomas. Hum Pathol 1984;15(11):1025–33.

24. Weiss SW, Rao VK. Well-differentiated liposarcoma (atypical lipoma) of deep soft tissue of the extremities, retroperitoneum, and miscellaneous sites. A follow-up study of 92 cases with analysis of the incidence of "dedifferention." Am J Surg Pathol 1992;16:1051–8.

Lipoma

25. Austin LR, Mack LC, Townsend CM, Lack EE. Infiltrating (intramuscular) lipomas and angiolipomas. A clinicopathologic study of six cases. Arch Surg 1980;115:281–4.

26. Bannayan GA. Lipomatosis, angiomatosis, and macroencephalia. A previously undescribed congenital syndrome. Arch Pathol 1971;92:1–5.

27. Bjerrgaard P, Hagen K, Daugaard S, Kofoed H. Intramuscular lipoma of the lower limb. Longterm follow-up after local resection. J Bone Joint Surg 1989;79:812–5.

28. Burgdorf WH, Doran CK, Worret WI. Folded skin with scarring: Michelin tire baby syndrome? J Amer Acad Dermatol 1982;7:90–3.

29. Demas BE, Avallone A, Hricak H. Pelvic lipomatosis: diagnosis and characterization by magnetic resonance imaging. Urol Radiol 1988;10:198–202.

30. Deschler DG, Lee K, Tami TA. Laryngeal infiltrating intramuscular lipoma. Otolaryngol Head Neck Surg 1993;108:374–7.

31. Dionne GP, Seemayer TA. Infiltrating lipomas and angiolipomas revisited. Cancer 1974;33:732–7.

32. Dotz W, Prioleau PG. Nevus lipomatosus cutaneus superficialis. A light and electron microscopic study. Arch Dermatol 1984;120:376–9.

33. Enzi G. Multiple symmetric lipomatosis: an updated clinical report. Medicine 1984;63:56–64.

34. Enzinger FM. Benign lipomatous tumors simulating a sarcoma. In: Management of primary bone and soft tissue tumors. Chicago: Year Book Medical Publishers, 1977.

35. Fletcher CD, Martin-Bates E. Intramuscular and intermuscular lipoma: neglected diagnoses. Histopathology 1988;12:275–87.

36. Garavaglia J, Gnepp DR. Intramuscular (infiltrating) lipoma of the tongue. Oral Surg Oral Med Oral Pathol 1987;63:348–50.

37. Grimmett GM, Hall MG Jr, Aird CC, Kurtz LH. Pelvic lipomatosis. Am J Surg 1973;125:347–9.

38. Hallel T, Lew S, Kfar-Saba I, Bansal M. Villous lipomatous proliferation of the synovial membrane (lipoma arborescens). J Bone Joint Surg 1988;70:264–9.

39. Heim S, Mandahl N, Rydholm A, Willén H, Mitelman F. Different karyotypic features characterize different clinicopathologic subgroups of benign lipogenic tumors. Int J Cancer 1988;42:863–7.

40. Held JL, Andrew JA, Kohn SR. Surgical amelioration of Dercum's disease: a report and review. J Dermatol Surg Oncol 1989;15:1294–6.

41. Hendricks WM, Limber GK. Nevus lipomatosus cutaneus superficialis. Cutis 1982;29:183–5.

42. Heyns CF. Pelvic lipomatosis: a review of its diagnosis and management. J Urol 1991;146:267–73.

43. Jones EW, Marks R, Pongsehirun D. Naevus superficialis lipomatosus. Br J Dermatol 1975;93:121–33.

44. Kindblom LG, Angervall L, Stener B, Wickbom I. Intermuscular and intramuscular lipomas and hibernomas. Cancer 1974;33:754–63.

45. Kindblom LG, Möller-Nielsen J. Diffuse lipomatosis in the leg after poliomyelitis. Acta Pathol Microbiol Scand 1975;83:339–44.

46. Klein FA, Smith MJ, Hasenetz I. Pelvic lipomatosis: 35 year experience. J Urol 1988;139:998–1001.

47. Lassman LP, Michael James CC. Lumbosacral lipomas. J Neurol Neurosurg Psych 1987;30:174–81.

48. Mandahl N, Heim S, Arheden K, Rydholm A, Willén H, Mitelman F. Three major cytogenetic subgroups can be identified among chromosomally abnormal solitary lipomas. Hum Genet 1988;79:203–8.

49. Murphy NB. Ossifying lipoma. Br J Radiol 1974;47:97–8.

49a. Murphy WM, Beckwith JB, Farrow GM. Tumors of the kidney, bladder, and related urinary structures. Atlas of Tumor Pathology. 3rd Series, Fascicle 11. Washington, D.C.: Armed Forces Institute of Pathology, 1994.

50. Myhre-Jensen O. A consecutive 7-year series of 1331 benign soft tissue tumors. Acta Orthop Scand 1981;52:287–93.

51. Phalen GS, Kendrick JI, Rodriguez JM. Lipomas of the upper extremity. A series of fifteen tumors in the hand and wrist and six tumors causing nerve compression. Am J Surg 1971;121:298–306.

52. Plaut GS, Salm R, Truscott DE. Three cases of ossifying lipoma. J Pathol Bacteriol 1959;78:292–5.

53. Rickwood AM, Hemalatha V, Zachary RB. Lipoma of the cauda equina (lumbosacral lipoma). Kinderchir 1979;27:159–69.

54. Ruzicka T, Vieluf D, Landthaler M, Braun-Falco O. Benign symmetric lipomatosis Launois-Bensaude. Report of 10 cases and review of the literature. J Am Acad Dermatol 1987;17:663–74.

55. Rydholm A, Berg NO. Size, site, and clinical incidence of lipoma. Factors in the differential diagnosis of the lipoma and sarcoma. Acta Orthop Scand 1983;54:929–34.

56. Shugar MA, Gavron JP. Benign symmetrical lipomatosis (Madelung's disease). Otolaryngol Head Neck Surg 1985;93:109–12.

57. Silverman TA, Enzinger FM. Fibrolipomatous hamartoma of nerve. A clinicopathologic analysis of 26 cases. Am J Surg Pathol 1985;9:7–14.

58. Sreekantaiah C, Leong SP, Karakousis CP, et al. Cytogenetic profile of 109 lipomas. Cancer Res 1991;51:422–33.
59. Sullivan CR, Dahlin DC, Bryan RS. Lipoma of the tendon sheath. J Bone Joint Surg 1956;38A:1275–9.
59a. Suster S, Fisher C. Immunoreactivity for the human hematopoietic progenitor cell antigen (CD34) in lipomatous tumors. Am J Surg Pathol 1997;21:195–200.
60. Weitzman G. Lipoma arborescens of the knee. J Bone Joint Surg 1965;47:1030–3.

Angiolipoma

61. Dixon AY, McGregor DH, Lee SH. Angiolipomas: an ultrastructural and clinicopathological study. Hum Pathol 1981;12:739–47.
61a. Fletcher CD, Akerman M, Dal Cin P, de Wever I, et al. Correlation between clinicopathologic features and karyotype in lipomatous tumors. Am J Pathol 1996;148:623–30.
62. Howard WR, Helwig EB. Angiolipoma. Arch Dermatol 1960;82:924–31.
63. Hunt SJ, Santa Cruz DJ, Barr RJ. Cellular angiolipoma. Am J Surg Pathol 1990;14:75–81.
63a. Rubin BP, Fletcher CD. The cytogenetics of lipomatous tumours. Histopathology 1997;30:507–11.

Myelolipoma

64. Chen KT, Felix EL, Flam MS. Extraadrenal myelolipoma. Am J Clin Pathol 1982;78:386–9.
65. Fowler MR, Alba JM, Williams RB, Byrd CR. Extraadrenal myelolipomas compared with extramedullary hematopoietic tumors: a case of presacral myelolipoma. Am J Surg Pathol 1982;6:363–74.
65a. Lack EE. Tumors of the adrenal gland and extra-adrenal paraganglia. Atlas of Tumor Pathology. 3rd Series, Fascicle 19. Washington, D.C.: Armed Forces Institute of Pathology, 1997.

Hibernoma

66. Angervall L, Björntorp P, Stener B. The lipid composition of hibernomas as compared with that of lipoma and mouse brown fat. Cancer Res 1965;25:408–9.
67. Fletcher CD, Akerman M, Dal Cin P, de Wever I, et al. Correlation between clinicopathologic features and karyotype in lipomatous tumors. Am J Pathol 1996;148:623–30.
68. Gaffney EF, Hargreaves HK, Semple E, Vellios F. Hibernoma: distinctive light and electron microscopic features and relationship to brown adipose tissue. Hum Pathol 1983;14:677–87.
68a. Levine GD. Hibernoma. An electron microscopic study. Hum Pathol 1972;3(3):351–9.

Lipoblastoma–Lipoblastomatosis

69. Arda IS, Senocak ME, Gögüs S, Büyükpamukçu N. A case of benign intrascrotal lipoblastoma clinically mimicking testicular torsion and review of the literature. J Pediatr Surg 1993;28(2):259–61.
70. Bolen JW, Thorning D. Benign lipoblastoma and myxoid liposarcoma: a comparative light and electron microscopic study. Am J Surg Pathol 1980;4:163–74.
71. Castleberry RP, Kelly DR, Wilson ER, Cain WS, Salter MR. Childhood liposarcoma. Report of a case and review of the literature. Cancer 1984;54:579–84.
72. Chung EB, Enzinger FM. Benign lipoblastomatosis. Cancer 1973;32:482–92.
73. Collins, MH, Chatten J. Lipoblastoma/lipoblastomatosis: a clinicopathologic study of 25 tumors. Am J Surg Pathol 1997;21:1131–7.
74. Fletcher CD, Akerman M, Dal Cin P, de Wever I, et al. Correlation between clinicopathologic features and karyotype in lipomatous tumors. Am J Pathol 1996;148:623–30.
75. Fletcher JA, Kozakewich HP, Schoenberg ML, Morton CC. Cytogenetic findings in pediatric adipose tumors: consistent rearrangement of chromosome 8 in lipoblastoma. Genes Chromosom Cancer 1993;6:24–9.
76. Létourneau L, Dufour M, Deschênes J. Shoulder lipoblastoma: magnetic resonance imaging characteristics. Can Assoc Radiol J 1993;44(3):211–4.
77. Mahour GH, Bryan BJ, Isaacs H. Lipoblastoma and lipoblastomatosis—a report of six cases. Surgery 1988;104:577–9.
78. Mentzel T, Calonje E, Fletcher CD. Lipoblastoma and lipoblastomatosis: a clinicopathological study of 14 cases. Histopathology 1993;23:527–33.
79. Merton DA, Needleman L, Alexander AA, Wolfson PJ, Goldberg BB. Lipoblastoma: diagnosis with computed tomography, ultrasonography, and color Doppler imaging. J Ultrasound Med 1992;11:549–52.
80. Ohjimi Y, Iwasaki H, Kaneko Y, Ishiguro M, Ohgami A, Kikuchi M. A case of lipoblastoma with t(3;8)(q12;q11.2). Cancer Genet Cytogenet 1992;62:103–5.
81. Schulman H, Barki Y, Hertzanu Y. Case report: mesenteric lipoblastoma. Clin Radiol 1992;46:57–8.
82. Shmookler BM, Enzinger FM. Liposarcoma occurring in children. An analysis of 17 cases and review of the literature. Cancer 1983;52:567–74.
83. Stringel G, Shandling B, Mancer K, Ein SH. Lipoblastoma in infants and children. J Pediatr Surg 1982;17:277–80.
84. Vellios F, Baez J, Shumacker HB. Lipoblastomatosis: a tumor of fetal fat different from hibernoma. Report of a case, with observations on the embryogenesis of human adipose tissue. Am J Pathol 1958;34:1149–59.

Chondroid Lipoma

85. Kindblom LG, Meis-Kindblom JM. Chondroid lipoma. An ultrastructural and immunohistochemical analysis with further observations regarding its differentiation. Hum Pathol 1995;26:706–15.
86. Meis JM, Enzinger FM. Chondroid lipoma. A unique tumor simulating liposarcoma and myxoid chondrosarcoma. Am J Surg Pathol 1993;17:1103–12.
87. Nielson GP, O'Connell JX, Dickersin GR, Rosenberg AE. Chondroid lipoma, a tumor of white fat cells. A brief report of two cases with ultrastructural analysis. Am J Surg Pathol 1995;19:1272–6.

Myolipoma

87a. Meis JM, Enzinger FM. Myolipoma of soft tissue. Am J Surg Pathol 1991;15:121–5.

Spindle Cell/Pleomorphic Lipoma

88. Angervall L, Dahl I, Kindblom LG, Save-Soderbergh J. Spindle cell lipoma. Acta Pathol Microbiol Scand 1976;84:477–87.
89. Azzopardi JG, Iocco J, Salm R. Pleomorphic lipoma: a tumor stimulating liposarcoma. Histopathology 1983;7:511–23.
90. Bartley GB, Yeatts RP, Garrity JA, Farrow GM, Campbell RJ. Spindle cell lipoma of the orbit. Am J Opthamol 1985;100:605–9.
91. Beham A, Schmid C, Hödl S, Fletcher CD. Spindle cell and pleomorphic lipoma: an immunohistochemical study and histogenetic analysis. J Pathol 1989;158:219–22.
92. Bolen JW, Thorning D. Spindle-cell lipoma. A clinical, light- and electron-microscopical study. Am J Surg Pathol 1981;5:435–41.
93. Christopoulos P, Nicolatou O, Patrikiou A. Oral spindle cell lipoma. Report of a case. Int J Oral Maxillofac Surg 1989;18:208–9.
94. Enzinger FM, Harvey DA. Spindle cell lipoma. Cancer 1975;36:1852–9.
94a. Fanburg-Smith JC, Devaney KO, Miettinen M, Weiss SW. Multiple spindle cell lipomas. A report of 7 familial and 11 nonfamilial cases. Am J Surg Pathol 1998;22:40–8.
94b. Fletcher CD, Akerman M, Dal Cin P, de Wever I, et al. Correlation between clinicopathologic features and karyotype in lipomatous tumors. Am J Pathol 1996;148:623–30.
95. Fletcher CD, Martin-Bates E. Spindle cell lipoma: a clinicopathological study with some original observations. Histopathology 1987;11:803–17.
96. Hawley IC, Krausz T, Evans DJ, Fletcher CD. Spindle-cell lipoma—a pseudoangiomatous variant. Histopathology 1994;24:565–9.
97. Jensen ML, Nielsen VT. Intramuscular (subfascial) vascular spindle cell lipoma. A case report. Tumori 1990;76:616–9.
98. Kitano M, Enjoji M, Iwasaki H. Spindle cell lipoma—a clinicopathologic analysis of twelve cases. Acta Pathol Jpn 1979;29:891–9.
99. Levy F, Goding GS. Spindle–cell lipoma: an unusual oral presentation. Otolaryngol Head Neck Surg 1989;101:601–3.
100. Mandahl N, Mertens F, Willen H, et al. A new cytogenetic subgroup in lipomas. Loss of chromosome 16. Clin Oncol 1994;120:707–11.
101. McDaniel RK, Newland JR, Chiles DG. Intraoral spindle cell lipoma: case report with correlated light and electron microscopy. Oral Surg 1984;57:52–7.
102. Nonaka S, Enomoto K, Kawabori S, Unno T, Muraoka S. Spindle cell lipoma within the larynx: a case report with correlated light and electron microscopy. ORL J Otorhinolaryngol Rel Spec 1993;55:147–9.
103. Robb JA, Jones RA. Spindle cell lipoma in a perianal location. Hum Pathol 1982;13:1052.
103a. Rubin BP, Fletcher CD. The cytogenetics of lipomatous tumours. Histopathology 1997;30:507–11.
104. Shmookler BM, Enzinger FM. Pleomorphic lipoma: a benign tumor simulating liposarcoma. A clinicopathologic analysis of 48 cases. Cancer 1981;47:126–33.
105. Sund S, Hordvik M, Mæhle B, Walle A, Myking A. Large intramuscular spindle-cell lipoma. With review of the literature. A case report. APMIS 1988;96:347–51.
105a. Suster S, Fisher C. Immunoreactivity for the human hematopoietic progenitor cell antigen (CD34) in lipomatous tumors. Am J Surg Pathol 1997;21:195–200.
106. Warkel RL, Rehme CG, Thompson WH. Vascular spindle cell lipoma. J Cutan Pathol 1982;9:113–8.

Atypical Lipomatous Tumors and Liposarcomas

107. Allsbrook WC Jr, Harmon DJ, Chongchitnant N, Erwin S. Liposarcoma of the larynx. Arch Pathol Lab Med 1985;109:294–6.
108. Argani P, Facchetti F, Irghirami G, Rosai J. Lymphocyte-rich well-differentiated liposarcoma: report of nine cases. Am J Surg Pathol 1997;21:884–95.
108a. Azumi N, Curtis J, Kempson RL, Hendrickson MR. Atypical and malignant neoplasms showing lipomatous differentiation. A study of 111 cases. Am J Surg Pathol 1987;11:161–83.
109. Bellinger MF, Gibbons MD, Koontz WW Jr, Graff M. Paratesticular liposarcoma. J Urol 1978;11:285–8.
110. Cicciarelli FE, Soule EH, McGoon DC. Lipoma and liposarcoma of the mediastinum: a report of 14 tumors including one lipoma of the thymus. J Thor Cardiovasc Surg 1964;47:411–29.
111. Coindre JM, de Loynes B, Bui ND, Stockle E, de Mascarel I, Trojani M. Dedifferentiated liposarcoma. A clinicopathological study of 6 cases. Ann Pathol 1992;12:20–8.

112. D'Abrera VS, Burfitt-Williams W. A giant scrotal liposarcoma. Med J Austr 1973;2:854–6.

112a. Dal Cin P, Sciot R, Panagopoulos I, et al. Additional evidence of a variant translocation t(12;22) with EWS/CHOP fusion in myxoid liposarcoma: clinicopathological features. J Pathol 1997;182:437–41.

113. Dei Tos AP, Mentzel T, Newman PL, Fletcher CD. Spindle cell liposarcoma, a hitherto unrecognized variant of liposarcoma. Am J Surg Pathol 1994;18:913–21.

113a. Dei Tos AP, Wadden C, Fletcher CD. S-100 protein staining in liposarcoma. Appl Immunohistochem 1996;4:95–101.

114. Eneroth M, Mandahl N, Heim S, et al. Localization of the chromosomal breakpoints of the t(12;16) in liposarcoma to subbands 12q13.3 and 16p11.2. Cancer Genet Cytogenet 1990;48:101–7.

115. Enterline HT, Culberson JD, Rocklin DB, Brady LW. Liposarcoma. A clinical and pathological study of 53 cases. Cancer 1960;13:932–50.

115a. Enzinger FM, Weiss SW. Soft tissue tumors. St. Louis: Mosby, 1988.

116. Enzinger FM, Winslow DJ. Liposarcoma. A study of 103 cases. Virch Arch [A] 1962;335:367–88.

117. Evans HL. Liposarcoma: a study of 55 cases with a reassessment of its classification. Am J Surg Pathol 1979;3:507–23.

117a. Evans HL. Liposarcomas and atypical lipomatous tumors. A study of 66 cases followed for a minimum of 10 years. Surg Pathol 1988;1:41–54.

117b. Evans HL. Smooth muscle in atypical lipomatous tumors. A report of three cases. Am J Surg Pathol 1990;14:714–8.

117c. Evans HL, Khurana KK, Kemp BL, Ayala AG. Heterologous elements in the dedifferentiated component of dedifferentiated liposarcoma. Am J Surg Pathol 1994;18:1150–7.

118. Evans HL, Soule EH, Winkelmann RK. Atypical lipoma, atypical intramuscular lipoma, and well-differentiated retroperitoneal liposarcoma: a reappraisal of 30 cases formerly classified as well-differentiated liposarcoma. Cancer 1979;43:574–84.

118a. Fanburg-Smith JC, Miettinen M. Liposarcoma with meningothelial-like whorls: a study of 17 cases of a distinctive histological pattern associated with dedifferentiated liposarcoma. Histopathology 1998;33:414–24.

118b. Farshid G, Weiss SW. Massive localized lymphedema of the morbidly obese. A histologically distinct reactive lesion simulating liposarcoma. Am J Surg Pathol 1998;22:1277–83.

118c. Fletcher CD, Akerman M, Dal Cin P, de Wever I, et al. Correlation between clinicopathologic features and karyotype in lipomatous tumors. Am J Pathol 1996;148:623–30.

119. Frierson HF, Cooper PH. Myxoid variant of dermatofibrosarcoma protuberans. Am J Surg Pathol 1983;7(5):445–50.

120. Hashimoto H, Enjoji M. Liposarcoma. A clinicopathologic subtyping of 52 cases. Acta Pathol Jpn 1982;32:933–48.

121. Henricks WH, Chu YC, Goldblum JR, Weiss SW. Dedifferentiated liposarcoma. A clinicopathological analysis of 155 cases with a proposal for an expanded definition of dedifferentiation. Am J Surg Pathol 1997;21:271–81.

122. Kilpatrick SE, Doyon J, Choong PF, Sim FH, Nascimento AG. The clinicopathologic spectrum of myxoid and round cell liposarcoma. A study of 95 cases. Cancer 1996;77:1450–8.

123. Kindblom LG, Angervall L, Fassina AS. Atypical lipoma. APMIS 1982;90:27–36.

124. Kindblom LG, Angervall L, Svendsen P. Liposarcoma: a clinicopathologic, radiographic, and prognostic study. Acta Pathol Microbiol Scand 1975;253:1–71.

125. Knight JC, Renwick PJ, Dal Cin P, Van Den Berghe H, Fletcher CD. Translocation t(12;16)(q13;p11) in myxoid liposarcoma and round cell liposarcoma: molecular and cytogenetic analysis. Cancer Res 1995;55:24–7.

126. Kraus MD, Guillou L, Fletcher CD. Well-differentiated inflammatory liposarcoma: an uncommon and easily overlooked variant of a common sarcoma. Am J Surg Pathol 1997;21:518–27.

127. Lucas DR, Nascimento AG, Sanjay BK, Rock MG. Well-differentiated liposarcoma. The Mayo Clinic experience with 58 cases. Am J Clin Pathol 1994;102:677–83.

128. McCormick D, Mentzel T, Beham A, Fletcher CD. Dedifferentiated liposarcoma. Clinicopathologic analysis of 32 cases suggesting a better prognostic subgroup among pleomorphic sarcomas. Am J Surg Pathol 1994;18:1213–23.

129. Mertens F, Johansson B, Mandahl N, et al. Clonal chromosome abnormalities in two liposarcomas. Cancer Genet Cytogenet 1987;28:137–44.

129a. Miettinen M, Enzinger FM. Epithelioid variant of pleomorphic liposarcoma: a study of 12 cases of a distinctive variant of high grade liposarcoma. Mod Pathol 1999;12:722–8.

129b. Nascimento AG, Kurtin PJ, Guillou L, Fletcher CD. Dedifferentiated liposarcoma: a report of nine cases with a peculiar neural like whorling pattern associated with metaplastic bone formation. Am J Surg Pathol 1998;22:945–55.

130. Palma PD, Barbazza R. Well-differentiated liposarcoma of the paratesticular area: report of a case with fine-needle aspiration preoperative diagnosis and review of the literature. Diag Cytopathol 1990;6:421–6.

130a. Reszel PA, Soule EH, Coventry MB. Liposarcoma of the extremities and limb girdles. A study of two hundred twenty-two cases. J Bone Joint Surg 1966;48:229–44.

131. Rosai J, Akerman M, Dal Cin P, De Wever I, et al. Combined morphologic and karyotypic study of 59 atypical lipomatous tumors. Evaluation of their relationship and differential diagnosis with other adipose tissue tumors (a report of CHAMP Study Group). Am J Surg Pathol 1996;20:1182–9.

131a. Rubin BP, Fletcher CD. The cytogenetics of lipomatous tumours. Histopathology 1997;30:507–11.

132. Salzano RP Jr, Tomkiewicz Z, Africano WA. Dedifferentiated liposarcoma with features of rhabdomyosarcoma. Conn Med 1991;55:200–2.

133. Saunders JR, Jaques DA, Casterline PF, Percarpio B, Goodloe S. Liposarcomas of the head and neck: a review of the literature and addition of four cases. Cancer 1979;43(1):162–8.

133a. Shimoda T, Yamashita H, Furusato M, et al. Liposarcoma. A light and electron microscopic study with comments on their relation to malignant fibrous histiocytoma and angiosarcoma. Acta Pathol Jap 1980;30(5):779–97.

134. Shmookler BM, Enzinger FM. Liposarcoma occurring in children. An analysis of 17 cases and review of the literature. Cancer 1983;52:567–74.

135. Siebert JD, Williams RP, Pulitzer DR. Myxoid liposarcoma with cartilaginous differentiation. Mod Pathol 1996;9:249–52.

136. Smith TA, Easley KA, Goldblum JR. Myxoid/round cell liposarcoma of the extremities. A clinicopathologic study of 29 cases with particular attention to the extent of round cell liposarcoma. Am J Surg Pathol 1996;20:171–80.

137. Snover DC, Sumner HW, Dehner LP. Variability of histologic pattern in recurrent soft tissue sarcomas originally diagnosed as liposarcoma. Cancer 1982;49:1005–15.

138. Sreekantaiah C, Karakousis CP, Leong SP, Sandberg AA. Trisomy 8 as a nonrandom secondary change in myxoid liposarcoma. Cancer Genet Cytogenet 1991;51:195–205.

138a. Suster S, Fisher C. Immunoreactivity for the human hematopoietic progenitor cell antigen (CD34) in lipomatous tumors. Am J Surg Pathol 1997;21:195–200.

139. Suster S, Wong TY, Moran CA. Sarcomas with combined features of liposarcoma and leiomyosarcoma. Study of two cases of an unusual soft-tissue tumor showing dual lineage differentiation. Am J Surg Pathol 1993;17:905–11.

140. Tallini G, Akerman M, Dal Cin P, De Wever I, et al. Combined morphologic and karyotypic study of 28 myxoid liposarcomas. Evaluation of their relationship and differential diagnosis with other adipose tissue tumors (a report of the CHAMP Study Group). Am J Surg Pathol 1996;20:1047–55.

141. Tallini G, Erlandson RA, Brennan MF, Woodruff JM. Divergent myosarcomatous differentiation in retroperitoneal liposarcoma. Am J Surg Pathol 1993;17:546–56.

142. Turc-Carel C, Limon J, Dal Cin P, Rao U, Karakousis C, Sandberg AA. Cytogenetic studies of adipose tissue tumors. II. Recurrent reciprocal translocation t(12;16) (q13;p11) in myxoid liposarcomas. Cancer Genet Cytogenet 1986;23:291–9.

142a. Weiss SW, Rao VK. Well-differentiated liposarcoma (atypical lipoma) of deep soft tissue of the extremities, retroperitoneum, and miscellaneous sites. A follow-up study of 92 cases with analysis of the incidence of "dedifferention." Am J Surg Pathol 1992;16:1051–8

143. Weiss SW, Sobin LH. WHO classification of soft tissue tumors, 2nd ed. New York: Springer-Verlag, 1994.

144. Wenig BM, Weiss SW, Gnepp DR. Laryngeal and hypopharyngeal liposarcoma. Am J Surg Pathol 1990;14:134–41.

145. Yoshikawa H, Ueda T, Mori S, et al. Dedifferentiated liposarcoma of the subcutis. Am J Surg Pathol 1996;20:1525–30.

❖❖❖

5

SMOOTH MUSCLE TUMORS

INTRODUCTION

There is no official intermediate or borderline category for smooth muscle tumors that have a significant incidence of recurrence but a negligible incidence of metastasis as there is for fibrous tumors, i.e., fibromatosis (Table 5-1). The only World Health Organization (WHO)-sanctioned morphologic categories currently available for smooth muscle tumors are leiomyoma (with this diagnosis clinicians usually assume nothing further will happen after excision) and leiomyosarcoma (which then includes tumors capable only of recurrence as well as those capable of metastasis). The reason for this classificatory situation is as follows. Bland soft tissue smooth muscle tumors are rare and some of them recur after such long periods of time that determining whether an intermediate or borderline category is clinically useful has not been possible because a large number of cases with long-term follow-up has not been available. Pathologists have circumvented this problem by using such artful terms as "of uncertain malignant potential," "potentially malignant," and "low malignant potential" for bland soft tissue smooth muscle tumors of a size that has been associated with recurrence. We prefer the first term and by it infer that the tumor might recur but we doubt it will metastasize, but in the final analysis there is too little information to accurately predict the outcome (Table 5-1).

Another problem should be appreciated. Because smooth muscle cells share many features with myofibroblasts, it is often difficult to be sure whether a soft tissue tumor composed of elongate cells is of smooth muscle type or whether it is fibroblastic, myofibroblastic, or fibrohistiocytic. The basic rule for identifying neoplastic smooth muscle cells is that they must cytologically "resemble" normal smooth muscle cells and be arranged, at least focally, in long bundles or fascicles (Table 5-2). That is, the cells should be fusiform; have easily visible, sometimes fibrillar, eosinophilic cytoplasm; and have a long cylindrical nucleus that has an inconspicuous nucleolus and is rounded at the ends (fig. 5-1). A cytoplas-

mic vacuole at one end of the nucleus is a feature of some smooth muscle cells.

Most often, collagen is sparse and delicate, if it is present at all between the smooth muscle cells. Unfortunately, during the process of neoplastic transformation, smooth muscle cells tend to lose cytoplasm and their nuclei often become thinner and their chromatin denser, causing the cells to resemble myofibroblasts and even fibroblasts. No generally recognized and accepted definitions have been established that draw a crisp line between the nuclear and cytoplasmic features that count as evidence of smooth muscle differentiation and those that would cause cells to be classified as myofibroblasts. Even when spindled tumor cells appear to have abundant cytoplasm by hematoxylin and eosin (H&E) staining, there can be uncertainty about whether the eosinophilic substance between the elongate nuclei is collagen or cytoplasm. Traditionally, the trichrome stain has been used to help solve this difficulty because it stains cytoplasm red and collagen blue or green. If the cells of a purported smooth muscle tumor have abundant red cytoplasm when stained with a trichrome preparation and there is little green or blue staining collagen between the cells, this

Table 5-1

SMOOTH MUSCLE TUMORS

Benign
(Managerial Groups Ia and Ib, Table 1-10)

Leiomyoma
Angiomyoma

Intermediate
Smooth Muscle Tumors of Uncertain
Malignant Potential *
(Managerial Group IIc, Table 1-10)

Malignant
(Managerial Group III, Table 1-10)

Leiomyosarcoma

---

* See the introduction for a definition of this term.

Table 5-2

CONTRASTING FEATURES OF SMOOTH MUSCLE CELLS, MYOFIBROBLASTS, AND FIBROBLASTS

Features	Smooth Muscle	Myofibroblast	Fibroblast
Architecture	Intersecting, tightly organized fascicles, at least focally	Often random arrangement of cells; if in fascicles the cells are usually loosely arranged; may be in storiform pattern	Any arrangement including tightly organized fascicles
Cytology Nuclear	Elongate, plump, rounded ends; chromatin often vesicular; nucleoli inconspicuous	Nuclei sometimes less elongate than smooth muscle and may be round, oval, or stellate but also may be identical to fibroblasts; chromatin usually vesicular	Long, thin, often with pointed ends; chromatin is dense and smooth
Cytoplasm	Elongate, eosinophilic, easily visible, and sometimes fibrillar	Visible but less abundant and less elongate than in smooth muscle	So scant it is very difficult to visualize; not fibrillar
Trichrome	Cytoplasm red, easily visible, and sometimes fibrillar	Less red cytoplasm	Cytoplasm so scant it is often not visible
Electron microscopy	Cytoplasm filled with fibrils containing dense bodies, pinocytotic vesicles, basal lamina; accordion shape of nuclei and arrangement of organelles around the nucleus are often features	Fewer cytoplasmic fibrils and fewer dense bodies; fibrils tend to be along cytoplasmic membranes; pinocytotic vesicles; RER more prominent than in smooth muscle cells and basal lamina less apparent	Scattered fibrils, dense bodies usually absent as is basal lamina; pinocytotic vesicles variable; organelles scattered throughout scant cytoplasm
Immunohistochemistry	Actin positive; almost all normal smooth muscle cells are also desmin positive; for desmin staining in tumors, see text	Actin positive; desmin variable	May be actin positive; rarely desmin positive

is considered to be supportive evidence of smooth muscle differentiation if the nuclear features are acceptable and the cells are arranged in fascicles, at least focally. However, even if the material between the tumor cell nuclei is cytoplasm by trichrome stain, not infrequently it is nonfibrillar and scant enough that the uncertainty about whether the tumor cells are of smooth muscle type or are myofibroblasts is not resolved.

When the electron microscope became available, pathologists turned to this technique because, ultrastructurally, normal smooth muscle cells contain a number of structures arranged in recognizable patterns that together allow identification as a smooth muscle cell. These include cytoplasmic microfilaments that practically fill the cytoplasm and are oriented parallel to the

long axis of the cell, dense contractile bodies among the myofilaments, basal lamina, pinocytotic vesicles, and mitochondria and rough endoplasmic reticulum localized around a nucleus which may have a serrated or "accordion"-like appearance. However, a variable number of these features are lost in neoplastic smooth muscle cells and no generally recognized definitional limit has been agreed upon as to how many must be present and in what arrangement before a cell is deemed to be of smooth muscle type (3). A large part of the problem, of course, is that myofibroblasts are partially endowed with some of these same structures, although rough endoplasmic reticulum is more prominent in myofibroblasts and basal lamina better developed in smooth muscle cells. Consequently, electron microscopy is of

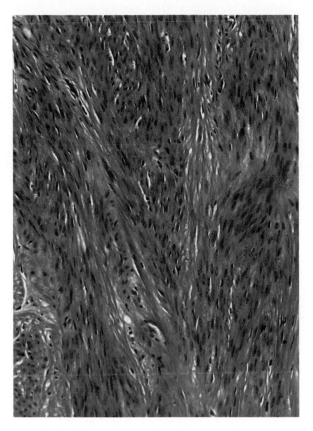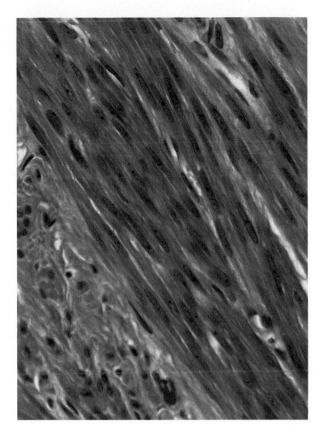

Figure 5-1
SMOOTH MUSCLE TUMOR
Left: Evidence for smooth muscle differentiation includes elongate cells with oblong nuclei and visible eosinophilic cytoplasm arranged at least focally in bundles.
Right: At higher magnification, oblong nuclei with rounded ends are characteristic of smooth muscle cells.

limited use in classifying tumors in which the neoplastic cells have some but not all the characteristics of a normal smooth muscle cell.

Immunohistochemistry can provide supportive evidence of smooth muscle differentiation. Normal smooth muscle cells express actin and desmin, and these antigens may also be expressed by the cells of a smooth muscle tumor (8,10). Unfortunately, fibroblasts and myofibroblasts also express muscle actin and occasionally even desmin so these stains are not specific (6).

The end result is a fairly high degree of nonreproducibility about the classification of smooth muscle tumors when the tumor cells do not display all or nearly all the features of normal smooth muscle. Our convention for interpreting a tumor as of smooth muscle type in the soft tissues (but not necessarily in the uterus) requires

that the cells have visible cytoplasm with a nucleus of the type found in normal smooth muscle cells, and at least focally, the cells be arranged in long fascicles (Table 5-2; fig. 5-1). If the desmin stain is positive, we consider it strongly supportive of smooth muscle differentiation as long as these minimal H&E requirements are met. We are wary of accepting actin-negative cells as smooth muscle type but, on the other hand, actin is not specific for smooth muscle differentiation (1). Although rare in soft tissue smooth muscle tumors, the situation gets even more difficult when neoplastic smooth muscle cells take on an epithelioid appearance or have clear cytoplasm. In this circumstance, finding areas of more conventional smooth muscle differentiation elsewhere in the tumor is the best way to solve the problem. Sometimes, the alternative cell types are desmin positive, but the incidence of desmin positivity in epithelioid and clear cells is less than in conventional spindled smooth muscle cells. In the final analysis, the important decision is the malignant potential of the neoplasm, and if there is doubt about whether a tumor in an adult is of smooth muscle or myofibroblastic type, we suggest evaluating it as a smooth muscle tumor.

Smooth muscle tumors occur much less frequently in the soft tissues than they do in the genitourinary and gastrointestinal tracts. As a result, one should consider the possibility of other tumor types when contemplating a diagnosis of a smooth muscle tumor in the soft tissue. In particular, myofibroblastic, fibroblastic, fibrohistiocytic, and neural tumors should always be in the differential diagnosis. Moreover, even when a smooth muscle tumor does develop in the soft tissues, estimating its potential for recurrence or metastasis is not always straightforward and often requires more information than just the histologic appearance (Table 5-1) (2,4,7,9). If the tumor is bland or low grade, the location must be known because the morphologic features that best predict aggressive behavior for bland smooth muscle tumors in the soft tissue are not necessarily the same as those for uterine or gastrointestinal smooth muscle tumors. Second, large size is a powerful predictor of aggressive behavior, even in the presence of bland morphology, for gastrointestinal and soft tissue smooth muscle tumors but not for uterine ones (9,11); in other words, bland histology is no assurance of a trouble-free course for patients with these tumors if they are large. Third, while marked pleomorphism, a high mitotic index, and tumor cell necrosis in a smooth muscle tumor should always elicit a diagnosis of leiomyosarcoma in any site, such tumors confined to the dermis essentially do not metastasize (metastasis rate of under 1 percent).

Children with the acquired immunodeficiency syndrome (AIDS) appear to have an increased incidence of leiomyoma and leiomyosarcoma involving organs, particularly within the abdomen, and the soft tissues. In situ hybridization has revealed Epstein-Barr virus (EBV) genomes in the tumor cells of these smooth muscle tumors (5,10a).

This chapter deals only with smooth muscle tumors of the soft tissues. A discussion of smooth muscle tumors in other sites, including the dermis, can be found in the appropriate Fascicles.

Glomus tumor is presented in the chapter on perivascular tumors.

BENIGN SMOOTH MUSCLE TUMORS (MANAGERIAL GROUPS Ia AND Ib, TABLE 1-10)

Angiomyoma (Vascular Leiomyoma)

Definition. Angiomyoma is a distinctive, relatively common, benign subcutaneous neoplasm composed of smooth muscle and thick-walled vessels. The smooth muscle in the vessel walls blends with that in the solid parts of the tumor.

Clinical Features. Patients with angiomyoma are most frequently between 30 and 60 years of age, and are most often women. The tumor usually occurs on the extremities, especially the lower extremity, and most often presents as a small (less than 2 cm), slowly growing mass of several years' duration. Angiomyoma is characteristically located in the subcutis, although the deep dermis is occasionally involved. This diagnosis is not used for deep smooth muscle tumors. In contrast to pilar leiomyomas, which are frequently multiple, almost all angiomyomas are solitary. Lesional pain is a prominent symptom in approximately half the patients.

Pathologic Findings. Grossly, angiomyoma forms a well-circumscribed, white-gray mass. Microscopically, it is made up of cells that have the features of mature, well-differentiated smooth muscle cells mixed among thick-walled vessels (fig. 5-2). Thin-walled vessels are also sometimes present. The smooth muscle in the walls of the thick-walled vessels blends with that in the remainder of the lesion. The nuclei are typically small and uniform but occasionally they are mildly enlarged and pleomorphic, probably the result of degeneration. Mitotic figures are usually absent or very rare. Areas of myxoid change, hyalinization, calcification, or fat may be present. Some authors have suggested that fat-containing angiomyomas be labeled "angiomyolipomas," and have even suggested a relationship with renal and retroperitoneal angiomyolipomas. We are unconvinced of any relationship and do not use the term angiomyolipoma for these subcutaneous lesions. The tumor border is characteristically well delimited, as would be expected from the gross circumscription.

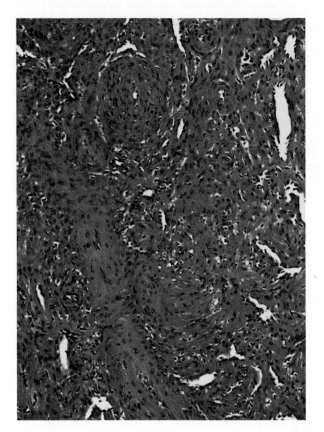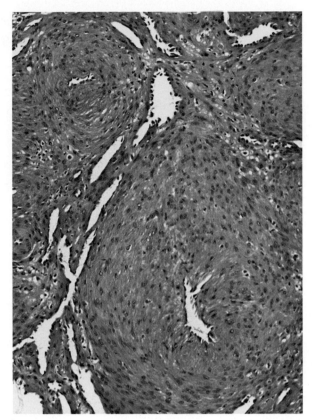

Figure 5-2
ANGIOMYOMA
Left: Angiomyomas contain numerous vessels, often thick-walled, in addition to a smooth muscle stroma.
Right: The smooth muscle in the walls of the vessels blends into the smooth muscle of the lesion.

Differential Diagnosis. Because of its distinctive histologic composition of well-differentiated smooth muscle and thick-walled vessels, angiomyoma is unlikely to be confused with other neoplasms. Those rare examples containing cells with some degree of nuclear pleomorphism can be distinguished from leiomyosarcoma by the characteristic vessels, lack of mitotic activity, and small size. Glomus tumor is usually subungual, the constituent cells are round rather than elongate, and the cytoplasm is not fibrillar. Fat may be found in angiomyomas, and this could cause confusion with angiolipoma. However, the latter lacks smooth muscle, and thrombi are commonly present in the vessels in angiolipoma.

Treatment and Prognosis. The tumor is benign, but very rarely can recur locally after simple excision.

Leiomyoma of Soft Tissue

Definition. Leiomyomas of the soft tissues are histologically bland, paucicellular smooth muscle tumors without mitotic figures.

General Considerations. It is our experience that leiomyomas of the deep soft tissue, including the retroperitoneum, are very rare except in the female pelvis. Moreover, some of these histologically bland, soft tissue smooth muscle tumors that are morphologic candidates for the category of leiomyoma recur or even spread, sometimes after long periods of time, further reducing the pool of harmless smooth muscle tumors in the soft tissue (12). Subcutaneous smooth muscle tumors are usually considered with the dermal ones because both are associated with normal smooth muscle in the lower

Table 5-3

GUIDELINES FOR EVALUATING SOFT TISSUE SMOOTH MUSCLE TUMORS*

Site	Leiomyoma	Smooth Muscle Tumor of Uncertain Malignant Potential	Leiomyosarcoma**
Retroperitoneum	Bland uniform nuclei and no mitotic figures and less than 5 cm; very rare if it exists at all (see text)	Bland uniform nuclei with division activity up to 4 mf/ 10 hpf or bland tumors without mitotic activity that are are >5 cm in diameter	Any one of the following: 1) >4 mf/10 hpf 2) tumor cell necrosis 3) pleomorphism at 10X magnification 4) nuclear atypia
Deep soft tissues, subcutaneous tissues, and vessels	Bland uniform nuclei and no mitotic figures; tumors may be larger than 5 cm but experience limited especially for larger tumors	Bland uniform nuclei with division activity up to 4 mf/10 hpf	Same as for retroperitoneum

*These guidelines are only for tumors in these sites. They may not be applicable to smooth muscle tumors in other locations.
**There is no specific category for soft tissue smooth muscle lesions that recur but do not metastasize. They are most often placed in the leiomyosarcoma category.

dermis. Both dermal and subcutaneous leiomyomas are divided into those associated with pilar arrector muscles, which can occur anywhere, and those that arise in the areola, nipple, scrotum, labium, penis, and vulva (15). The latter group are referred to as *genital leiomyomas*. Dermal and subcutaneous leiomyomas are discussed in the Fascicle, Non-Melanocytic Tumors of the Skin (14). The following discussion pertains only to leiomyomas that occur in the deep soft tissues, and is divided into retroperitoneal tumors and those that occur in other deep soft tissue sites.

Leiomyomas of the Retroperitoneum

General Considerations. It is doubtful whether the term leiomyoma should ever be applied to a retroperitoneal smooth muscle tumor over 4 cm because bland smooth muscle tumors in this site larger than this size can recur and spread. The available evidence indicates that any retroperitoneal smooth muscle tumor with 5 or more mitotic figures per 10 high-power fields should be considered malignant regardless of the cytologic features (16,18). We consider those with bland histology and 1 to 4 mitotic figures per 10 high-power fields as of uncertain malignant potential, as we do bland smooth muscle tumors that are mitotically inactive and over 5 cm in diameter (Table 5-3). Retroperitoneal smooth muscle tumors characterized by pleomorphism, tumor cell necrosis, or nuclear atypia should be interpreted as leiomyosarcoma no matter what the mitotic index. This leaves only bland tumors with no mitotic activity and a diameter of less than 5 cm for the category of leiomyoma. Such tumors are vanishingly rare.

The possibility of *parasitic leiomyoma* is often raised when a woman is found to have a bland retroperitoneal smooth muscle tumor. We are wary of this concept and classify all retroperitoneal smooth muscle tumors as primary unless they are clearly attached to the genitalia or other structures outside the retroperitoneum. Morphologically bland but clinically malignant gastrointestinal stromal tumors also may spread to the retroperitoneum and mimic a primary smooth muscle tumor in that site.

Leiomyomas do occur in the pelvis of women. In our experience, most develop in areas where smooth muscle is present, such as the broad and round ligaments. Although experience is limited, we have found that the criteria we use to predict malignancy for uterine tumors seems to accurately predict the aggressive potential of pelvic smooth muscle tumors. When contemplating a diagnosis of pelvic leiomyoma, care should be taken to exclude a smooth muscle tumor arising from the muscularis propria of the large or small bowel because all of these should be considered potentially malignant no matter how bland. Excluded from this cautionary note are leiomyomatous polyps arising in the muscularis mucosae of the large bowel; they are benign.

The following discussion pertains only to retroperitoneal smooth muscle tumors that might be candidates for a diagnosis of leiomyoma of the retroperitoneum.

Clinical and Pathologic Findings. Because the definition of retroperitoneal leiomyoma requires it to be of small size, it would be an incidental finding in this location (18). The pathologic features are those of a well-differentiated, cytologically bland smooth muscle tumor in which the mitotic count is zero, the tumor is no greater than 5 cm in diameter, and pleomorphism is absent. The constituent cells should have easily seen eosinophilic cytoplasm with the H&E stain or red-staining cytoplasm by trichrome; the nuclei are vesicular or evenly dense. At least focally, the cells should be arranged in fascicles, and positive actin and desmin stains are helpful. Histologically benign retroperitoneal smooth muscle tumors with identifiable division figures are considered by us to be of uncertain malignant potential, as are those morphologically bland tumors that are greater than 5 cm in diameter but with less than 1 mitotic figure per 10 high-power fields (Table 5-3).

Differential Diagnosis. See Retroperitoneal Leiomyosarcoma below. The diagnosis of retroperitoneal leiomyoma probably should be made only after consultation (see General Considerations above).

Treatment and Prognosis. Tumors categorized as retroperitoneal leiomyomas should be cured by conservative excision; if they recur, the recurrence should be nondestructive.

Leiomyomas in the Deep Soft Tissue Other Than the Retroperitoneum and Pelvis, Including Leiomyomas Arising in Vessels

General Considerations. Soft tissue leiomyomas are very rare neoplasms and the recent series of 11 cases reported by Kilpatrick and associates (13) is probably the largest in the literature. Initially, these investigators suggested that any smooth muscle tumor in the deep soft tissue with more than 1 mitotic figure per 20 high-power fields be considered at least potentially malignant and not labeled as leiomyoma. In a subsequent letter, the authors reported that one of the cytologically bland tumors in this series with 1 mitotic figure per 50 high-power fields recurred and they now advocate that bland smooth muscle tumors in the soft tissues with any mitotic activity be considered potentially malignant (of uncertain malignant potential) (12). The follow-up time in this series is fairly short so it is possible more of the tumors will recur because bland retroperitoneal smooth muscle tumors and gastrointestinal stromal (smooth muscle) tumors can recur many years after the primary tumor has been removed. We think a diagnosis of leiomyoma of the deep soft tissue should be made with great caution and only for tumors that are bland, have no mitotic figures, and are preferably not much larger than 5 cm. Because experience with bland soft tissue and vascular smooth muscle tumors is limited, the prudent pathologist will point out in the pathology report that a diagnosis of soft tissue leiomyoma is problematic. These remarks also apply to bland smooth muscle tumors arising in vessels and deep smooth muscle tumors with prominent vessels.

Clinical Features. The few cases reported indicate that both sexes are equally affected. Most patients are young adults and most tumors develop in the extremities.

Pathologic Findings. Leiomyomas of the deep soft tissues are characteristically circumscribed and lobulated grossly. The cut surface is usually whorled, although myxoid and cystic change is common (13). Calcification is occasionally found. Microscopically, leiomyomas are composed, at least focally, of cells that demonstrate obvious smooth muscle differentiation, i.e., they closely resemble normal smooth muscle because the cells are elongate, have eosinophilic cytoplasm and oblong rounded nuclei, and are arranged in fascicles, at least focally. Most are paucicellular, although some cellular smooth muscle tumors of the soft tissues have been classified as leiomyoma (13). The definition of soft tissue leiomyoma excludes tumors demonstrating mitotic activity.

Focal myxoid change and hyalinization are almost universal, while calcification, sometimes in the form of psammoma bodies, and ossification are found in fewer tumors. However, tumor cell necrosis is not a feature of leiomyoma, and if present in a smooth muscle tumor should arouse immediate suspicion of leiomyosarcoma. Nuclear palisading in a Verocay body–like pattern, clear cell change, focal epithelioid histology, fibrosis, fatty differentiation, and hyalinization have been seen in some tumors (13,13a,17). Cells with enlarged, hyperchromatic, bizarre-shaped nuclei resembling the cells that populate "ancient schwannoma" may be found focally in an otherwise characteristic leiomyoma. When these are present, special care must be taken to be sure mitotic figures are absent. Leiomyomas containing such cells are almost always hypocellular, and hypercellular examples are best considered to be at least of uncertain malignant potential.

Desmin was expressed by the tumor cells in all 11 cases of Kilpatrick and associates (13) and it is probably best not to diagnose a deep soft tissue tumor as a leiomyoma unless the desmin stain is positive. S-100 protein stains have been negative in the rare cases in which the stain was used (13).

Differential Diagnosis. The differential diagnosis of soft tissue leiomyoma includes neural tumors, fibrous and myofibroblastic tumors, fibrous histiocytomas, and leiomyosarcoma. Insistence upon easily recognized smooth muscle cells, positive actin and desmin stains, and negative S-100 protein stain before diagnosing a soft tissue tumor as a leiomyoma will eliminate practically all these other considerations except leiomyosarcoma. When the patient is a woman and the smooth muscle tumor is in the abdominal wall, pelvis, or buttock, care must be taken to be sure that the tumor is not extending from the uterus. The definitional features we use to distinguish soft tissue leiomyoma from leiomyosarcoma are presented in the General Considerations section above.

Treatment and Prognosis. Soft tissue leiomyomas are cured by a conservative excision. If they recur, the recurrence is not aggressive or uncontrolled. A recurring bland soft tissue smooth muscle tumor should be labeled as of "uncertain malignant potential."

MALIGNANT SMOOTH MUSCLE TUMORS (MANAGERIAL GROUP III, TABLE 1-10)

Leiomyosarcoma

Definition. Leiomyosarcoma is a malignant tumor composed, at least focally, of cells that demonstrate smooth muscle differentiation.

General Considerations. Two problems plague the recognition of leiomyosarcoma of the soft tissues. First, the more poorly differentiated the leiomyosarcoma, the less obvious is the evidence of smooth muscle differentiation and the greater the resemblance to other poorly differentiated spindle cell sarcomas. Second, morphologically bland smooth muscle tumors can recur and sometimes cause patient death as a result of uncontrolled growth, or even metastasize (19,20). A discussion of this classificatory dilemma and our definition of smooth muscle differentiation is presented in the Introduction to this chapter. Our conventions for predicting the aggressive potential of soft tissue smooth muscle tumors are presented in the General Considerations section of the previous section on leiomyoma, the Pathologic Features in this section, and Table 5-3. It is useful for diagnostic and prognostic purposes to divide leiomyosarcomas by location into the following sites: retroperitoneum, deep soft tissues, subcutaneous tissue, and those arising from vessels.

About half of all soft tissue leiomyosarcomas occur in the retroperitoneum. Included in this group are leiomyosarcomas that arise in the mesentery and omentum, but not gastrointestinal stromal (smooth muscle) tumors.

Leiomyosarcoma of the Retroperitoneum

Clinical Features. Retroperitoneal leiomyosarcomas are usually discovered in middle-aged and older adults (27a,29). About two thirds of the patients are women (35). Leiomyosarcomas in the retroperitoneum rarely cause symptoms until they are quite large, and most are detected because of abdominal swelling or discovery of a mass which may be painful. Imaging studies are very useful in localizing the mass. At surgery, the usual retroperitoneal leiomyosarcoma is huge, averaging about 1500 g and measuring over 10 cm (27a,28,29,35).

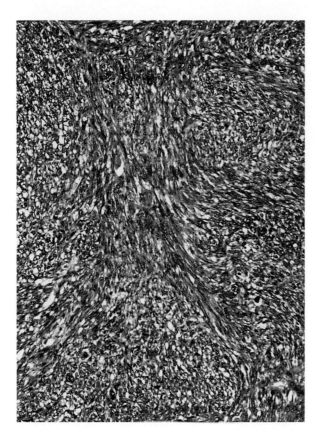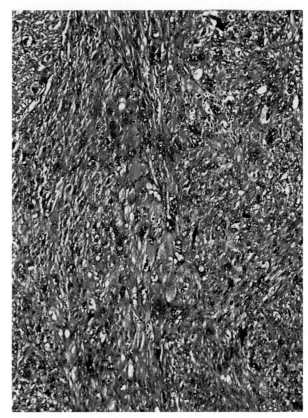

Figure 5-3
LEIOMYOSARCOMA OF THE RETROPERITONEUM

Leiomyosarcomas of the retroperitoneum and soft tissues range from well-differentiated smooth muscle tumors with obvious smooth muscle differentiation (left) to pleomorphic sarcomas in which smooth muscle differentiation is difficult to discern (right). Desmin staining is often useful in recognizing smooth muscle differentiation.

Pathologic Findings. Grossly, the tumors are usually gray-white to flesh colored; focally cystic change, hemorrhage, and necrosis are common. Microscopically, retroperitoneal leiomyosarcomas vary from well-differentiated tumors composed of cells that display obvious smooth muscle differentiation to those so poorly differentiated that they resemble pleomorphic malignant fibrous histiocytoma (MFH) (fig. 5-3) (24,27a,29,35). The former may be so bland and paucicellular that they are morphologically indistinguishable from leiomyoma and are recognized because mitotic figures are present or because they are large; the latter are recognized as leiomyosarcoma on the basis of focal areas of smooth muscle differentiation. The prototypic leiomyosarcoma of the retroperitoneum is moderately cellular and composed of elongate cells with easily seen eosinophilic cytoplasm and elongate nuclei with rounded ends. Nucleoli may

be prominent and the cells are arranged, at least focally, in fascicles (fig. 5-3, left). More poorly differentiated cases are marked by less cytoplasm, denser and more granular chromatin, and greater nuclear pleomorphism (fig. 5-3, right).

Other histologic features mark some retroperitoneal leiomyosarcomas (27a,29,35). Multinucleated tumor giant cells, including osteoclastlike giant cells, are common, and some tumors are composed in part of epithelioid cells which may or may not demonstrate cytoplasmic clearing (clear cell pattern) (22,25,27a). An inflammatory infiltrate, sometimes massive, is found in some leiomyosarcomas (26). A few tumors are composed predominantly or exclusively of epithelioid cells, and when this occurs, finding areas of typical smooth muscle differentiation or positive desmin staining of the epithelioid cells, coupled with negative mucin and keratin stains,

247

help identify the tumor as of smooth muscle type (29). In some tumors, the nuclei align themselves in Verocay-like bodies (35). Rare anaplastic leiomyosarcomas feature large strap-like cells with eosinophilic cytoplasm that does not contain cross-striations and occasionally, tumors are composed predominantly of cells with granular cytoplasm (29). Mitotic figures are usually numerous but may be difficult to find in well-differentiated examples.

The stroma may be hyalinized or, less frequently, focally myxoid (35). Rarely, a tumor will be predominantly or exclusively myxoid and only focally will smooth muscle cells be recognized. Obviously, a myxoid neoplasm cannot be recognized as of smooth muscle type unless some tumor cells are differentiated as smooth muscle. Necrosis and hemorrhage are common, and coagulative tumor cell necrosis in a smooth muscle tumor is, for practical purposes, limited to leiomyosarcoma. Occasional retroperitoneal leiomyosarcomas have prominent hyalinized vessels, and in a few the vessels are arranged in a pericytic pattern (29,35). Leiomyosarcoma has been reported as the sarcomatous portion of dedifferentiated liposarcoma (30,33).

As discussed above in the section Leiomyomas of the Retroperitoneum, predicting the malignant potential of a morphologically bland smooth muscle tumor in the retroperitoneum has a large potential for error (28,29). We depend primarily on size and mitotic activity (Table 5-3). We think all retroperitoneal smooth muscle tumors with greater than 5 mitotic figures per 10 high-power fields, as well as those with significant pleomorphism regardless of the mitotic index, should be interpreted as leiomyosarcoma (28). We consider retroperitoneal smooth muscle tumors to be of uncertain malignant potential if they are bland and contain 1 to 4 mitotic figures per 10 high-power fields or if they are bland, mitotically inactive, and greater than 5 cm in diameter (see also Leiomyoma section above) (fig. 5-4). We wish to stress again that the criteria for malignancy that are valid for uterine smooth muscle tumors do not necessarily apply to retroperitoneal tumors because these criteria will significantly under-recognize retroperitoneal smooth muscle tumors capable of at least recurrence.

Retroperitoneal leiomyosarcomas have been graded both on the basis of the degree of nuclear atypia and anaplasia as well as the extent of necrosis. Histologic grading does not predict outcome particularly well, but if morphologically low-grade neoplasms recur, they usually take a longer time to do so than high-grade leiomyosarcomas (35).

Special Studies. Almost all leiomyosarcomas contain cells that express one or more muscle actins, and desmin is reported to be positive in 50 to 100 percent of tumors (21,27a,31,32). This variability in desmin reactivity most likely reflects the different definitions of what counts as evidence of smooth muscle differentiation used by various investigators. However, crisp definitions are seldom provided so the cause of this variability remains uncertain. In our experience, 70 to 80 percent of leiomyosarcomas contain desmin-positive cells and 90 to 95 percent contain actin-positive cells. We think it doubtful that a sarcoma should be interpreted as leiomyosarcoma when both actin and desmin stains are negative. On the other hand, many other types of tumor cells express antigens recognized by muscle actin, and focal desmin staining has also been reported in a wide variety of neoplasms other than those of smooth muscle type. Normal smooth muscle cells sometimes express an antigen recognized by antibodies against cytokeratin, usually CAM5.2, and positive staining for keratin and epithelial membrane antigen has been reported in smooth muscle tumors (27). A few leiomyosarcomas contain cells that express S-100 protein and CD34 (31,34). Therefore, the possibility of a smooth muscle tumor containing cells positive for one or the other of these antibodies should be kept in mind when considering the differential diagnostic possibilities. We consider the presence of muscle actin and desmin in tumor cells to be strongly supportive of smooth muscle differentiation as long as the histologic features are those of a smooth muscle tumor. Actin alone provides less support because it frequently decorates myofibroblasts, which may also be desmin positive.

Differential Diagnosis. Many benign and malignant neoplasms in the retroperitoneum are composed of cells that resemble smooth muscle cells so the differential diagnosis of retroperitoneal leiomyosarcoma is extensive and important. Among the benign neoplasms, the most important are cellular schwannoma, because it is a spindle cell tumor that can grow to large size,

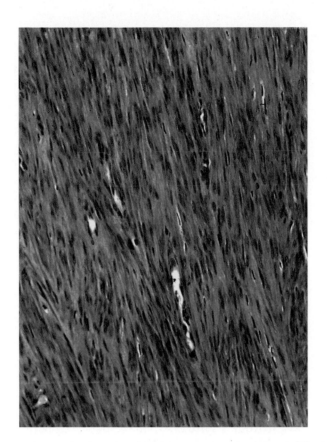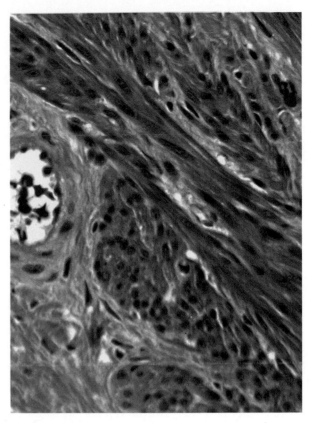

Figure 5-4
RETROPERITONEAL SMOOTH MUSCLE TUMOR OF UNCERTAIN MALIGNANT POTENTIAL
This bland retroperitoneal tumor was 8 cm in diameter and contained less than 1 mitotic figure per 10 high-power fields.
In this location a completely tumor-free course cannot be guaranteed even when the tumor is this bland.

and angiomyolipoma, because it contains smooth muscle. By definition, cellular schwannoma is an S-100 protein–positive neoplasm that can recur locally, so this stain is always indicated when a retroperitoneal spindle cell neoplasm might be neural. Cellular schwannomas are negative for desmin, feature hyalinized vessels, have areas frequently recognizable as schwannoma, and foam cells are present. Neurofibromas and ordinary schwannomas are also S-100 protein positive. Angiomyolipoma contains fat cells and large tangled vessels, many of which lack an internal elastic lamina. The smooth muscle cells of the tumor radiate from these abnormal vessels and in some tumors can become so predominant that fat is hard to find. Moreover, a few angiomyolipomas contain atypical pleomorphic cells and mitotic figures may be numerous. However, the smooth muscle cells in angiomyolipoma are HMB45 positive, in contrast

to the cells in leiomyosarcoma. Almost all angiomyolipomas arise in the kidney, although a few may be predominantly or rarely, exclusively in the retroperitoneum, and leiomyosarcomas do not contain the abnormal vessels that are the hallmark of angiomyolipoma.

Mesenteric fibromatosis is a consideration when leiomyosarcoma involves the mesentery. While the cells in mesenteric fibromatosis may be actin positive, they are not usually desmin positive and the stroma is more diffusely myxoid than the stroma in the usual leiomyosarcoma. Most importantly, the cells do not display smooth muscle features; rather they have fibroblastic characteristics, including uniform, small nuclei and sparse cytoplasm. The cells in retroperitoneal fibrosis are also fibroblasts, this lesion almost always causes medial deviation of the ureters, and there is a chronic inflammatory component.

Inflammatory myofibroblastic tumor (inflammatory fibrosarcoma, inflammatory pseudotumor) is composed of myofibroblasts and these sometimes can have features indistinguishable from smooth muscle cells. However, chronic inflammation is prominent and the lesions occur almost exclusively in children and young adults, an age when leiomyosarcoma essentially does not develop in the retroperitoneum.

Many malignant neoplasms enter the differential diagnosis of retroperitoneal leiomyosarcoma. One of the most important is sarcomatoid renal cell carcinoma. Because some leiomyosarcomas contain keratin- and epithelial membrane antigen–positive cells, keratin stains cannot be entirely relied upon to distinguish renal cell carcinoma from leiomyosarcoma. However, a diffusely positive keratin stain and imaging studies localizing the tumor to the kidney are good evidence that a spindled neoplasm is a renal cell carcinoma. Moreover, CAM5.2 rather than AE1 is the keratin most often positive in smooth muscle tumors. Epithelioid leiomyosarcoma must be distinguished from carcinoma; mucin stains may be useful in this regard, as is taking numerous sections to determine if the tumor has more characteristic smooth muscle features in other areas. Melanoma cells almost always express S-100 protein, HMB45, or both. Leiomyosarcoma can have areas indistinguishable from pleomorphic MFH, but somewhere in a leiomyosarcoma the tumor cells must be differentiated as smooth muscle. The cells in fibrosarcomas are arranged in fascicles but they lack the amount of cytoplasm that is required for smooth muscle cells. Fibrosarcoma is rare in the retroperitoneum except as the dedifferentiated component of a dedifferentiated liposarcoma. Malignant peripheral nerve sheath tumor (MPNST) is a sarcoma that arises from a nerve or in a patient with neurofibromatosis. About half of MPNSTs are S-100 protein positive; they are desmin negative. Rarely, focal areas of metaplastic smooth muscle can be found in atypical lipomatous tumors (well-differentiated liposarcoma) but these are tumors of adult fat so fat is also present in the tumor (23). An even rarer occurrence is leiomyosarcoma as the dedifferentiated component of dedifferentiated liposarcoma (30,33).

Treatment and Prognosis. Almost all retroperitoneal leiomyosarcomas are large when discovered and many invade adjacent organs. Their size and invasive properties cause a significant number to be unresectable at the time of surgery; consequently, mortality is very high. In the series reported by Shmookler and Lauer (29), 75 percent of the patients were dead of tumor at a mean follow-up of 3.5 years, and Ranchod and Kempson (28) report that only 1 of 13 patients did not die of tumor and that patient died of unrelated causes. Morphologic features correlate poorly with ultimate outcome but low-grade leiomyosarcomas tend to take a longer time to recur than do high-grade ones. Even so, ultimately almost all patients die as a result of their tumor (35). The most common sites of metastasis are the lung and liver but metastasis to bone, soft tissues, and skin is frequent (27a). Adjuvant therapy has not proven to be effective.

The outcome of tumors with features that cause them to be classified as "of uncertain malignant potential" is largely unknown but some can recur.

Leiomyosarcoma of Deep Soft Tissues Outside the Retroperitoneum

Clinical Features. These, like retroperitoneal leiomyosarcomas, affect women more often than men (38). A small subset occur in children some of whom, but not all, have AIDS (36). They usually arise in the extremities, particularly the lower extremity, and are discovered because of their mass effect. Deep soft tissue leiomyosarcomas are usually smaller at diagnosis than their retroperitoneal counterparts.

Pathologic Findings. The gross, microscopic, and immunohistologic features are identical to retroperitoneal leiomyosarcoma as described above, and the same problems arise in predicting the malignant potential of these tumors. As noted earlier in this chapter, leiomyoma of the deep soft tissues is much less common than leiomyosarcoma. We use the same rules for predicting malignancy for deep soft tissue smooth muscle tumors as we do for the retroperitoneal ones (see above and Table 5-3; figs. 5-5, 5-6). Tumors with morphologic features that are borderline are best considered to be of uncertain malignant potential. Epithelioid cells, clear cells, granular cells, multinucleated giant cells, and strap-like cells have been reported in leiomyosarcomas of the deep soft tissues (fig. 5-7) (36a,39,40,42,44). The giant cells often resemble osteoclasts and are negative

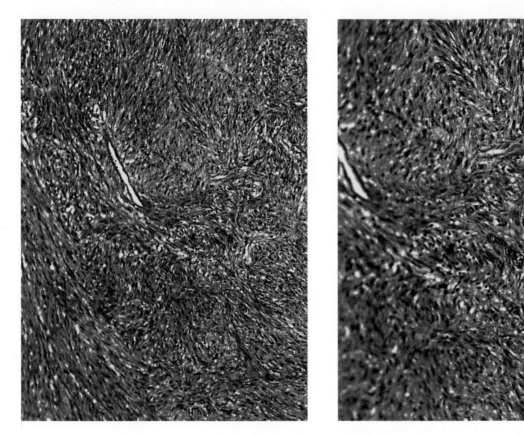

Figure 5-5
SOFT TISSUE LEIOMYOSARCOMA

Left: When pleomorphism is apparent at low magnification, a soft tissue or retroperitoneal smooth muscle tumor should not be interpreted as benign.

Right: The pleomorphism and smooth muscle differentiation are apparent at higher magnification.

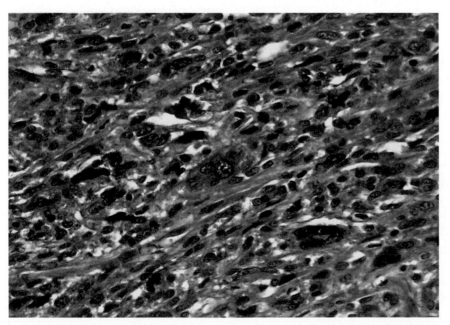

Figure 5-6
SOFT TISSUE
LEIOMYOSARCOMA

Many soft tissue leiomyosarcomas are markedly pleomorphic and so poorly differentiated that evidence of smooth muscle differentiation is present only focally.

for muscle markers but positive for CD68 (40). A dense inflammatory infiltrate is found in some tumors (41).

Differential Diagnosis. This is essentially the same as for retroperitoneal leiomyosarcoma (see above) except that direct extension of renal cell carcinoma is not a problem, although metastatic renal cell carcinoma certainly is a major differential diagnostic consideration, and monophasic synovial sarcoma is added to the differential diagnostic list. However, synovial sarcoma cells do not have the elongated round-ended nuclei of smooth muscle cells; rather their nuclei are stubby and their cytoplasm sparse. Synovial sarcomas lack the nuclear pleomorphism that is common in leiomyosarcomas; also, they are often microscopically lobulated and ropy eosinophilic collagen is commonly present. Both tumors may have a pericytic vascular pattern although it is far more common in synovial sarcoma. About half of monophasic synovial sarcomas contain cells that express cytokeratin but this is not a particularly useful observation because leiomyosarcoma may contain such cells. However, desmin is negative and CD99 may be positive in synovial sarcomas.

Treatment and Prognosis. The tumor-free survival rate of patients with extremity leiomyosarcoma is better than that for those with retroperitoneal lesions and in most series is around 50 percent. This probably reflects the smaller size at which these tumors are discovered rather than any inherent biologic differences in the neoplasms. Age 60 years or older, vascular invasion, deep site, and size over 5 cm have been reported to be independent risk factors for a fatal outcome (37,38,43). Children with soft tissue leiomyosarcoma have an excellent prognosis and are most often cured by excision (36).

Leiomyosarcoma of the Subcutaneous Tissue

General Considerations. These tumors, which occur more commonly in men, have a predilection for the extremities, and because they are superficial they are usually discovered when they are relatively small, although they are not typically as small as dermal leiomyosarcomas.

Pathologic Findings. The gross and histologic features are essentially the same as for retroperitoneal leiomyosarcoma except that hemor-

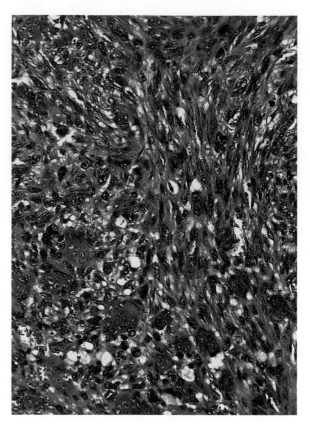

Figure 5-7
SOFT TISSUE LEIOMYOSARCOMA
An example with multinucleated giant cells.

rhage and necrosis are less commonly present. We use the same mitotic counts and size criteria to predict malignancy (see above and Table 5-3).

Differential Diagnosis. The differential diagnosis includes spindle cell neoplasms that involve the dermis and subcutaneous tissues. In addition, subcutaneous leiomyosarcoma must be sharply distinguished from dermal leiomyosarcoma because of significant differences in outcome. Spindle cell carcinoma, primary and metastatic; malignant melanoma, both spindle cell and desmoplastic; neural tumors; pleomorphic MFH; fibrosarcoma; benign fibrous histiocytoma containing prominent myofibroblastic cells; and nodular fasciitis all figure in the differential diagnosis. Unless the sarcoma in question is composed of obvious smooth muscle cells, immunohistochemical stains are almost always warranted when leiomyosarcoma of the subcutaneous tissues is a diagnostic possibility. A useful panel includes keratin, epithelial membrane antigen, S-100 protein, actin, and desmin. Keratin is usually strongly and diffusely positive in carcinoma and, if positive in leiomyosarcoma, is almost always focal and weak and recognized by CAM5.2 but usually not AE1. S-100 protein is rarely positive in leiomyosarcoma. If the tumor has the H&E morphology of leiomyosarcoma, positive actin and desmin stains coupled with negative S-100 protein and keratin stains provides good support for the diagnosis. Benign fibrous histiocytomas often contain foam cells, and giant cells are common. The cells of fibrosarcoma possess sparse pale cytoplasm and the nuclei tend to be thinner and more hyperchromatic than those in smooth muscle cells, giving an overall basophilic appearance to the tumor. Malignant peripheral nerve sheath tumor (MPNST) arises from a nerve or a neurofibroma, or in neurofibromatosis, and about half contain cells which express S-100 protein. Its cells also have paler cytoplasm than the cells of leiomyosarcoma. Essentially all neurofibromas and schwannomas are S-100 protein positive. Nodular fasciitis features myofibroblasts and fibroblasts that are nearly always smooth muscle actin positive; however, the constituent cells are arranged loosely in bundles rather than tightly in fascicles and the stroma has a "torn" appearance rarely seen in leiomyosarcoma. Desmin is infrequently positive in nodular fasciitis. The cells in nodular fasciitis are uniform and the chromatin is delicate and often vesicular. The diagnosis of pleomorphic MFH implies a tumor composed of pleomorphic cells not demonstrating any direction of differentiation other than fibroblastic, myofibroblastic, and histiocyte-like. Actin and CD68 may be positive but desmin, keratin, and S-100 protein are almost always negative.

Leiomyosarcoma confined to the dermis essentially does not metastasize so it must be sharply distinguished from subcutaneous leiomyosarcoma. For a histologically malignant smooth muscle tumor to be deemed dermal, we think at least 90 percent of it must be in the dermis.

Treatment and Prognosis. As befits its usual small size and relatively superficial location, subcutaneous leiomyosarcoma in most series has a significantly lower metastatic rate than its counterparts in the deep soft tissues and retroperitoneum. Size is an important predictor of metastasis and leiomyosarcomas of the subcutis less than 5 cm rarely metastasize (45).

Leiomyosarcoma Arising in Vessels

General Considerations. Leiomyosarcoma can arise from vessels, but such tumors are very rare. The inferior vena cava is the vessel most commonly involved and other veins are the next most common site (46). The pulmonary artery is the most common site of arterial leiomyosarcoma and all other arteries together are somewhat less frequently involved than that artery. Of course, some reported examples of deep soft tissue and subcutaneous leiomyosarcomas may, in fact, be examples of leiomyosarcoma arising in vessels in which the vessel of origin has been destroyed.

Clinical Features. Nearly 90 percent of patients with leiomyosarcoma of the inferior vena cava are middle-aged or older women. Most of the tumors arise in the upper third of this vein, and when the hepatic veins become invaded and blocked by tumor the patients may develop the Budd-Chiari syndrome with hepatomegaly, jaundice, and ascites. Leiomyosarcomas developing lower in the vena cava may obstruct the renal veins and cause renal dysfunction, including the nephrotic syndrome and renal failure. Leiomyosarcomas involving the upper third of the vena cava are almost always unresectable but tumors located in a more inferior location sometimes can be completely removed. Vena cavograms can confirm the presence of an intraluminal mass (46).

Leiomyosarcomas of veins other than the vena cava are very rare. When leiomyosarcoma does occur outside the vena cava, veins of the lower extremity are most commonly involved, especially the saphenous, iliac, and femoral veins, although there are reports of rare cases arising from smaller veins (47). The sex incidence of leiomyosarcoma originating from veins other than the inferior vena cava is approximately 1 to 1. Venous leiomyosarcomas usually present as mass lesions, although lower leg edema may be the initial symptom. The pulmonary artery is the most common site of arterial leiomyosarcoma. Almost all of the patients with pulmonary artery leiomyosarcoma are adults and the symptoms relate to decreased pulmonary flow and infiltration of the heart and the smaller pulmonary arteries.

Pathologic Findings. Within veins, leiomyosarcoma may develop as a localized mass and then grow along the luminal surface but it also frequently invades through the wall of the vein into surrounding structures. Arterial leiomyosarcomas tend to be restricted to the lumen and wall of the artery. The histologic features of leiomyosarcoma arising in veins or arteries are identical to those of leiomyosarcoma of the retroperitoneum, and we use the same mitotic index and size criteria to predict behavior for these lesions as we do for retroperitoneal ones (see above). As in the retroperitoneum, leiomyoma of the vessels is a very rare neoplasm and we are not convinced it actually exists. Even if one is tempted to make a diagnosis of leiomyoma of a vessel because the tumor is so small, bland, and mitotically inactive, a disclaimer in the comment section of the pathology report about the lack of experience with bland mitotically inactive smooth muscle tumors arising in vessels is in order.

Differential Diagnosis. The differential diagnosis is essentially the same as for retroperitoneal leiomyosarcoma except that intravenous leiomyomatosis (IV leiomyomatosis) has to be considered for smooth muscle tumors involving the inferior vena cava and the femoral veins in women. IV leiomyomatosis begins in the uterus, and while it can extend up the lumen of the vena cava and other veins, it does not infiltrate through the wall of the vein as do most leiomyosarcomas. There is often extensive hyalinization in IV leiomyomatosis and the cells are frequently epithelioid. Although atypia may be seen in some examples of IV leiomyomatosis, in most examples the cells are bland and mitotically inactive.

While leiomyosarcoma may rarely arise from the pulmonary artery and even the aorta, most sarcomas arising in the great arteries are anaplastic and do not have cells displaying smooth muscle features. They usually have morphologic features that fit the definition of pleomorphic MFH, but a few large artery sarcomas show skeletal, smooth muscle, osseous, cartilaginous, or vascular differentiation.

Treatment and Prognosis. The majority of patients with leiomyosarcoma of the vessels die of their disease. The only hope for cure is complete resection but most tumors are far advanced by the time of diagnosis (46).

REFERENCES

Introduction

1. Azumi N, Ben EJ, Battifora H. Immunophenotypic diagnosis of leiomyosarcomas and rhabdomyosarcomas with monoclonal antibodies to muscle-specific actin and desmin in formalin-fixed tissue. Mod Pathol 1988;1:469–74.
2. Enzinger FM, Weiss SW. Soft tissue tumors. St. Louis: Mosby 1995:1067–74.
3. Hashimoto H, Daimaru Y, Tsuneyoshi M, Enjoji M. Leiomyosarcoma of the external soft tissues. A clinicopathologic, immunohistochemical, and electron microscopic study. Cancer 1986;57:2077–88.
4. Kilpatrick SE, Mentzel T, Fletcher CD. Leiomyoma of deep soft tissue. Clinicopathologic analysis of a series. Am J Surg Pathol 1994;18:576–82.
5. McClain KL, Leach CT, Jenson HB, et al. Association of Epstein-Barr virus with leiomyosarcomas in children with AIDS. N Engl J Med 1995;332:12–8.
6. Merchant W, Calonje E, Fletcher CD. Inflammatory leiomyosarcoma: a morphological subgroup within the heterogeneous family of so-called inflammatory malignant fibrous histiocytoma. Histopathology 1995;27:525–32.
7. Ranchod M, Kempson RL. Smooth muscle tumors of the gastrointestinal tract and retroperitoneum: a pathologic analysis of 100 cases. Cancer 1977;39:255–62.
8. Rangdaeng S, Truong LD. Comparative immunohistochemical staining for desmin and muscle-specific actin. A study of 576 cases. Am J Clin Pathol 1991;96:32–45.
9. Shmookler BM, Lauer DH. Retroperitoneal leiomyosarcoma. A clinicopathologic analysis of 36 cases. Am J Surg Pathol 1983;7:269–80.
10. Swanson PE, Wick MR, Dehner LP. Leiomyosarcoma of somatic soft tissues in childhood: an immunohistochemical analysis of six cases with ultrastructural correlation. Hum Pathol 1991;22:569–77.
10a. van Hoeven KH, Factor SM, Kress Y, Woodruff JM. Visceral myogenic tumors. A manifestation of HIV infection in children. Am J Surg Pathol 1993;17:1176–81.
11. Wile AG, Evans HL, Romsdahl MM. Leiomyosarcoma of soft tissue: a clinicopathologic study. Cancer 1981;48:1022–32.

Leiomyoma of Soft Tissues

12. Fletcher CD, Kilpatrick SE, Mentzel T. The difficulty in predicting behavior of smooth-muscle tumors in deep soft tissue. Am J Surg Pathol 1995;19:116–7.
13. Kilpatrick SE, Mentzel T, Fletcher CD. Leiomyoma of deep soft tissue. Clinicopathologic analysis of a series. Am J Surg Pathol 1994;18:576–82.
13a. Meis JM, Enzinger FM. Myolipoma of soft tissue. Am J Surg Pathol 1991;15:121–5.
14. Murphy GF, Elder DE. Non-melanocytic tumors of the skin. Atlas of Tumor Pathology. 3rd Series, Fascicle 1. Washington, D.C.: Armed Forces Institute of Pathology, 1991.
15. Newman PL, Fletcher CD. Smooth muscle tumours of the external genitalia: clinicopathological analysis of a series. Histopathology 1991;18:523–9.
16. Ranchod M, Kempson RL. Smooth muscle tumors of the gastrointestinal tract and retroperitoneum: a pathologic analysis of 100 cases. Cancer 1977;39:255–62.
17. Scurry JP, Carey MP, Targett CS, Dowling JP. Soft tissue lipoleiomyoma. Pathology 1991;23:360–2.
18. Shmookler BM, Lauer DH. Retroperitoneal leiomyosarcoma. A clinicopathologic analysis of 36 cases. Am J Surg Pathol 1983;7:269–80.

Leiomyosarcoma

19. Enzinger FM, Weiss SW. Soft tissue tumors. St. Louis: Mosby, 1995:1067–74.
20. Fletcher CD, Kilpatrick SE, Mentzel T. The difficulty in predicting behavior of smooth-muscle tumors in deep soft tissue. Am J Surg Pathol 1995;19:116–7.

Leiomyosarcoma of the Retroperitoneum

21. Azumi N, Ben EJ, Battifora H. Immunophenotypic diagnosis of leiomyosarcomas and rhabdomyosarcomas with monoclonal antibodies to muscle-specific actin and desmin in formalin-fixed tissue. Mod Pathol 1988;1:469–74.
22. Enzinger FM, Weiss SW. Soft tissue tumors. St. Louis: Mosby, 1995:1067–74.
23. Evans HL. Smooth muscle in atypical lipomatous tumors. A report of three cases. Am J Surg Pathol 1990;14:714–8.
24. Hashimoto H, Daimaru Y, Tsuneyoshi M, Enjoji M. Leiomyosarcoma of the external soft tissues. A clinicopathologic, immunohistochemical, and electron microscopic study. Cancer 1986;57:2077–88.
25. Mentzel T, Calonje E, Fletcher CD. Leiomyosarcoma with prominent osteoclast-like giant cells. Analysis of eight cases closely mimicking the so-called giant cell variant of malignant fibrous histiocytoma. Am J Surg Pathol 1994;18:258–65.
26. Merchant W, Calonje E, Fletcher CD. Inflammatory leiomyosarcoma: a morphological subgroup within the heterogeneous family of so-called inflammatory malignant fibrous histiocytoma. Histopathology 1995;27:525–32.
27. Miettinen M. Immunoreactivity for cytokeratin and epithelial membrane antigen in leiomyosarcoma. Arch Pathol Lab Med 1988;112:637–40.
27a. Rajani B, Smith TA, Reith JD, Goldblum JR. Retroperitoneal leiomyosarcomas unassociated with the gastrointestinal tract: a clinicopathologic analysis of 17 cases. Mod Pathol 1999;12:21–8.
28. Ranchod M, Kempson RL. Smooth muscle tumors of the gastrointestinal tract and retroperitoneum: a pathologic analysis of 100 cases. Cancer 1977;39:255–62.
29. Shmookler BM, Lauer DH. Retroperitoneal leiomyosarcoma. A clinicopathologic analysis of 36 cases. Am J Surg Pathol 1983;7:269–80.
30. Suster S, Wong TY, Moran CA. Sarcomas with combined features of liposarcoma and leiomyosarcoma. Study of two cases of an unusual soft-tissue tumor showing dual lineage differentiation. Am J Surg Pathol 1993;17:905–11.
31. Swanson PE, Stanley MW, Scheithauer BW, Wick MR. Primary cutaneous leiomyosarcoma. A histological and immunohistochemical study of 9 cases, with ultrastructural correlation. J Cutan Pathol 1988;15:129–41.
32. Swanson PE, Wick MR, Dehner LP. Leiomyosarcoma of somatic soft tissues in childhood: an immunohistochemical analysis of six cases with ultrastructural correlation. Hum Pathol 1991;22:569–77.
33. Tallini G, Erlandson RA, Brennan MF, Woodruff JM. Divergent myosarcomatous differentiation in retroperitoneal liposarcoma. Am J Surg Pathol 1993;17:546–56.
34. Van de Rijn M, Rouse RV. CD34: a review. Appl Immunohistochem 1994;2:71–80.
35. Wile AG, Evans HL, Romsdahl MM. Leiomyosarcoma of soft tissue: a clinicopathologic study. Cancer 1981;48:1022–32.

Leiomyosarcoma of Deep Soft Tissues Outside the Retroperitoneum

36. de Saint Aubain Somerhausen N, Fletcher CD. Leiomyosarcoma of soft tissue in children: clinicopathologic analysis of 20 cases. Am J Surg Pathol 1999;23:755–63.
36a. Enzinger FM, Weiss SW. Soft tissue tumors. St. Louis: Mosby, 1995:1067–74.
37. Gustafson P, Willen H, Baldetorp B, Ferno M, Akerman M, Rydholm A. Soft tissue leiomyosarcoma. A population-based epidemiologic and prognostic study of 48 patients, including cellular DNA content. Cancer 1992;70:114–9.
38. Hashimoto H, Daimaru Y, Tsuneyoshi M, Enjoji M. Leiomyosarcoma of the external soft tissues. A clinicopathologic, immunohistochemical, and electron microscopic study. Cancer 1986;57:2077–88.

39. Matthews TJ, Fisher C. Leiomyosarcoma of soft tissue and pulmonary metastasis, both with osteoclast-like giant cells. J Clin Pathol 1994;47:370–1.

40. Mentzel T, Calonje E, Fletcher CD. Leiomyosarcoma with prominent osteoclast-like giant cells. Analysis of eight cases closely mimicking the so-called giant cell variant of malignant fibrous histiocytoma. Am J Surg Pathol 1994;18:258–65.

41. Merchant W, Calonje E, Fletcher CD. Inflammatory leiomyosarcoma: a morphological subgroup within the heterogeneous family of so-called inflammatory malignant fibrous histiocytoma. Histopathology 1995;27:525–32.

42. Suster S. Epithelioid leiomyosarcoma of the skin and subcutaneous tissue. Clinicopathologic, immunohistochemical, and ultrastructural study of five cases. Am J Surg Pathol 1994;18:232–40.

43. Wile AG, Evans HL, Romsdahl MM. Leiomyosarcoma of soft tissue: a clinicopathologic study. Cancer 1981;48:1022–32.

44. Wilkinson N, Fitzmaurice RJ, Turner PG, Freemont AJ. Leiomyosarcoma with osteoclast-like giant cells. Histopathology 1992;20:446–9.

Leiomyosarcoma of the Subcutaneous Tissue

45. Hashimoto H, Daimaru Y, Tsuneyoshi M, Enjoji M. Leiomyosarcoma of the external soft tissues. A clinicopathologic, immunohistochemical, and electron microscopic study. Cancer 1986;57:2077–88.

Leiomyosarcomas Arising in Vessels

46. Demers ML, Curley SA, Romsdahl MM. Inferior vena cava leiomyosarcoma. J Surg Oncol 1992;51:89–92.

47. Varela-Duran J, Oliva H, Rosai J. Vascular leiomyosarcoma: the malignant counterpart of vascular leiomyoma. Cancer 1979;44:1684–91.

6

SKELETAL MUSCLE TUMORS

BENIGN SKELETAL MUSCLE TUMORS (MANAGERIAL GROUPS Ia AND Ib, TABLE 1-10)

Rhabdomyoma

Definition. Rhabdomyomas are benign tumors in which at least some cells are differentiated as skeletal muscle cells with cytoplasmic cross-striations. Actin and desmin stains are definitionally positive.

General Considerations. Most benign soft tissue tumors outnumber their malignant counterparts considerably, but this situation is reversed for skeletal muscle tumors; rhabdomyomas account for only 2 percent of all skeletal muscle neoplasms (3). There are three clinical and histologic subtypes of rhabdomyomas: *adult, fetal,* and *genital,* accounting for about 50, 40, and 10 percent of these tumors, respectively (Table 6-1). The adult and fetal subtypes primarily occur in the soft tissue of the head and neck and the submucosa of the oropharynx, nasopharynx, and larynx,

Table 6-1

SKELETAL MUSCLE TUMORS

Benign
(Managerial Groups Ia and Ib, Table 1-10)

Rhabdomyoma
    Adult
    Fetal
    Genital

Malignant
(Managerial Groups III and IV, Table 1-10)

Embryonal*
    Botryoid—Superior prognosis
    Spindled—Superior prognosis
    NOS**—Intermediate prognosis
    Anaplastic—Poor prognosis
Alveolar*
    Typical—Poor prognosis
    Solid—Poor prognosis
    Adult Pleomorphic—Poor prognosis

---

*See text for discussion of tumor type and prognosis.
**NOS, not otherwise specified.

whereas genital rhabdomyomas almost exclusively occur in the vulva and vagina. Nearly 50 percent of fetal rhabdomyomas develop in the first year of life while the adult and genital types occur mostly in middle-aged and older individuals.

Clinical Features. Two thirds of fetal rhabdomyomas arise in the soft tissues of the face, preauricular and postauricular regions, neck, and periorbital area; about one third arise in the mucosal regions of the nasopharynx, oropharynx, and larynx (4,9,15). Very rare examples have been reported in the mediastinum (5), retroperitoneum (5), thigh (2), chest wall (2), abdominal wall (15), stomach (15), and anus (15). The patients most commonly present with a solitary polypoid mass, but other symptoms depend on location and include proptosis, nasal cavity and airway obstruction, and hoarseness. The male to female ratio is 3 to 1. The median duration of symptoms is about 8 months but varies from a few days to up to 19 years. About 25 percent of the cases are congenital and an additional 15 percent occur before the age of 1 year. Nearly 45 percent occur after the age of 15 years. The mean age at presentation is 19 years (1,3,4,9,15). Multicentric fetal rhabdomyomas have been reported in association with multiple basal cell carcinomas and various osseous anomalies (2,5).

Two thirds of adult rhabdomyomas arise in the mucosa of the oropharynx, nasopharynx, and larynx, and about one third arise in the branchial musculature of the neck in the distribution of the third and fourth branchial arches. Rare examples have been reported in the musculature of the lip, cheek, orbit, mediastinum, prostate, and stomach (15). Most patients present with a single round or polypoid mass of 2 weeks' to 3 years' duration, but about 15 percent have multicentric masses (10,15). Depending upon the site and size of the tumor the patient may also present with nasal or airway obstruction, or dysphagia. The male to female ratio is 3–4 to 1. Most patients are between 40 and 70 years old, with a mean age of 55 years (4,8,10), but this tumor has been reported in patients as young as 2 years and as old as 82 years.

Genital rhabdomyomas are very rare, benign, skeletal muscle tumors which almost exclusively occur in the vagina or vulva of young or middle-aged women (mean age, 40 years; range, 8 to 52 years). The lesions present as a slowly growing polypoid mass or cyst. Most of the patients are asymptomatic but dyspareunia, mucosal erosion, and hemorrhage have been reported. One case each has been described in the prostate (12), the tunica vaginalis of the testis (12a), and the uterine cervix (13).

Gross Findings. Fetal rhabdomyomas are well circumscribed, soft, and tan, pink, red, or gray-white, and have a glistening, often mucoid cut surface (3,9). Submucosal lesions are usually polypoid but may be sessile and have a smooth surface. They measure from 1 to 12 cm, but most are around 4 to 5 cm in diameter.

Adult rhabdomyomas are also well demarcated and on cut surface usually are deep tan to red-brown, lobulated, and rubbery, soft, or fleshy. Submucosal tumors are usually polypoid but may be sessile and have a smooth surface (10,15). They are usually smaller than fetal rhabdomyomas, with an average size of 3 to 4 cm and a maximum of 7 to 8 cm.

Genital rhabdomyoma usually presents as a 1- to 3-cm, lobulated, firm, polypoid, and pink, tan, or gray-white mass in the wall of the vagina or vulva (15).

Microscopic Findings. Fetal rhabdomyoma is characterized by two different histologic subtypes, myxoid and cellular. The central portion of *myxoid fetal rhabdomyoma* is composed of immature, slender skeletal muscle cells with delicate cytoplasmic cross-striations and undifferentiated oval, round, and spindled mesenchymal cells. Both cell types are set within abundant myxoid to fibromyxoid stroma (fig. 6-1) (3,9). The skeletal muscle cells, which closely resemble those of the myotubular stage of striated muscle development, are usually bipolar; have thin, tapered, eosinophilic cytoplasmic processes (fig. 6-2); and are arranged in narrow fascicles or short bundles (fig. 6-1) (3). The nuclei have smooth contours, fine chromatin, and inconspicuous nucleoli. The undifferentiated cells have oval or angulated hyperchromatic nuclei, fine chromatin, and scant, wispy cytoplasm (fig. 6-2). Toward the periphery, the muscle cells tend to mature and come to resemble fully differentiated skeletal

muscle cells while still mixed with undifferentiated cells (figs. 6-1, 6-3) (3,9). A "pseudocambium" layer, largely consisting of plasma cells and lymphocytes, is often found under the epithelium in mucosal fetal rhabdomyoma (fig. 6-4).

The *cellular type*, as would be expected, features less conspicuous stroma (fig. 6-5A) and what little stroma is present is collagenous or myxoid (fig. 6-5B,C). At low magnification, the tumor cells are arranged in interlacing bundles and fascicles in parallel or plexiform architecture (fig. 6-5C). The constituent cells of the cellular subtype demonstrate a broad range of skeletal muscle differentiation. Some tumors feature immature skeletal muscle cells similar to those found in the myxoid variant (fig. 6-6), but by definition these are present in larger numbers than in that variant. In others, ganglion cell–like rhabdomyoblasts with large vesicular central nuclei and prominent eosinophilic nucleoli (fig. 6-6B,C), or strap cells with abundant basophilic to deeply eosinophilic cytoplasm containing easy to see cross-striations predominate (fig. 6-6C) (1,4,9,15). Sometimes the tumor cells of cellular fetal rhabdomyoma contain glycogen, and when this is abundant the cytoplasm may be vacuolated. Clusters of differentiated cells may intermingle with adjacent adipose tissue and skeletal muscle. In the latter circumstance, it may be impossible to determine where the tumor ends and normal skeletal muscle begins. Mitotic activity is usually absent but occasional cellular tumors contain easily found mitotic figures which are always normal (1,4,9, 15). Because of the large number of differentiated muscle cells that is always present, there is little difficulty in recognizing the cellular type as a skeletal muscle tumor. The problem is distinguishing cellular fetal rhabdomyoma from rhabdomyosarcoma. This is discussed in the Differential Diagnosis section below.

Adult rhabdomyoma features distinct, well-demarcated, variably sized lobules (fig. 6-7) composed of closely packed, large, polygonal cells measuring 15 to 150 μm (fig. 6-8) (4,9). These strikingly large cells have small, round, centrally or peripherally situated nuclei, with one or two prominent nucleoli, and abundant eosinophilic, granular or peripherally vacuolated cytoplasm; the latter may impart a spider web appearance to the cells (fig. 6-9). The cells are rich in glycogen and contain haphazardly arranged crystalline material which

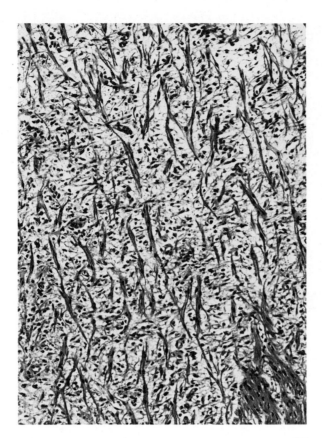 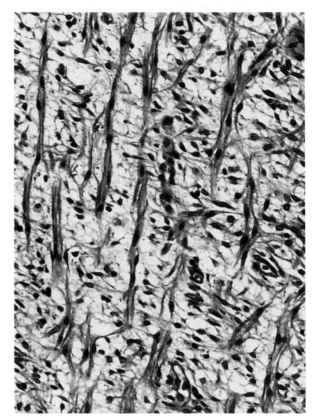

Figure 6-1
MYXOID FETAL RHABDOMYOMA
At low power, fetal rhabdomyoma is composed of an admixture of undifferentiated round mesenchymal cells and immature skeletal muscle cells set within a richly myxoid or edematous stroma.

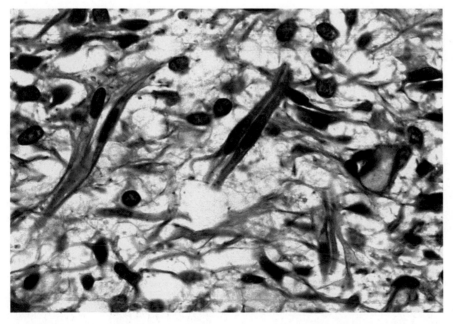

Figure 6-2
MYXOID FETAL
RHABDOMYOMA
The bipolar, immature skeletal muscle cells of fetal rhabdomyoma have tapered eosinophilic cytoplasmic processes and closely resemble the myotubular stage of striated muscle development. The undifferentiated cells have round or oval nuclei and inconspicuous cytoplasm.

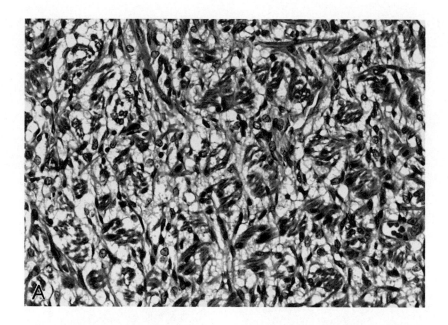

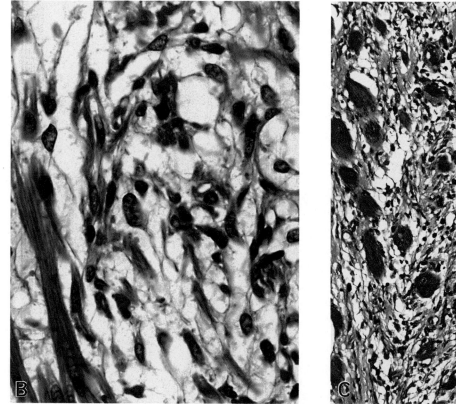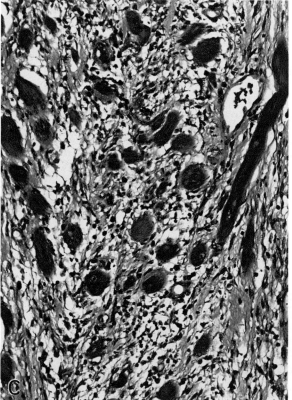

Figure 6-3
MYXOID FETAL RHABDOMYOMA
While immature muscle cells and mesenchymal cells predominate in the central portion of the tumor, better differentiated skeletal muscle cells are often found at the periphery. The bland, undifferentiated small round and oval mesenchymal cells are still admixed with these better differentiated cells.

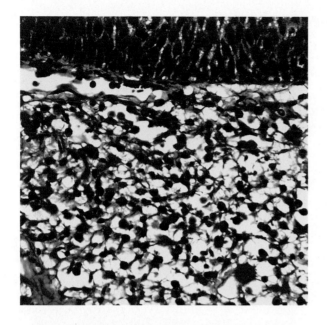

Figure 6-4
MYXOID FETAL RHABDOMYOMA

Fetal rhabdomyomas which originate in mucosal locations can be confused with embryonal rhabdomyosarcoma because of the presence of a pseudocambium layer composed predominantly of plasma cells and lymphocytes. The lack of mitoses and cytologic atypia are helpful in distinguishing rhabdomyoma from rhabdomyosarcoma.

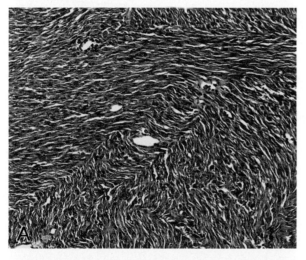

Figure 6-5
CELLULAR FETAL RHABDOMYOMA

In the cellular subtype of fetal rhabdomyoma, the stroma is typically less conspicuous than in the myxoid subtype (A,B). The tumor cells are arranged in interlacing fascicles (A) or in patternless arrangements (B,C). Undifferentiated mesenchymal cells may be difficult to discern (A) or are admixed with ganglion cell-like rhabdomyoblasts or strap cells with deeply eosinophilic cytoplasm with cross-striations (B,C). Distinction from rhabdomyosarcoma may sometimes be difficult.

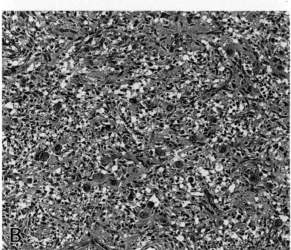

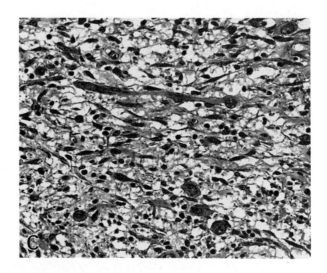

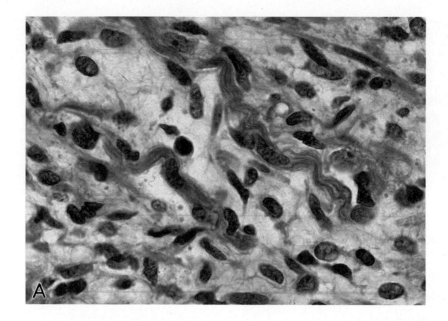

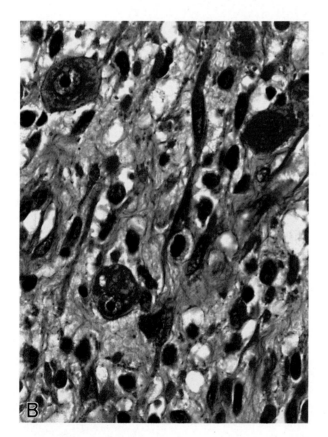
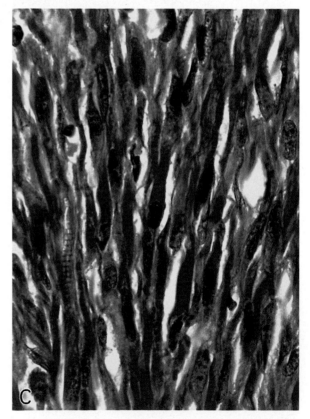

Figure 6-6
CELLULAR FETAL RHABDOMYOMA

A broad range of skeletal muscle differentiation including immature skeletal muscle cells (A), ganglion cell-like rhabdomyoblasts (B), and strap cells with abundant eosinophilic cytoplasm and numerous cross-striations (C) characterize cellular fetal rhabdomyoma.

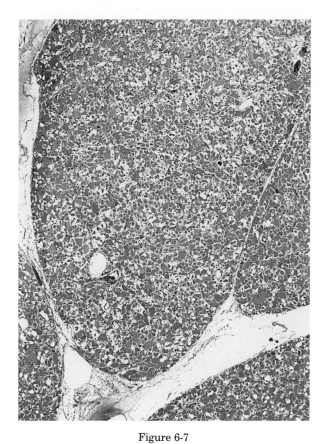

Figure 6-7
ADULT RHABDOMYOMA
Adult rhabdomyoma consists of distinct, well demarcated, variably sized lobules of polygonal cells.

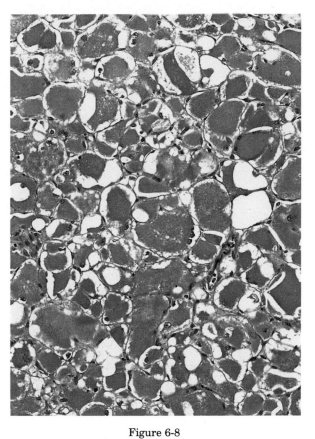

Figure 6-8
ADULT RHABDOMYOMA
Large, closely packed polygonal cells measuring up to 150 μm in diameter characterize adult rhabdomyoma.

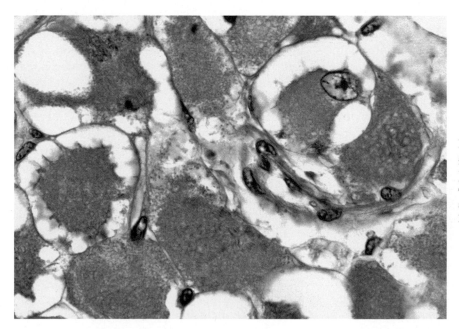

Figure 6-9
ADULT RHABDOMYOMA
The cells of adult rhabdomyoma have an abundant, eosinophilic, granular, often peripherally vacuolated cytoplasm, imparting a spiderweb appearance to some cells. The nuclei are round and have vesicular chromatin and one or more prominent nucleoli.

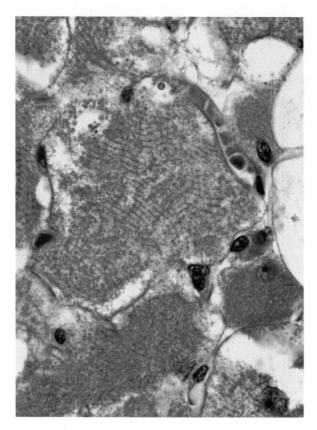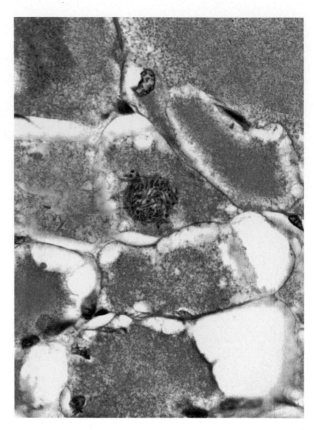

Figure 6-10
ADULT RHABDOMYOMA
The cells of adult rhabdomyoma characteristically contain haphazardly arranged crystalline material reminiscent of sarcomeric bands (left) and rod-like configurations (right).

may have a rod-like configuration (fig. 6-10). Cross-striations are present in some cells but may be absent or difficult to find in others. The cells are separated by a scant stroma containing collapsed and dilated vascular channels. Mitoses are almost never found in adult rhabdomyomas.

Genital rhabdomyoma is characterized by a submucosal proliferation of haphazardly arranged, interlacing bundles of elongated, strap-shaped, spindled, and polygonal cells which have abundant eosinophilic cytoplasm with easily discernible cross-striations. (fig. 6-11). The cells are set in abundant myxoid or collagenous stroma, with a scattering of lymphocytes (4,15). The nuclei are round or oval, have fine chromatin, and have a prominent eosinophilic nucleolus. Some cells are binucleate or even multinucleated and nuclear pseudoinclusions can be found. Nuclear pleomorphism, mitoses, and tumor cell necrosis are not features of genital rhabdomyoma.

Special Studies. Although phosphotungstic acid hematoxylin (PTAH) and trichrome stains may highlight the cross-striations and crystalline rod-like structures in the cytoplasm of the cells of rhabdomyoma, desmin and muscle-specific actin even more vividly highlight these structures. Both actin and desmin stains are positive in rhabdomyomas, and monoclonal myoglobin and fast myosin antibodies also decorate the cells (7). Some cells also stain with CD56 and CD57, S-100 protein, and alpha-smooth muscle actin (8–10). Glial fibrillary acid protein (GFAP) stains the cells of 40 percent of fetal rhabdomyomas (9).

Electron microscopy is not necessary for the diagnosis of rhabdomyoma, but if performed fine structural examination demonstrates striated muscle differentiation with variable sarcomeric formations. Hypertrophic Z-bands account for the rod-like inclusions seen by light microscopy

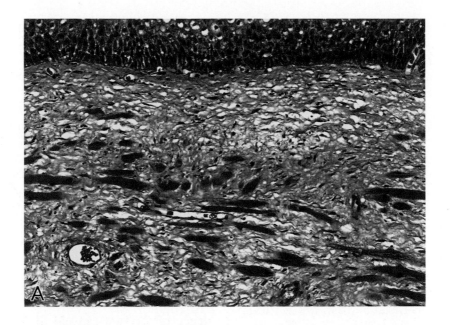

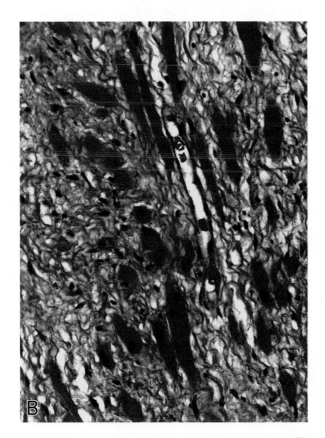

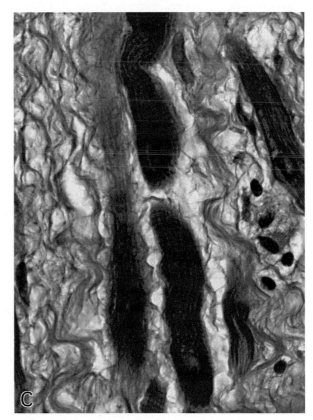

Figure 6-11
GENITAL RHABDOMYOMA
The genital rhabdomyoma consists of a submucosal proliferation of haphazardly arranged skeletal muscle cells with easily discernible cross-striations set within an abundant myxoid or fibrous stroma.

and are similar in appearance to those observed in nemaline myopathy (8,10).

Differential Diagnosis. The differential diagnosis of fetal rhabdomyoma includes the spindle cell and botryoid variants of embryonal rhabdomyosarcoma, infantile (desmoid type) fibromatosis, and neuromuscular hamartoma.

Because the two have many similarities, such as a myxoid stroma and primitive cells, the principal lesion which must be distinguished from the myxoid variant of fetal rhabdomyoma is the botryoid variant of embryonal rhabdomyosarcoma. The lack of a true cambium layer composed of tumor cells, the dearth of mitotic figures, the absence of cytologic atypia and tumor cell necrosis, the maturation of skeletal muscle cells at the periphery of the tumor, the usually noninfiltrative margins, and a superficial location are features which distinguish fetal rhabdomyoma from embryonal rhabdomyosarcoma. However, occasional fetal rhabdomyomas contain normal mitotic figures and demonstrate superficial infiltration of the surrounding skeletal muscle and adipose tissue. In this circumstance, the other features of fetal rhabdomyoma listed above point to the correct diagnosis. The cellular subtype is particularly treacherous because it shares many similarities with the spindle cell variant of embryonal rhabdomyosarcoma. Easily found mitotic figures may be present in both, but tumor cell necrosis and cellular pleomorphism are features of rhabdomyosarcoma, not cellular fetal rhabdomyoma. There are reports of possible malignant transformation of the cellular subtype to rhabdomyosarcoma (6,11). In our opinion these cases more likely represent spindle cell embryonal rhabdomyosarcoma from the outset and are illustrative of the difficulty in differentiating "cellular" fetal rhabdomyoma from some cases of the spindle cell variant of embryonal rhabdomyosarcoma. Consultation is warranted in cases where this distinction is difficult.

Infantile (desmoid type) fibromatosis and fetal rhabdomyoma both infiltrate skeletal muscle and adipose tissue, and this may cause diagnostic difficulties. However, infantile (desmoid type) fibromatosis is characterized by fascicles of spindle cells, is usually more deeply situated than fetal rhabdomyoma, and lacks the slender cells with cross-striations and the undifferenti-

ated cells in a myxoid stroma that characterize fetal rhabdomyoma.

Neuromuscular hamartoma is characterized by S-100 protein–positive nerve fibers admixed with well-defined bundles of skeletal muscle, all contained in the same perimysial sheath. Some neuromuscular hamartomas contain a more cellular stroma with small spindled cells, resulting in loss of the typical nodular pattern of growth, and may be confused with a fetal rhabdomyoma.

The histologic appearance of adult rhabdomyoma with its large, polygonal skeletal muscle cells is so distinctive that it should not be mistaken for any other tumor. However, alveolar soft part sarcoma, granular cell tumor, and hibernoma might be considered in the differential diagnosis. Both granular cell tumor and hibernoma lack light microscopic and immunohistologic evidence of striated muscle differentiation. Furthermore, the cells of granular cell tumor and hibernoma are much smaller than those of adult rhabdomyoma, and they lack cytoplasmic glycogen. Granular cell tumor also has poorly defined cell borders, and the epithelium overlying the adult rhabdomyoma is normal or thinned whereas granular cell tumor is usually associated with pseudoepitheliomatous hyperplasia. Granular cell tumor is almost always strongly S-100 protein positive whereas the cells in adult rhabdomyoma are negative or only weakly positive for this stain. Alveolar soft part sarcoma is composed of discohesive round or oval cells with eosinophilic cytoplasm which grow in an alveolar pattern unlike the cells in adult rhabdomyoma; periodic acid–Schiff (PAS)/diastase stains often demonstrate intracytoplasmic crystalline rods and granules rather than the intracytoplasmic glycogen characteristic of rhabdomyoma. Moreover, the clusters of cells in alveolar soft part sarcoma are surrounded by sinusoidal thin walled vessels, a pattern not present in rhabdomyoma. Alveolar soft part sarcomas may be desmin, muscle-specific actin, and S-100 protein positive, and thus can have an immunologic profile identical to that of adult rhabdomyoma. However, they do not express nuclear myogenin or MyoD1 suggesting that they do not represent tumors of skeletal muscle origin (14).

Vaginal polyps and, most importantly, the botryoid variant of embryonal rhabdomyosarcoma are the principal lesions to be considered in the differential diagnosis of genital rhabdomyoma. Age at presentation (less than 25 years for patients with embryonal rhabdomyosarcoma versus greater than 40 years for patients with genital rhabdomyoma); cytologic atypia, significant mitotic activity, and a "cambium" layer (features of embryonal rhabdomyosarcoma); and a history of an asymptomatic, slowly growing tumor (rhabdomyoma) rather than a rapidly growing mass (rhabdomyosarcoma) are features useful in establishing the correct diagnosis. There are no immunohistologic features that are helpful in this differential diagnosis. Spindle cells with cross-striations are not a feature of vaginal polyps, and the cytologic atypia that may be found in vaginal polyps is not a feature of genital rhabdomyoma.

Treatment and Prognosis. The treatment of choice for all types of rhabdomyoma is surgical excision. About 5 percent of fetal rhabdomyomas and about 15 percent of adult rhabdomyomas recur at an average of 6 years (range, 1 month to 35 years) after the original excision. Recurrent tumor is thought to be due to incomplete excision (10). Local recurrence has not been reported in genital rhabdomyoma. There are no reported instances of uncontrolled local growth, metastases, or death due to fetal, adult, or genital rhabdomyoma.

Neuromuscular Hamartoma

Definition. Neuromuscular hamartoma (*neuromuscular choristoma, benign Triton tumor*) is a rare developmental lesion composed of mature skeletal muscle and nerve.

General Considerations. Tumors composed of striated muscle and neural elements are referred to as Triton tumors. Malignant Triton tumor refers to rhabdomyosarcoma and malignant peripheral nerve sheath sarcoma while benign Triton tumor usually refers to a lesion which appears to be developmental and thus represents a hamartoma or choristoma. Fewer than 20 cases have been reported. The lesion usually presents as a mass related to the brachial plexus or sciatic nerve during the first 2 years of life.

Clinical Features. Two thirds of neuromuscular hamartomas arise from or are closely related to either the brachial plexus or sciatic nerves (19, 20,23,24). Other sites include the intercostal, median, trigeminal, spinal, and optic nerves.

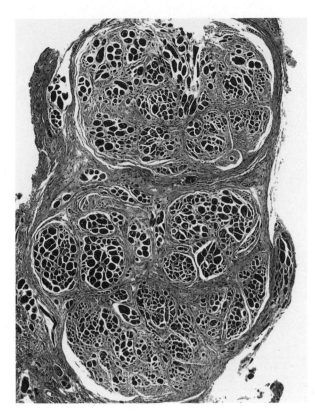

Figure 6-12
NEUROMUSCULAR HAMARTOMA
Neuromuscular hamartoma consists of nodules, most of which are further subdivided into smaller nodules by narrow bands of connective tissue.

Cutaneous and tongue primary sites have also been reported (21,23). Two thirds of the patients present before 2 years of age with an asymptomatic, palpable mass or with a florid neurologic disability (19,20,23,24). A few cases of neuromuscular hamartoma were noted at birth and two cases have been reported in adults (22,23).

Gross Findings. Neuromuscular hamartomas appear as circumscribed, firm, multinodular, gray-brown-white masses which are usually attached to or intimately associated with a nerve (16,19,20). Postoperative hard, gray-white, firm masses measuring from 3 to 14 cm have been reported in several cases (17,18,20).

Microscopic Findings. Microscopically, neuromuscular hamartomas consist of multiple, 3- to 5-mm nodules, most of which are further subdivided into smaller nodules by narrow bands of connective tissue (fig. 6-12) (17,19,20,24). The

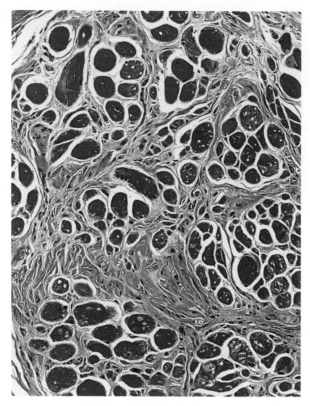

Figure 6-13
NEUROMUSCULAR HAMARTOMA

The nodules of the neuromuscular hamartoma contain fascicles of striated muscle fibers of varying size and myelinated and nonmyelinated nerve fibers, all of which are contained within the same perimysial fibrous sheath.

nodules are composed of fascicles of striated muscle fibers of varying size, and myelinated and nonmyelinated nerve fibers all of which are contained within the same perimysial fibrous sheath (fig. 6-13). Smooth muscle fibers were evident in one case (24). The connective tissue which invests the nodules may be more abundant and crowd out and replace the bundles of muscle and nerve fibers. In other cases the nodular arrangement of striated muscle and nerve may be focally lost. In this circumstance the stroma is more cellular and contains bland spindle cells with oval nuclei and scant cytoplasm, and there is a haphazard distribution of striated muscle and nerve fibers (fig. 6-14). Microscopic examination of postoperative lesions may show residual neuromuscular hamartoma, but most lesions have the appearance of an extra-abdominal desmoid (17,18,20).

Special Studies. The striated muscle of neuromuscular hamartoma is clearly identifiable by light microscopy and stains with desmin, skeletal muscle myosin, and muscle-specific actin (20,24). The nerves may be more difficult to appreciate but these can be highlighted with an S-100 protein stain (fig. 6-15), and GFAP stains many of these cells as well.

Differential Diagnosis. Neuromuscular hamartoma should be readily identifiable because of its relationship with a nerve and the

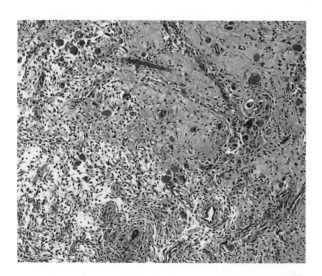

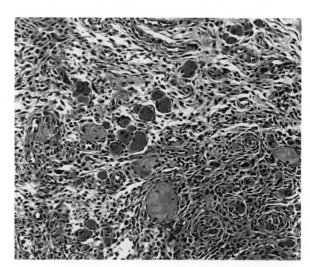

Figure 6-14
NEUROMUSCULAR HAMARTOMA

Exceptionally, the stroma of neuromuscular hamartomas is more cellular and contains bland spindle cells with oval nuclei and scant cytoplasm. There is a haphazard distribution of striated muscle and nerve fibers.

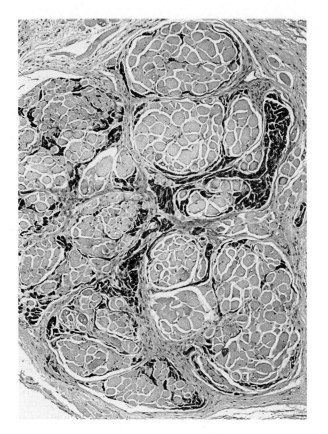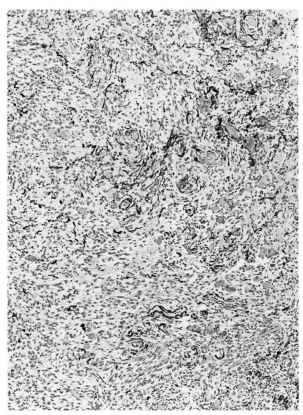

Figure 6-15
NEUROMUSCULAR HAMARTOMA
The nerve fibers of neuromuscular hamartomas may be difficult to appreciate but can be highlighted with stains for S-100 protein.

characteristic nodules of mature skeletal muscle admixed with nerve fibers. However, when the lobular pattern is combined with a diffuse proliferation of small spindle cells, fetal rhabdomyoma or embryonal rhabdomyosarcoma may be considered. The S-100 protein stain, which stains nerve fibers, should allow separation of neuromuscular hamartoma from the other considerations, as does the lack of mitotic activity and cellular atypia.

Treatment and Prognosis. Spontaneous involution has followed partial excision in a few cases. Complete excision may be curative but may also result in further neurologic complications. Thus, a conservative approach of biopsy for diagnosis followed by observation has been recommended (18,20). Biopsy or complete excision may, however, be followed by a sizable recurrence due to postoperative fibromatosis (17,18,20).

MALIGNANT SKELETAL MUSCLE TUMORS (MANAGERIAL GROUPS III AND IV, TABLE 1-10)

Introduction

Malignant tumors composed of cells with light microscopic, electron microscopic, or immunologic evidence of skeletal muscle differentiation form the category of rhabdomyosarcoma. The definitional light microscopic feature is cytoplasmic cross-striations while ultrastructurally the diagnostic feature is evidence of sarcomeric differentiation. Immunologically, at least some cells in a rhabdomyosarcoma must express desmin, myoglobin, MyoD1, or myogenin. The presence of fusion genes PAX3-FKHR and PAX7-FKHR appears to be specific for alveolar rhabdomyosarcoma.

In the past, four major morphologic categories of rhabdomyosarcoma have been recognized:

embryonal, botryoid, alveolar, and pleomorphic (25). This classification has been subsequently modified (Table 6-1) (25a). Embryonal rhabdomyosarcoma, the most common type, accounts for 70 to 75 percent of all rhabdomyosarcomas, occurs predominantly in children, and is presently subdivided morphologically into embryonal not otherwise specified (NOS), spindled, anaplastic, and botryoid, which is now also considered to be a variant of embryonal rhabdomyosarcoma. Alveolar rhabdomyosarcoma occurs predominantly in children and adolescents, and accounts for 20 to 25 percent of all rhabdomyosarcomas. Patients with the alveolar type have a much worse prognosis than those with embryonal rhabdomyosarcoma. Tumors thought to have features of both embryonal and alveolar rhabdomyosarcomas, diagnosed as mixed rhabdomyosarcomas in the past, likely represent solid forms of alveolar rhabdomyosarcoma; because they behave like alveolar rhabdomyosarcoma, they should be classified as such for therapeutic, staging, and prognostic purposes. When confronted with a "small blue cell tumor," a small fragment of fresh tissue should be routinely snap frozen for potential molecular analysis since characteristic translocations and fusion genes have been identified not only in alveolar rhabdomyosarcoma, but in many other soft tissue neoplasms, as discussed in this Fascicle. Pleomorphic rhabdomyosarcoma is very rare, accounting for less than 5 percent of rhabdomyosarcomas, and rarely occurs in individuals younger than 40 years. Morphologically, it is high grade and has features indistinguishable from pleomorphic malignant fibrous histiocytoma except that some tumor cells display evidence of skeletal muscle differentiation.

Embryonal Rhabdomyosarcoma

Definition. Embryonal rhabdomyosarcoma is a malignant small blue cell tumor with a predilection for children and certain anatomic sites; variable numbers of cells demonstrate evidence of skeletal muscle differentiation by light microscopy, immunohistochemistry, or electron microscopy.

General Considerations. Embryonal rhabdomyosarcoma is by far the most common malignant soft tissue tumor in pediatric patients, accounting for 8 to 10 percent of all childhood neoplasms. The vast majority of these neoplasms develop in the first two decades of life, but they can be found in any age group. Neonatal rhabdomyosarcomas are very rare and account for less than 0.5 percent of cases. About 10 percent of embryonal rhabdomyosarcomas occur during the first year of life, nearly 35 percent between 1 and 4 years of age, 45 percent between 5 and 15 years (29), and the majority of the remaining 10 percent between 15 and 25 years. Cases presenting after the age of 40 years are extraordinarily rare (53).

Embryonal rhabdomyosarcoma is divided into four histologic subtypes: embryonal not otherwise specified, botryoid, spindle cell, and anaplastic. Histologic subtyping is very important because patients with the various subtypes have different prognoses and may require different therapies. Hence, pathologists are expected to specify the subtype in the diagnosis line of the surgical pathology report. Surgery and multidrug chemotherapy, with or without irradiation, have resulted in a striking improvement in patient survival over the past 20 years (29).

Clinical Features. A mass, with or without pain, is the most common presentation for a patient with any of the histologic subtypes of embryonal rhabdomyosarcoma. If the primary site happens to be a hollow organ, the patient may present with signs of obstruction and bleeding. There are differences in the most frequent site of presentation, mean age of the patient at presentation, sex predilection, and long-term prognosis among the histologic subtypes.

Embryonal rhabdomyosarcoma not otherwise specified (NOS), is the most frequent subtype, accounting for about three quarters of all embryonal rhabdomyosarcomas (46). The mean age for patients with this subtype is about 7 years (46), and the male to female ratio 1.75 to 1. The most common primary sites are head and neck (47 percent), genitourinary tract (28 percent), and extremities (9 percent); less common sites include the pelvis (5 percent), retroperitoneum (5 percent), and trunk (3 percent). All other locations are rare and account for the remaining 3 percent (46).

The *botryoid variant* accounts for about 10 percent of all cases of embryonal rhabdomyosarcoma, occurs at a somewhat younger mean age of 5.6 years, and is found most commonly in the genitourinary tract (80 percent), followed by the

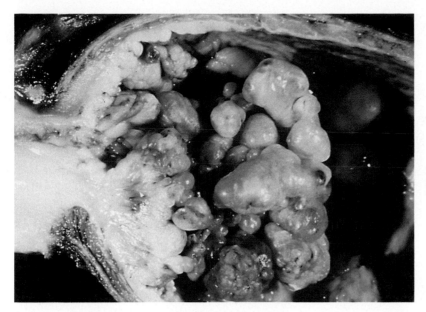

Figure 6-16
EMBRYONAL
RHABDOMYOSARCOMA,
BOTRYOID TYPE
Embryonal rhabdomyosarcoma is characterized by clusters of edematous, grape-like masses which protrude into cavities or lumens of hollow organs.

head and neck (15 percent), gastrointestinal tract (4.5 percent), and perianal region (0.5 percent) (46). Exceptional examples have been reported in the seventh and eighth decades of life as well (53). Because of its site of origin, patients with botryoid tumors usually present with signs of obstruction and bleeding.

The *spindle cell variant,* which accounts for about 6 percent of embryonal rhabdomyosarcomas, occurs more frequently in males, probably because this histologic subtype is often paratesticular (28,39). In one series, the age at presentation ranged from 7 months to 23 years (mean, 15.5 years) (28). In another report, the mean age at presentation was about 6 years (39). A review of 800 rhabdomyosarcomas revealed 46 cases of the spindle variant, of which 33 percent were paratesticular, 16 percent involved the head and neck, 12 percent involved the orbit, 9 percent the retroperitoneum, and the remainder originated in the trunk, prostate, and intra-abdominal soft tissue (39).

The *anaplastic variant* represents 3.5 percent of the tumors entered in the Intergroup Rhabdomyosarcoma Studies (46). This variant most frequently involves the lower extremity (25 percent), followed by the paratesticular region (16 percent), head and neck (9 percent), and retroperitoneum and pelvis (9 percent) (37). The mean age at presentation was 6 years and the male to female sex ratio was 1.7 to 1.

Gross Findings. Most embryonal rhabdomyosarcomas are fleshy, solid, and well circumscribed, and exhibit a gray-yellow-tan to white color spectrum. They may be soft or firm, and focally hemorrhagic and necrotic. Almost all measure between 1 and 32 cm, with a mean size in the Intergroup Rhabdomyosarcoma Studies of about 5 cm (46). The botryoid variant is usually softer than other variants and is gray-tan and gelatinous. Typically it grows as numerous, small, grape-like vesicles which protrude into the lumen of the organ or tissue of origin (fig. 6-16) (34,46). Although the subtypes of embryonal rhabdomyosarcoma are defined histologically, the botryoid variant is also partially defined by its gross appearance and location. The spindled variant often resembles a leiomyoma and has a lobular, whorled, firm, gray-white cut surface (39).

Microscopic Findings. By light microscopy, embryonal rhabdomyosarcoma NOS is a "small blue cell" neoplasm composed of varying numbers of round, oval, and polygonal to elongate cells, most often arranged in nondescript sheets, but also in broad anastomosing fascicles, or sometimes as dispersed individual cells (fig. 6-17). The cells may be tightly packed with little intercellular substance (fig. 6-17A,B) or can be scattered in an abundant fibrotic (fig. 6-18, left), edematous, or myxoid stroma (fig. 6-18, right). Occasionally they are arranged in nests or strands.

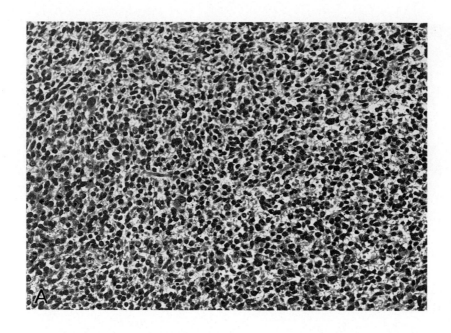

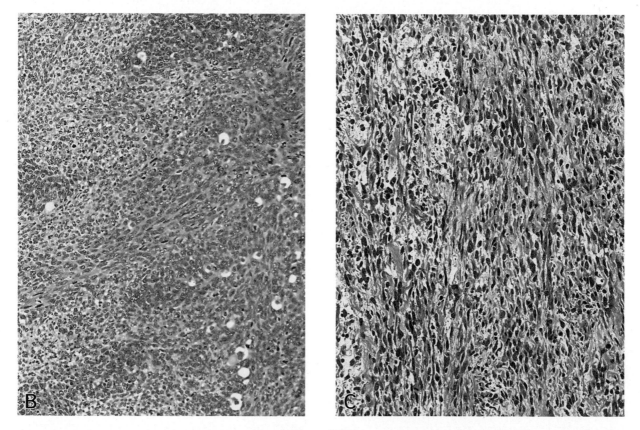

Figure 6-17
EMBRYONAL RHABDOMYOSARCOMA, NOS
The cells in embryonal rhabdomyosarcoma may be arranged in nondescript sheets (A) or anastomosing fascicles (B), or are individually dispersed (C) within varying amounts of stroma.

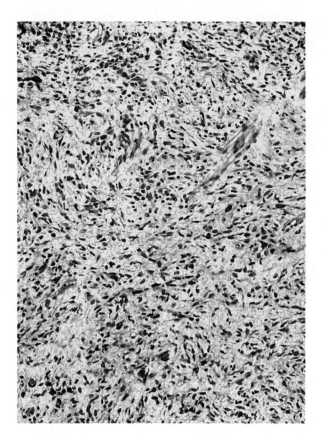 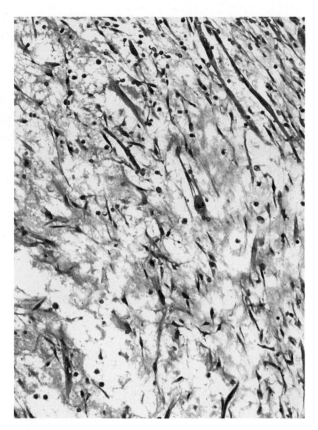

Figure 6-18
EMBRYONAL RHABDOMYOSARCOMA NOS
Left: In embryonal rhabdomyosarcoma the cells are often found in association with an abundant fibromyxoid stroma.
Right: Sometimes the tumor is paucicellular, due to massively edematous or myxoid stroma.

The cells comprising embryonal rhabdomyosarcoma are categorized as undifferentiated, differentiating, or well differentiated depending on their cytoplasmic features (45,46). Undifferentiated cells have scant, delicate, wispy, pale cytoplasm without evidence of skeletal muscle differentiation and round to spindled, centrally placed nuclei (fig. 6-19). Differentiating cells contain more abundant amphophilic to eosinophilic, sometimes fibrillar cytoplasm, which often pushes the usually rounded nucleus aside (fig. 6-20). Such cells are very characteristic of embryonal rhabdomyosarcoma. Other differentiating cells may have tapering bipolar cytoplasm or a tadpole configuration, with the nucleus located at one end of the cell (fig. 6-21). Tadpole cells may have multiple nuclei arranged in tandem, a feature that is unique to embryonal rhabdomyosarcomas and rhabdomyomas (fig. 6-21). Well-differentiated rhabdomyoblasts have cytoplasmic cross-stria-

tions (figs. 6-21A,C, 6-22). Most often the differentiating and differentiated cells are set within a collagenous matrix while the undifferentiated cells tend to be in a myxoid matrix. These three cell types, present in varying numbers, are the constituent cells of embryonal rhabdomyosarcoma.

The tumor cell nuclei vary from round to polygonal to spindled, and their contours are either smooth (figs. 6-19B, 6-20, left), jagged, or crenelated (figs. 6-19C, 6-20, right). Most often, the nuclei contain dense smooth chromatin and the nucleolus is usually not visible or is at most small and inconspicuous (figs. 6-19–6-21). These nuclear features are so characteristic of embryonal rhabdomyosarcoma that they should alert the observer to this possibility whenever a small round blue cell tumor is encountered. However, in some cases the cells have more vesicular nuclei with prominent nucleoli (fig. 6-23). Nuclear pleomorphism can be moderate but falls short of that

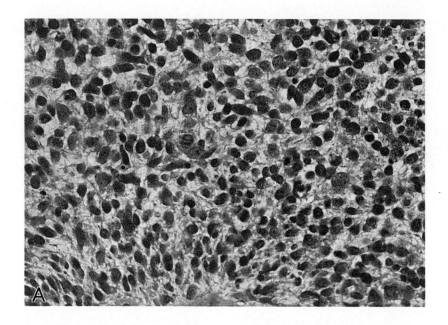

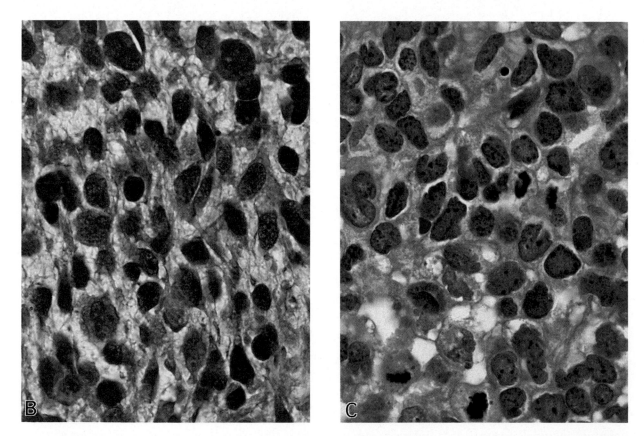

Figure 6-19
EMBRYONAL RHABDOMYOSARCOMA NOS

Most embryonal rhabdomyosarcomas contain as one component undifferentiated round or oval cells having a sparse clear or amphophilic wispy cytoplasm, very dense nuclear chromatin, and irregular nuclear membranes.

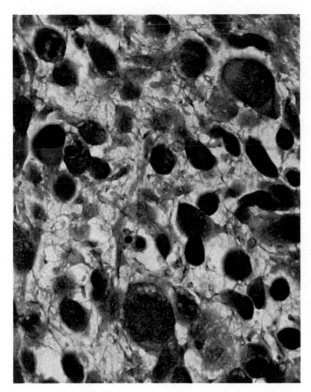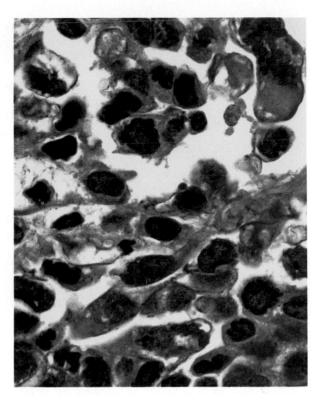

Figure 6-20
EMBRYONAL RHABDOMYOSARCOMA NOS
Cells with increased amounts of eosinophilic or basophilic cytoplasm which displace the densely hyperchromatic nucleus are characteristic of embryonal rhabdomyosarcoma. These are rare in other types of round blue cell tumors and so are very helpful diagnostically.

found in the anaplastic variant (see below). Few if any mitotic figures are found in embryonal rhabdomyosarcomas composed predominantly or exclusively of well-differentiated cells, while up to 20 to 30 mitoses per 10 high-power fields are not uncommon in lesions with less-differentiated cells. In fine needle aspiration biopsies the undifferentiated cells are noncohesive, with little or no cytoplasm, while the differentiating cells have variable amounts of dense eosinophilic cytoplasm. The nuclei of both cell types have dense chromatin and small nucleoli. Cross-striations are not found in the cytoplasm unless the cells are well differentiated (fig. 6-24).

Cells containing cytoplasmic cross-striations visible by light microscopy occur in only a third of embryonal rhabdomyosarcomas (figs. 6-21A,C, 6-22) (27,34,41), but when present allow diagnosis and distinguish rhabdomyosarcoma from other small blue cell neoplasms, except for the rare ectomesenchymoma. When cross-striations

are not identified, tadpole-shaped cells and cells with eosinophilic cytoplasm and eccentric dense nuclei (figs. 6-20, 6-21), along with clinical information such as the age of patient and site of the primary tumor, allow diagnosis, but today immunohistologic stains are almost always obtained for confirmation. About 1 percent of embryonal rhabdomyosarcomas contain cells which have rhabdoid features (36) characterized by circumscribed, pink, ground glass-like or finely fibrillar, round to oval cytoplasmic inclusion bodies which usually displace the nucleus (fig. 6-25). They may be as large as the nucleus. Cells containing such inclusions may have obvious cross-striations, but others do not and some are smaller with scant cytoplasm. These latter cells may have vesicular nuclei with prominent nucleoli furthering their mimicry of the cells that comprise malignant rhabdoid tumor, a neoplasm that must be distinguished from embryonal rhabdomyosarcoma with rhabdoid features (see Differential Diagnosis).

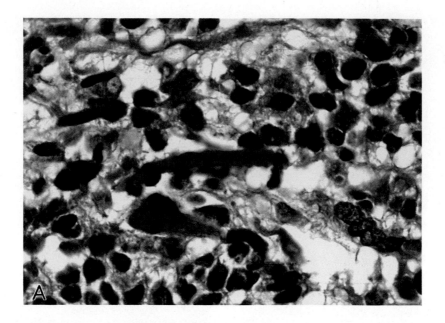

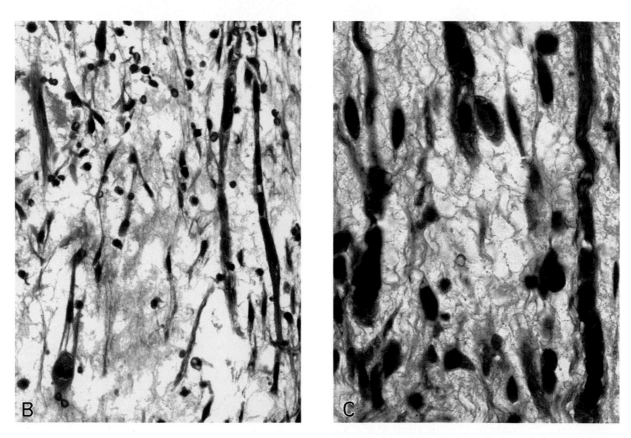

Figure 6-21
EMBRYONAL RHABDOMYOSARCOMA NOS

Differentiating cells of embryonal rhabdomyosarcoma have tapered, bipolar cytoplasm or a tadpole configuration with the nuclei located at one end of the cell. The arrangement of nuclei in tandem, like cars on a train, is illustrated in all three photomicrographs and is a feature unique to skeletal muscle neoplasms.

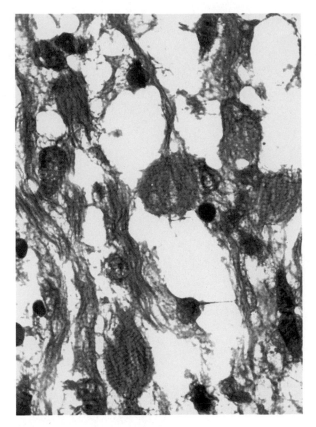

Figure 6-22
EMBRYONAL RHABDOMYOSARCOMA NOS

Well-differentiated rhabdomyoblasts are found in approximately one third of embryonal rhabdomyosarcomas. The cells have eosinophilic cytoplasm with cytoplasmic cross-striations.

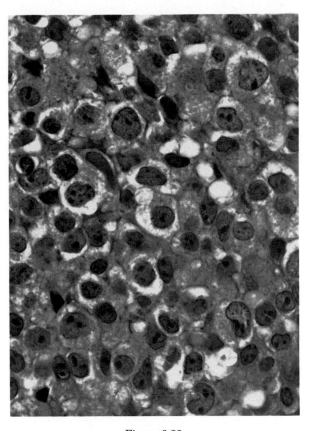

Figure 6-23
EMBRYONAL RHABDOMYOSARCOMA NOS

The cells in some embryonal rhabdomyosarcomas have nuclei with fine chromatin and small nucleoli, and an abundant amphophilic to clear cytoplasm. These cases can be confused with PPNET and malignant lymphoma.

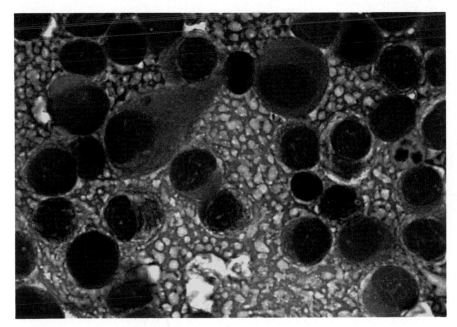

Figure 6-24
EMBRYONAL
RHABDOMYOSARCOMA NOS

Fine needle aspiration biopsy specimens of embryonal rhabdomyosarcoma may contain noncohesive, poorly differentiated cells with little or no cytoplasm and, in some cases, differentiating cells with varying amounts of dense eosinophilic cytoplasm. Support for embryonal rhabdomyosarcoma can be obtained by positive actin and desmin stains.

277

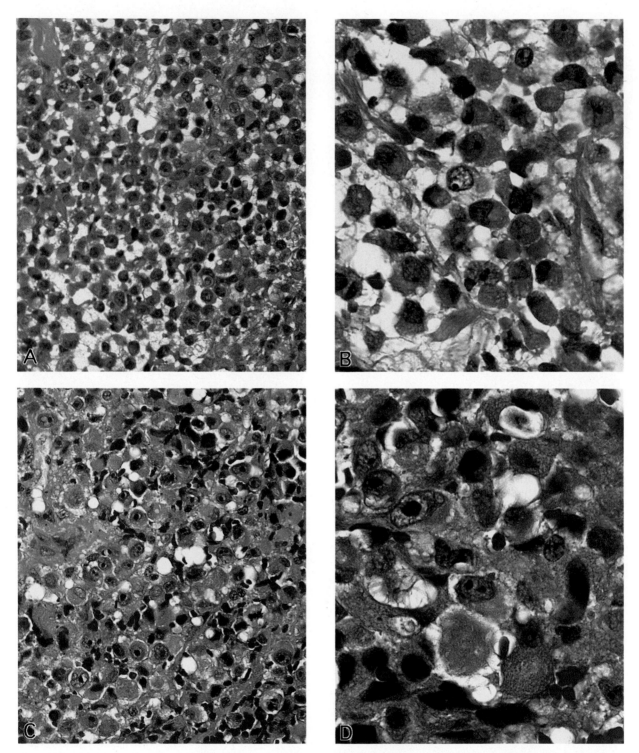

Figure 6-25
EMBRYONAL RHABDOMYOSARCOMA NOS

Embryonal rhabdomyosarcomas consisting predominantly of cells with circumscribed, pink, ground glass or fibrillar, round to oval cytoplasmic inclusions are very rare. Obvious cross-striations are seldom evident. The nuclei are typically more vesicular and have more prominent nucleoli than in the usual embryonal rhabdomyosarcoma. Immunohistochemical stains with a panel antibody approach, as outlined in the text, are necessary to establish the diagnosis and to distinguish this tumor from malignant rhabdoid tumor or other mimics.

A PAS stain will reveal variable amounts of cytoplasmic glycogen in the majority of embryonal rhabdomyosarcomas, and tumor cells with abundant glycogen can have a clear or vacuolated cytoplasm, the latter suggesting a spiderweb if the glycogen has been washed out during tissue processing (fig. 6-26). However, abundant glycogen is also a feature of peripheral primitive neuroectodermal tumor (PPNET)/Ewing's sarcoma and thus should not be used as a diagnostic tool to distinguish these two neoplasms.

Tumors removed from patients who have had preoperative chemotherapy or radiation therapy may show evidence of skeletal muscle differentiation to the point that the entire tumor consists of well-differentiated, bland, mature skeletal muscle cells (27,43). In this circumstance, further therapy should not be given because fully differentiated cells apparently lose their ability to divide, proliferate, and metastasize. However, undifferentiated and differentiating cells may be focal and if present are an indication for further therapy. Therefore, thorough sampling is indicated.

The botryoid variant is defined microscopically by a hypercellular zone of undifferentiated, short, spindled and round cells with little cytoplasm lying in a parallel band beneath the epithelium (fig. 6-27)(30,34,45,46,53). This hypercellular zone is the much heralded "cambium" layer and the cells

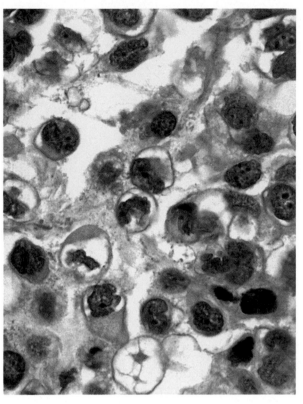

Figure 6-26
EMBRYONAL RHABDOMYOSARCOMA NOS
Abundant cytoplasmic glycogen occurs in many embryonal rhabdomyosarcomas and may impart a clear cytoplasm. Sometimes the glycogen-rich cells have a spiderweb appearance due to the fixation process, as seen here.

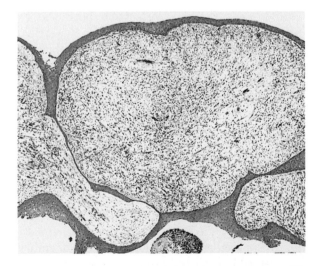

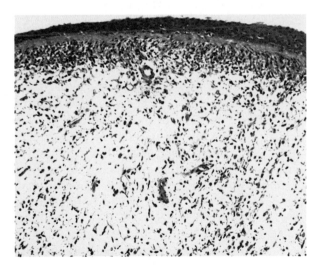

Figure 6-27
EMBRYONAL RHABDOMYOSARCOMA, BOTRYOID TYPE
At low-power magnification, the botryoid variant of embryonal rhabdomyosarcoma is characterized by polypoid or lobulated masses of cells covered by mucosa with an underlying hypercellular zone of poorly differentiated cells, the so called cambium layer, which is characteristic of this subtype.

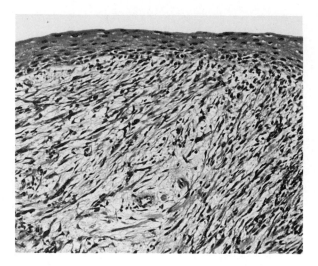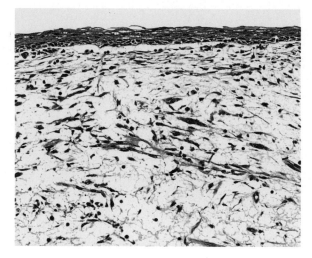

Figure 6-28
EMBRYONAL RHABDOMYOSARCOMA, BOTRYOID TYPE
The cambium layer may be only focally evident, so that some tumors consist mainly of paucicellular, edematous tissue with scattered undifferentiated and atypical larger cells (left) or sheets of round or spindled cells which might be mistaken for a benign polyp or a fibroinflammatory lesion (right).

composing it typically have a high mitotic rate. In many cases the cambium layer is only focally evident. Deep to the cambium layer, the lesion typically becomes less cellular and is composed of scattered undifferentiated and differentiating cells growing as sheets of round or spindle cells, as in classic embryonal rhabdomyosarcoma (figs. 6-27, 6-28, 6-29, left). The cytologic features of the cells in the botryoid variant are the same as those of classic embryonal rhabdomyosarcoma, described above, and thus botryoid tumors contain variable numbers of undifferentiated, differentiating, and well-differentiated cells (fig. 6-29).

While spindle-shaped cells occur in most embryonal rhabdomyosarcomas, tumors composed of greater than 50 percent spindled cells are subcategorized as the spindle cell variant (28, 39). The spindle-shaped cells often have eosinophilic, variably fibrillar cytoplasm and may be arranged in a storiform pattern but in about half the cases the cells are found in bundles more akin to leiomyosarcoma (fig. 6-30). Intercellular collagen is often scant (figs. 6-30A, 6-31, left), however, a few tumors feature individual spindle cells set in a very abundant collagenous stroma (figs. 6-30B, 6-31, right). Cells with cytoplasmic cross-striations, while present in most spindle cell rhabdomyosarcomas, are sparse (fig. 6-32). The nuclei are cigar shaped and may have prominent

nucleoli. Mitotic activity is most often low to absent, especially in paucicellular tumors with prominent fibrous stroma.

Anaplastic embryonal rhabdomyosarcoma features scattered cells with lobated, hyperchromatic nuclei that are definitionally three times larger than the nuclei of the surrounding tumor cells (fig. 6-33). The histologic features are otherwise those of the classic type of embryonal rhabdomyosarcoma. Cells with both the required nuclear enlargement and the hyperchromasia must be present before an embryonal rhabdomyosarcoma can be characterized as anaplastic. Moreover, the anaplasia must be multifocal or diffuse. Minor foci of anaplasia do not adversely affect prognosis and should not be considered sufficient to classify the tumor as anaplastic. In the usual example, the anaplastic cells occur as loosely scattered cells in a myxoid stroma, aggregate in clusters, or grow in solid continuous sheets. Abnormal mitotic figures are commonly present (fig. 6-33B,D) (37).

Special Studies. Immunohistochemistry plays a pivotal role in the identification of embryonal rhabdomyosarcomas because over 90 percent contain cells that are desmin and actin positive. A panel approach is best, in our opinion, and our current initial panel for evaluating small blue cell tumors usually includes desmin, muscle-specific

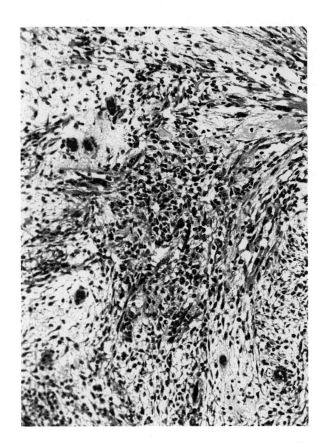 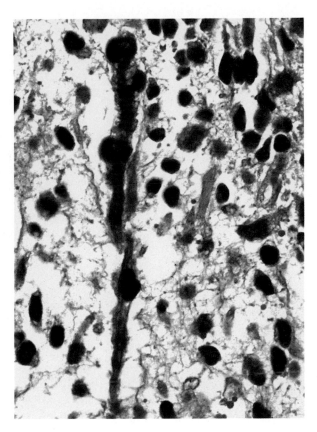

Figure 6-29
EMBRYONAL RHABDOMYOSARCOMA, BOTRYOID TYPE
Most embryonal rhabdomyosarcomas of the botryoid subtype also contain deep foci of hypercellularity (left) in which round and spindled undifferentiated cells are admixed with differentiating rhabdomyoblasts (right).

actin, low molecular weight cytokeratin, CD99, common leukocyte antigen, S-100 protein, and epithelial membrane antigen. When such a panel is used, up to one third of cases initially categorized as "undifferentiated small round cell sarcoma of childhood" can be reclassified as embryonal rhabdomyosarcoma, based on a characteristic histologic pattern and the identification of desmin-positive tumor cells (35,54).

The intermediate filament desmin has been reported to be expressed by the constituent cells of at least 95 percent of embryonal rhabdomyosarcomas NOS and botryoid rhabdomyosarcomas (fig. 6-34) (26,32). As few as 5 percent of the cells may be positive for desmin in embryonal rhabdomyosarcomas composed solely of undifferentiated cells, while diffuse and strong staining of a larger proportion of the neoplastic cells is almost always found in tumors containing differentiating and well-differentiated cells.

Desmin expression is so highly characteristic of the classic and botryoid variants of embryonal rhabdomyosarcoma that when it is absent great care should be taken, and probably consultation obtained, before interpreting a tumor as either of these types of embryonal rhabdomyosarcoma. In fact, the small number of classic rhabdomyosarcomas that have been reported to be desmin negative may represent false negatives because of technical problems, or undifferentiated malignant neoplasms that should not have been classified as rhabdomyosarcoma. Immunostains for myogenic regulatory proteins MyoD1 and myogenin decorate the nuclei of the tumor cells in 90 percent of embryonal rhabdomyosarcomas. These appear to be specific and sensitive markers of skeletal muscle differentiation and are increasingly used for diagnosis (29a,60). In our opinion, all embryonal rhabdomyosarcomas should contain cells that stain for desmin, MyoD1, or myogenin; those that

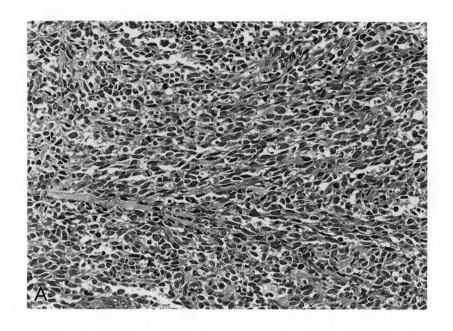

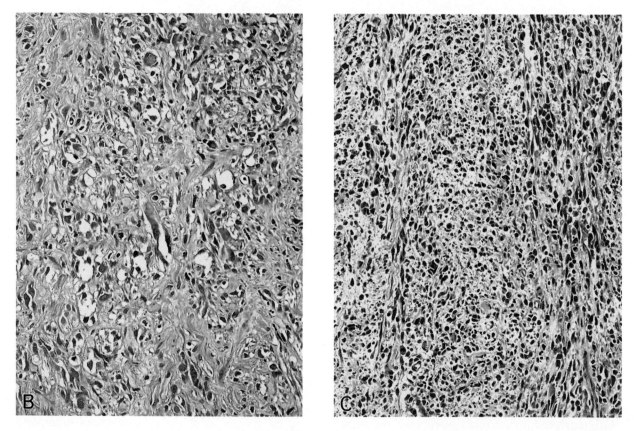

Figure 6-30
EMBRYONAL RHABDOMYOSARCOMA, SPINDLE CELL TYPE

Spindle-shaped cells are usually found in embryonal rhabdomyosarcomas and when 50 percent or more of the tumor is composed of these, the sarcoma is subcategorized as the spindle cell type. The cells may be arranged in patterns reminiscent of leiomyosarcoma (A) and malignant fibrous histiocytoma (B,C).

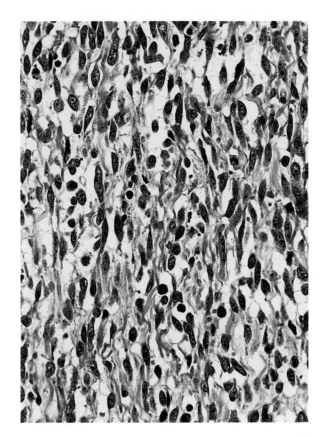 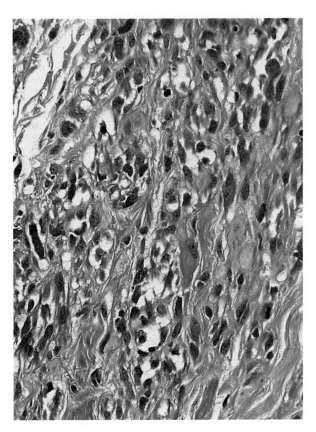

Figure 6-31
EMBRYONAL RHABDOMYOSARCOMA, SPINDLE CELL TYPE
Left: These nondescript spindle-shaped cells are characteristic of many spindle cell embryonal rhabdomyosarcomas and must be distinguished from other forms of spindle cell sarcoma because of the excellent prognosis associated with this subtype.
Right: Some cases are quite paucicellular and have a very fibrotic stroma in which undifferentiated round and spindled cells are admixed with differentiating rhabdomyoblasts with more abundant eosinophilic cytoplasm.

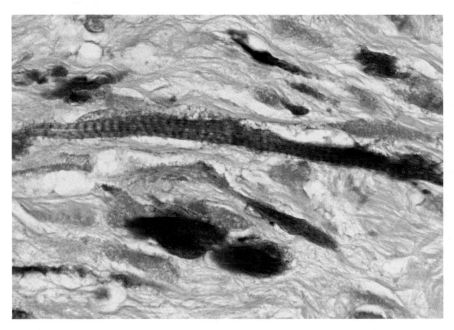

Figure 6-32
EMBRYONAL
RHABDOMYOSARCOMA,
SPINDLE CELL TYPE
Rhabdomyoblasts with cytoplasmic cross-striations can be found in most spindle cell variants of embryonal rhabdomyosarcoma but are sparse and difficult to find. Immunohistologic staining for desmin often highlights these cells.

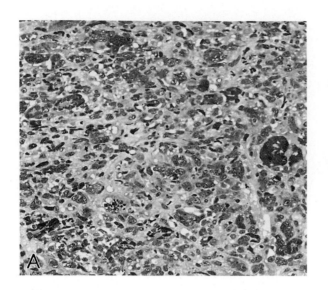

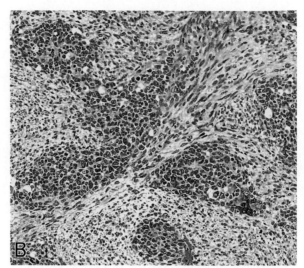

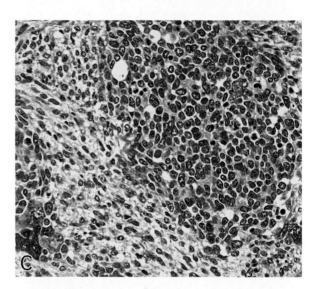

Figure 6-33
EMBRYONAL RHABDOMYOSARCOMA,
ANAPLASTIC TYPE

The cells in anaplastic embryonal rhabdomyosarcoma contain extremely hyperchromatic nuclei that are three times larger than the nuclei of surrounding tumor cells. These cells are admixed with smaller, undifferentiated, round and spindle-shaped cells (A–C). Bizarre mitotic figures (D) and rare cells suggesting skeletal muscle differentiation (E) are found in this subtype.

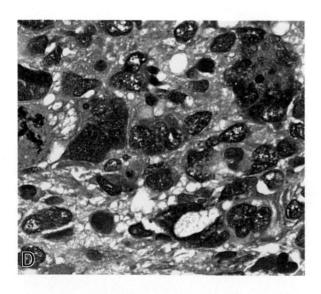

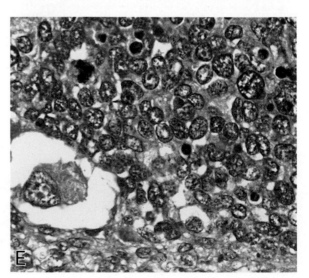

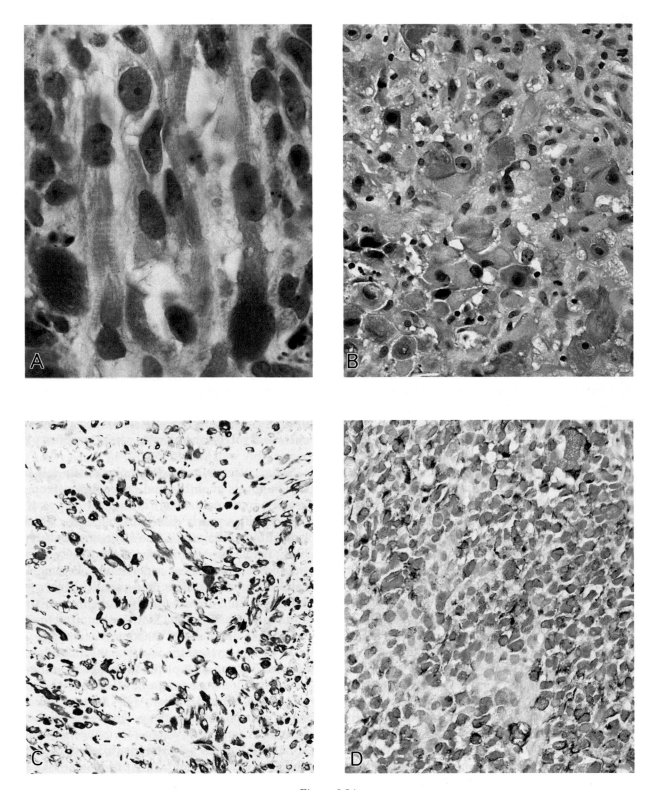

Figure 6-34
EMBRYONAL RHABDOMYOSARCOMA

Immunohistochemical staining is very helpful in distinguishing embryonal rhabdomyosarcoma from other malignancies. Desmin stains are especially helpful in identifying cells with cytoplasmic cross-striations (A), muscle differentiation in rhabdoid cells (B), and the spindle cell (C) and anaplastic (D) variants.

Embryonal rhabdomyosarcoma may be difficult to distinguish from fetal rhabdomyoma. Fetal rhabdomyoma is usually well demarcated, more often superficially located than rhabdomyosarcoma, has rare if any mitoses, and has tumor cells that demonstrate insignificant cytologic atypia, pleomorphism, and no necrosis. Unlike embryonal rhabdomyosarcoma, fetal rhabdomyoma has cells which tend to be better differentiated at the periphery of the tumor. The differentiated cells of rhabdomyoma also have more delicate, less dense nuclei and more numerous cross-striations than do the cells of most embryonal rhabdomyosarcomas. Distinguishing fetal rhabdomyoma from the spindle cell and botryoid variants of embryonal rhabdomyosarcoma can be difficult. A pseudocambium layer, consisting of plasma cells and lymphocytes lacking mitoses, occurs in some cases of mucosal fetal rhabdomyoma. This could lead to the mistaken diagnosis of the botryoid variant, while the hypercellularity and overall lack of a mixture of small primitive cells and differentiating rhabdomyoblasts in cellular fetal rhabdomyoma could be interpreted as evidence of the spindle cell variant. This differential is also discussed under Rhabdomyoma in this chapter.

Embryonal rhabdomyosarcoma with extensive maturation can be confused with an adult rhabdomyoma. However, adult rhabdomyomas are composed of large, polygonal to round, tightly packed cells which have abundant eosinophilic, granular, or vacuolated cytoplasm. These have been given the moniker "spider" cells. As is the case with embryonal rhabdomyosarcoma, cross-striations may be difficult to find; however, mitotic figures are rarely present and the undifferentiated and differentiating cells, which are mixed in varying numbers with the differentiated cells in embryonal rhabdomyosarcoma, are not found in adult rhabdomyoma.

Upper respiratory tract and genitourinary tract polyps characteristically have an edematous stroma and occasionally may contain cells which demonstrate considerable cytologic atypia. When the latter occurs, they can resemble the botryoid type of embryonal rhabdomyosarcoma. However, polyps lack a subepithelial cambium layer and are diffusely paucicellular rather than focally hypercellular (47), features that point to the correct diagnosis. Cells with cross-striations and cells positive for desmin are not found in polyps. This distinction can be difficult in small, traumatized specimens and a repeat biopsy should be performed if the lesion is clinically suspicious for malignancy but the histologic features are equivocal.

Another lesion that might be confused with a vaginal, vulvar, or cervical botryoid embryonal rhabdomyosarcoma is genital rhabdomyoma. The latter grows as a polypoid mass, is rarely more than 3 cm, and contains mature skeletal muscle cells with distinct cross-striations. The stroma is variably collagenous and myxoid. Unlike embryonal rhabdomyosarcoma, genital rhabdomyoma lacks a subepithelial cambium layer, and the constituent cells demonstrate little or no cytologic atypia.

Leiomyosarcoma, fibrosarcoma, and malignant fibrous histiocytoma with a predominance of spindle cells might be mistaken for the spindle cell variant of embryonal rhabdomyosarcoma, although these three occur predominantly in older adults, an age in which embryonal rhabdomyosarcoma is rare. Most spindle variants of embryonal rhabdomyosarcoma contain cells with cytoplasmic cross-striations discernible by light microscopy, although they may be hard to find. A paratesticular site and an age less than 25 years also point toward spindle cell rhabdomyosarcoma. Since desmin and muscle-specific actin are found in both rhabdomyosarcoma and leiomyosarcoma these stains are not useful in distinguishing these two tumors. However, monoclonal myoglobin has been reported to be positive in most spindle cell variants of embryonal rhabdomyosarcoma and MyoD1 and myogenin should be positive also; all three of these stains are negative in leiomyosarcoma. The cells of fibrosarcoma do not express desmin, MyoD1, or myogenin (58).

Myofibroma (myofibromatosis) and infantile fibromatosis are also important diagnostic considerations. Neither demonstrates the nuclear atypia of the spindle cell variant of embryonal rhabdomyosarcoma, and the former often features a pericytic vascular pattern in areas where the cells have a "small blue cell" appearance.

Distinction of the rhabdoid variant of embryonal rhabdomyosarcoma, NOS, from malignant rhabdoid tumor is extremely important because the treatment and prognosis are so different for the two tumors. Malignant rhabdoid tumors typically contain cells with vesicular nuclei and prominent nucleoli, while the rhabdoid variant of rhabdomyosarcoma characteristically is composed of cells with hyperchromatic nuclei of more variable size and shape, and smaller and less conspicuous nucleoli. Immunohistology can be of assistance because the eosinophilic cytoplasmic inclusions in the rhabdoid variant of rhabdomyosarcoma are composed of desmin-positive filaments and the cells nearly always stain for muscle-specific actin, while the inclusions in malignant rhabdoid tumor are usually cytokeratin positive and, in our experience, are desmin and actin negative. The cells in malignant rhabdoid tumor do not show evidence of sarcomeric differentiation by electron microscopy and they are also almost always epithelial membrane antigen positive, a stain that is negative in embryonal rhabdomyosarcoma cells.

Whenever a diagnosis of pleomorphic liposarcoma, pleomorphic malignant fibrous histiocytoma, or pleomorphic rhabdomyosarcoma is entertained for a pediatric age patient, the anaplastic variant of embryonal rhabdomyosarcoma should be considered, because the former tumors are so rare in the young. Pleomorphic rhabdomyosarcoma accounted for only 0.8 percent of the cases in the pediatric Intergroup Rhabdomyosarcoma Studies I, II, and III (46) and is typically found in patients over the age of 50 years. Distinguishing pleomorphic rhabdomyosarcoma from anaplastic embryonal rhabdomyosarcoma may not be of critical importance since both respond poorly to treatment; however, those few pleomorphic rhabdomyosarcomas reported in children appear to have a better prognosis than the anaplastic variant of embryonal rhabdomyosarcoma (46). The anaplastic variant always has a background of classic embryonal rhabdomyosarcoma with foci, either multifocal or diffuse, composed of anaplastic cells as defined in the pathology section above. Such a background is absent in the three other pleomorphic sarcomas.

Treatment and Prognosis. Overall, disease-free survival for patients with embryonal rhabdomyosarcoma has improved from 20 percent to 70 percent since the introduction of current chemotherapy, modern radiotherapy, and improved surgical procedures. Individual patient survival depends primarily on three fac-

Table 6-2

INTERGROUP RHABDOMYOSARCOMA STUDY GROUPS*

Group 1	Localized disease, completely resected (regional nodes not involved) Confined to organ or muscle of origin Contiguous involvement, with infiltration outside the muscle or organ of origin, as through fascial planes
Group 2	Grossly resected tumor with microscopic residual disease; no evidence of gross residual tumor; no evidence of regional node involvement Regional disease, completely resected (no microscopic residual tumor); regional nodes involved and/or tumor extends into adjacent organ Regional disease with involved nodes; grossly resected, but with evidence of microscopic residual
Group 3	Incomplete resection or biopsy with gross residual disease
Group 4	Distant metastases, present at onset (lung, liver, bones, bone marrow, brain, and distant muscles and nodes)

*Modified from: Maurer HM, Beltangady M, Gehan EA, et al. The Intergroup Rhabdomyosarcoma Study, I. A final report. Cancer 1988;61:209–20.

tors: the histologic subtype, the primary site of the neoplasm, and the Intergroup Rhabdomyosarcoma Study clinical group (stage) (Table 6-2). Treatment of patients with embryonal rhabdomyosarcoma is primarily determined by the clinical group of the tumor (40).

The histologic type of the embryonal rhabdomyosarcoma distinctly influences outcome so all embryonal rhabdomyosarcomas should be subtyped using the definitions provided in the pathology section above and this information should be included in the pathology report. The Intergroup Rhabdomyosarcoma Study has designated each histologic subtype as belonging to a good, intermediate, or poor prognostic category (29). Within the good prognostic category are the botryoid (overall patient survival more than 90 percent) and the paratesticular spindle cell (overall patient survival more than 95 percent) rhabdomyosarcomas. The intermediate prognostic category includes embryonal rhabdomyosarcoma NOS and nonparatesticular spindle cell variants (about 70 percent patient survival overall). Embryonal rhabdomyosarcomas that demonstrate multifocal or diffuse anaplasia as defined in the pathology section above are placed in the poor prognostic category because overall survival is no higher than 45 to 50 percent. Tumors with focal anaplasia are associated with patient survival that is similar to embryonal rhabdomyosarcoma NOS; consequently, they are placed in the intermediate category.

Given identical stage (clinical group) and histologic subtype, the site of the primary tumor may affect patient outcome. Patients with head and neck, genitourinary, and orbital lesions have a better overall prognosis than those with parameningeal, extremity, trunk, and retroperitoneal tumors (38).

Disease-free survival is also significantly influenced by the stage or clinical group of the tumor (29). These clinical groups are presented in Table 6-2 and are determined by both the clinical and pathologic findings. Consequently, the pathology report should always contain sufficient information for clinicians to determine the clinical group (stage). The Intergroup Rhabdomyosarcoma Study reports an overall survival of 92 percent for patients whose tumors fall into group 1, 82 percent for group 2, 70 percent for group 3, and 32 percent for group 4. The prognosis of adults with embryonal rhabdomyosarcoma is extremely poor as compared to the pediatric patient, with a less than 10 percent 5-year survival rate (44,53).

The most common sites for metastases are lung (58 percent), lymph nodes (33 percent), liver (22 percent), and brain (20 percent) (56).

Alveolar Rhabdomyosarcoma

Definition. Alveolar rhabdomyosarcoma is a high-grade sarcoma characterized by solid and alveolar growth of cells, some of which demonstrate evidence of skeletal muscle differentiation by light microscopy, electron microscopy, or immunohistology.

General Considerations. Alveolar rhabdomyosarcoma accounts for about 20 to 25 percent of childhood rhabdomyosarcomas. Any rhabdomyosarcoma with an alveolar pattern, no matter

how focal, should be classified as an alveolar rhabdomyosarcoma rather than a mixed alveolar/embryonal rhabdomyosarcoma. Unlike embryonal rhabdomyosarcoma, alveolar rhabdomyosarcoma does not respond well to current therapy and is still associated with a poor prognosis. As a result, distinction from embryonal rhabdomyosarcoma is very important. Unlike embryonal rhabdomyosarcoma, characteristic chromosomal translocations t(2;13) and t(1;13) have been reported in most alveolar rhabdomyosarcomas.

Clinical Features. Alveolar rhabdomyosarcoma occurs in individuals of all ages but most are between 2 and 25 years old. The mean age was 9 years for cases submitted to the Intergroup Rhabdomyosarcoma Studies (80); almost 70 percent of children in an international oncology study were 10 years old or younger at presentation (83). The male to female ratio is 1.2 to 1. The tumors most commonly involve the extremities (45 percent), followed by the head/neck (20 percent), trunk (12 percent), pelvis (6 percent), anus (6 percent), retroperitoneum (5 percent), genitourinary tract (2 percent), and intrathoracic locations (2 percent) (80).

Pathologic Findings. Macroscopically, alveolar rhabdomyosarcomas are pale yellow to white, soft, and hemorrhagic (64). The mean size is about 5 cm and ranges from 2 to 8 cm (79,80).

By light microscopy, the tumor cells comprising the usual alveolar rhabdomyosarcoma grow, at least focally, as nests or clusters (fig. 6-35) separated by fibrous septa. Towards the center of the nests the cells are discohesive and seem to be loose within a space, while the cells at the edge are attached, a pattern that simulates lung and gives the tumor its name (74,86,90). However, most alveolar rhabdomyosarcomas also contain foci of more solid tumor growth and some are predominantly solid. Needless to say, the latter have been categorized as the *solid variant* (fig. 6-35F,G) (86,90).

Several types of cells can be found in the alveolar areas. One type is round with sparse cytoplasm, measures 10 to 15 μm, is centrally located, and floats freely within the alveolar spaces (fig. 6-36). These cells do not demonstrate evidence of skeletal muscle differentiation by light microscopy. A second cell type is larger, 15 to 30 μm (72); polygonal, pyramidal, or elongate; and rests on a basement membrane and protrudes into the lumen of the alveolar space (fig. 6-36). These larger peripheral cells usually have more abundant fibrillar eosinophilic cytoplasm, sometimes with cross-striations, and may contain an abundant amount of cytoplasmic glycogen. They have round, oval, or reniform densely hyperchromatic nuclei with 1 to 3 small round nucleoli. In addition to these two cell types, variable numbers of multinucleated giant cells (figs. 6-35E, 6-37) and larger cells with more abundant eosinophilic, sometimes vacuolated cytoplasm (fig. 6-38) are usually evident; tadpole- and strap-shaped myoblasts occur in some cases as well. Finding multinucleated giant cells in an fine needle aspiration specimen from a soft tissue mass in a child should raise the question of alveolar rhabdomyosarcoma. Foci of coagulative tumor cell necrosis are frequently encountered. Rhabdomyoblasts containing diagnostic cytoplasmic cross-striations by light microscopy are found in up to one third of tumors (74,87).

In the solid variant, an alveolar pattern is present only in focal areas (figs. 6-35F,G, 6-39); this can be missed in small biopsy specimens. Rare cases may be exclusively solid. Most solid lesions also consist of nests of cells surrounded by narrow rims of vascularized fibrous tissue, but unlike the alveolar variant the centers of the nests are solidly filled with round and oval cells with little cytoplasm, to polygonal cells with more abundant eosinophilic cytoplasm, rather than the mixed population of loosely cohesive cells described above. In addition, a centrally desquamated component is lacking. Distinction from embryonal rhabdomyosarcoma is possible in most (but not all) cases, based on the more consistently rounded cells and larger, more uniform nuclei in the alveolar variant.

Only a few cases of alveolar rhabdomyosarcoma with *anaplastic features* have been reported and patients with these seem to have an even worse prognosis (77). Like anaplastic embryonal rhabdomyosarcoma, the anaplastic cells in this form of alveolar rhabdomyosarcoma definitionally have lobate, hyperchromatic nuclei three times larger than the nuclei of surrounding cells (fig. 6-40). Moreover, multipolar atypical mitoses are often identified. The multinucleate cells in the usual alveolar variant may be large, but their nuclei do not meet either the size or the hyperchromasia requirement for anaplasia. As

in anaplastic embryonal lesions, the anaplastic cells in alveolar rhabdomyosarcoma are loosely scattered or are found aggregated in clusters or sheets within a background of cells otherwise characteristic of alveolar rhabdomyosarcoma.

A small number of alveolar rhabdomyosarcomas with *rhabdoid features* have been reported (76). The rhabdoid cells occur focally in otherwise typical alveolar rhabdomyosarcoma. They have circumscribed, pink, ground-glass–like or finely fibrillar, round to oval cytoplasmic bodies (fig. 6-41) and their nuclei often have large eosinophilic nucleoli.

Special Studies. The usual alveolar rhabdomyosarcoma can easily be recognized by light microscopic examination; however, immunohistology should be used to confirm the diagnosis if the tumor has unusual features. Immunohistochemistry is especially helpful in recognizing the solid variant because it so often mimics other types of soft tissue neoplasms. Although a rather large number of skeletal muscle proteins have been identified in rhabdomyosarcomas, the best categorized, most useful diagnostically, and ones we use routinely are desmin and muscle-specific actin. Like embryonal rhabdomyosarcoma, at least 95 percent of alveolar rhabdomyosarcomas contain desmin-positive cells (fig. 6-42), and muscle-specific actin is positive in over 90 percent of tumors (68,85,87,91). Myogenin and MyoD1 are also positive in most alveolar rhabdomyosarcomas (65a,93). We do not think a tumor should be diagnosed as alveolar rhabdomyosarcoma if the muscle-specific actin, desmin, MyoD1, or myogenin stains are all negative unless cytogenetic or molecular genetic examination demonstrates one of the translocations or fusion proteins characteristic of alveolar rhabdomyosarcoma. Vimentin is positive in nearly 60 percent of tumors (68,85,87), cytokeratin (CAM5.2) in 13 percent, and myoglobin in almost 60 percent (85,87). A high percentage of alveolar rhabdomyosarcomas also stain for neuron-specific enolase (70 percent) and S-100 protein (40 percent) (85). S-100 protein is diffusely and strongly positive in some cases, especially in the solid areas, whereas in others only scattered cells are positive. The staining is both cytoplasmic and nuclear. In the few cases studied, dystrophin (78) and creatinine kinase-MM (91), both skeletal muscle proteins, were positive.

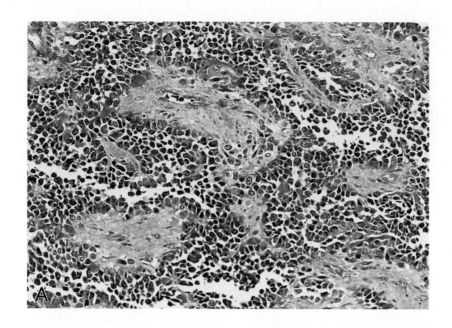

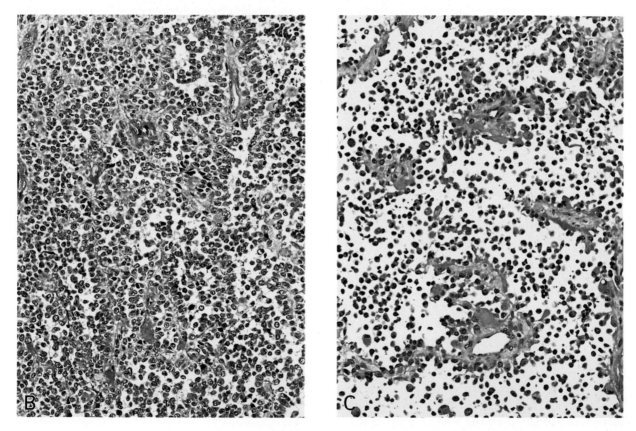

Figure 6-35
ALVEOLAR RHABDOMYOSARCOMA

Tumor cells in alveolar rhabdomyosarcoma typically grow in nests or clusters separated by fibrous septa, with central desquamated cells (A–C) but this tumor also can contain foci of more solid growth (D,E), or may be predominantly solid (F,G). The latter cases may be mistaken for other types of small cell neoplasm, including embryonal rhabdomyosarcoma. Multinucleated giant cells, illustrated in E, are often present.

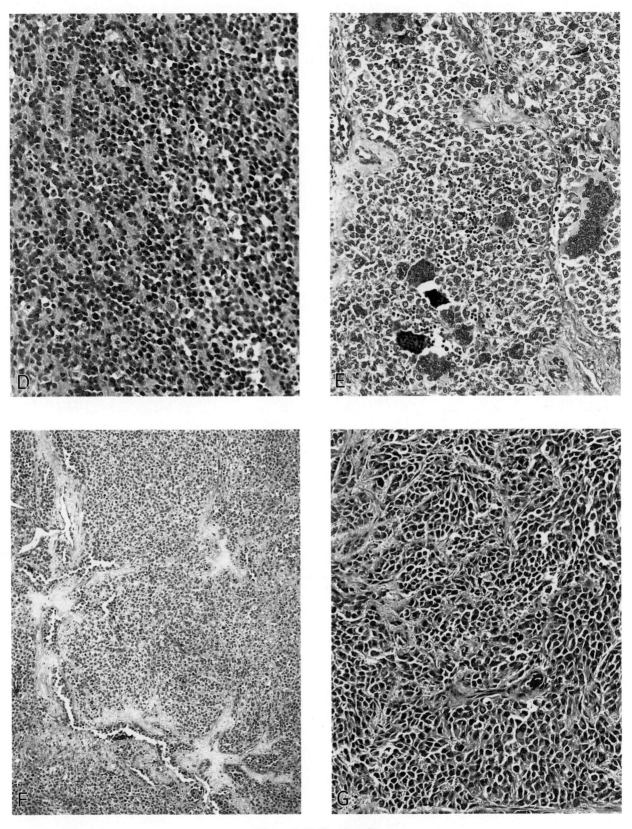

Figure 6-35 (Continued)

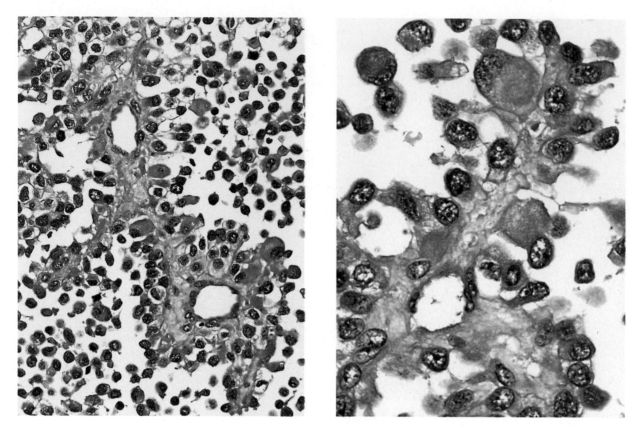

Figure 6-36
ALVEOLAR RHABDOMYOSARCOMA

The characteristic features of alveolar rhabdomyosarcoma are the alveolar spaces containing desquamated small, round and poorly differentiated skeletal muscle cells and the fibrovascular stroma lined by both undifferentiated round cells and differentiating cells with abundant eosinophilic cytoplasm. Cross-striations are rarely identified.

Figure 6-37
ALVEOLAR
RHABDOMYOSARCOMA

Some cases of alveolar rhabdomyosarcoma also contain desquamated multinucleated giant cells.

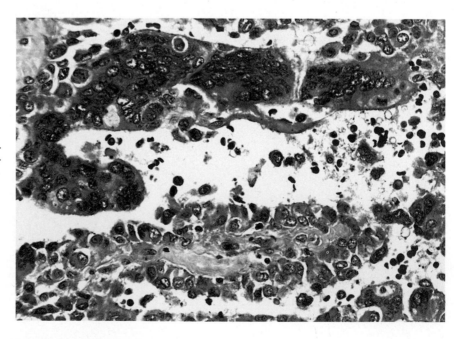

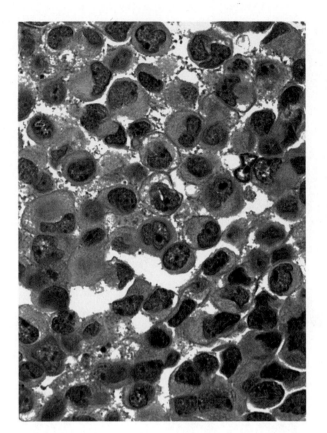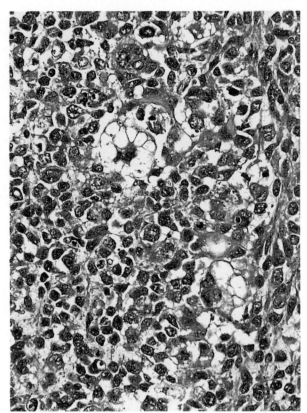

Figure 6-38
ALVEOLAR RHABDOMYOSARCOMA

In some examples of alveolar rhabdomyosarcoma, the cytologic features of the neoplastic cells are similar to those found in embryonal rhabdomyosarcoma (left), including small, round and spindle-shaped cells with hyperchromatic, variably shaped nuclei and vacuolated spiderweb cells (right). The latter are also suggestive of lipoblasts, which could lead to an erroneous diagnosis.

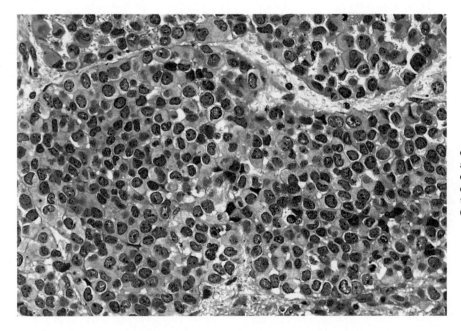

Figure 6-39
ALVEOLAR
RHABDOMYOSARCOMA

The alveolar pattern may be only focally evident in some cases of alveolar rhabdomyosarcoma. This can lead to a misdiagnosis of embryonal rhabdomyosarcoma, based upon a needle or excisional biopsy (see figure 6-35F,G).

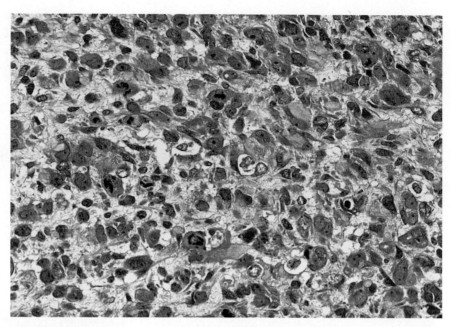

Figure 6-40
ALVEOLAR
RHABDOMYOSARCOMA,
ANAPLASTIC VARIANT
Some alveolar rhabdomyosarcomas contain foci of anaplastic cells. These hyperchromatic nuclei must be three times larger than the nuclei of surrounding cells. This variant apparently has a worse prognosis than the typical alveolar rhabdomyosarcoma.

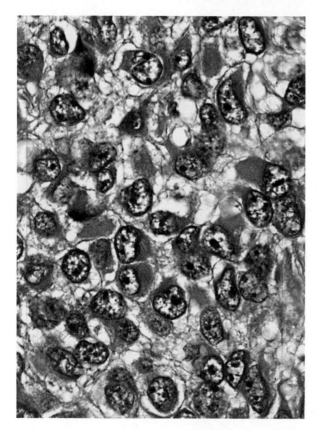

Figure 6-41
ALVEOLAR RHABDOMYOSARCOMA,
RHABDOID FEATURES
On rare occasions, alveolar rhabdomyosarcomas contain a large number of rhabdoid cells in what is otherwise a typical alveolar rhabdomyosarcoma.

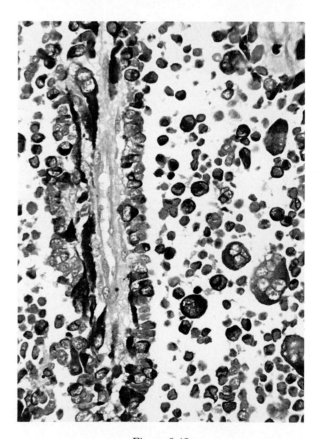

Figure 6-42
ALVEOLAR RHABDOMYOSARCOMA
Cytoplasmic staining for desmin distinguishes alveolar rhabdomyosarcoma from other tumors that grow in an alveolar pattern.

CD99 is rarely positive and when positive, only weakly and focally so (61,82).

Fine structural examination can confirm the presence of skeletal muscle differentiation, but is not necessary in establishing the diagnosis. The ultrastructural features that count as evidence of skeletal muscle differentiation are identical to those described for embryonal rhabdomyosarcoma.

Chromosome analysis has demonstrated two characteristic cytogenetic aberrations in alveolar rhabdomyosarcoma: the translocation t(2;13)(q35-37;q14) in nearly 85 percent of alveolar rhabdomyosarcoma and the translocation t(1;13)(p36;q14) in the remainder (81,94). *PAX3*, a human gene–containing sequence homologous to the paired box on chromosome 2, a conserved domain implicated in transcriptional control of skeletal muscle development, is the locus which is rearranged in the t(2;13) translocation (63), whereas *PAX7* on chromosome 1, expressed during the differentiation of trunk and limb muscular development, is rearranged in the t(1;13) translocation (66). The *FKHR* gene has been found to be the locus on chromosome 13 to which the *PAX3* (62,71,88) and *PAX7* (66,67) genes fuse. It is likely that the cases of embryonal rhabdomyosarcoma with the *PAX3/FKHR* fusion gene reported by Downing et al. (70) actually represent the solid form of alveolar rhabdomyosarcoma. Identification of these fusion genes by reverse transcription polymerase chain reaction may come to be definitional for solid forms of alveolar rhabdomyosarcoma, but more cases need to be examined. This test may be especially useful for needle core or fine needle aspiration biopsy specimens in which the typical features of alveolar rhabdomyosarcoma are not evident.

Differential Diagnosis. The alveolar pattern, with discohesive cells and multinucleated giant cells in the center of spaces, is so characteristic that the diagnosis of alveolar rhabdomyosarcoma is seldom in doubt in representative biopsies, even in the presence of rhabdoid features or anaplasia (71). However, when most of the tumor consists of solid nests of cells, PPNET/Ewing's sarcoma, neuroblastoma, and malignant rhabdoid tumor should be considered in the differential diagnosis. Taking an adequate number of sections, followed by careful search for an alveolar pattern, are the best and most cost-effective means to establish the diagnosis.

Positive immunostaining for desmin and muscle-specific actin, MyoD1, or myogenin, which we require before diagnosing any type of rhabdomyosarcoma, serves to distinguish alveolar rhabdomyosarcoma from the PPNET/Ewing's sarcoma family, neuroblastoma, and malignant rhabdoid tumor but not from embryonal rhabdomyosarcoma and desmoplastic small cell tumor. Examples of the PPNET/Ewing's sarcoma family with an alveolar pattern and divergent skeletal muscle differentiation (primitive malignant ectomesenchymoma), moreover, will be misdiagnosed if one relies solely upon the light microscopic pattern and antibodies capable of detecting skeletal muscle differentiation. Furthermore, one biphenotypic tumor not only stained with CD99 and desmin, but also showed simultaneous expression of *PAX3-FKHR* and *EWS-FLI1* transcripts (67a). For this reason, a panel of antibodies should always be used whenever the diagnosis of alveolar rhabdomyosarcoma is uncertain by light microscopy. Our current initial panel includes muscle-specific actin, desmin, S-100 protein, CD99, low molecular weight (CAM5.2) keratin, and epithelial membrane antigen.

S-100 protein may be focally positive in embryonal rhabdomyosarcoma, PPNET/Ewing's sarcoma family, and neuroblastoma, but diffuse strong staining is evident in nearly 40 percent of alveolar rhabdomyosarcomas and thus S-100 protein, if present, can help distinguish the latter from the former. Strong S-100 protein staining can lead to a mistaken diagnosis of malignant melanoma because the latter often grows in alveolar as well as solid patterns, and the neoplastic cells may have brightly eosinophilic cytoplasm. Malignant melanoma is desmin and muscle-specific antigen negative and often HMB45 positive. CD99 is usually diffusely and strongly positive in PPNET/Ewing's sarcoma; CD99 staining in alveolar rhabdomyosarcoma is rare, focal, and weak.

Other soft tissue tumors that may present with an alveolar pattern include alveolar soft part sarcoma and metastatic poorly differentiated carcinomas. It has been suggested that alveolar soft part sarcoma is a tumor with skeletal muscle differentiation because the constituent cells in some tumors stain for desmin and muscle-specific actin, and MyoD1 stains may be positive (84). While 50 percent of alveolar soft part sarcomas in one study (92) stained with desmin, none stained with muscle-specific actin or myoglobin, there was no nuclear staining for MyoD1 or myogenin, and a specific protein band on Western blot analysis for MyoD1 was not seen, so the issue is unresolved. Like alveolar rhabdomyosarcoma, alveolar soft part sarcomas are composed of discohesive round or oval cells with eosinophilic cytoplasm which grow in an alveolar pattern, but in contrast, have PAS-diastase–positive intracytoplasmic crystalline rods and granules rather than intracytoplasmic glycogen, and they lack the pleomorphism, multiple cell types, and giant cells of alveolar rhabdomyosarcoma. Moreover, in alveolar soft part sarcoma the clusters of tumor cells are surrounded by thin walled sinusoidal blood vessels, not fibrous tissue as in alveolar rhabdomyosarcoma. Metastatic carcinomas are usually readily identified with positive immunostaining for cytokeratins and epithelial membrane antigen, and negative staining for desmin and muscle-specific actin.

Treatment and Prognosis. Stage for stage, the prognosis is worse for patients with alveolar rhabdomyosarcoma than for those with embryonal rhabdomyosarcoma and its variants. The 3-year disease-free survival rate was 53 percent when all clinical groups and subtypes were evaluated together in a study of 344 cases (80). The Intergroup Rhabdomyosarcoma Study uses the same clinical groups for alveolar rhabdomyosarcoma as they do for embryonal rhabdomyosarcoma. The 5-year disease-free survival for all patients with group 1 alveolar rhabdomyosarcoma was 57 percent; for group 2, 75 percent; for group 3, 56 percent; and for group 4, 20 percent (65). There was an improvement in the survival rate between the Intergroup Rhabdomyosarcoma Studies I and II with 3-year disease-free survival for all groups increasing from 43 to 69 percent (73). In a French series, the 5-year survival rate was only 5 percent among patients with clinically positive lymph nodes and there were no survivors among patients with distant metastases (80); the overall survival rate for all stages at 5 years was 44 percent. There are reports which suggest that identification of the fusion gene status may be associated with distinct clinical features and outcome (69,75). The PAX3-FKHR gene protein was found more commonly among patients with metastases at multiple sites at presentation while the PAX7-FKHR gene protein was found more commonly in younger patients with group 1 or 2 tumors presenting in an extremity (69,75). Metastases are similar in distribution but twice as common for alveolar rhabdomyosarcoma compared to embryonal rhabdomyosarcoma; the most common sites are lung (60 percent), lymph nodes (50 percent), bone (40 percent), and brain and liver (25 percent each) (89).

Pleomorphic Rhabdomyosarcoma

Definition. Pleomorphic rhabdomyosarcoma is a high-grade sarcoma composed of large, bizarre, polygonal, round and spindle-shaped cells, some of which demonstrate evidence of skeletal muscle differentiation.

General Considerations. In the distant past, many otherwise undifferentiated pleomorphic sarcomas were classified as pleomorphic rhabdomyosarcoma, even though the constituent cells rarely contained cytoplasmic cross-striations, the only evidence of skeletal muscle differentiation available by light microscopy. With the advent of the fibrous histiocytoma concept, these pleomorphic sarcomas were reclassified as pleomorphic malignant fibrous histiocytoma unless cytoplasmic cross-striations were found, an extremely rare event. When antibodies against skeletal muscle proteins became available, there was renewed interest in determining if a subset of the tumors classified as a pleomorphic malignant fibrous histiocytoma contained cells that expressed skeletal muscle antigens, thus qualifying them as pleomorphic rhabdomyosarcoma. Some success in this endeavor has been reported, but whether patient care resources should be spent to distinguish among sarcomas that will be treated the same and have the same outcome is controversial. This issue is further explored in chapter 1 and the introduction to the chapter devoted to the fibrous histiocytomas (chapter 3).

Clinical Features. The most common primary site is the deep soft tissue of the lower extremity (97). Other sites include the chest wall, upper extremity, pelvis, and retroperitoneum (98). The tumor occurs predominantly in middle-aged and elderly males. Patients present with a rapidly growing, sometimes painful mass.

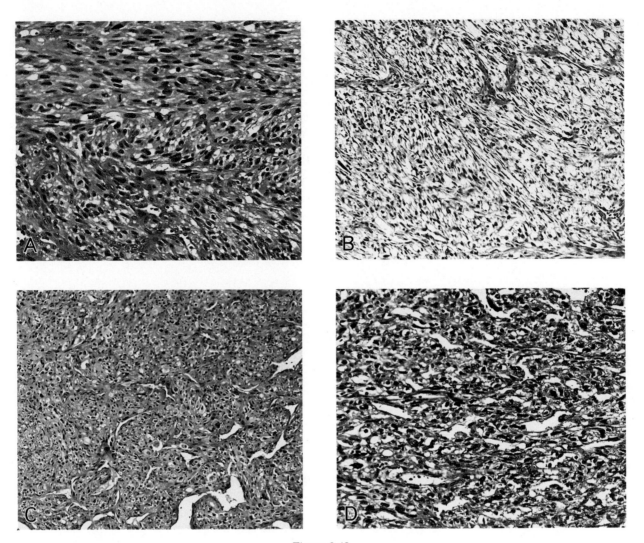

Figure 6-43
ADULT PLEOMORPHIC RHABDOMYOSARCOMA
The cells in pleomorphic rhabdomyosarcoma may be arranged in fascicular, storiform, hemangiopericytoma-like, and patternless patterns, identical to patterns seen in other pleomorphic sarcomas.

Pathologic Findings. The tumors are typically large, usually measuring between 10 and 30 cm, are often lobulated and seemingly well circumscribed, red-gray, and firm. Hemorrhagic and yellow-white areas of necrosis are common.

The microscopic appearance is essentially identical to that of pleomorphic malignant fibrous histiocytoma, with an admixture of spindle-shaped and pleomorphic polygonal and round, often bizarre cells arranged in fascicular, storiform, hemangiopericytoma-like, and patternless patterns (figs. 6-43) (95,97,98). Large areas of necrosis and dense lymphohistiocytic infiltrates

are evident in the majority of cases. In some cases there are large myxoid areas containing pleomorphic cells which simulate myxoid malignant fibrous histiocytoma. Large polygonal and spindle-, tadpole-, and racquet-shaped cells are present and usually prominent. These are indistinguishable from the cells found in other types of adult pleomorphic sarcomas unless cytoplasmic cross-striations are identified, an occurrence so rare that it is hardly worthwhile searching for (fig. 6-44) (95,97,98). The nuclei typically are oval or round and vesicular or hyperchromatic, with large, sometimes multiple nucleoli. The

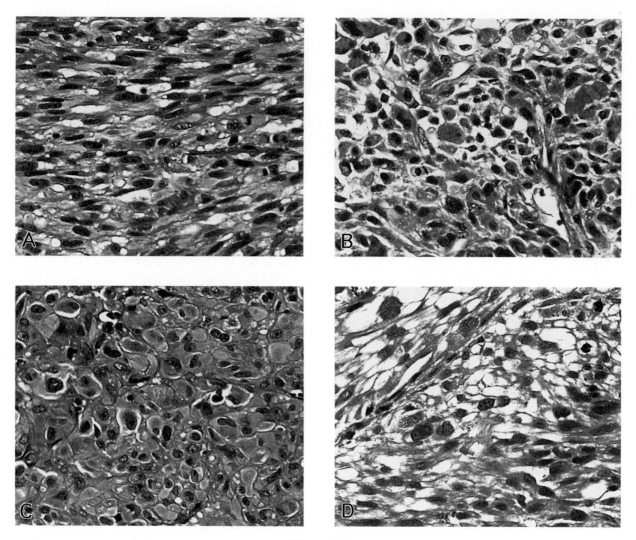

Figure 6-44
ADULT PLEOMORPHIC RHABDOMYOSARCOMA
The cells in pleomorphic rhabdomyosarcoma may be spindled (A), pleomorphic and polygonal (B), contain abundant eosinophilic cytoplasm (C), or have clear cytoplasm due to artifactual washing out of glycogen (D). Similar cells are seen in leiomyosarcoma, liposarcoma, and malignant fibrous histiocytoma. The diagnosis is based upon immunohistologic and ultrastructural features of skeletal muscle differentiation.

cytoplasm is abundant in many cells and is most often deeply eosinophilic and granular (fig. 6-44C). Because cells with cross-striations are essentially not found by light microscopy, evidence of skeletal muscle differentiation must be sought by immunohistology or electron microscopy. The tumor cells may contain abundant glycogen which can result in a clear, foamy, or coarsely vacuolated cytoplasm (fig. 6-44D). Most pleomorphic rhabdomyosarcomas contain more than 10 mitoses per 10 high-power fields and abnormal mitotic figures, often bizarre, are easily found in most tumors.

Special Studies. Because cross-striations, emblematic of skeletal muscle, are almost never found in hematoxylin and eosin–stained sections of pleomorphic rhabdomyosarcoma, the diagnosis is essentially always made by immunohistologic or fine structural techniques. In our opinion, for a diagnosis of pleomorphic rhabdomyosarcoma based on immunohistochemistry, at least some tumor cells must express desmin and muscle-specific actin (96–98) and one or more of the following: monoclonal myoglobin, MyoD1, myogenin, or fast myosin (94a,99,100). As far as is known currently, these latter four are specific skeletal muscle proteins not expressed by other types of cells. Alpha-sarcomeric actin is also expressed by the tumor cells of pleomorphic rhabdomyosarcoma (97,98) but is much less specific and is not used by us. Smooth muscle actin is also often expressed, but its nonspecificity makes it less useful.

Electron microscopy can also reveal evidence of skeletal muscle differentiation and can be used either as an adjunct to immunologic techniques or as the sole evidence of such differentiation. Ultrastructurally, the features pointing to skeletal muscle differentiation (97,98) are identical to those described in the section concerning embryonal rhabdomyosarcoma.

No consistent cytogenetic abnormality has been described in pleomorphic rhabdomyosarcoma.

Differential Diagnosis. The differential diagnosis of pleomorphic rhabdomyosarcoma is essentially the same as that for pleomorphic malignant fibrous histiocytoma (see chapter 3). When confronted with a pleomorphic sarcomatous-appearing neoplasm in the soft tissue, we often use a small panel of antibodies to determine whether the tumor is metastatic carcinoma or melanoma. Whether this should be performed in every case of pleomorphic sarcoma is currently controversial, but if there is any doubt it is better to perform the stains. The initial panel most often includes antibodies against cytokeratin, epithelial membrane antigen, S-100 protein, desmin, and muscle-specific actin, assuming lymphoma is not a consideration. On occasion, anaplastic large cell lymphoma can simulate a pleomorphic sarcoma, and the constituent lymphoma cells may be CD45 negative. Consequently, T- and B-cell markers should be utilized if lymphoma is possible and the CD45 stain is negative.

The next step is consideration of other pleomorphic sarcomas, particularly malignant fibrous histiocytoma, pleomorphic liposarcoma (requires identification of lipoblasts), pleomorphic leiomyosarcoma (requires spindle cells with evidence of smooth muscle differentiation arranged at least focally in fascicles), and malignant peripheral nervous sheath tumor (requires origin from a nerve or a neurofibroma). Myxoid malignant fibrous histiocytoma enters the differential diagnosis because the stroma of pleomorphic rhabdomyosarcoma may be myxoid as well. Desmin, muscle specific actin, alpha-sarcomeric actin, MyoD1, and monoclonal myoglobin antibodies can be used to identify pleomorphic rhabdomyosarcoma (desmin is positive also in smooth muscle tumors), and CD68 often marks malignant fibrous histiocytoma, although it also marks many other types of cells.

The possibility of a rhabdomyosarcomatous component in a tumor of another type should be kept in mind. In particular, Triton tumor should be considered when there is evidence of nerve origin or neurofibromatosis, and dedifferentiated liposarcoma when there is a large retroperitoneal neoplasm. Study of other areas of the tumor may resolve the question.

Treatment and Prognosis. There are very few studies which have examined the long-term course and prognosis of patients who develop this pleomorphic neoplasm, because it is rare and because diagnostic criteria have been in flux. However, in reported cases with follow-up, a majority of patients died of disseminated neoplasm within 1 year of presentation (97,98). The lung is the most common site of metastatic disease (97,98).

REFERENCES

Rhabdomyoma

1. Crotty PL, Nakhleh RE, Dehner LP. Juvenile rhabdomyoma. An intermediate form of skeletal muscle tumor in children. Arch Pathol Lab Med 1993;117:43–7.
2. Dahl I, Angervall L, Save-Soderbergh J. Foetal rhabdomyoma. Case report of a patient with two tumours. Acta Pathol Microbiol Scand [A] 1976;84:107–12.
3. Dehner LP, Enzinger FM, Font RL. Fetal rhabdomyoma. An analysis of nine cases. Cancer 1972;30:160–6.
4. Di Sant'Agnese PA, Knowles DM. Extracardiac rhabdomyoma: a clinicopathologic study and review of the literature. Cancer 1980;46:780–9.
5. Di Santo S, Abt AB, Boal DK, Krummel TM. Fetal rhabdomyoma and nevoid basal cell carcinoma syndrome. Pediatr Pathol 1992;12:441–7.
6. Enzinger FM, Weiss SW. Soft tissue tumors. 3rd ed. St. Louis: Mosby, 1995:1084–5.
7. Eusebi V, Ceccarelli C, Daniele E, Collina G, Viale G, Mancini AM. Extracardiac rhabdomyoma: an immunocytochemical study and review of the literature. Appl Pathol 1988;6:197–207.
8. Helliwell TR, Sissons MC, Stoney PJ, Ashworth MT. Immunochemistry and electron microscopy of head and neck rhabdomyoma. J Clin Pathol 1988;41:1058–63.
9. Kapadia SB, Meis JM, Frisman DM, Ellis GL, Heffner DK. Fetal rhabdomyoma of the head and neck: a clinicopathologic and immunophenotypic study of 24 cases. Hum Pathol 1993;24:754–65.
10. Kapadia SB, Meis JM, Frisman DM, Ellis GL, Heffner DK, Hyams VJ. Adult rhabdomyoma of the head and neck: a clinicopathologic and immunophenotypic study. Hum Pathol 1993;24:608–17.
11. Kodet R, Fajstavr J, Kabelka Z, Koutecky J, Eckschlager T, Newton WA Jr. Is fetal cellular rhabdomyoma an entity or a differentiated rhabdomyosarcoma? A study of patients with rhabdomyoma of the tongue and sarcoma of the tongue enrolled in the intergroup rhabdomyosarcoma studies I, II, and III. Cancer 1991;67:2907–13.
12. Morra MN, Manson AL, Gavrell GJ, Quinn AD. Rhabdomyoma of prostate. Urology 1992;39:271–3.
12a. Tanda F, Rocca PC, Bosincu L, Massarelli G, Cossu A, Manca A. Rhabdomyoma of the tunica vaginalis of the testis: a histologic, immunohistochemical, and ultrastructural study. Mod Pathol 1997;10:608–11.
13. Urbanke VA. Reines rhabdomyom der gebarmutter. Zbl Allg Path Bd 1962;103:241–3.
14. Wang NP, Marx J, McNutt MA, Rutledge JC, Gown AM. Expression of myogenic regulatory proteins (myogenin and MyoD1) in small blue round cell tumors of childhood. Am J Pathol 1995;147:1799–810.
15. Willis J, Abdul-Karim FW, di Sant'Agnese PA. Extracardiac rhabdomyomas. Semin Diagn Pathol 1994;11:15–25.

Neuromuscular Hamartoma

16. Boman F, Palau C, Floquet A, Floquet J, Lascombes P. Neuromuscular hamartoma. Ann Pathol 1991;11:36–41.
17. Bonneau R, Brochu P. Neuromuscular choristoma. A clinicopathologic study of two cases. Am J Surg Pathol 1983;7:521–8.
18. Chen KT. Neuromuscular hamartoma. J Surg Oncol 1984;26:158–60.
19. Markel SF, Enzinger FM. Neuromuscular hamartoma—a benign "triton tumor" composed of mature neural and striated muscle elements. Cancer 1982;49:140–4.
20. Mitchell A, Scheithauer BW, Ostertag H, Sepehrnia A, Sav A. Neuromuscular choristoma. Am J Clin Pathol 1995;103:460–5.
21. O'Connell JX, Rosenberg AE. Multiple cutaneous neuromuscular choristomas. Report of a case and a review of the literature. Am J Surg Pathol 1990;14:93–6.
22. Orlandi E. Sopra un caso di rhabdomioma del nervo ischiatico. Arch Sci Med (Torino) 1895;19:113–37.
23. Tiffee JC, Barnes EL. Neuromuscular hamartomas of the head and neck. Arch Otolaryngol Head Neck Surg 1998;124:212–6.
24. Van Dorpe J, Sciot R, De Vos R, Uyttebroeck A, Stas M, Van Damme B. Neuromuscular choristoma (hamartoma) with smooth and striated muscle component: case report with immunohistochemical and ultrastructural analysis. Am J Surg Pathol 1997;21:1090–5.

Rhabdomyosarcoma: Introduction

25. Horn RC, Enterline HT. Rhabdomyosarcoma: a clinicopathological study and classification of 39 cases. Cancer 1958;11:181–99.
25a. Qualman SJ, Coffin CM, Newton WA, et al. Intergroup Rhabdomyosarcoma Study: update for pathologists. Pediatr Dev Pathol 1998;1:550–61.

Embryonal Rhabdomyosarcoma

26. Altmannsberger M, Weber K, Droste R, Osborn M. Desmin is a specific marker for rhabdomyosarcomas of human and rat origin. Am J Pathol 1985;118:85–95.
27. Bale PM, Reye RD. Rhabdomyosarcoma in childhood. Pathology 1975;7:101–11.
28. Cavazzana AO, Schmidt D, Ninfo V, et al. Spindle cell rhabdomyosarcoma. A prognostically favorable variant of rhabdomyosarcoma. Am J Surg Pathol 1992;16:229–35.
29. Crist W, Gehan EA, Ragab AH, et al. The Third Intergroup Rhabdomyosarcoma Study. J Clin Oncol 1995;13:610–30.
29a. Cui S, Hano H, Harada T, Takai S, Masui F, Ushigome S. Evaluation of new monoclonal anti-MyoD1 and antimyogenin antibodies for the diagnosis of rhabdomyosarcoma. Pathol Int 1999;29:62–8.

30. Daya DA, Scully RE. Sarcoma botryoides of the uterine cervix in young women: a clinicopathological study of 13 cases. Gynecol Oncol 1988;29:290–304.

31. de Alava E, Ladanyi M, Rosai J, Gerald WL. Detection of chimeric transcripts in desmoplastic small round cell tumor and related developmental tumors by reverse transcriptase polymerase chain reaction. A specific diagnostic assay. Am J Pathol 1995;147:1584–91.

32. Dodd S, Malone M, McCulloch W. Rhabdomyosarcoma in children: a histological and immunohistochemical study of 59 cases. J Pathol 1989;158:13–8.

33. Douglass EC, Shapiro DN, Valentine M, et al. Alveolar rhabdomyosarcoma with the t(2;13): cytogenetic findings and clinicopathologic correlations. Med Pediatr Oncol 1993;21:83–7.

34. Horn RC, Enterline HT. Rhabdomyosarcoma: a clinicopathological study and classification of 39 cases. Cancer 1958;11:181–99.

35. Kodet R. Rhabdomyosarcoma in childhood. An immunohistological analysis with myoglobin, desmin and vimentin. Pathol Res Pract 1989;185:207–13.

36. Kodet R, Newton WJ, Hamoudi AB, Asmar L. Rhabdomyosarcomas with intermediate–filament inclusions and features of rhabdoid tumors. Light microscopic and immunohistochemical study. Am J Surg Pathol 1991;15:257–67.

37. Kodet R, Newton WJ, Hamoudi AB, Asmar L, Jacobs DL, Maurer HM. Childhood rhabdomyosarcoma with anaplastic (pleomorphic) features. A report of the Intergroup Rhabdomyosarcoma Study. Am J Surg Pathol 1993;17:443–53.

38. Lawrence W, Gehan EA, Hays DM, Beltangady M, Maurer HM. Prognostic significance of staging factors of the UICC staging system in childhood rhabdomyosarcoma: a report from the Intergroup Rhabdomyosarcoma Study (IRS–II). J Clin Oncol 1987;5:46–54.

39. Leuschner I, Newton WJ Jr, Schmidt D, et al. Spindle cell variants of embryonal rhabdomyosarcoma in the paratesticular region. A report of the Intergroup Rhabdomyosarcoma Study. Am J Surg Pathol 1993;17:221–30.

40. Maurer HM, Beltangady M, Gehan EA, et al. The Intergroup Rhabdomyosarcoma Study–I. A final report. Cancer 1988;61:209–20.

41. Mierau GW, Favara BE. Rhabdomyosaracoma in children. Ultrastructural study of 31 cases. Cancer 1980;46:2035–40.

42. Molenaar WM, Dam-Meiring A, Kamps WA, Cornelisse CJ. DNA-aneuploidy in rhabdomyosarcomas as compared with other sarcomas of childhood and adolescence. Hum Pathol 1988;19:573–9.

43. Molenaar WM, Oosterhuis JW, Kamps WA. Cytologic "differentiation" in childhood rhabdomyosarcomas following polychemotherapy. Hum Pathol 1984;15:973–9.

44. Nayar RC, Prudhomme F, Parise O Jr, Gandia D, Luboinski B, Schwaab G. Rhabdomyosarcoma of the head and neck in adults: a study of 26 patients. Laryngoscope 1993;103:1362–6.

45. Newton WA Jr, Gehan EA, Webber BL, et al. Classification of rhabdomyosarcomas and related sarcomas. Pathologic aspects and proposal for a new classification—an Intergroup Rhabdomyosarcoma Study. Cancer 1995;76:1073–85.

46. Newton WA Jr, Soule EH, Hamoudi AB, et al. Histopathology of childhood sarcomas, Intergroup Rhabdomyosarcoma Studies I and II: clinicopathologic correlation. J Clin Oncol 1988;6:67–75.

47. Norris HJ, Taylor HB. Polyps of the vagina. A benign lesion resembling sarcoma botryoides. Cancer 1966;19:227–32.

48. Pappo AS, Crist WM, Kuttesch J, et al. Tumor-cell DNA content predicts outcome in children and adolescents with clinical group III embryonal rhabdomyosarcoma. The Intergroup Rhabdomyosarcoma Study Committee of the Children's Cancer Group and the Pediatric Oncology Group. J Clin Oncol 1993;11:1901–5.

48a. Pawel BR, Hamoui AB, Asmar L, et al. Undifferentiated sarcoma of children: pathology and clinical behavior—an Intergroup Rhabdomyosarcoma Study. Med Pediatr Oncol 1997;29:170–80.

49. Pinto A, Paslawski D, Sarnat HB, Parham DM. Immunohistochemical evaluation of dystrophin expression in small round cell tumors of childhood. Mod Pathol 1993;6:679–83.

50. Ramani P, Rampling D, Link M. Immunocytochemical study of 12E7 in small round-cell tumours of childhood: an assessment of its sensitivity and specificity. Histopathology 1993;23:557–61.

51. Schmidt D, Leuschner I, Moeller R, Harms D. Immunohistochemical findings in rhabdomyosarcoma. Pathologe 1990;11:283–9.

52. Schmidt RA, Cone R, Haas JE, Gown AM. Diagnosis of rhabdomyosarcomas with HHF35, a monoclonal antibody directed against muscle actins. Am J Pathol 1988;131:19–28.

53. Seidal T, Kindblom LG, Angervall L. Rhabdomyosarcoma in middle-aged and elderly individuals. APMIS 1989;97:236–48.

54. Seidal T, Walaas L, Kindblom LG, Angervall L. Cytology of embryonal rhabdomyosarcoma: a cytologic, light microscopic, electron microscopic, and immunohistochemical study of seven cases. Diagn Cytopathol 1988;4:292–9.

55. Shapiro DN, Sublett JE, Li B, Downing JR, Naeve CW. Fusion of PAX3 to a member of the forkhead family of transcription factors in human alveolar rhabdomyosarcoma. Cancer Res 1993;53:5108–12.

56. Shimada H, Newton WJ, Soule EH, Beltangady MS, Maurer HM. Pathology of fatal rhabdomyosarcoma. Report from Intergroup Rhabdomyosarcoma Study (IRS-I and IRS-II). Cancer 1987;59:459–65.

57. Sorensen PH, Shimada H, Liu XF, Lim JF, Thomas G, Triche TJ. Biphenotypic sarcomas with myogenic and neural differentiation express the Ewing's sarcoma EWS/FLI1 fusion gene. Cancer Res 1995;55:1385–92.

58. Tallini G, Parham DM, Dias P, Cordon-Cardo C, Houghton PJ, Rosai J. Myogenic regulatory protein expression in adult soft tissue sarcomas. A sensitive and specific marker of skeletal muscle differentiation. Am J Pathol 1994;144:693–701.

59. Triche TJ. Pathology of pediatric malignancies. In: Pizzo PA, Poplack DG, ed. Principles and practice of pediatric oncology. Philadelphia: JB Lippincott, 1993:115–52.

60. Wang NP, Marx J, McNutt MA, Rutledge JC, Gown AM. Expression of myogenic regulatory proteins (myogenin and MyoD1) in small blue round cell tumors of childhood. Am J Pathol 1995;147:1799–810.

Alveolar Rhabdomyosarcoma

61. Ambros IM, Ambros PF, Strehl S, Kovar H, Gadner H, Salzer KM. MIC2 is a specific marker for Ewing's sarcoma and peripheral primitive neuroectodermal tumors. Evidence for a common histogenesis of Ewing's sarcoma and peripheral primitive neuroectodermal tumors from MIC2 expression and specific chromosome aberration. Cancer 1991;67:1886–93.

62. Barr FG, Galili N, Holick J, Biegel JA, Rovera G, Emanuel BS. Rearrangement of the PAX3 paired box gene in the paediatric solid tumour alveolar rhabdomyosarcoma. Nat Genet 1993;3:113–7.

63. Barr FG, Holick J, Nycum L, Biegel JA, Emanuel BS. Localization of the t(2;13) breakpoint of alveolar rhabdomyosarcoma on a physical map of chromosome 2. Genomics 1992;13:1150–6.

64. Churg A, Ringus J. Ultrastructural observations on the histogenesis of alveolar rhabdomyosarcoma. Cancer 1978;41:1355–61.

65. Crist WM, Garnsey L, Beltangady MS, et al. Prognosis in children with rhabdomyosarcoma: a report of the Intergroup Rhabdomyosarcoma Studies I and II. Intergroup Rhabdomyosarcoma Committee. J Clin Oncol 1990;8:443–52.

65a. Cui S, Hano H, Harada T, Takai S, Masui F, Ushigome S. Evaluation of new monoclonal anti-MyoD1 and anti-myogenin antibodies for the diagnosis of rhabdomyosarcoma. Pathol Int 1999;29:62–8.

66. Davis RJ, D'Cruz CM, Lovell MA, Biegel JA, Barr FG. Fusion of PAX7 to FKHR by the variant t(1;13) (p36;q14) translocation in alveolar rhabdomyosarcoma. Cancer Res 1994;54:2869–72.

67. de Alava E, Ladanyi M, Rosai J, Gerald WL. Detection of chimeric transcripts in desmoplastic small round cell tumor and related developmental tumors by reverse transcriptase polymerase chain reaction. A specific diagnostic assay. Am J Pathol 1995;147:1584–91.

67a. de Alava E, Lozano MD, Sola I, et al. Molecular features in a biphenotypic small cell sarcoma with neuroectodermal and muscle differentiation. Hum Pathol 1998;29:181–4.

68. Dodd S, Malone M, McCulloch W. Rhabdomyosarcoma in children: a histological and immunohistochemical study of 59 cases. J Pathol 1989;158:13–8.

69. Douglass EC, Shapiro DN, Valentine M, et al. Alveolar rhabdomyosarcoma with the t(2;13): cytogenetic findings and clinicopathologic correlations. Med Pediatr Oncol 1993;21:83–7.

70. Downing JR, Khandekar A, Shurtleff SA, et al. Multiplex RT-PCR assay for the differential diagnosis of alveolar rhabdomyosarcoma and Ewing's sarcoma. Am J Pathol 1995;146:626–34.

70a. Flamant F, Rodary C, Rey A, et al. Treatment of non-metastatic rhabdomyosarcomas in childhood and adolescence. Results of the second study of the International Society of Paediatric Oncology: MMT84. Eur J Cancer 1998;32:1050–62.

71. Fredericks WJ, Galili N, Mukhopadhyay S, et al. The PAX3-FKHR fusion protein created by the t(2;13) translocation in alveolar rhabdomyosarcomas is a more potent transcriptional activator than PAX3. Mol Cell Biol 1995;15:1522–35.

72. Gonzalez-Crussi F, Black-Schaffer S. Rhabdomyosarcoma of infancy and childhood. Problems of morphologic classification. Am J Surg Pathol 1979;3:157–71.

73. Heyn R, Beltangady M, Hays D, et al. Results of intensive therapy in children with localized alveolar extremity rhabdomyosarcoma: a report from the Intergroup Rhabdomyosarcoma Study. J Clin Oncol 1989;7:200–7.

74. Horn RC, Enterline HT. Rhabdomyosarcoma: a clinicopathological study and classification of 39 cases. Cancer 1958;11:181–99.

75. Kelly KM, Womer RB, Sorensen PH, Xiong QB, Barr FG. Common and variant gene fusions predict distinct clinical phenotypes in rhabdomyosarcoma. J Clin Oncol 1997;15:1831–6.

76. Kodet R, Newton WA Jr, Hamoudi AB, Asmar L. Rhabdomyosarcomas with intermediate-filament inclusions and features of rhabdoid tumors. Light microscopic and immunohistochemical study. Am J Surg Pathol 1991;15:257–67.

77. Kodet R, Newton WA Jr, Hamoudi AB, Asmar L, Jacobs DL, Maurer HM. Childhood rhabdomyosarcoma with anaplastic (pleomorphic) features. A report of the Intergroup Rhabdomyosarcoma Study. Am J Surg Pathol 1993;17:443–53.

78. Miettinen M, Rapola J. Immunohistochemical spectrum of rhabdomyosarcoma and rhabdomyosarcoma–like tumors. Expression of cytokeratin and the 68-kD neurofilament protein. Am J Surg Pathol 1989;13:120–32.

79. Newton WA Jr, Gehan EA, Webber BL, et al. Classification of rhabdomyosarcomas and related sarcomas. Pathologic aspects and proposal for a new classification–an Intergroup Rhabdomyosarcoma Study. Cancer 1995;76:1073–85.

80. Newton WA Jr, Soule EH, Hamoudi AB, et al. Histopathology of childhood sarcomas, Intergroup Rhabdomyosarcoma Studies I and II: clinicopathologic correlation. J Clin Oncol 1988;6:67–75.

81. Parham DM, Shapiro DN, Downing JR, Webber BL, Douglass EC. Solid alveolar rhabdomyosarcomas with the t(2;13). Report of two cases with diagnostic implications. Am J Surg Pathol 1994;18:474–8.

82. Ramani P, Rampling D, Link M. Immunocytochemical study of 12E7 in small round-cell tumours of childhood: an assessment of its sensitivity and specificity. Histopathology 1993;23:557–61.

83. Reboul MJ, Quintana E, Mosseri V, et al. Prognostic factors of alveolar rhabdomyosarcoma in childhood. An International Society of Pediatric Oncology study. Cancer 1991;68:493–8.

84. Rosai J, Dias P, Parham DM, Shapiro DN, Houghton P. MyoD1 protein expression in alveolar soft part sarcomas as confirmatory evidence of its skeletal muscle nature. Am J Surg Pathol 1991;15:974–81.

85. Schmidt D, Leuschner I, Moeller R, Harms D. [Immunohistochemical findings in rhabdomyosarcoma]. Pathologe 1990;11:283–289.

86. Seidal T, Kindblom LG, Angervall L. Alveolar and poorly differentiated rhabdomyosarcoma. A clinicopathologic, light-microscopic, ultrastructural and immunohistochemical analysis. APMIS 1988;96:825–38.

87. Seidal T, Mark J, Hagmar B, Angervall L. Alveolar rhabdomyosarcoma: a cytogenetic and correlated cytological and histological study. Acta Pathol Microbiol Immunol Scand 1982;90:345–54.

88. Shapiro DN, Sublett JE, Li B, Downing JR, Naeve CW. Fusion of PAX3 to a member of the forkhead family of transcription factors in human alveolar rhabdomyosarcoma. Cancer Res 1993;53:5108–12.

89. Shimada H, Newton WA Jr, Soule EH, Beltangady MS, Maurer HM. Pathology of fatal rhabdomyosarcoma. Report from Intergroup Rhabdomyosarcoma Study (IRS-I and IRS-II). Cancer 1987;59:459–65.

90. Triche TJ. Pathology of pediatric malignancies. In: Pizzo PA, Poplack DG, eds. Principles and practice of pediatric oncology. Philadelphia: JB Lippincott, 1993:115–52.

91. Tsokos M, Howard R, Costa J. Immunohistochemical study of alveolar and embryonal rhabdomyosarcoma. Lab Invest 1983;48:148–55.

92. Wang N, Bacchi C, Jiang J, McNutt M, Gown A. Does alveolar soft-part sarcoma exhibit skeletal muscle differentiation? An immunocytochemical and biochemical study of myogenic regulatory protein expression. Mod Pathol 1996;9:496–506.

93. Wang NP, Marx J, McNutt MA, Rutledge JC, Gown AM. Expression of myogenic regulatory proteins (myogenin and MyoD1) in small blue round cell tumors of childhood. Am J Pathol 1995;147:1799–810.

94. Whang PJ, Knutsen T, Theil K, Horowitz ME, Triche T. Cytogenetic studies in subgroups of rhabdomyosarcoma. Genes Chromosom Cancer 1992;5:299–310.

Pleomorphic Rhabdomyosarcoma

94a. Cui S, Hano H, Harada T, Takai S, Masui F, Ushigome S. Evaluation of new monoclonal anti-MyoD1 and anti-myogenin antibodies for the diagnosis of rhabdomyosarcoma. Pathol Int 1999;29:62–8.

95. Enzinger FM, Weiss SW. Soft tissue tumors. 3rd ed. St. Louis: Mosby, 1995:1084–5.

96. Fletcher CD. Pleomorphic malignant fibrous histiocytoma: fact or fiction? Am J Surg Pathol 1992;16:213–28.

97. Gaffney EF, Dervan PA, Fletcher CD. Pleomorphic rhabdomyosarcoma in adulthood. Analysis of 11 cases with definition of diagnostic criteria. Am J Surg Pathol 1993;17:601–9.

98. Schürch W, Bégin LR, Seemayer TA, et al. Pleomorphic soft tissue myogenic sarcomas of adulthood. A reappraisal in the mid-1990s. Am J Surg Pathol 1996;20:131–47.

99. Tallini G, Parham DM, Dias P, Cordon-Cardo C, Houghton PJ, Rosai J. Myogenic regulatory protein expression in adult soft tissue sarcomas. A sensitive and specific marker of skeletal muscle differentiation. Am J Pathol 1994;144:693–701.

100. Wesche WA, Fletcher CD, Dias P, Houghton PJ, Parham DM. Immunohistochemistry of MyoD1 in adult pleomorphic soft tissue sarcomas. Am J Surg Pathol 1995;19:261–9.

7
VASCULAR TUMORS

INTRODUCTION

Vascular tumors represent one of the largest groups of soft tissue tumors. A classification scheme is shown in Table 7-1. The tumors are histologically and clinically heterogeneous and, considering their ubiquity, are not at all well understood. The majority of vascular lesions are clinically benign. Angiosarcomas as well as the group of lesions that might be regarded as of low-grade or intermediate malignancy are rare, yet the capacity of benign lesions to mimic more aggressive tumors, both clinically and morphologically, is considerable and hence pathologists often find themselves having to rule out a malignant diagnosis. Frequently, this is not as straightforward as it sounds. As a rule (within which there are inevitably occasional exceptions), the presence of a lobular growth pattern favors benignity, while the presence of endothelial multilayering, particularly if accompanied by nuclear hyperchromasia, pleomorphism, and mitotic activity, favors malignancy. Endothelial atypia alone (without multilayering) or the presence of a dissecting growth pattern alone does not equate with angiosarcoma and may be seen in a variety of benign lesions, as is discussed in the following text.

Given the morphologic heterogeneity of endothelial tumors it is worth noting that vascular differentiation may take many forms, ranging from the development of obvious canalized vessels, to the presence only of intracytoplasmic lumina, to a solid, sheet-like or spindle cell growth pattern. Electron microscopy is often not adequate for proving endothelial differentiation in the more anaplastic lesions, due to the problems of sampling error and the frequent scarcity of Weibel-Palade bodies (the pathognomonic ultrastructural feature of endothelial cells). So long as tissue is suitably fixed, probably the most sensitive and reliable way of proving that a lesion is endothelial is by immunohistochemistry, particularly using antibodies to CD31 or von Willebrand factor (VWF).

Quite a range of agents has been used over the past 15 years for the immunohistochemical analysis of vascular tumors and the following comments reflect our general experience. Antibodies directed against CD31 and VWF are, for all practical purposes, specific for endothelial cells (in the setting of a soft tissue neoplasm). However, they differ in that CD31 is very sensitive whereas VWF stains a smaller proportion of cases. Among angiosarcomas, more than 95 percent are CD31 positive, whereas VWF stains no more than 50 to 60 percent (with a higher percentage among epithelioid lesions). CD34 also stains a high proportion of cases but is nonspecific, being also expressed in a wide variety of spindle cell tumors, such as dermatofibrosarcoma, solitary fibrous tumor, schwannoma, and gastrointestinal stromal tumors to name but a small selection. The lectin *Ulex europaeus* I, although popular in the past, has largely been superceded due both to its marked nonspecificity as well as the requirement for using a different direct technique. Although CD31 is the best endothelial marker (1a), there are some tumors which stain for only one (or perhaps two) of the most popular antigens (CD31, VWF, and CD34); therefore, in occasional cases in which a vascular neoplasm is strongly suspected but is CD31 negative, it is worth using antibodies to VWF and CD34 also. In practice, other endothelial antigens have failed to gain widespread popularity, either because they work only in specially fixed or frozen tissue, or because of relative nonspecificity. Until recently, no antibody (at least in paraffin sections) has been able to distinguish reliably between blood vascular and lymphatic endothelium, but vascular endothelial growth factor receptor-3 (VEGFR-3) shows considerable promise in this regard (1b).

There are three main areas which remain largely unresolved concerning vascular tumors. First, it remains uncertain whether some of the more common benign lesions are or are not neoplastic. Specifically, it is unclear whether juvenile capillary hemangiomas are malformations (hamartomas) or benign clonal (neoplastic) proliferations, although the former seems most likely. Similarly, it is unknown whether the ubiquitous pyogenic granuloma (lobular capillary

Table 7-1

VASCULAR TUMORS

BLOOD VESSELS

Benign
(Managerial Categories Ia and Ib, Table 1-10)

Reactive vascular proliferations
  Papillary endothelial hyperplasia (Masson's tumor)
  Reactive angioendotheliomatosis
  Glomeruloid hemangioma
  Bacillary angiomatosis
Vascular ectasias
  Nevus flammeus (salmon patch, port-wine stain)
  Nevus araneus
  Venous lake
  Angioma serpiginosum
  Hereditary hemorrhagic telangiectasia (Osler-Weber-Rendu disease)
  Angiokeratoma
Capillary hemangioma
  Tufted angioma

Verrucous hemangioma
Cherry angioma
Lobular hemangioma (pyogenic granuloma)
Cavernous hemangioma
  Sinusoidal hemangioma
Arteriovenous hemangioma
  Superficial (cirsoid aneurysm)
  Deep
Epithelioid hemangioma (angiolymphoid hyperplasia with eosinophilia)
Microvenular hemangioma
Targetoid hemosiderotic hemangioma ("hobnail" hemangioma)
Venous hemangioma
Spindle cell hemangioma

Intermediate
(Managerial Categories IIa and IIc, Table 1-10)

Deep hemangiomas
  Intramuscular
  Synovial
Angiomatosis
Retiform hemangioendothelioma

Malignant endovascular papillary angioendothelioma of lymph node
Kaposiform hemangioendothelioma
Polymorphous hemangioendothelioma
Giant cell angioblastoma
Kaposi's sarcoma*

Malignant
(Managerial Category III, Table 1-10)

Epithelioid hemangioendothelioma

Angiosarcoma (includes lymphangiosarcoma)
  Associated with lymphedema ("lymphangiosarcoma")
  Epithelioid

LYMPH VESSELS

Lymphangioma
  Lymphangioma circumscriptum
  Cystic hygroma
  Progressive lymphangioma

Lymphangiomatosis

---

*For the reasons why Kaposi's sarcoma is placed in the Intermediate Tumor Category, see General Considerations in the Intermediate Tumor section of the text.

---

hemangioma) is a reactive lesion or a benign neoplasm: there are items of evidence that could point in either direction, which suggests that perhaps the same morphologic pattern can arise by different pathogenetic routes.

Second, there exists a group of vascular tumors that are often labeled "intermediate" or "borderline malignant" in some classifications but have very different biologies, ranging from the certainly benign behavior of spindle cell hemangioma, formerly known as spindle cell hemangioendothelioma (reflected in its position among the benign tumors in Table 7-1), to the malignant (albeit often low grade) behavior of epithelioid hemangioendothelioma, which we have moved to the malignant category based on our current studies. The nosologic status of the remainder of these lesions is under current scrutiny and ongoing review, and much of the remaining uncertainty is due to the relatively small case numbers available for study and the comparatively limited follow-up data. This is an area of continuing conceptual shift and the classification of vascular tumors is likely to be remodified in coming years.

The third major area of persistent difficulty is our inability to reliably distinguish between blood vascular and lymphatic endothelium in normal tissues and in vascular tumors. Despite a wide variety of claims made over the years, there are no definitive ultrastructural differences between such cells nor are there reproducible means of making the distinction immunohistochemically. Certainly, the adage that the presence of intraluminal red blood cells excludes such vessels from being lymphatic in type is mistaken and of no practical value. Because the histogenetic concept of mesenchymal neoplasia has largely fallen from favor, identification of a precise vessel type usually need not worry the pathologist, especially since it seems that some vascular lesions (e.g., intramuscular angioma) often show mixed features. However, lymphatic lesions do exist and general clues to their recognition are the usual presence, at least focally, of vessels with an imperceptibly thin wall as well as vessels with irregular, jagged outlines.

With regard to the above-mentioned unresolved conceptual difficulties, the following text adopts a pragmatic viewpoint, with the principal aim of facilitating accurate diagnosis while avoiding entanglement in presently insoluble controversies. The subclassification of benign vascular lesions has become complex and detailed (see Table 7-1). In general, confusion between benign entities will not have major clinical repercussions; however, some lesions (e.g., microvenular and hobnail hemangiomas or progressive lymphangioma) are easily mistaken for a malignant lesion, with obviously serious clinical implications. Similarly, retiform hemangioendothelioma is often mistaken for angiosarcoma, despite its much less aggressive course. It is for the purpose of separating out these different clinical behaviors that the classification scheme favors a "splitting" rather than "lumping" philosophy. So called intimal sarcomas are covered in the Fascicle, Tumors of the Heart and Great Vessels (1).

BENIGN VASCULAR TUMORS AND TUMOR-LIKE CONDITIONS (MANAGERIAL GROUPS Ia AND Ib, TABLE 1-10)

REACTIVE VASCULAR PROLIFERATIONS

Under this heading are described those lesions that are accepted generally to be non-neoplastic but which clinically and histologically often simulate tumor(s).

Papillary Endothelial Hyperplasia

Definition. Papillary endothelial hyperplasia is a form of organizing thrombus characterized by hyaline papillae covered by an endothelial monolayer. It is also known as *intravascular papillary endothelial hyperplasia, Masson's tumor,* and *Masson's vegetant intravascular hemangioendothelioma.*

Clinical Features. Papillary endothelial hyperplasia is relatively common when associated with thrombosis, either in a normal vessel, a preexisting vascular lesion (e.g., hemorrhoidal vein or hemangioma) or, least often, in an extravascular hematoma (1c–3). The so called *primary type,* occurring in normal vessels, is most common in the fingers or neck, in young adults of either sex; it presents as a painless or occasionally tender nodule. Most examples measure less than 2 cm in diameter. The clinical features of those cases developing in association with a preexistent vascular lesion (*secondary type*) are determined by the nature of the prior pathology. Probably the two most common lesions of this type are cavernous hemangioma and hemorrhoidal veins. Only very rare examples of papillary endothelial hyperplasia are multiple (5) and this usually reflects the multifocality of a preexisting process with superimposed thrombosis; papillary endothelial hyperplasia arising in an extravascular thrombus is extremely uncommon (4).

Pathologic Findings. Most examples of papillary endothelial hyperplasia are obviously intravascular, whether or not the vessel is normal or part of an angioma. Irrespective of the clinical setting in which papillary endothelial hyperplasia arises, its morphologic features are similar and consist primarily of innumerable small papillae with hyaline cores associated with

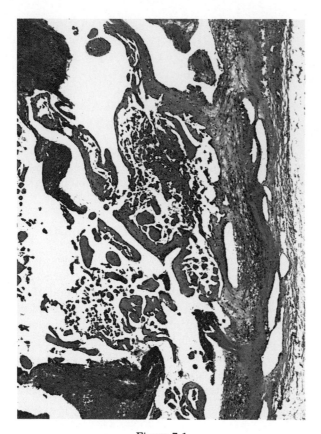

Figure 7-1
PAPILLARY ENDOTHELIAL HYPERPLASIA
Within the lumen of this cavernous angioma there are multiple papillary structures and an adjacent thrombus.

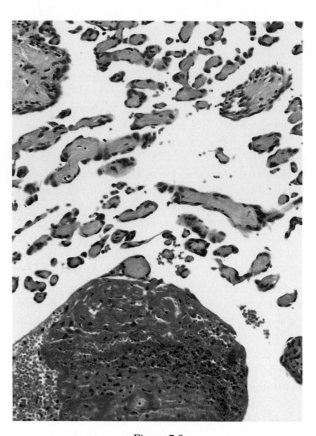

Figure 7-2
PAPILLARY ENDOTHELIAL HYPERPLASIA
The papillae generally have a hyaline core, representing organized thrombus, and are covered by an endothelial monolayer.

an adjacent thrombus (fig. 7-1). Often one can see transition from organizing fibrin thrombus into the papillae, which then seem to fall away from the thrombus. Papillae often have eosinophilic fibrin in their cores. Each papilla appears to develop by a process of hyalinization and the simultaneous development of an attenuated endothelial covering (fig. 7-2). The papillary core generally is acellular but may contain rare thin-walled capillaries. The endothelial cells are always bland and monolayered, and mitotic figures are rare. The characteristic papillae may appear to lie free within vascular lumens or may be attached to the vessel wall.

Special Studies. Stains for fibrin highlight the thrombus and the cores of "younger" papillae, and elastic stains may assist in the identification of any preexisting vessel walls. Additional stains play no real role in this diagnosis.

Differential Diagnosis. The appearance and intravascular location are usually so distinctive that there is no real differential diagnosis. Angiosarcoma is almost never purely intravascular and rarely, if ever, has the same degree of papillarity. The rare examples of angiosarcoma with an intravascular component show endothelial atypia, hyperchromasia, and multilayering. Spindle cell hemangioma (see page 332) may have papillary structures but these are much more cellular and are associated with solid spindle cell areas.

Treatment and Prognosis. This is a benign, nonrecurring process. Any evidence of recurrence after excision, which is exceptional, reflects persistence or regrowth of the preexisting lesion in which the papillary endothelial hyperplasia had occurred.

Reactive Angioendotheliomatosis

Definition. Reactive angioendotheliomatosis is a rare condition of varied etiology which results in a multifocal, benign capillary proliferation, most often (but not exclusively) in the skin. This condition is unrelated to so called malignant angioendotheliomatosis, which is a form of angiotropic lymphoma.

Clinical Features. The clinical features of reactive angioendotheliomatosis are varied, likely reflecting the small case numbers and differing etiologies (8). However, the majority of patients are adults who present with highly variable, cutaneous, erythematous lesions, ranging in appearance from ecchymoses through macules to plaques. Associated clinical conditions include bacterial endocarditis, hepatic or renal failure, peripheral vascular disease (6), paraproteinemia, and cryoglobulinemia (7), although it remains unknown to what extent any of these are truly causative. In the majority of cases the condition is self-limiting within a period of months.

Pathologic Findings. Irrespective of etiology, this process is characterized by a multifocal, discontinuous proliferation of small, close-packed capillaries in the dermis (fig. 7-3) and less often in subcutis. Extravasation of red blood cells is common but there is no endothelial atypia and usually no associated inflammatory response. In those cases associated with abnormal circulating proteins, eosinophilic or hyaline globules (resembling small fibrin thrombi but more refractile) may be seen.

Differential Diagnosis. Diagnosis depends heavily on clinicopathologic correlation since the histologic features may closely resemble the effects of venous stasis in the lower limb. Multifocal Kaposi's sarcoma may be considered in the differential diagnosis but in its patch stage, shows endothelial atypia and a dissecting growth pattern, and in its plaque stage, has a notable spindle cell component as well as plasma cells and hemosiderin deposition.

Glomeruloid Hemangioma

Definition. Glomeruloid hemangioma is a rare, multifocal, usually intravascular capillary proliferation associated, in most cases, with multicentric Castleman's disease.

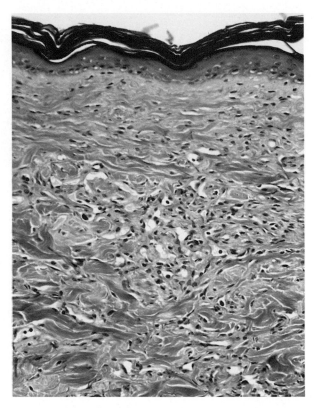

Figure 7-3
REACTIVE ANGIOENDOTHELIOMATOSIS
Within the dermis is a diffuse capillary proliferation. This biopsy comes from a patient in renal failure with multiple erythematous cutaneous macules.

Clinical Features. Glomeruloid hemangioma represents one of the cutaneous manifestations of multicentric Castleman's disease associated with POEMS syndrome (polyneuropathy, organomegaly, endocrinopathy, M-protein, skin changes) (9). Clinically, patients have multiple, cutaneous, angiomatous or bruise-like lesions, many of which histologically resemble ordinary cherry angiomas.

Pathologic Findings. As the name suggests, this lesion is characterized principally by intravascular glomerulus-like proliferations of capillaries within dermal blood vessels (fig. 7-4). These capillaries are clustered to form tufts, with an outer layer of pericytes, and commonly, some of the endothelial cells show cytoplasmic vacuolation (fig. 7-5). Hyaline droplets composed of immunoglobulin are commonly noted in the stroma or within blood vessels. Comparable changes may be seen in vessels in deep soft tissue or visceral locations.

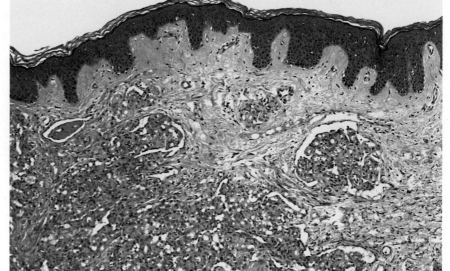

Figure 7-4
GLOMERULOID
HEMANGIOMA
Note the characteristic intra-vascular proliferation of capillary vessels.

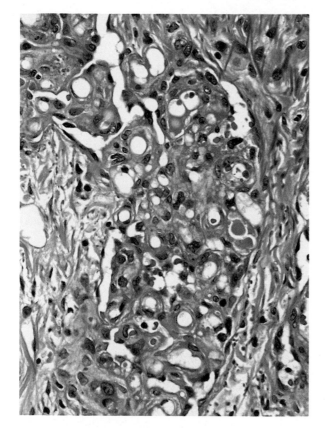

Figure 7-5
GLOMERULOID HEMANGIOMA
A closer view reveals endothelial cytoplasmic vacuoliza-tion and hyaline droplets composed of immunoglobulin.

Differential Diagnosis. Clinically, glomeru-loid hemangioma may resemble Kaposi's sarcoma but there is no histomorphologic overlap (see page 345). There is some similarity to intravascular pyogenic granuloma but the latter occurs as a solitary lesion within a single larger vein.

Bacillary Angiomatosis

This reactive vascular proliferation, which has an infective etiology, is detailed in the Fas-cicle, Non-Melanocytic Tumors of the Skin (9a). Interestingly, due to antimycobacterial prophy-laxis in patients with acquired immunodefi-ciency syndrome (AIDS), its incidence has di-minished both rapidly and considerably.

VASCULAR ECTASIAS

Under this heading, a selection of vascular abnormalities are described which are charac-terized by dilatation of preexisting vessels rather than true proliferation (10,11,14,16). It is highly unlikely that these are true neoplasms.

Nevus Flammeus

Definition. Nevus flammeus (*salmon patch, port-wine stain, nevus telangiectaticus*) is the most common form of birthmark, and is characterized usually by dilatation of thin-walled dermal vessels.

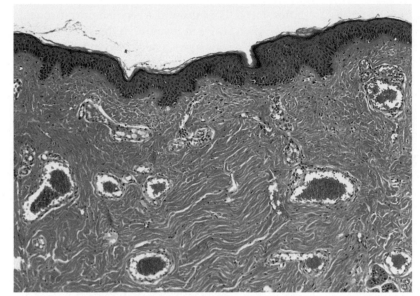

Figure 7-6
PORT-WINE STAIN
Dilated and congested dermal vessels
are the sole histologic abnormality.

Clinical Features. Nevus flammeus is said to occur in 30 to 50 percent of newborn infants, usually on the head, and takes two principal forms (12). The more common is the salmon patch which is a pinkish red, flat macule that regresses spontaneously over time. Those on the face regress more rapidly than those on the neck. Less often, the lesion becomes large, raised, and more deeply colored and is then known as a port-wine stain. This latter subset tends not to regress and, more importantly, may be associated with an underlying, usually ipsilateral, intracranial vascular malformation (*Sturge-Weber syndrome*). When the same phenomenon occurs in a limb (the underlying malformation usually leading to significant limb hypertrophy), this is known as *Klippel-Trenaunay syndrome*.

Pathologic Findings. Irrespective of the clinical form, the histologic features are quite subtle and often minimal, being characterized simply by dilation and congestion of thin-walled vessels in the dermis (fig. 7-6) and, less often, the subcutis. These vessels are otherwise entirely normal in appearance and hence clinicopathologic correlation is required.

Nevus Araneus

Definition. Nevus araneus (*spider nevus, arterial spider*) is a small, cutaneous, acquired vascular ectasia, most often located on the trunk.

Clinical Features. Nevus araneus is a very common lesion, occurring in small numbers in many adults and in increased numbers in association with pregnancy, alcoholism, and (less often) hyperthyroidism. Each lesion comprises a tiny, cutaneous, red papule from which small tortuous vessels often radiate. Spontaneous regression is common.

Pathologic Findings. Nevus araneus consists simply of a thick-walled dilated arteriole in the dermis, which branches into smaller superficial capillaries.

Venous Lake

Definition. Venous lake is a common vascular ectasia of acquired type, usually occurring in sun-damaged skin.

Clinical Features. Venous lake is the name given for purplish, papular vascular ectasias which occur mainly in the head and neck region of the elderly (10). Such lesions generally measure less than 0.5 cm, show a predilection for the ears and lips, and have no tendency to regress.

Pathologic Features. Venous lake appears to consist of a single, dilated and congested venous varicosity located in the superficial dermis.

Angioma Serpiginosum

Definition. Angioma serpiginosum is a rare, acquired vascular ectasia affecting mainly the lower limb(s).

Clinical Features. This is a slowly progressive form of vascular ectasia, usually starting in childhood, with a predilection for females (13, 15). It is characterized by the development of pinkish red papules or macules which spread over the lower limb (or limbs) in a serpiginous or gyrate fashion. There is no tendency for spontaneous regression.

Pathologic Findings. Again, clinical correlation is required since, histologically, all that is seen are small dilated vessels in the superficial dermis.

Hereditary Hemorrhagic Telangiectasia (Osler-Weber-Rendu Disease) Angiokeratoma

These two usually multifocal vascular ectasias, which often form part of an inherited disorder, are covered in the Fascicle, Non-Melanocytic Tumors of the Skin (14a).

Capillary Hemangioma

Definition. Capillary hemangioma is a benign vascular proliferation composed of small, capillary-sized blood vessels and most often has a lobular architecture.

General Considerations. The term capillary hemangioma encompasses a group of histologically similar but clinically distinct hemangiomas (21,23a,25,27a). Its best known and prototypical form is *juvenile capillary hemangioma,* also known as *infantile hemangioendothelioma, cellular hemangioma of infancy,* or *strawberry nevus.* Variants of capillary hemangioma include *pyogenic granuloma, tufted angioma, verrucous hemangioma,* and *cherry angioma.* All are clinically benign but, in their most cellular forms, are sometimes misdiagnosed as malignant. As stated in the Introduction to this chapter, the single most useful clue to benignity in this setting is the presence of a lobular growth pattern.

Clinical Features. The prototypical juvenile form of capillary hemangioma accounts for up to a third of the vascular tumors in infants and children and has an incidence of 1 to 2 per 100 live births (23a). Although it may arise at almost any location, the skin and soft tissues of the head and neck region are by far the sites of predilection. Females are affected more than males. These lesions typically are present at, or soon

after, birth. They grow as a reddish purple macule which then starts to involute in the second year of life. Most lesions have involuted totally by the time the patient is 6 or 7 years of age, with a minority persisting 2 to 3 years beyond this (27,28).

Pyogenic granuloma (also known as *granuloma pyogenicum* or *lobular capillary hemangioma*) is a very common type of capillary hemangioma, formerly thought to be infective in origin, which may develop at any age or location but which is especially common on the fingers and the oral or nasal mucous membranes (17,29,30,34,35). Oral lesions in pregnancy are sometimes known as *granuloma gravidarum.* Pyogenic granuloma usually grows rapidly to form a solitary, hemorrhagic, cutaneous or mucosal nodule up to 2 cm in size; there may be a history of preceding trauma. Rare cases are subcutaneous (23), multiple ("eruptive") (32,38), or intravascular (usually intravenous) (22). Up to 10 percent of lesions recur locally, usually after incomplete excision, and this is especially frequent in nasal cases. A rare subset of lesions, mainly in children, recurs with adjacent satellitosis (37).

Tufted angioma (also known as *angioblastoma of Nakagawa*) is an acquired form of capillary hemangioma which occurs much more often in children than adults, and is most common on the neck or upper trunk (20,32,39). This is a progressive lesion which expands through the development of seemingly discontinuous, reddish purple macules and papules. Regression is rare (30) but growth generally ceases when the patient ceases to grow.

Verrucous hemangioma most often presents in the distal lower extremities of young children as a warty cutaneous lesion, easily mistaken for a primarily epidermal growth (19,24). In its earliest stages, usually in neonatal life, it more often resembles an ordinary hemangioma, being characterized by a reddish blue macule. Local nondestructive recurrence is quite common.

Cherry angioma (also known as *senile angioma* or *Campbell de Morgan spot*) is a very common cutaneous lesion, affecting almost all adults and presenting as one or more red papules on the trunk or upper limb girdle (25). Such lesions increase in number with age and have no clinical significance.

Pathologic Findings. The histologic appearances of juvenile capillary hemangioma depend upon the age of the lesion. In the earliest

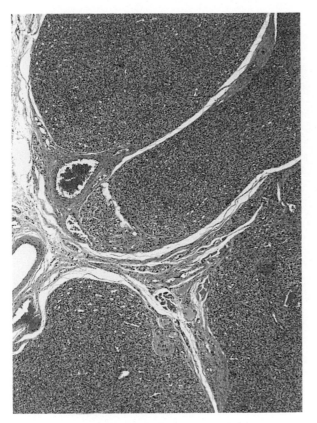

Figure 7-7
JUVENILE CAPILLARY HEMANGIOMA
Note the well-formed lobular growth pattern.

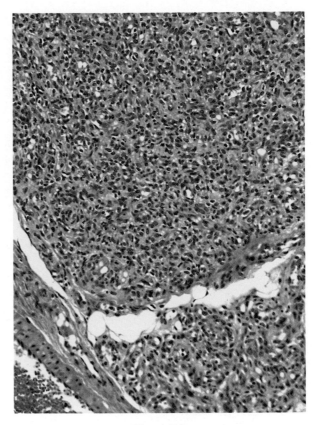

Figure 7-8
JUVENILE CAPILLARY HEMANGIOMA
Individual lobules are composed of closely packed capillaries with inconspicuous lumina.

(growth) phase, when most biopsies are taken, this is a floridly cellular lesion which at low-power microscopy has a well-formed lobular architecture (fig. 7-7). Tissues of the dermis, subcutis, and deeper may be involved. Individual lobules are composed of closely packed, small capillaries showing little or no luminal canalization (fig. 7-8). Endothelial cells may have frequent normal mitoses. At this stage, the vascular nature of the tumor may not be immediately apparent. As time passes, there is progressive vascular canalization and dilation (fig. 7-9). As regression begins there is a relative increase in fibrotic stroma which then separates ectatic vascular channels, and eventually both components largely involute. In many cases, at any stage of evolution, a larger feeding vessel (or vessels) can be identified. Especially in the active growth phase, it is not unusual to find perineurial (or even endoneurial) invasion by tumor (fig. 7-10) (18,35).

Pyogenic granuloma is morphologically very similar to juvenile capillary hemangioma but is confined to the dermis in the majority of cases and is generally exophytic (fig. 7-11), often with surface ulceration. Occasional cases are subcutaneous (23). By the time of excision, lesional capillaries are usually well canalized and there may be striking mitotic activity in both endothelial and stromal cells (fig. 7-12). Following ulceration, which is not invariable, the stroma becomes inflamed and edematous, and the lobular architecture may become blurred. Stromal neutrophils are not a feature of nonulcerated cases. Late stage lesions with irregular or ectatic vascular spaces may be confused with a more sinister lesion, in which case residual lobular architecture and a feeding vessel are usually most easily identified towards the base, and these are helpful, reassuring features. The same features are helpful in those cases, especially from mucous

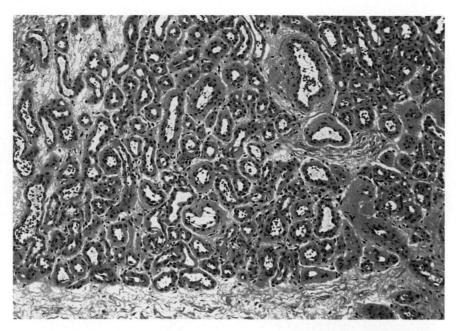

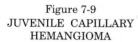
Figure 7-9
JUVENILE CAPILLARY
HEMANGIOMA
This lesion, from a 2-year-old child, shows well-developed vascular lumina.

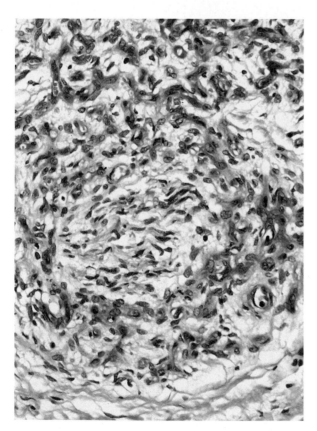

Figure 7-10
JUVENILE CAPILLARY HEMANGIOMA
Perineurial spread is a feature of around 10 percent of cases.

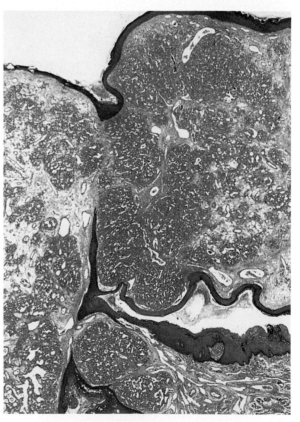

Figure 7-11
PYOGENIC GRANULOMA
(LOBULAR CAPILLARY HEMANGIOMA)
A typical polypoid, exophytic lesion with a lobular architecture is seen. Capillary lobules are most easily identified towards the base.

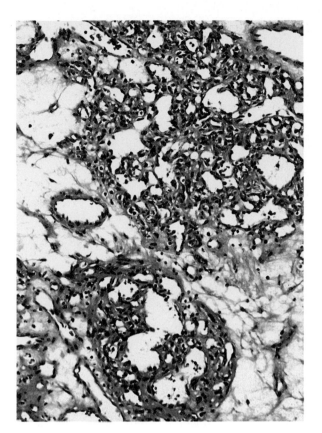 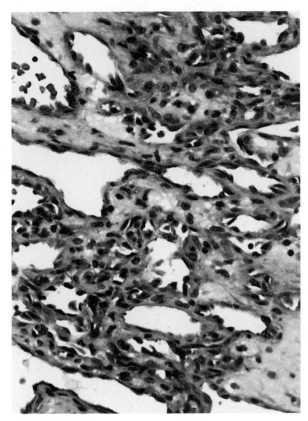

Figure 7-12
PYOGENIC GRANULOMA (LOBULAR CAPILLARY HEMANGIOMA)
Left: Excised lesions usually show stromal edema and dilated vessels.
Right: Lining endothelium is bland but mitoses may be frequent both in endothelial and stromal cells.

membranes, which tend to show pseudosarcomatous reactive or degenerative endothelial atypia (fig. 7-13) (36). Subcutaneous or intravascular examples do not show secondary stromal inflammation and edema (fig. 7-14).

Tufted angioma closely resembles the cellular phase of juvenile capillary hemangioma (fig. 7-15) but with several specific differences: 1) the individual lobules are discontinuous and dispersed, producing a so called cannon-ball distribution in the dermis (fig. 7-16); 2) some of the individual lobules tend to have a thin-walled semilunar or crescentic lymphatic channel at their periphery (fig. 7-17); and 3) in some cases the endothelial cells contain crystalline cytoplasmic inclusions of uncertain nature (26). Some cases have a spindle cell appearance, due to a relative predominance of pericytes.

Verrucous hemangioma, in its subcutaneous component, resembles the other lobular capillary

hemangiomas (see above) but is distinguished partly by the fact that its dermal component has a mixture of cavernous and capillary vessels (fig. 7-18), and more especially by the distinctive overlying epidermal changes, specifically acanthosis, papillomatosis, and hyperkeratosis, thus simulating a warty lesion (fig. 7-19). Adjacent to the subcutaneous capillary lobules, capillary-sized vessels also ramify into adjacent adipose tissue.

Cherry angioma is a mature form of lobular capillary hemangioma, and is comprised of thin-walled, canalized capillary vessels forming a small number of lobules in the papillary dermis (fig. 7-20). The appearance resembles a late-stage pyogenic granuloma without ulceration and the secondary effects thereof.

Special Studies. In most cases additional stains are unnecessary. However, in the very cellular juvenile cases, reticulin staining helps to highlight the underlying vasoformative architecture

317

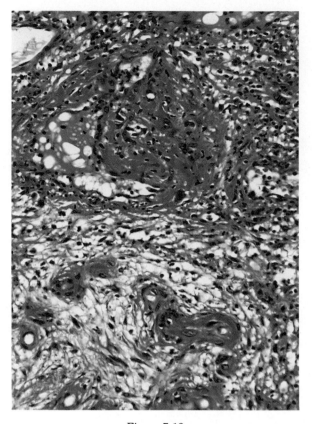

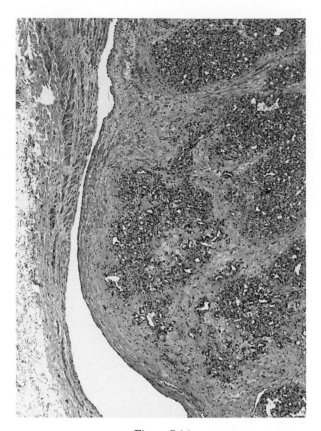

Figure 7-13
PYOGENIC GRANULOMA
(LOBULAR CAPILLARY HEMANGIOMA)
This ulcerated lesion from the lip shows marked reactive endothelial pleomorphism.

Figure 7-14
INTRAVASCULAR PYOGENIC GRANULOMA
This lobular, uninflamed lesion is located in the lumen of a vein from the neck of a young female.

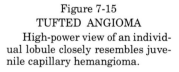

Figure 7-15
TUFTED ANGIOMA
High-power view of an individual lobule closely resembles juvenile capillary hemangioma.

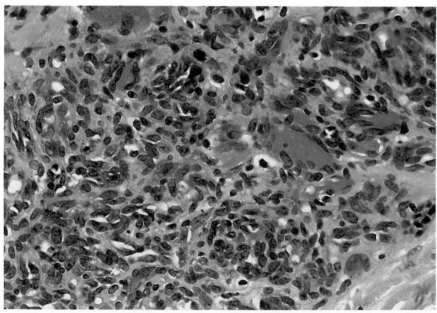

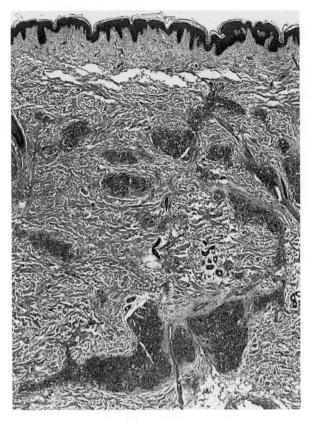

Figure 7-16
TUFTED ANGIOMA
Low-power view reveals the characteristic discontinuous distribution of capillary lobules.

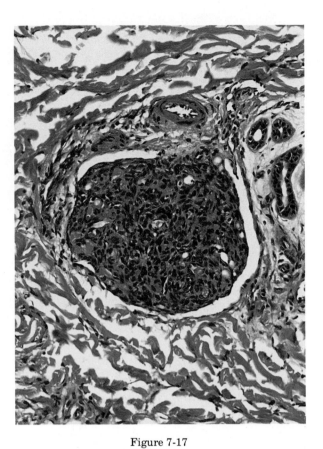

Figure 7-17
TUFTED ANGIOMA
Semilunar or crescentic vascular spaces are commonly present at the periphery of individual lobules.

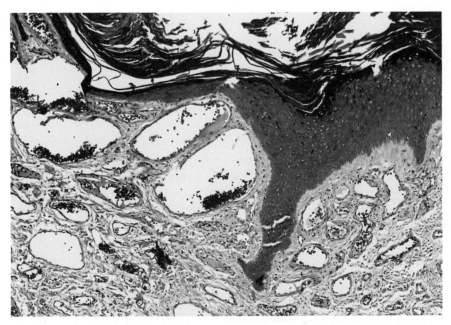

Figure 7-18
VERRUCOUS HEMANGIOMA
The dermal component usually shows mixed capillary and cavernous features. Note the overlying hyperkeratosis.

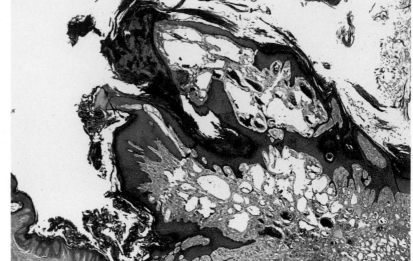

Figure 7-19
VERRUCOUS HEMANGIOMA
The marked overlying epidermal changes closely simulate a warty lesion at low power.

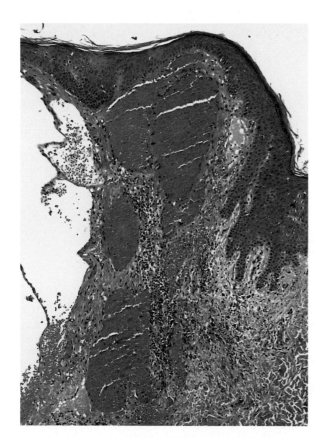

Figure 7-20
CHERRY ANGIOMA
These rarely biopsied lesions consist of dilated capillary lobules in the papillary dermis.

and a CD31 or VWF stain can confirm endothelial differentiation. Some cases of pyogenic granuloma overlap morphologically with bacillary angiomatosis, so a Warthin-Starry stain to check for bacilli may be useful. In cases of tufted angioma in which the cells are more spindled, immunopositivity for actin and negativity for CD34 may aid in the distinction from Kaposi's sarcoma.

Differential Diagnosis. Many of the differential diagnostic considerations lie in differentiating the individual variants of capillary hemangioma and are detailed above. It is important to distinguish between juvenile capillary hemangioma and tufted angioma since they may present in a similar clinical setting but the latter does not regress spontaneously. The rapid growth, high cellularity, and frequent mitoses in some lesions, especially in juvenile cases and mucosal pyogenic granulomas, may require the exclusion of angiosarcoma. As stated earlier, the presence of a lobular architecture, often with feeder vessels, and the absence of endothelial multilayering or atypia are key distinguishing features. Angiosarcoma essentially never has a lobular architecture or feeder vessels. Highly cellular capillary hemangiomas with little or no luminal canalization may be hard to distinguish from other spindle cell neoplasms but the reticulin pattern (fig. 7-21) and immunopositivity for CD31 and VWF are usually discriminatory.

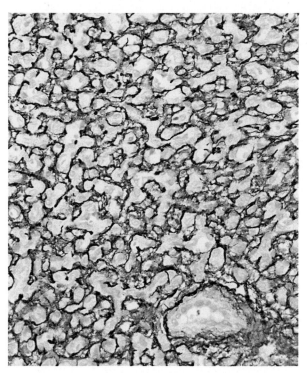

Figure 7-21
JUVENILE CAPILLARY HEMANGIOMA
Even in solidly cellular lesions, reticulin staining highlights the vasoformative architecture.

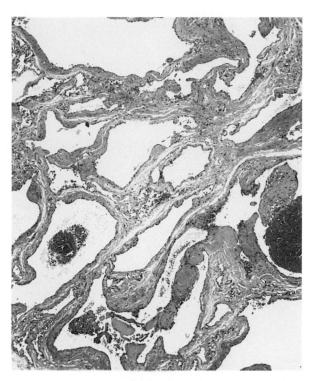

Figure 7-22
CAVERNOUS HEMANGIOMA
Lesional vessels are large with dilated lumina.

Treatment and Prognosis. The usual course of the individual subtypes is detailed under the clinical subheadings above. As a general rule, only the juvenile type of capillary hemangioma regresses spontaneously, while the other variants generally do not. Juvenile type capillary hemangiomas are therefore only excised if they threaten vital structures or fail to regress. Each of the variants is prone to nondestructive local recurrence unless completely excised.

Cavernous Hemangioma

Definition. Cavernous hemangioma is a benign vascular proliferation composed of dilated, generally thin-walled blood vessels.

Clinical Features. Cavernous hemangioma has a clinical distribution similar, in terms of age, sex, and location, to juvenile capillary hemangioma (see above) (41,42,45,47). When superficially located, lesions tend to be bluer than capillary hemangiomas; other important differences include being significantly less common, often involving deeper tissues, being more poorly cir-

cumscribed and, most notably, showing little or no tendency to regress spontaneously. Clinical associations, in a minority of cases, include consumption coagulopathy (Kasabach-Merritt syndrome) (44), association with comparable bluish cutaneous cavernous hemangiomas in the gastrointestinal tract (blue rubber bleb nevus syndrome [43,46]), and association with multiple enchondromas (Maffucci's syndrome). In the latter syndrome some of the vascular lesions are spindle cell hemangiomas (see page 332).

Sinusoidal hemangioma, a distinct variant of cavernous hemangioma, presents usually as a solitary, purplish blue nodule on the trunk (including breast) or upper limb of middle-aged to older adults, with a slight predominance in females (40). Clinically, it may be mistaken for melanoma or, especially in the breast, for angiosarcoma.

Pathologic Findings. Ordinary cavernous hemangioma is a poorly circumscribed lesion composed of dilated, usually thin-walled vessels lined by flattened endothelium (fig. 7-22). These vessels are often congested and may show

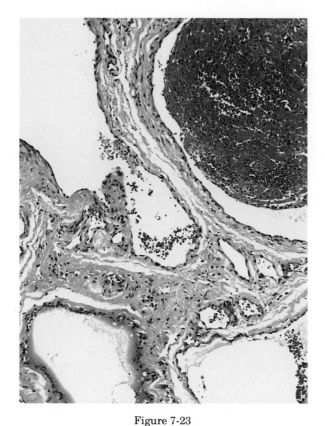

Figure 7-23
CAVERNOUS HEMANGIOMA
Individual vessels have a bland endothelial lining and are often focally thrombosed.

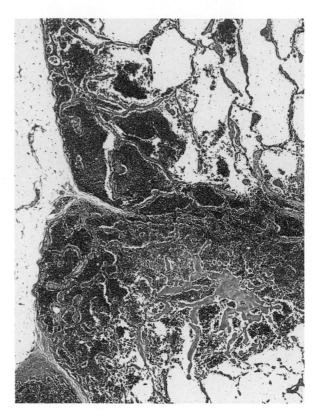

Figure 7-24
SINUSOIDAL HEMANGIOMA
In contrast to usual cavernous hemangioma, these lesions are lobulated.

thrombosis (fig. 7-23), sometimes with phleboliths. Variation in vessel size is common and there may be areas with more capillary type vessels as well as larger, thick-walled vessels. Stromal chronic inflammation is common.

Sinusoidal hemangioma differs from the usual type by being circumscribed and often lobulated, and by having thin-walled vessels which intercommunicate in a complex fashion (fig. 7-24). Cross-cutting of these thin walls often produces a pseudopapillary appearance (fig. 7-25). Thrombosis, infarction, and sometimes dystrophic calcification may be seen. The endothelium is always monolayered but rarely may show mild atypia and pleomorphism, perhaps as a reaction to thrombosis. Repeated thrombosis, with organization, progressively leads, in some cases, to a more solid, cellular-looking appearance (fig. 7-26).

Special Studies. On occasion, an elastic stain may facilitate distinction from an arteriovenous hemangioma (see below). Additional stains or other techniques have little or no role in the diagnosis of cavernous hemangioma.

Differential Diagnosis. Usual type cavernous hemangioma really has no differential diagnosis, except perhaps for arteriovenous hemangioma which has a thicker muscle coat as well as an internal elastic lamina in the arterial component. Sinusoidal hemangioma on occasion may need to be distinguished from well-differentiated angiosarcoma. However, the latter has a dissecting rather than lobular growth pattern and invariably shows more endothelial atypia with at least focal multilayering. Furthermore, in the setting of a breast lesion, angiosarcoma develops in the parenchyma whereas sinusoidal hemangioma is subcutaneous.

Treatment and Prognosis. Neither type of cavernous hemangioma recurs after complete excision. However larger examples of the conventional type may be hard to excise in sensitive head and neck locations and alternative, more

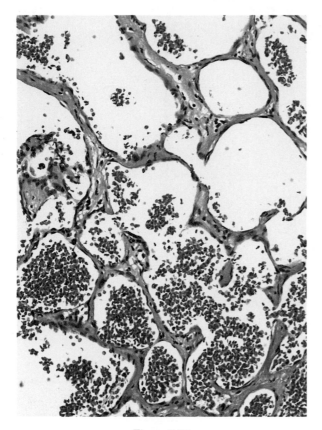

Figure 7-25
SINUSOIDAL HEMANGIOMA
Individual vessels are thin-walled, producing a pseudo-papillary or sieve-like appearance.

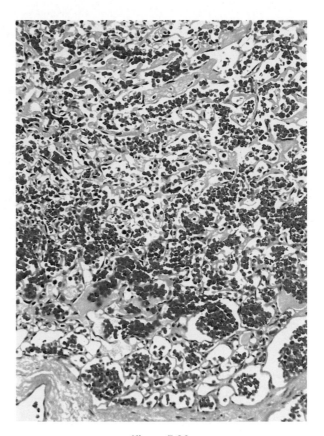

Figure 7-26
SINUSOIDAL HEMANGIOMA
Some cases have more solid, collapsed areas which likely are the result of repeated thrombosis.

conservative therapies (e.g., use of steroids or interferon) are under constant review.

Arteriovenous Hemangioma

Definition. Arteriovenous hemangioma is a benign vascular hamartoma or malformation characterized by the presence of arteriovenous shunts.

Clinical Features. There are two main types of arteriovenous hemangioma: those which are deep-seated and those which are cutaneous (48–51). Both are uncommon but the cutaneous form is more frequent than the deep form.

Cutaneous arteriovenous hemangiomas, which are also known as *cirsoid aneurysm* or *acral arteriovenous tumor (*49*)*, are most common in the head and neck region of middle-aged adults and show a predilection for the lips and oral region. They present as a red-blue papule which quite commonly is painful. Manifestations of arteriovenous shunting are minimal or (usually) absent.

More deep-seated arteriovenous hemangiomas are clinically significant lesions which usually occur in the limbs or head and neck region of children, adolescents, and young adults. They are commonly associated with a significant degree of arteriovenous shunting, detectable by auscultation and angiography, and this in turn can lead to complications such as limb hypertrophy, high-output cardiac failure, and consumption coagulopathy, as well as considerable pain in the affected location.

Pathologic Findings. Whether superficial (fig. 7-27) or deep (fig. 7-28), these lesions consist of a variably circumscribed admixture of different vessel types, notable among which are thick-walled veins and arterial vessels, with the former usually predominant. Areas of ordinary capillary or cavernous hemangioma are frequent. Reliable characterization of such vessels often requires the use of elastic stains (fig. 7-29) and obvious

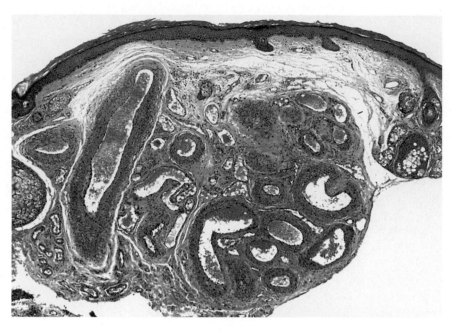

Figure 7-27
CUTANEOUS
ARTERIOVENOUS
HEMANGIOMA
This lesion from the face is composed of typically thick-walled vessels.

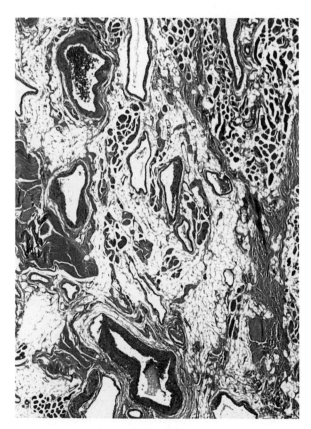

Figure 7-28
INTRAMUSCULAR ARTERIOVENOUS HEMANGIOMA
Similarly large but more widely distributed vessels are evident.

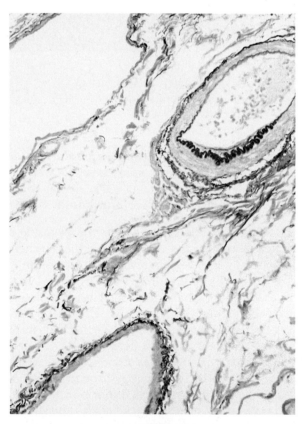

Figure 7-29
INTRAMUSCULAR ARTERIOVENOUS HEMANGIOMA
Certain designation of the vessel types may require the use of elastic stains (Elastic van Gieson).

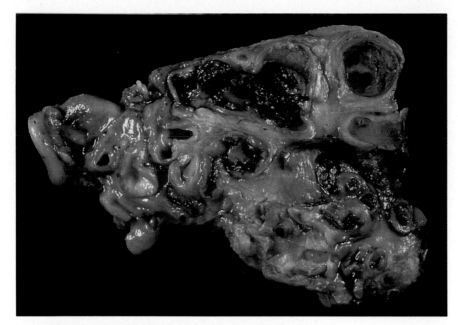

Figure 7-30
ARTERIOVENOUS
HEMANGIOMA
This deep-seated mass from the thigh is composed of large vessels with extensive thrombosis.

arteriovenous shunts may not be demonstrable without viewing multiple levels in the tissue block. Deep-seated lesions may be best characterized by angiography, as mentioned above. However, the diagnosis also can be reached in most cases by demonstrating the appropriate vessel types and then finding marked fibrointimal thickening in the venous component, indicative of the effect of high pressure flow. Like cavernous hemangioma, these lesions often show thrombosis and dystrophic calcification (fig. 7-30).

Special Studies. As mentioned above, elastic stains may be helpful in identification of the different vessel types.

Differential Diagnosis. Possible differential diagnoses might include cavernous hemangioma (see above) or angiomatosis (see below).

Treatment and Prognosis. Arteriovenous hemangiomas show no tendency to regress spontaneously. Superficially located lesions do not recur following local excision. Large deep-seated lesions may be harder to control surgically purely because of their anatomic extent and their tendency to be associated with complex malformed vasculature throughout the affected location. In general, wide or even radical excision, based upon the angiographically defined extent of the lesion, provides the most favorable results.

Epithelioid Hemangioma

Definition. Epithelioid hemangioma (*angiolymphoid hyperplasia with eosinophilia, histiocytoid hemangioma*) is a benign hemangioma characterized by well-formed vessels lined by endothelial cells, with copious eosinophilic and sometimes vacuolated cytoplasm and plump vesicular nuclei.

General Considerations. A variety of vascular tumors or pseudotumors are characterized by epithelioid endothelial cells (64). Such lesions, in the past, have also been labeled as histiocytoid hemangiomas (61,63), but it is now clear that several different entities were included in that category. In biologic terms, these range from the infective process, bacillary (epithelioid) angiomatosis, through epithelioid hemangioma, to epithelioid hemangioendothelioma, a low-grade malignancy, and epithelioid angiosarcoma, a high-grade malignancy. The extent to which these latter three lesions form a continuous spectrum, both clinically and morphologically, is not absolutely settled, but it does seem that there exists a few cases that have features intermediate between each category. It is important to appreciate that the focal presence of epithelioid endothelial cells alone does not imply a diagnosis of an epithelioid vascular neoplasm. Such cells may be present, but usually only in very small areas (albeit with no sharply defined cutoff point), in almost any vascular lesion, ranging from pyogenic granuloma through intramuscular hemangioma to conventional angiosarcoma.

Clinical Features. Epithelioid hemangioma most often presents as a cutaneous or subcutaneous, quite often multicentric lesion in the head and neck region of young to middle-aged adults; sex incidence is approximately equal (52,55,59, 66,67). However, the overall age range and anatomic distribution is wide, including not only soft tissue locations but also, occasionally, visceral sites. Occasional cases involve both soft tissue and underlying bone, and rare cases arise in the lumen of major blood vessels (58,60). In the past this entity was confused with or merged with Kimura's disease (53,56,65), which led to some erroneous conceptions; in reality, epithelioid hemangioma is almost never associated with lymphadenopathy and the incidence of circulating eosinophilia is no more than 10 percent. Individual lesions appear as reddish brown nodules or plaques, and lesion duration in most cases is less than 6 to 9 months.

Pathologic Findings. When occurring in the dermis, these lesions are poorly circumscribed, whereas when subcutaneous, they are more sharply demarcated. In either location they consist of a variably lobular proliferation of small, sometimes thick-walled vessels with patent lumens which are lined by plump, eosinophilic, epithelioid endothelial cells (fig. 7-31). Endothelial cell cytoplasm, which is often vacuolated, is often copious enough to fill the vascular lumens. The endothelial cell nuclei are plump and vesicular, with nonvisible or inconspicuous nucleoli, generally no atypia, and scarce mitoses. Lesional vessels are well formed and do not show the more linear or sheet-like endothelial growth of more aggressive epithelioid endothelial tumors. However, small solid clusters of epithelioid endothelial cells may be present. Those few cases that extend to involve underlying bone tend to be highly cellular (fig. 7-32).

The appearance of the stroma is variable and, despite the older name of angiolymphoid hyperplasia with eosinophilia, no more than about 50 percent of cases have a prominent inflammatory component; this is usually more common in subcutaneous lesions. When present, the inflamma-

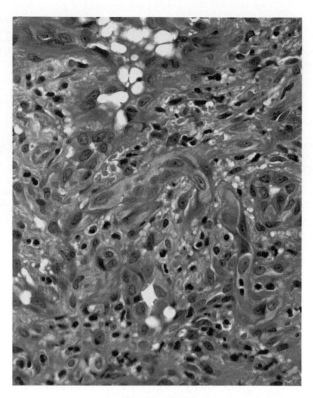

Figure 7-31
EPITHELIOID HEMANGIOMA
Lesional vessels have plump endothelial cells with copious, sometimes vacuolated, eosinophilic cytoplasm.

tory element consists mainly of lymphocytes, with variably prominent follicles, and eosinophils (fig. 7-33). Some lesions have such a prominent inflammatory component that the vascular proliferation is largely obscured, leading to a mistaken diagnosis as an inflammatory process (fig. 7-34). In older lesions the stroma is often fibrotic (fig. 7-35) and even somewhat myxoid.

An important feature, not widely appreciated in the early reports, is that around 50 percent of lesions involve a small artery or muscular vein. This involvement ranges from mural disruption to total luminal occlusion and, in fact, a significant proportion of cases are entirely intravascular (fig. 7-36) (62).

Special Studies. Immunohistochemically, the majority of lesional endothelial cells stain as those in other benign lesions: usually positive for von Willebrand factor, CD31, and CD34. Although epithelioid hemangiomas in bone are often keratin positive, this is rarely the case in soft tissue examples (which contrasts with malignant epithelioid

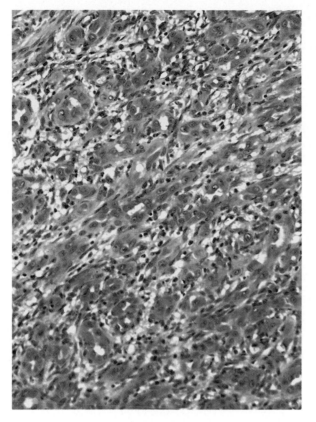

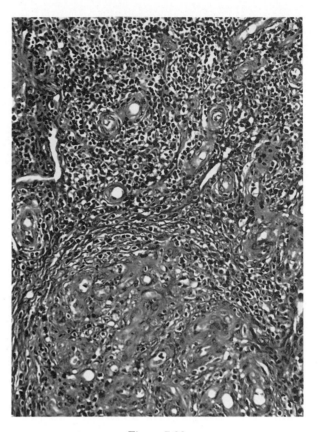

Figure 7-32
EPITHELIOID HEMANGIOMA
This lesion from the foot shows a very cellular vascular proliferation. The lesion involved skin, subcutis, and underlying bone.

Figure 7-33
EPITHELIOID HEMANGIOMA
When present, the inflammatory component consists of eosinophils and lymphocytes.

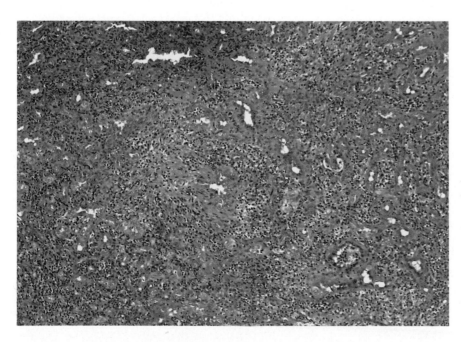

Figure 7-34
EPITHELIOID HEMANGIOMA
In very inflamed lesions the vessels may be largely obscured, especially at low power.

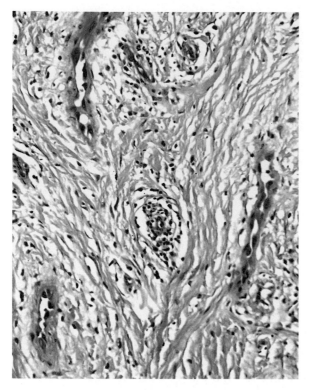

Figure 7-35
EPITHELIOID HEMANGIOMA
This longstanding lesion has a very fibrotic stroma with widely dispersed blood vessels (showing typically plump endothelium).

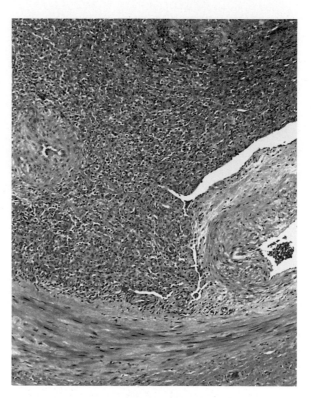

Figure 7-36
EPITHELIOID HEMANGIOMA
This lesion from the forehead is confined within the lumen of a thick-walled muscular vessel.

endothelial lesions [see below]). The ultrastructural correlate of copious eosinophilic cytoplasm is the presence of prominent intracytoplasmic intermediate filaments.

Differential Diagnosis. Kimura's disease is an IgE-mediated allergic disorder which lacks epithelioid endothelial cells but is notable for marked fibrosis, prominent germinal centers with folliculolysis, eosinophil microabscesses, and high endothelial venules (fig. 7-37) (53,56,65). Lymph node involvement is common. Epithelioid hemangioendothelioma does not have such well-formed vessels and is usually characterized by a linear and more nested endothelial growth pattern, associated with myxohyaline stroma and less inflammation. Bacillary angiomatosis may look very similar to epithelioid hemangioma but is notable for the presence of stromal neutrophils and aggregates of amphophilic or basophilic nuclear debris and bacilli. Injection-site granulomas may superficially resemble epithelioid hemangioma

but closer examination usually shows that the endothelial cells, while plump and reactive, are not epithelioid (54,57).

Treatment and Prognosis. Up to a third of cases recur locally (52,59) but it is possible that these fall more strictly into the category of multicentric lesions. Local recurrence is generally not destructive and there is no evidence that these lesions metastasize.

Microvenular Hemangioma

Definition. Microvenular hemangioma is an uncommon, benign, dermal vascular tumor characterized by small angulated venules without atypia.

Clinical Features. Microvenular hemangioma, which has only been recognized in recent years, presents as a solitary, elevated, reddish-purple cutaneous nodule or plaque at almost any location (68,69). Young adults are most often affected and there may be a clinical resemblance to Kaposi's sarcoma.

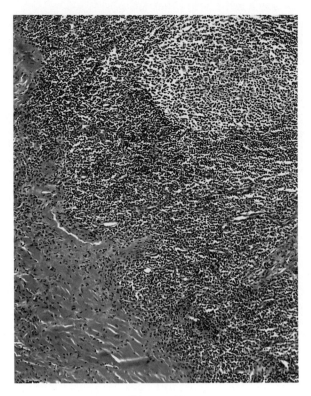

Figure 7-37
KIMURA'S DISEASE
This entity differs from epithelioid hemangioma principally by showing stromal fibrosis and well-formed germinal centers, and by lacking epithelioid endothelium.

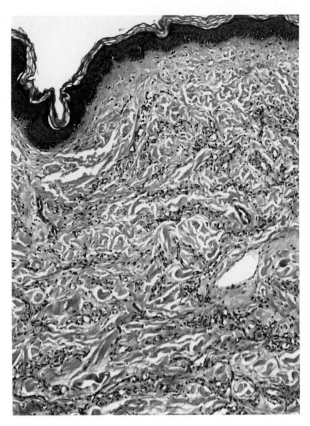

Figure 7-38
MICROVENULAR HEMANGIOMA
Lesional vessels ramify through the dermis, and are mainly distributed parallel to the epidermis.

Pathologic Findings. This distinctive lesion is characterized by small thin-walled vessels, likely venules, which arborize through the full thickness of the dermis (fig. 7-38), often culminating at the dermal-subcutaneous junction in small capillary tufts or lobules. The lateral margins are not well demarcated. Individual vessels seem usually to have two cell layers: luminal endothelial cells with plump, hyperchromatic nuclei and little cytoplasm, and a surrounding outer layer of pericytes (fig. 7-39). Adjacent dermal collagen usually appears sclerotic and there is usually little or no inflammation.

Special Studies. Special stains play no role in this diagnosis.

Differential Diagnosis. The principal differential diagnosis is patch-stage Kaposi's sarcoma. However, the latter shows more irregular collagen dissection, tends mainly to affect the superficial dermis, and is generally associated with stromal plasma cells and a minor spindle cell component.

Hobnail Hemangioma

Definition. Hobnail hemangioma (*targetoid hemosiderotic hemangioma*) is an uncommon, benign, dermal vascular tumor characterized by plump, protuberant endothelial cell nuclei, often with small endothelial papillae.

Clinical Features. Hobnail hemangioma is a recently recognized lesion which affects mainly young to middle-aged adults. It may arise at a wide variety of cutaneous or mucosal sites, but is seen mainly on the lower limb or trunk (70–72). Duration is variable. Many cases appear as a reddish brown papule or macule, and the presence of an ecchymotic-like ring of cutaneous discoloration in some cases led to the original designation as targetoid hemosiderotic hemangioma (71). Since this is a clinical description and one which is not always applicable, the term hobnail hemangioma is preferred (70a).

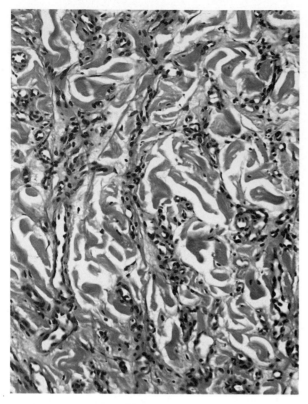

Figure 7-39
MICROVENULAR HEMANGIOMA
Individual vessels have plump endothelial nuclei and an outer layer of pericytes. Note the sclerotic appearance of the dermal collagen.

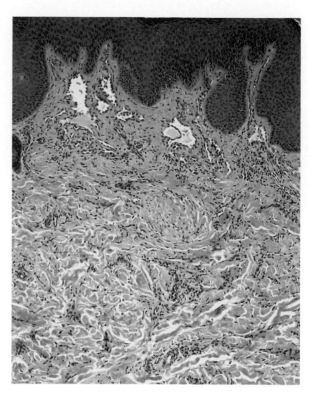

Figure 7-40
HOBNAIL HEMANGIOMA
Distinctively, at low power, the papillary dermal vessels are dilated while the deeper component is inconspicuous.

Pathologic Findings. Hobnail hemangioma typically affects mainly the papillary dermis but extends also into the deeper reticular dermis. At low-power microscopy it has a wedge-shaped outline and the vessels become progressively less conspicuous with increasing dermal depth (fig. 7-40). The more prominent superficial vessels are thin-walled, variably ectatic, and variably angulated. Distinctively, they are lined, at least in large part, by small, hyperchromatic, protuberant (hence hobnail) endothelial nuclei with little or no associated cytoplasm (fig. 7-41). Small papillary structures composed of such nuclei are common but generalized multilayering is absent. As the vessels extend deeper into the dermis they become narrower and more attenuated, with inconspicuous nuclei (fig. 7-42). In the deeper portions of the lesion there is often, but not invariably, stromal hemosiderin deposition and a sprinkling of lymphocytes.

Special Studies. Stromal hemosiderin can be highlighted, if necessary, with an iron stain. Additional stains play no real role in this diagnosis.

Differential Diagnosis. Retiform hemangioendothelioma is distinguished by its more prominent arborizing vasculature and its larger, more striking endothelial nuclei (70). Progressive lymphangioma clinically presents as a larger macule and lacks hobnail endothelial nuclei. Angiosarcoma shows irregular dissection of collagen and more overt endothelial atypia and multilayering. Epithelioid hemangioma, while sharing protuberant endothelial cells, is characterized by copious eosinophilic or vacuolated endothelial cytoplasm, in sharp contrast to the almost bare nuclei of hobnail hemangioma. Lesions almost identical to hobnail hemangioma may occur in the skin after radiotherapy, in which circumstance clinical correlation is necessary.

Treatment and Prognosis. Hobnail hemangioma appears entirely benign, with no tendency to recur following simple excision.

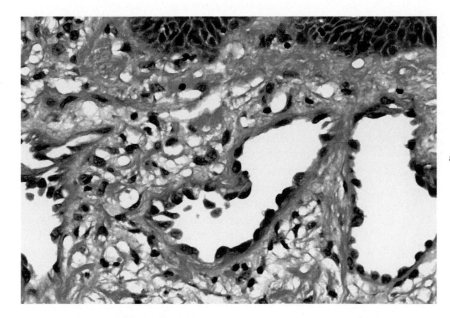

Figure 7-41
HOBNAIL HEMANGIOMA
The superficial vessels are ectatic
and have protuberant (hobnail) nuclei.

Venous Hemangioma

Definition. Venous hemangioma is an uncommon benign vascular tumor composed of variably sized veins, usually having thick muscular walls.

Clinical Features. Venous hemangioma is not well characterized as a discrete entity but seems to occur mainly in deep soft tissues, where it is usually best regarded as a subset of intramuscular angioma (see Angiomatosis). Comparable lesions also occur in the subcutis, usually in the limbs. Overall age range is wide but adults are most often affected. It is possible, however, that these are longstanding malformative type lesions which take many years to come to clinical attention.

Pathologic Findings. Venous hemangioma is characterized by large, thick-walled vessels (fig. 7-43), usually having a dilated lumen and well-developed muscular walls without an internal elastic lamina. Fibrointimal thickening, suggestive of arteriovenous shunting, is not usually seen. There may be luminal thrombosis, sometimes with phleboliths. In deep-seated locations there may be an admixture of other vessel types, supporting redesignation of those cases as intramuscular angioma.

Special Studies. Elastic stains may be helpful in excluding an arteriovenous hemangioma. Additional stains play no role in this diagnosis.

Differential Diagnosis. Arteriovenous hemangioma is composed of mixed vessel types

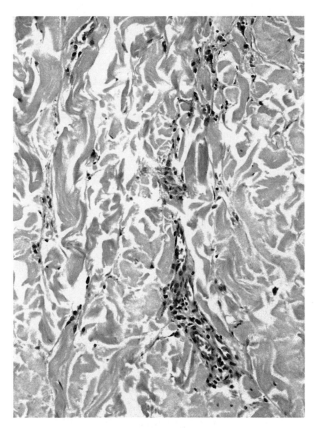

Figure 7-42
HOBNAIL HEMANGIOMA
Vessels in the deep dermis are angulated and inconspicuous, often being associated with a scattering of lymphocytes and hemosiderin deposition.

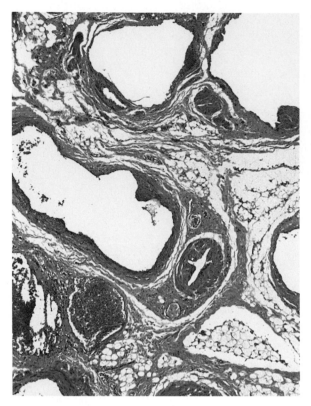

Figure 7-43
VENOUS HEMANGIOMA
Most cases are composed mainly of large thick-walled veins.

with a definable arterial component (most easily demonstrated by elastic stains). Cavernous hemangioma generally lacks the thick muscular walls of venous hemangioma.

Treatment and Prognosis. Available data are limited but deep-seated lesions may be hard to excise completely and thus recur in the same way as intramuscular angiomas. Subcutaneous lesions generally do not recur.

Spindle Cell Hemangioma

Definition. Spindle cell hemangioma, also known as *spindle cell hemangioendothelioma,* is a benign, usually superficial vascular tumor composed of cavernous spaces and solid spindle cell areas with vacuolated endothelial cells.

General Considerations. Spindle cell hemangioma was first described under the rubric spindle cell hemangioendothelioma and, at that time, was thought to represent a distinctive low-grade form of angiosarcoma with potential for frequent

recurrence and rare metastasis (79). Time and the study of more cases has shown this not to be the case. Rather, this lesion appears to be either a benign neoplasm or perhaps a reactive process engrafted on abnormal, often malformed vessels (73,75–77). Its tendency for multicentricity likely reflects a field change effect.

Clinical Features. Spindle cell hemangioma may present over a very wide age range; many lesions are first noticed in childhood or early adulthood but may not come to medical attention for many years thereafter (75,77–79). Sex incidence is approximately equal. The majority of cases develop in the skin and subcutis of the distal extremities; more proximal or deep-seated examples are uncommon. Up to 50 percent of patients develop multiple lesions, usually in the same general anatomic region, and this process may occur over a period of decades. Individual lesions appear as small (less than 2 cm), sometimes painful nodules which produce bluish skin if located in the dermis. Up to 10 percent of patients have associated clinical anomalies which might contribute to an altered vasculature or blood flow in the affected limb; specifically, these are lymphedema, enchondromatosis (hence Maffucci's syndrome) (74), Klippel-Trenaunay syndrome, and early onset varicose veins (presumed due to a venous valve defect).

Pathologic Findings. Grossly, these lesions appear as small hemorrhagic nodules in deep dermal or subcutaneous tissue. Histologically, they are unencapsulated but reasonably circumscribed and up to 50 percent involve a large preexisting vessel (usually a vein) (fig. 7-44). Perhaps 20 to 30 percent are entirely intravascular. At low-power magnification most lesions have two main components: solid spindle cell areas and dilated cavernous vascular spaces (fig. 7-45). The latter may contain thrombi, phleboliths, or cellular papillary structures resembling strands of the more solid spindled tissue. An additional low-power feature, evident in the majority of cases, is the presence of nearby, abnormal, thick-walled vessels which often show features of a localized arteriovenous shunt.

Closer examination of the spindle cell areas reveals slit-like spaces that represent either poorly formed or collapsed vascular channels, surrounded by pericytic and fibroblastic spindle cells. In these areas there are typically admixed plump

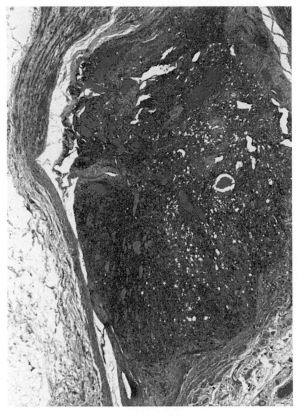

Figure 7-44
SPINDLE CELL HEMANGIOMA
This tumor from the forearm is located entirely within a vein.

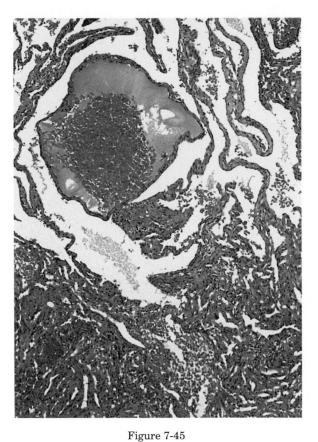

Figure 7-45
SPINDLE CELL HEMANGIOMA
Medium-power view reveals solid areas and cavernous spaces with associated papillary structures.

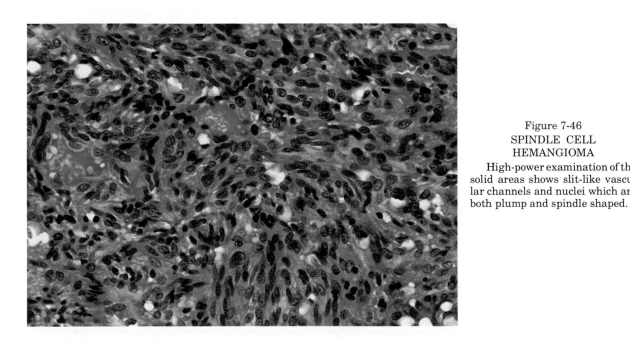

Figure 7-46
SPINDLE CELL
HEMANGIOMA
High-power examination of the solid areas shows slit-like vascular channels and nuclei which are both plump and spindle shaped.

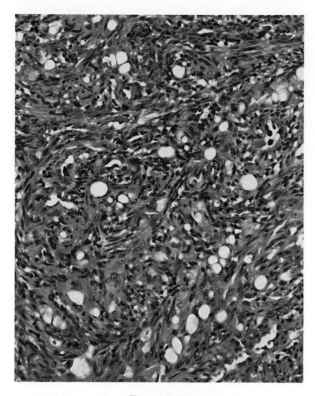

Figure 7-47
SPINDLE CELL HEMANGIOMA
Endothelial cytoplasmic vacuolation is a characteristic feature.

and spindled endothelial nuclei as well as spindled nuclei of supportive cells (fig. 7-46). Endothelial cells with plump, more rounded nuclei often show striking cytoplasmic vacuolation (reminiscent of that seen in epithelioid hemangioendothelioma) and this is an important diagnostic clue (fig. 7-47). With very rare exceptions, there is no nuclear atypia and mitoses are scarce; however, occasional cases have nuclear atypia and hyperchromasia which most likely are degenerative or reactive in nature. Isolated cases have been associated with coexistent features of epithelioid hemangioendothelioma (80).

Special Studies. Reticulin stains demonstrate that the solid spindled areas are actually composed of vascular channels. Immunohistochemistry serves only to demonstrate that the cell population in the spindled areas is mixed, comprising some endothelial cells (CD31 or CD34 positive), some pericytes (actin positive), and some fibroblasts.

Differential Diagnosis. The principal lesion in the differential diagnosis is Kaposi's sarcoma,

which rarely contains cavernous spaces, lacks vacuolated endothelial cells, has hyaline globules (not seen in spindle cell hemangioma), and has spindle cells that are more uniformly immunopositive for CD34 and CD31. In addition, Kaposi's sarcoma is rarely, if ever, intravascular. Kaposiform hemangioendothelioma lacks cavernous spaces or vacuolated endothelial cells and has a lobular growth pattern. Occasionally, aneurysmal benign fibrous histiocytoma (see chapter 3) is mistaken for spindle cell hemangioma. However, the former shows much greater cytologic polymorphism, a generally storiform growth pattern, and overlying epidermal hyperplasia, and it lacks vacuolated endothelial cells or immunopositivity for endothelial antigens.

Treatment and Prognosis. Solitary lesions are cured by simple local excision. Patients with multiple lesions often continue to develop new lesions, usually in the same general area in the manner of a field defect, over many years but true recurrence in a previous excision site is rare. The originally reported metastasizing case is now generally accepted to have been an irradiation-induced sarcoma and there is no evidence that spindle cell hemangioma affects life expectancy or has any significant morbidity whatever. These facts contributed significantly to the decision to drop the term "hemangioendothelioma" for this entity.

INTERMEDIATE VASCULAR TUMORS (MANAGERIAL GROUPS II AND IIa, TABLE 1-10)

Grouped under this heading are those lesions that can recur destructively and those that rarely metastasize. Although intramuscular angioma and angiomatosis are in the "benign" category in the World Health Organization (WHO) classification and have not previously been regarded as "intermediate," we think the incidence of poorly controlled recurrences associated with these lesions is sufficient grounds to move them to this category (managerial category IIa). Although not often acknowledged, the recurrence rate of these lesions and the frequent need for radical surgery easily parallels that for desmoid fibromatoses. On the other hand, epithelioid hemangioendothelioma is often classified as an intermediate tumor, but recent evidence, including our own (128), reveals a metastatic rate that makes classification as a malignant neoplasm (managerial category III) more appropriate. Kaposi's sarcoma presents special managerial classificatory problems. Classic (elderly endemic) Kaposi's sarcoma may recur, but recurrences are not destructive and development of systemic disease is rare. Such lesions are best classified as benign (managerial category Ib). On the other hand, patients with AIDS-related Kaposi's sarcoma and some patients with the African form develop systemic disease often enough for such an event to be assumed at the onset (managerial category IV). We classify Kaposi's sarcoma as an intermediate tumor, but readers should be aware of this variable biologic potential which depends on the clinical setting.

Deeply Located Hemangiomas

Deeply located hemangiomas occur principally in skeletal muscle but also in joints, bone, nerves, and lymph nodes. The principal relevance of such lesions is that, when compared to their more common cutaneous counterparts, they tend to reach a larger size; to be more often symptomatic; to have greater morbidity in terms of clinical effects, local control, and complications; and to recur more often. Hemangiomas of bone, peripheral nerve, and lymph node are described in their respective Fascicles, as are visceral and organ-based hemangiomas where relevant.

Intramuscular Angioma

Definition. Intramuscular angioma is a lesion composed of morphologically benign vascular channels occurring within skeletal muscle, and is almost always associated with variable amounts of adipose tissue. Also known as *intramuscular hemangioma* and *intramuscular angiolipoma,* the term angioma is preferred to hemangioma since the vessels are often of mixed type.

Clinical Features. Intramuscular angioma is one of the more common deep-seated soft tissue tumors and may present at any age, although adolescents and young adults are affected most frequently, with approximately equal sex distribution (81–83). Anatomic distribution is both varied and wide but, in order of frequency, the lower limb is the most common site, followed by head and neck region, upper limb, and trunk. Retroperitoneal and mediastinal examples are

rare. Patients present with a slowly enlarging and often longstanding mass which, particularly in limb lesions, is often painful. The pain may be worse after exercise. The pathologic features (see below) suggest that many of these lesions may represent malformations and, as such, their true onset may be congenital or in early infancy. Radiologically, the lesions often show calcification, due either to phleboliths or stromal bone formation.

Pathologic Findings. Intramuscular angiomas are most often large, poorly demarcated lesions which grossly may appear yellowish (due to their usual component of adipose tissue) and which often have obviously vascular or hemorrhagic areas (fig. 7-48). Focal calcification or ossification is common. Size depends heavily on anatomic location but examples arising in the lower limb commonly measure greater than 10 cm.

In histologic terms, the appearance is very variable and we do not find that classification by vessel type is either practical or meaningful in most cases since, almost invariably, the vessel types are mixed (82). In fact, in some cases there appears to be an admixture of both blood vessels and lymphatic channels, underscoring the likely malformative nature of many of these lesions. In terms of predominant vessel type, lesions with prominent, thick-walled, muscular veins and lesions showing a complex mixture of capillary and cavernous-size vessels, as well as an arteriovenous component, are the most common (fig. 7-49). A small subset of cases are of pure capillary type and have a highly cellular lobular appearance mimicking that seen in capillary hemangioma; these lesions are most common in the head and neck region. A similarly small subset has the appearance of a cavernous lymphangioma (see below) (fig. 7-50), often associated with lymphocytic aggregates, and such lesions seem to be largely confined to the trunk, upper limb girdle, and head. Virtually all forms of intramuscular angioma diffusely infiltrate the muscle and entrap residual skeletal muscle cells, leading to bizarre degenerative or reactive sarcolemmal forms (fig. 7-51). In addition, almost all cases have a prominent adipocytic stromal component (fig. 7-49), sometimes much larger in volume than the vessels, hence the old term "infiltrating angiolipoma" (84). Whether this fat is an intrinsic part of the lesion, which is more likely, or whether it is the result of muscular atrophy

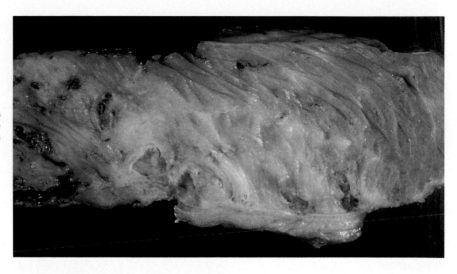

Figure 7-48
INTRAMUSCULAR ANGIOMA
A typically ill-defined mass from the soleus muscle. Notice the yellowish fatty component and the relatively inconspicuous vessels.

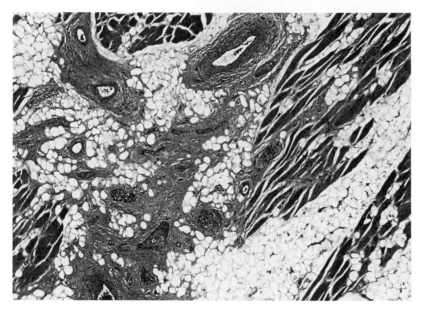

Figure 7-49
INTRAMUSCULAR ANGIOMA
Note the complex mixture of vessel types as well as the very prominent adipocytic component.

cannot be ascertained with absolute certainty, but lesions composed of both fat and angiomatous vessels are classified as intramuscular angioma. Metaplastic ossification is also a frequent, and sometimes prominent, stromal feature, especially in cases of very mixed or malformed vessel types.

Special Studies. Aside from elastic stains, which may be used to demonstrate an arteriovenous component, additional diagnostic techniques play no role in this diagnosis.

Differential Diagnosis. The most common entity in the differential diagnosis is intramuscular lipoma, which is distinguished by its far

fewer vessels. The distinction is clinically relevant since intramuscular lipomas recur less often. Occasionally, solidly cellular cases of predominantly capillary type intramuscular angioma are mistaken for a malignant vascular tumor, especially if mitoses are frequent and there are reactive sarcolemmal nuclei. Principal clues to the benign diagnosis, aside from the rarity of deep-seated angiosarcoma, are the lobular architecture and the lack of endothelial multilayering or atypia.

Treatment and Prognosis. Intramuscular angiomas show no tendency to regress spontaneously and have a high local recurrence rate (at least 50 percent) unless widely excised. Recurrences can

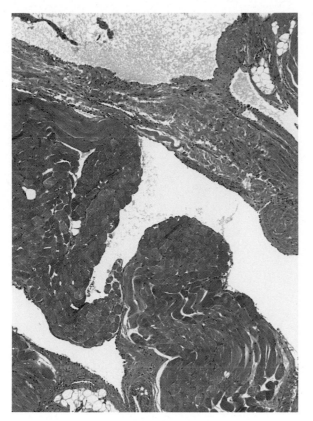

Figure 7-50
INTRAMUSCULAR ANGIOMA
This tumor from the chest wall consists mainly of large, thin-walled lymphatic spaces.

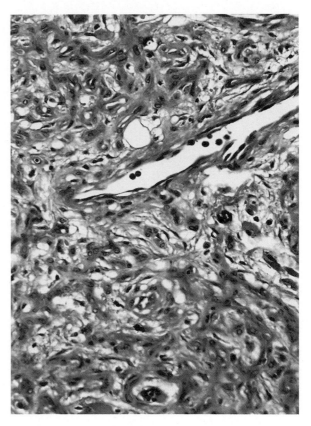

Figure 7-51
INTRAMUSCULAR ANGIOMA
This cellular lesion of mainly capillary type is associated with hyperchromatic reactive sarcolemmal nuclei in entrapped muscle cells.

be infiltrative and destructive so, in general, wide excision of the type undertaken for desmoid fibromatosis is usually appropriate. The recurrence rate shows no correlation with vessel type.

Synovial Hemangioma

Definition. Synovial hemangioma is a proliferation of benign blood vessels occurring within a synovial-lined joint or bursa.

Clinical Features. Synovial hemangiomas are uncommon. The knee is affected in the majority of cases, and presentation includes joint swelling, pain, and sometimes hemarthrosis (85). Less common sites are the elbow or hand. Most examples present during childhood or adolescence, suggesting a malformative origin.

Pathologic Findings. Most cases resemble cavernous hemangioma (see Cavernous Hemangioma) as at other locations and a smaller propor-

tion are of capillary or arteriovenous type. In general, the lesional vessels are found immediately beneath the synovial surface (fig. 7-52), and adjacent stromal scarring and hemosiderin deposition, likely due to trauma, are common. In some cases, especially those of longer standing, there may be villous hyperplasia of the overlying synovium.

Special Studies. Special stains usually play no role in this diagnosis.

Differential Diagnosis. There is no real differential diagnosis for such lesions. Cases in which there is contiguous growth of vessels into adjacent soft tissues and bone are better regarded as a form of angiomatosis (see below).

Angiomatosis

Definition. Angiomatosis is a diffuse proliferation of benign vascular structures in multiple tissue planes.

337

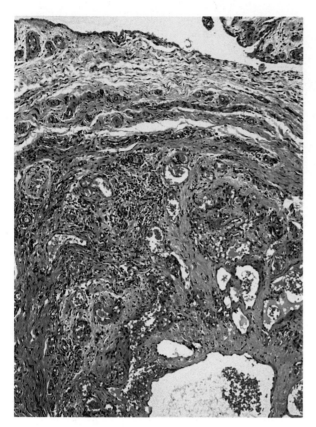

Figure 7-52
SYNOVIAL HEMANGIOMA
This mixed cavernous and capillary lesion is located immediately beneath the synovial lining of the knee joint.

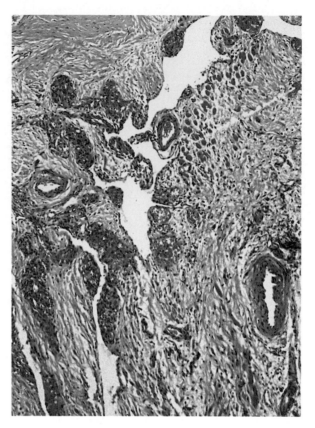

Figure 7-53
ANGIOMATOSIS
In this field skeletal muscle and fascia are diffusely infiltrated by vessels of varying type.

Clinical Features. Angiomatosis is rare and not well characterized. Most patients present in childhood or adolescence with diffuse soft tissue swelling, usually affecting all or a large part of a limb, especially the lower limb, although smaller examples do occur (86,87). The trunk may also be affected and there is an approximately equal sex incidence. The swelling may be painful and, in some patients, is associated with hypertrophy of the affected limb. As discussed for several of the lesions above, the early age at presentation and the pathologic features suggest that this is a developmental or malformative process. Gaining local control of these diffuse lesions can be extremely difficult (see below).

Pathologic Findings. The cardinal feature of angiomatosis is diffuse proliferation of vessels in multiple tissue planes, most often skin, subcutis, and underlying muscle, although bone also may be involved. There appear to be two main histo-

logic patterns: a *mixed vessel type* (fig. 7-53), as is often seen in intramuscular angioma (see above) and a *capillary-predominant type,* often having a somewhat lobular architecture (fig. 7-54). Either form is characteristically accompanied by increased amounts of adipose tissue.

Special Studies. Special stains and other pathologic techniques play no role in the diagnosis but angiography may be helpful in delineating the clinical extent of the lesion.

Differential Diagnosis. The diagnosis is based largely on clinicopathologic correlation. On purely morphologic grounds, the lesion may be indistinguishable from juvenile capillary hemangioma, arteriovenous hemangioma, or intramuscular angioma.

Treatment and Prognosis. Because of the difficulty either in identifying lesional margins or in undertaking a wide enough resection (bearing in mind that very radical surgery may not be

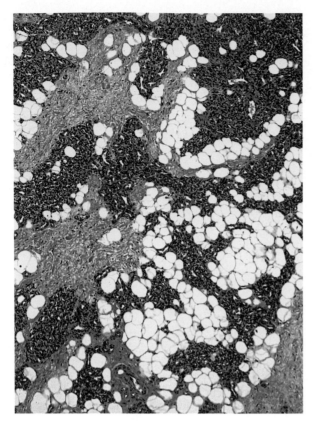

Figure 7-54
ANGIOMATOSIS
This capillary-predominant lesion involved the subcutis and underlying muscle of the entire lower leg of an 18-month-old child.

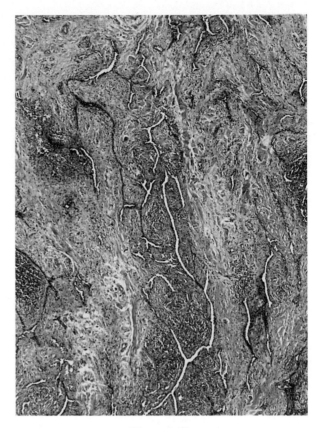

Figure 7-55
RETIFORM HEMANGIOENDOTHELIOMA
Note the characteristic arborizing vascular pattern.

indicated for an asymptomatic diffuse vascular anomaly such as this), repeated local recurrence is very common and reliable local control is hard to obtain in many patients. However, surgeons may be compelled to treat these lesions due to the pain and cosmetic disfigurement which often result.

Retiform Hemangioendothelioma

Definition. Retiform hemangioendothelioma is a rare endothelial neoplasm characterized by arborizing vessels and a hobnail endothelial morphology.

Clinical Features. Retiform hemangioendothelioma is a recently characterized tumor, formerly co-classified with angiosarcoma, which arises in the skin, mainly of the distal extremities, and usually affects young adults of either sex, although cases occur in older patients (88–91). The lesion usually presents as a slowly growing plaque, sometimes with a reddish purple

hue. One patient with multiple lesions has been described (90). Occasional cases occur in the setting of preceding lymphedema or irradiation (88). Lesional size rarely exceeds 2 to 3 cm.

Pathologic Findings. The tumor is centered mainly in the reticular dermis but often extends into both the papillary dermis and subcutis. It is characterized, at low-power magnification, by arborizing, elongated and generally narrow vessels (fig. 7-55) with hyperchromatic protuberant endothelial nuclei (fig. 7-56), hence the resemblance to rete testis, as is implied in the name. Approximately 50 percent of cases show a prominent lymphoid infiltrate which may be both stromal and intraluminal (fig. 7-57).

Closer examination of the neoplastic vessels, as they ramify through the dermis, reveals protuberant (hobnail or tombstone) endothelial nuclei with basal cytoplasm which merges imperceptibly with the vascular basement membrane. Some endothelial cells may form papillae reminiscent of

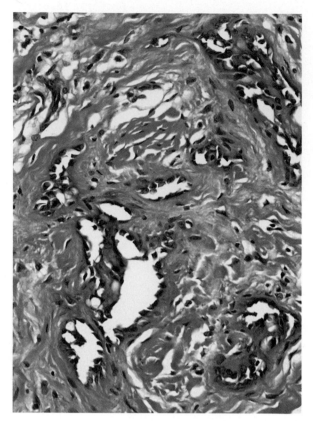

Figure 7-56
RETIFORM HEMANGIOENDOTHELIOMA
Note the protuberant (hobnail) endothelial nuclei.

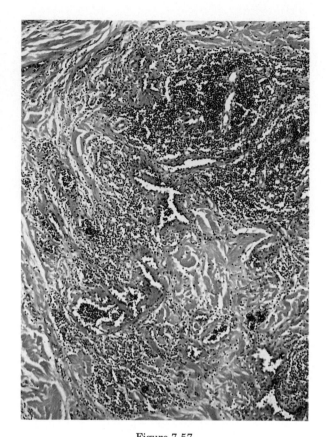

Figure 7-57
RETIFORM HEMANGIOENDOTHELIOMA
This case has a prominent lymphocytic infiltrate both in the stroma and in the lumen of vessels.

malignant endovascular papillary angioendothelioma (fig. 7-58) (see below) and rare cells may be vacuolated. Most tumors have variably prominent, but usually small, more solid areas composed of plumper endothelial cells arranged in sheets (fig. 7-59). In exceptional cases these solid areas may be more spindled. There is no endothelial pleomorphism and mitoses are scarce. In the single lymph node metastasis described so far the tumor cells were spindled (88).

Special Studies. The neoplastic endothelial cells stain with usual vascular markers, generally marking more strongly with CD34 than with CD31 or VWF. Keratin positivity is not a feature.

Differential Diagnosis. Hobnail hemangioma is a smaller, more superficial and more localized lesion in which the vessels in the papillary dermis are more dilated but narrow and disappear in the reticular dermis. Angiosarcoma generally affects older patients, and shows more irregular infiltration and collagen dissection, a greater endothelial pleomorphism, multilayering, and mitotic activity. Malignant endovascular papillary endothelioma (see below), while cytologically similar to retiform hemangioendothelioma, generally forms endovascular papillae within cavernous lymphatic-like spaces.

Treatment and Prognosis. Unless widely excised, these lesions recur locally and often do so repeatedly over a period of many years. The development of persistent uncontrolled disease in a distal location (wherein good margins are hard to obtain) sometimes leads to a digital (or ray) amputation. To date, only a single patient developed metastatic disease and this was to a groin lymph node (88). At the time of writing no patient is known to have died of retiform hemangioendothelioma but we do not exclude this as a possibility in the future.

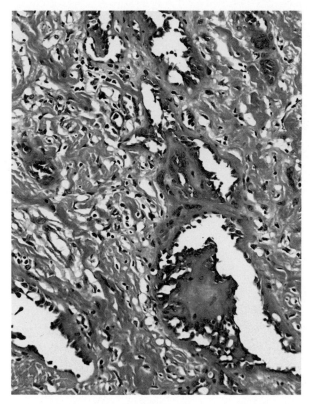

Figure 7-58
RETIFORM HEMANGIOENDOTHELIOMA
Intraluminal tufts or papillae, reminiscent of Dabska's tumor, are present focally in some cases.

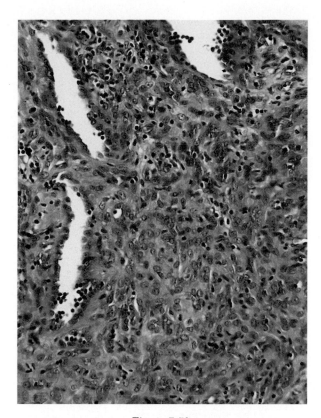

Figure 7-59
RETIFORM HEMANGIOENDOTHELIOMA
Many cases have small areas with a more solid, sheet-like growth pattern.

Malignant Endovascular Papillary Angioendothelioma (Dabska's Tumor, Papillary Intralymphatic Angioendothelioma)

General Considerations. Since the first formal description of this tumor type in 1969 (92), less than ten convincing additional case reports had been published, and not all were morphologically homogeneous, until the recent publication of Fanburg-Smith et al. (92a). These authors have relabeled the lesion papillary intralymphatic angioendothelioma and reported 12 cases.

Clinical Features. Based on available data, malignant endovascular papillary angioendothelioma (Dabska's tumor) affects mainly, but not exclusively, infants and children and shows a wide anatomic distribution, with predilection for the skin (92–94). It seems to present most often as a slowly growing, indurated plaque.

Pathologic Findings. With the confines of very limited data (92–94), not least because histo-

logic review of some of the originally reported cases suggests that at least a subset were in fact retiform hemangioendothelioma (91a), this lesion most often seems to be characterized by dilated, thin-walled, intradermal vessels, reminiscent of lymphatics, within which are cellular papillary structures composed of endothelial cells and admixed lymphocytes (fig. 7-60). Stromal lymphocytes are also a feature in some cases. The endothelial cells tend to be small and rounded, with a small amount of eosinophilic cytoplasm and hobnail type nuclei lacking significant atypia (fig. 7-61). The papillary tufts of endothelial cells may have a hyaline core. Lymphocytes tend to cluster around these papillae.

Special Studies. No reproducible data on more than a few cases are available.

Differential Diagnosis. The differential diagnosis of malignant endovascular papillary angioendothelioma is the same as for retiform hemangioendothelioma (see above).

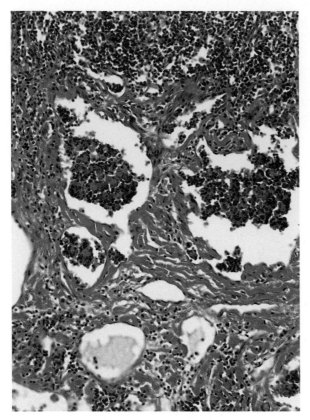

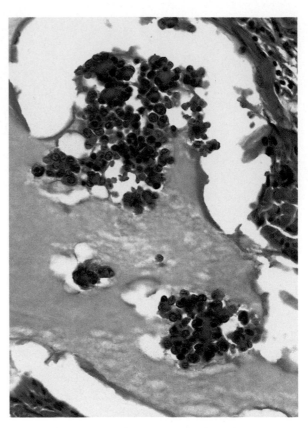

Figure 7-60
DABSKA'S TUMOR
Dilated lymphatic-like spaces contain papillary clusters of endothelial cells. Note the adjacent lymphocytes.

Figure 7-61
DABSKA'S TUMOR
The endothelial papillae often have a hyaline core. Individual endothelial cells are rounded.

Treatment and Prognosis. In the original series it was suggested that these lesions recur locally and rarely may spread to lymph nodes without systemic metastasis. However, it seems that at least one of the originally reported patients later died with metastatic disease so the issue of how malignant these lesions really are remains unresolved. In this circumstance it would seem advisable to widely excise any lesion that shows a reasonable morphologic fit.

Kaposiform Hemangioendothelioma

Definition. Kaposiform hemangioendothelioma, also known as *Kaposi-like infantile hemangioendothelioma,* is a locally aggressive vascular neoplasm affecting mainly children and having a lobular spindle cell growth pattern.

Clinical Features. Kaposiform hemangioendothelioma occurs most often in infants and children, especially those under the age of 2 years, but may also occur in adults (97) and, while it was originally thought to occur mainly in the retroperitoneum, can also arise in the limbs (95–100). Sex distribution is equal. It presents as a poorly marginated, multinodular, infiltrative mass which may reach a considerable size, especially in the retroperitoneum. Clinical effects are due mainly to its infiltrative growth as well as a common association with consumption coagulopathy (Kasabach-Merritt syndrome), which seems to be an almost consistent feature of retroperitoneal cases (95,96,100). Up to 20 percent of cases also are associated with lymphangiomatosis of the adjacent soft tissue (100).

Pathologic Findings. Macroscopically, the lesions consist initially of multiple hemorrhagic nodules, each measuring no more than 1 to 2 cm in most cases. The nodules and intervening fibrous tissue then coalesce to form a firm mass.

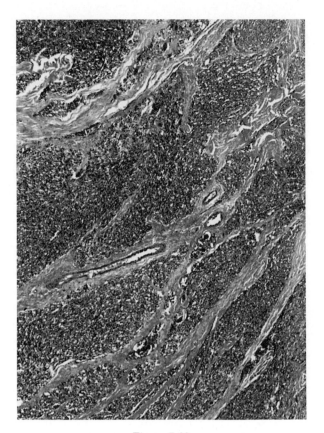

Figure 7-62
KAPOSIFORM HEMANGIOENDOTHELIOMA
Note the distinctive lobularity at low power, a feature not seen in Kaposi's sarcoma.

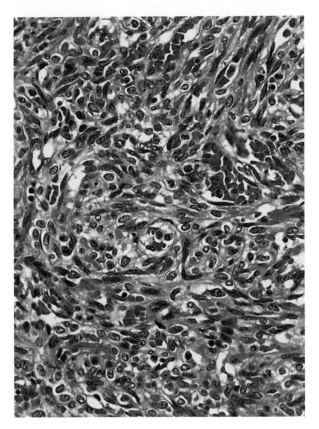

Figure 7-63
KAPOSIFORM HEMANGIOENDOTHELIOMA
Individual lobules are composed of palely eosinophilic spindle cells, some of which have plump nuclei.

Histologically, the striking features at low-power microscopy are high cellularity and a lobular architecture with poorly defined margins (fig. 7-62). Individual lobules closely resemble Kaposi's sarcoma in being composed of uniform spindle cells with pale eosinophilic cytoplasm and elongated nuclei (fig. 7-63). However, these are associated, especially at the lobular periphery, with rounded, thin-walled capillaries and frequent fibrin microthrombi (fig. 7-64). Atypia is absent and mitoses are scarce. Some cases contain clusters of more epithelioid endothelial cells which may show cytoplasmic vacuolation. Hyaline globules are an occasional feature. Especially in deep-seated lesions, the margins can be very infiltrative and destroy adjacent normal tissue, such as pancreas.

Special Studies. A significant proportion of the spindle cells stain with endothelial markers, while some are also actin positive in keeping with the nature of pericytes.

Differential Diagnosis. On morphologic grounds, Kaposi's sarcoma is the main entity in the differential diagnosis. In young children, however, this is exceptionally rare outside lymph nodes. In addition, Kaposi's sarcoma generally lacks the lobularity, dilated capillaries, and fibrin microthrombi of kaposiform hemangioendothelioma. Spindle cell hemangioma differs by rarely being deep-seated and by the presence of cavernous spaces, frequent papillary structures, and prominently vacuolated epithelioid endothelial cells. Tufted angioma is a dermal lesion in which the lobules are smaller, more widely dispersed, and usually less spindled in cytologic terms, often with a crescentic lymphatic vessel at their periphery.

Treatment and Prognosis. Kaposiform hemangioendothelioma is fatal in perhaps 20 percent of cases but this seems only to occur in retroperitoneal lesions or those associated with

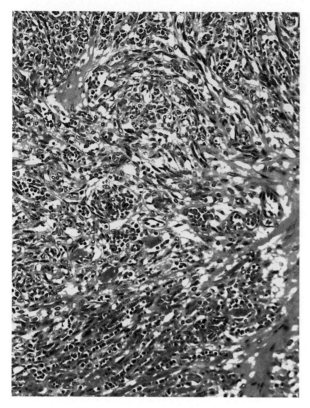

Figure 7-64
KAPOSIFORM HEMANGIOENDOTHELIOMA
Fibrin microthrombi are numerous.

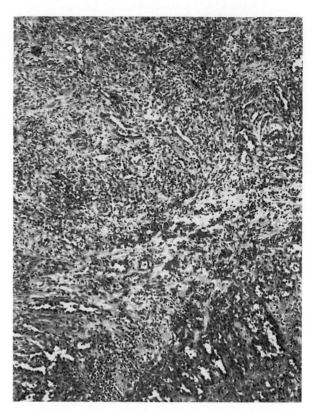

Figure 7-65
POLYMORPHOUS HEMANGIOENDOTHELIOMA
Low-power view shows mixed angiomatous and solid areas.

consumption coagulopathy. At any location recurrence is frequent and control of local disease is often difficult, sometimes necessitating radical surgery. Although one limb lesion involved adjacent lymph nodes (96), no case with systemic metastasis has been reported as yet.

Polymorphous Hemangioendothelioma

Definition. Polymorphous hemangioendothelioma is a very rare, low-grade endothelial malignancy with a complex variety of growth patterns.

Clinical Features. Few cases of polymorphous hemangioendothelioma have been reported. It occurs mainly in lymph nodes (101), usually in adults (see the Fascicle, Tumors of the Lymph Nodes and Spleen [102a]). Isolated cases also exist in soft tissue (102). Although data are limited, it seems that these lesions have the potential to metastasize as well as recur (102).

Pathologic Findings. Polymorphous hemangioendothelioma is a complex mixture of solid,

primitive vascular and more angiomatous endothelial areas (fig. 7-65). Tumor cells are consistently plump and even epithelioid, with occasional vacuoles. Solid areas have a sheet-like, nested, or trabecular growth pattern. The angiomatous component may have a retiform appearance (see Retiform Hemangioendothelioma above) (fig. 7-66). Nuclear atypia is not a feature and mitoses are rare.

Giant Cell Angioblastoma

A single case of giant cell angioblastoma has been reported (103) and we have seen one other convincing example (courtesy of Dr. H. Kozakewich, Boston, MA). Both were congenital lesions, one in the upper limb and one in the palate, and both were characterized by progressive, infiltrative local growth, leading to amputation in the first case. Histologically, both cases consisted of diffusely infiltrating vascular channels, lined by a plump endothelial monolayer associated with

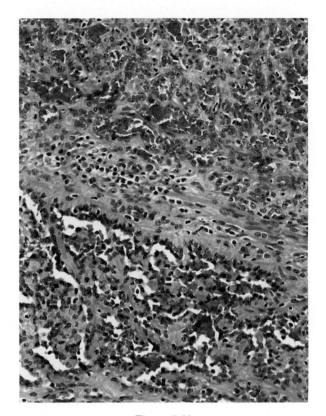

Figure 7-66
POLYMORPHOUS HEMANGIOENDOTHELIOMA
In this field a solid epithelioid area abuts a retiform angiomatous area.

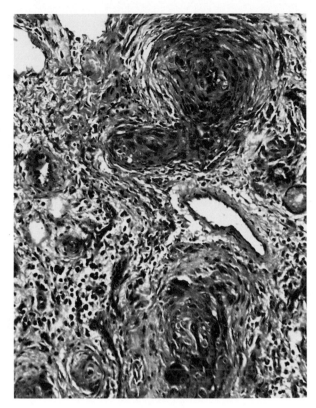

Figure 7-67
GIANT CELL ANGIOBLASTOMA
Associated with this vascular proliferation are nodular clusters of histiocyte-like cells and osteoclasts. These nodules seem to be angiocentric.

whorled nodules of histiocyte-like cells and osteoclastic giant cells; these nodules are reminiscent of plexiform fibrohistiocytic tumor. In areas, the histiocyte-like nodules seem to be centered around the lesional vessels (fig. 7-67).

Kaposi's Sarcoma

Definition. Kaposi's sarcoma (KS) is a low-grade clonal endothelial proliferation with a variably vasoformative or spindle cell growth and often is associated with immunodeficiency.

General Considerations. KS has been the subject of great attention and research in the past two decades. Prior to that time it occurred in two main forms: elderly endemic and African (see below). But then the advent of a large number of AIDS-related cases (113), seemingly with a more aggressive course, focused attention on this, up to that time, somewhat neglected entity (106,108, 113,116,123,124). There has been considerable

dispute as to whether KS is a multifocal reactive vascular lesion or a true neoplasm but the pendulum is now swinging back to the latter (original) viewpoint, based on recent evidence of clonality (121) and the demonstrated ability of lesional cells for independent growth in vitro. Recently, it has been convincingly shown that most cases in each clinical subset (see below) are likely etiologically related to HHV8 (KSHV) infection (119,120), although absolute proof is lacking.

Clinical Features. KS is most easily understood if subclassified into clinical groups (106, 116,123) as follows:

Classic KS presents typically as one or more, indolent, red-brown vascular lesions in the distal extremities of elderly patients, with a notable predilection for patients of Mediterranean or Ashkenazi Jewish origin. Preexisting edema in the affected limb(s) is common. Development of systemic (visceral) involvement is exceptionally rare and this type of KS seems to have no impact on life expectancy. However, patients with classic KS are at increased risk for developing a hematolymphoid malignancy, both processes possibly reflecting an age-related defect in the immune system.

AIDS-related KS presents most often as disseminated, multi-organ disease, with a predilection for mucocutaneous sites as well as the lungs, gastrointestinal tract, and lymph nodes (106, 113,116,123). Widespread skin lesions as well as oral mucosal involvement are most common but almost any site may be affected, with the notable exceptions of bone, skeletal muscle, and cerebral tissue (114,117,118). The overwhelming majority of cases occur in male patients and, among Western patients, most cases occur in homosexuals. In African patients with AIDS, KS is also common in the heterosexual group. In the absence of sex-related risk factors, KS is extremely uncommon in either the drug abuse or hemophilia-related risk groups.

KS associated with iatrogenic immunosuppression is very uncommon but occurs mainly in patients on long-term immunosuppressive therapy, usually related to organ transplantation (105,106,111,116,122). To date, most cases have been described in renal transplant recipients, likely reflecting their comparatively large numbers and the longer time period over which this surgical technique has been used. The clinical course is variable but is more often indolent than aggressive. Some cases regress spontaneously if immunosuppressive therapy is withdrawn.

African KS is a separate endemic form of KS, likely related to chronic immunosuppression, to which factors such as malaria and tropical splenomegaly contribute (104,109,110,117). It has been known for many years but its clinical picture has been confused by the advent of the AIDS epidemic. Prior to the AIDS-related cases there were two main clinical groups: adult males with progressive cutaneous disease of the lower limbs but very rare systemic involvement and a childhood form, affecting mainly lymph nodes in patients of either sex, and associated usually with systemic spread and a fatal outcome if left untreated.

Pathologic Findings. Although they form a morphologic continuum, the histologic features of KS in skin and soft tissue are traditionally divided into patch, plaque, and nodular forms.

Only the nodular type is really obvious macroscopically, being characterized by a reddish purple, usually elevated dermal nodule, most often less than 2 to 3 cm in diameter. In histologic terms, the clinical subsets described above are indistinguishable, although the classic (endemic) type is rarely diagnosed before it reaches the nodular stage, whereas early detection in AIDS patients leads to a high proportion of biopsies in the patch stage. The appearance of visceral or nodal disease is covered in their respective volumes of this Fascicle series.

Patch stage KS is characterized by thin-walled, narrow vascular channels dissecting through dermal collagen, usually parallel to the epidermis (fig. 7-68). These vessels have plump, hyperchromatic endothelial nuclei with little associated cytoplasm and no endothelial multilayering, and are associated with scattered plasma cells, small numbers of spindle cells, extravasated red blood cells, and hemosiderin in the stroma. Often, the process wraps around preexisting dermal structures (larger vessels or adnexal structures), the so called promontory sign (fig. 7-69). Cases in which the dissecting channels are notably ectatic are sometimes referred to as *lymphangiomatous KS* (107,112).

Plaque stage KS differs from patch stage by the development of a more prominent spindle cell component (fig. 7-70), both around vessels and also ramifying in bundles through the full thickness of the dermis. Spindle cells are uniform in appearance with eosinophilic cytoplasm (fig. 7-71), are associated with more prominent stromal hemorrhage, and may extend into the subcutis. Extracellular or cytoplasmic refractile hyaline globules are usually easily found (106,113). Their precise nature is uncertain but they may represent degenerate red blood cells, sometimes located within phagolysosomes.

Nodular KS consists of a well-circumscribed but unencapsulated mass of eosinophilic spindle cells, arranged in whorls and fascicles, with intervening slit-like spaces (fig. 7-72). When cut in cross section the fascicles have a sieve-like appearance. Nuclei are ovoid to elongated and generally bland with frequent mitoses (fig. 7-73). Within the slit-like spaces extravasated red blood cells are numerous and hyaline globules are generally easily found (fig. 7-74), especially in AIDS-related and African cases (115). Very

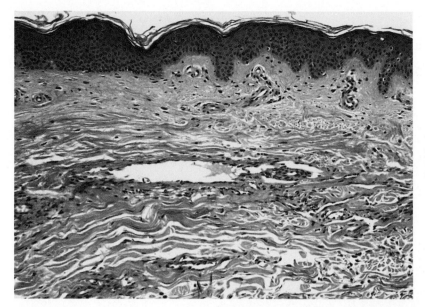

Figure 7-68
KAPOSI'S SARCOMA
This patch stage lesion shows thin-walled dissecting vessels parallel to the epidermis. Note also extravasated red blood cells and scattered perivascular spindle cells.

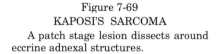

Figure 7-69
KAPOSI'S SARCOMA
A patch stage lesion dissects around eccrine adnexal structures.

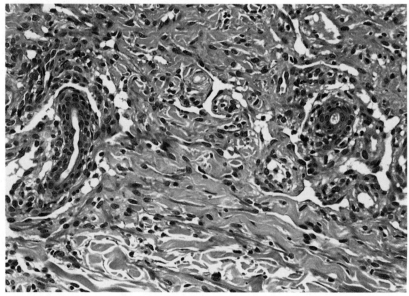

rare examples of nodular KS show marked nuclear atypia and pleomorphism (so called *anaplastic KS*); most cases so diagnosed in the past likely represented other tumor types. Necrosis and vascular invasion are exceedingly rare.

Special Studies. The dissecting vessels seen in patch and plaque stage disease stain with usual endothelial markers. The spindle cells in nodular KS typically stain strongly for CD34 (fig. 7-75) and CD31 but only focally and weakly for VWF or *Ulex europaeus* I. Virtually all cases show nu-

clear immunoreactivity for HHV-8. The hyaline globules can be highlighted by their diastase-PAS or trichrome positivity. Electron microscopy confirms that at least some of the spindle cells have usual endothelial features.

Differential Diagnosis. Patch stage KS needs to be distinguished from angiosarcoma, progressive lymphangioma, and hobnail hemangioma. Angiosarcoma shows more endothelial atypia and multilayering, and generally develops in a different clinical context (see below). Progressive

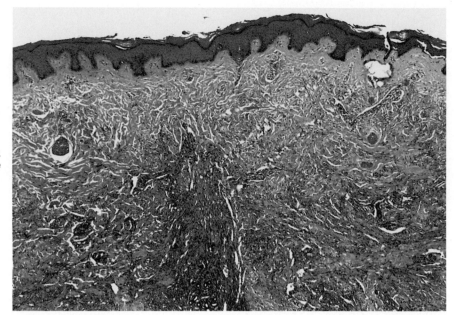

Figure 7-70
KAPOSI'S SARCOMA
Plaque stage lesions are much more cellular and extend more deeply.

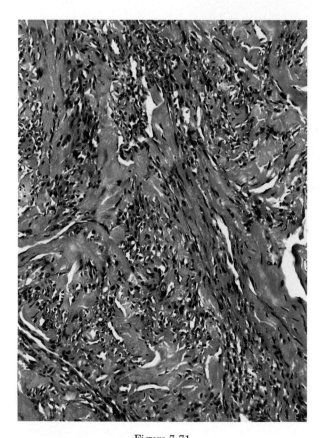

Figure 7-71
KAPOSI'S SARCOMA
In this plaque stage lesion the spindle cells ramify in bundles through the dermis.

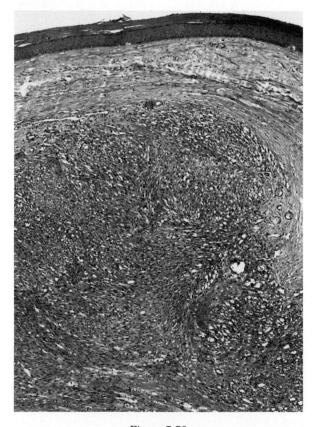

Figure 7-72
KAPOSI'S SARCOMA
The lesions in nodular stage disease are usually well circumscribed.

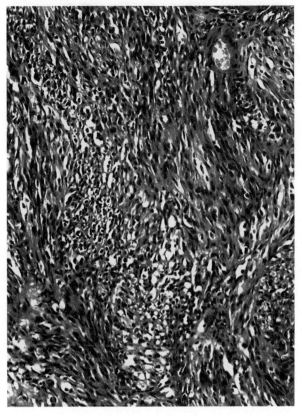

Figure 7-73
KAPOSI'S SARCOMA
The fascicles are composed of uniform eosinophilic spindle cells with slit-like spaces. When cut in cross section they have the appearance of a sieve.

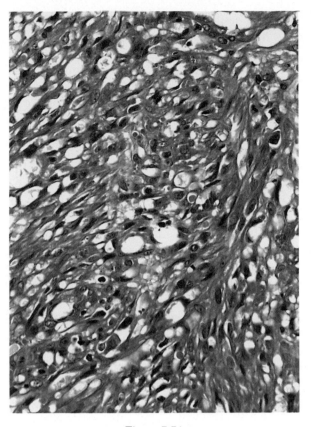

Figure 7-74
KAPOSI'S SARCOMA
The typically bland spindle cell morphology and associated hyaline droplets are evident in this field.

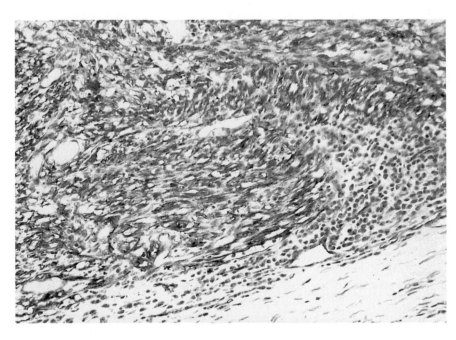

Figure 7-75
KAPOSI'S SARCOMA
Lesional spindle cells are consistently immunopositive for CD34 (ABC method).

lymphangioma is clinically different (see page 360) and lacks atypical endothelial nuclei or inflammatory cells. Hobnail hemangioma, at least in the superficial dermis, has more dilated vessels and a less irregular, dissecting pattern. Nodular KS must be distinguished from spindle cell hemangioma, kaposiform hemangioendothelioma, and aneurysmal benign fibrous histiocytoma. Spindle cell hemangioma has cavernous spaces, often has papillary structures, and always contains vacuolated endothelial cells. Kaposiform hemangioendothelioma affects mainly children and has a multilobular growth pattern, usually with fibrin microthrombi. Aneurysmal fibrous histiocytoma shows cytologic polymorphism, lateral entrapment of dermal collagen, overlying epidermal hyperplasia, and a storiform growth pattern. Plaque stage KS, which is the least often biopsied, really has no differential diagnosis.

Treatment and Prognosis. Indolent endemic lesions may be persistent, recurrent, and complicated by bleeding but are nondestructive and generally nonaggressive. AIDS-related and African childhood lesions most often result in progressive disease, eventually with systemic (visceral) involvement. In the absence of treatment this may lead to severe compromise of lung function as well as gastrointestinal hemorrhage. As mentioned earlier, whether this represents conventional "metastatic" spread remains controversial since the absence of bone or brain involvement is hard to explain when compared to other malignant neoplasms.

MALIGNANT VASCULAR TUMORS (MANAGERIAL GROUP III, TABLE 1-10)

Epithelioid Hemangioendothelioma

Definition. Epithelioid hemangioendothelioma (EHE) is a morphologically low-grade malignant endothelial neoplasm characterized by epithelioid endothelial cytomorphology and a unicellular or linear, as opposed to a canalized, pattern of vascular differentiation.

Clinical Features. Although well known to occur in lung, liver, bone, and, less often, other organs (132), the focus here is on EHE arising primarily in soft tissue. Readers are referred to other volumes of this series as appropriate. In contrast to other locations, EHE arising in soft

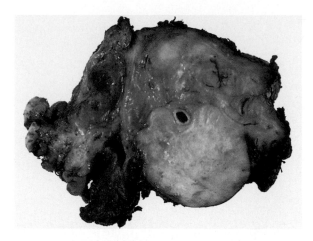

Figure 7-76
EPITHELIOID HEMANGIOENDOTHELIOMA
This tumor from the groin, which had largely obliterated the femoral vein, has a pale, fibrous cut surface with an ill-defined margin. (Courtesy of Dr. E.A. Sankey, London, U.K.)

tissue is most often, at least initially, a solitary lesion and occurs mainly in mid-adult life, affecting patients of either sex equally (125,128,129, 131,132). Examples in children are distinctly rare. Almost any anatomic location may be affected and more cases are subfascial than subcutaneous; up to 10 percent are dermal in location. The usual presenting feature is an enlarging mass; a significant proportion of patients complain of pain, likely resulting from lesional angiocentricity (see below). When excised, most tumors measure less than 5 cm and examples greater than 10 cm are uncommon. Importantly, a subset of patients (perhaps 10 percent at most) are found to have had, or later develop, multiorgan EHE over a very prolonged period, often decades. This may include any combination and order of soft tissue, lung, bone, liver, and other involvement. Whether or not this truly represents indolent metastasis or whether it is indicative of field change disease is as yet unelucidated. No etiologic associations have been identified so far in EHE of soft tissue.

Pathologic Findings. Macroscopically, these lesions tend to be firm, fibrous or gritty, with a pale cut surface and a variably delimited margin (fig. 7-76). Occasional cases may show obvious involvement of a large vessel. There is usually no gross evidence of hemorrhage or necrosis.

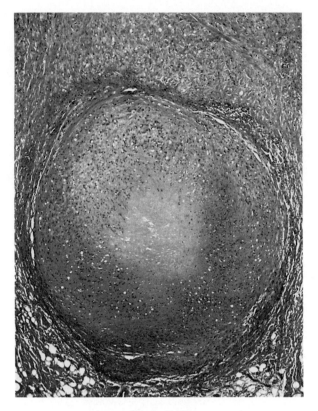

Figure 7-77
EPITHELIOID HEMANGIOENDOTHELIOMA
The tumor has filled this vein and has spread into surrounding soft tissue in an eccentrically, apparently centrifugal fashion.

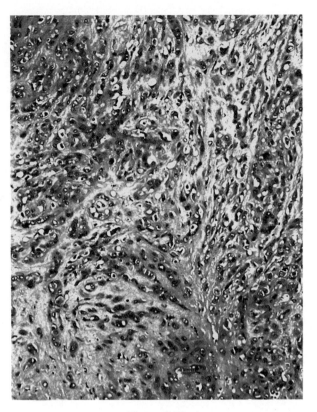

Figure 7-78
EPITHELIOID HEMANGIOENDOTHELIOMA
A typical case composed of cords of epithelioid cells in a myxohyaline matrix.

Histologically, most examples of EHE are poorly marginated, infiltrative lesions while occasional cases are multinodular. Approximately one third appear to originate from a vessel, usually a vein, and to spread centrifugally within a myxohyaline stroma (fig. 7-77). Other examples have an entirely diffuse growth pattern with no evidence of a specialized stroma. For the most part, tumor cells are arranged in cords, strands, small nests, or singly, with little or no evidence of overt vessel formation (fig. 7-78). Individual cells are plump, rounded or, less often, spindled, with palely eosinophilic cytoplasm and a vesicular nucleus with an inconspicuous nucleolus. A variable proportion of cells typically show striking cytoplasmic vacuolation (fig. 7-79), known as intracytoplasmic lumina, within which red blood cells are occasionally seen. Adjacent stroma may show recent or old hemorrhage, hyalinization, focal chronic inflammation, and, in up to 15 per-

cent of cases, metaplastic ossification (fig. 7-80) (128). Some cases, particularly those in the mediastinum, show an osteoclastic giant cell reaction in the stroma (127,129,133).

Most cases have little or no cytologic atypia and few mitoses (generally less than 2 per 10 high-power fields), but 10 to 15 percent of these tumors have worrisome features in the form of either nuclear atypia and pleomorphism, more spindle cell type cytology, higher mitotic activity, or focally more solid sheet-like growth reminiscent of epithelioid angiosarcoma (fig. 7-81). At the individual case level, these features do not correlate reliably with more aggressive behavior (128); nevertheless, there is a trend in this regard which suggests the existence of a morphologic and biologic continuum between EHE and epithelioid angiosarcoma. Rare cases may be very hard to subclassify in this context. It is our practice, when a lesion shows predominant characteristics of EHE but with obvious solid foci

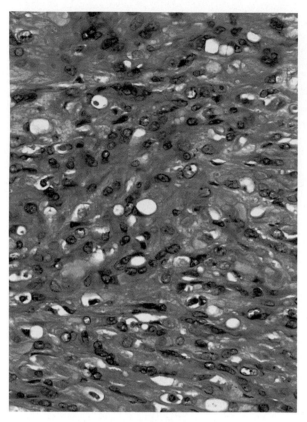

Figure 7-79
EPITHELIOID HEMANGIOENDOTHELIOMA
Lesional cells have vesicular nuclei, eosinophilic cytoplasm, and frequent cytoplasmic vacuoles ("lumina").

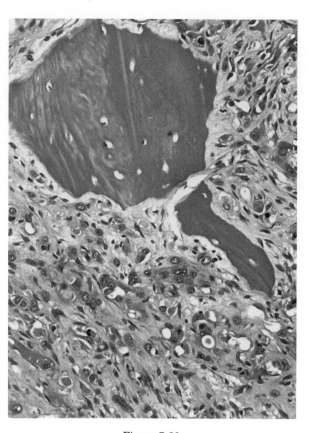

Figure 7-80
EPITHELIOID HEMANGIOENDOTHELIOMA
Metaplastic ossification in the stroma is a relatively frequent finding.

Figure 7-81
EPITHELIOID
HEMANGIOENDOTHELIOMA
This case shows marked nuclear atypia and focally is forming more solid nests and sheets. These are features which suggest an increased risk of clinical aggression.

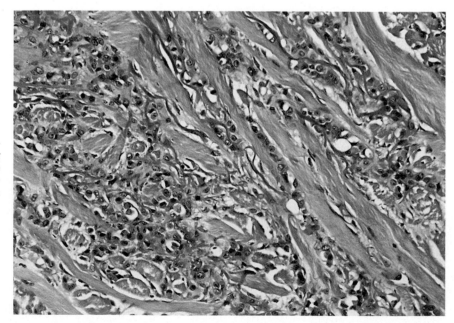

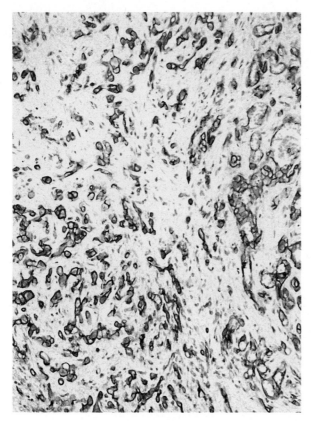

Figure 7-82
EPITHELIOID HEMANGIOENDOTHELIOMA
Almost all the lesional cells are strongly immunopositive
for CD31 (ABC method).

and increased atypia, to use the designation "malignant epithelioid hemangioendothelioma" in order to convey greater concern about the likely clinical behavior.

Special Studies. In the absence of fixation, or other artefacts, essentially all cases are immunopositive for one or more endothelial antigens, among which CD31 (fig. 7-82) and VWF are the most specific. In addition, up to a third are positive for keratin, which is usually only focal but can be potentially misleading (126,128,130). A significant proportion of cases are also positive for actin in the endothelial cells. If there is a need to establish vascular differentiation by other means, a reticulin stain reveals that the nests and cords are invested by a reticulin sheath in the manner of a tubular (vascular) structure and, by electron microscopy, tumor cells show usual endothelial features in the form of scattered Weibel-Palade bodies, prominent pinocytosis, and usu-

ally a well-formed external lamina. Additional features seen in EHE are prominent sheets of cytoplasmic filaments, hence the epithelioid appearance, as well as intracytoplasmic lumina.

Differential Diagnosis. EHE is distinguished by its well-formed, canalized vessels and often lobular architecture. Epithelioid angiosarcoma, by contrast, tends to grow in diffuse sheets and the tumor cells tend to be larger than those of EHE, with a prominent amphophilic nucleolus. Frankly vasoformative foci may be present. Cellular myxoid liposarcoma (round cell liposarcoma) is sometimes mistaken for EHE but differs by the presence of thin-walled, arborizing vessels, the usual presence of multivacuolated (as well as monovacuolated) lipoblasts, and negativity for endothelial markers. Metastatic carcinoma or epithelioid sarcoma are separable by their usually strong and diffuse positivity for keratin and epithelial membrane antigen while CD31 and VWF are negative. CD34 is less helpful in this context since up to 50 percent of epithelioid sarcomas are positive. Vacuolated cells in a carcinoma commonly contain mucin; conversely, vacuolated cells are usually sparse in epithelioid sarcoma. The distinctive necrosis and eosinophilic collagen of epithelioid sarcoma are not features of EHE.

Treatment and Prognosis. Aside from those rare patients who develop indolent multiorgan disease (mentioned above), up to a third of patients with EHE of soft tissue develop nodal or systemic metastases and overall mortality is about 20 percent, hence the designation as borderline seems inappropriate (128). Predicting behavior reliably on histologic grounds is not possible since very bland lesions may metastasize, although there is a trend for more atypical lesions to be more aggressive. The local recurrence rate is only 10 to 15 percent, likely reflecting the comparative ease of obtaining adequate margins around relatively small tumors.

Angiosarcoma

Definition. Angiosarcoma, also known as *hemangiosarcoma, lymphangiosarcoma,* and *malignant hemangioendothelioma,* is a malignant endothelial neoplasm characterized by an atypical, multilayered or solid endothelial proliferation and a vasoformative architecture.

General Considerations. Angiosarcoma is the preferred term since there are no reliable means to distinguish (or prove) blood vascular or lymphatic endothelial origin or differentiation. Use of the term hemangioendothelioma, other than with a specific qualifier relating to a defined entity, is discouraged since this word has been used over the past 40 years to describe a wide variety of lesions which span the full spectrum of vascular tumor biology. Angiosarcomas of the breast and visceral organs are described in their respective Fascicles.

Clinical Features. Classically, angiosarcoma in skin and soft tissue was said to occur in two main forms: most often in the head and neck region of elderly individuals (138,141,143,147,152,156) and much less often in a lymphedematous limb (135, 137,138,153,157) (irrespective of etiology), as was first described in postmastectomy patients (Stewart-Treves syndrome) (153). The majority of cases in both groups are cutaneous in origin and have usually a reddish brown or bruise-like appearance. However, over time, other, albeit smaller, clinical subsets have emerged, specifically a group arising in deep soft tissue, including the abdominal cavity, which is often of the epithelioid type (140,150a), and a group arising at the site of prior irradiation (139,142,148). Hence, angiosarcoma is widely distributed, although skin of the breast (139) and anterior abdominal wall seem the most common areas of predilection. Angiosarcomas in deep soft tissue probably account for 15 to 20 percent of cases, a higher proportion than previously believed. Angiosarcomas may also in exceptional cases arise from a large vessel (134,140) or nerve, or as part of a nerve sheath neoplasm (154). Although formerly regarded as a tumor of the elderly, an increasing number of cases are now recognized in younger adults and even children (145,146), at least in our experience. The reason for this changing (or broadening) distribution is unclear, but it remains most sensible to think twice and perhaps seek consultative opinion before diagnosing angiosarcoma outside its most common clinical settings.

In contrast to hepatosplenic angiosarcomas, there is very little evidence to suggest a role for chemical agents in the etiology of cutaneous or soft tissue angiosarcoma, but rare cases arise at the site of a foreign body or previous trauma (136,144). Some authors have postulated that

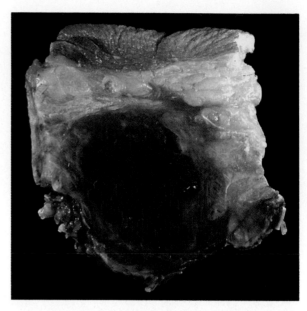

Figure 7-83
ANGIOSARCOMA
This epithelioid angiosarcoma, involving fascia and deep subcutis, has a very hemorrhagic cut surface.

ultraviolet irradiation (sunlight) may be etiologically important (156).

Pathologic Findings. Macroscopically, angiosarcomas are not generally distinctive, at least in usual biopsy form, despite the often dramatic blue-red skin lesions seen clinically. Larger deep-seated masses may be hemorrhagic (fig. 7-83) but this is not a consistent feature.

Histologically, the appearance of angiosarcoma is both very variable and often mixed within an individual lesion, usually reflecting different degrees of vascular differentiation. Better differentiated lesions or areas (fig. 7-84) are characterized by irregularly infiltrative or dissecting vascular channels lined by endothelial cells showing variable degrees of cytologic pleomorphism, nuclear atypia, mitotic activity, and multilayering, often with tufts or papillae. The neoplastic vessels commonly have a complex, irregularly anastomosing growth pattern. In the most innocent-looking cases, the combination of nuclear hyperchromasia and multilayering is the best clue to malignancy, although nucleomegaly is not always a feature and nucleoli are not always present. With increasing anaplasia tumor cells become more atypical, close-packed, and often spindle-shaped (fig. 7-85), with progressive loss

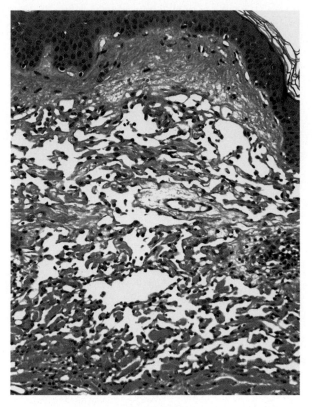

Figure 7-84
ANGIOSARCOMA
This well-differentiated example from a lymphedematous
limb shows marked collagen dissection and papillary growth.

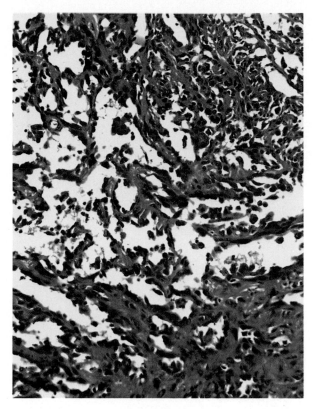

Figure 7-85
ANGIOSARCOMA
This moderately differentiated lesion shows greater en-
dothelial nuclear atypia and a more variable growth pattern.

of evident vascular channels, such that the most poorly differentiated examples usually appear as a high-grade spindle cell malignancy (fig. 7-86) with no distinguishing features on H&E examination. Very rare examples have granular cytoplasm (150). Cases with a very infiltrative, dissecting pattern of growth, especially those in the head and neck, often extend over a wide area both laterally and deeply, permeating subcutis, muscle, and even bone, and commonly extend beyond clinically evident margins or even beyond what is clinically resectable (fig. 7-87). In addition, angiosarcoma often seems to have a discontinuous or multifocal growth pattern, suggestive of a field change phenomenon. The sometimes subtle nuclear features, delicate dissecting growth pattern, and tendency for discontinuous tumor growth render frozen section useless in the reliable assessment of resection margins in better differentiated angiosarcomas. Some cases of angiosarcoma show a prominent lymphocytic in-

filtrate and this has been suggested as a favorable prognostic factor (143).

It has long been recognized that angiosarcoma may focally be composed of larger, more rounded epithelioid cells (152) but only over the past 10 years has the purely epithelioid form been fully characterized (132,140). Epithelioid lesions more often arise in deep soft tissue (140, 150a) than skin (149,151), and in the abdominal cavity were formerly confused with carcinoma or mesothelioma. They tend to have a sheet-like rather than obviously vasoformative architecture (fig. 7-88). Tumor cells typically are large, amphophilic (often rather hepatoid), and have a large vesicular nucleus with a prominent nucleolus (fig. 7-89), reminiscent of malignant melanoma. Intracytoplasmic lumina are usually evident in some cells and may contain occasional erythrocytes. There is usually little pleomorphism but mitoses are frequent and hemorrhage and necrosis are common.

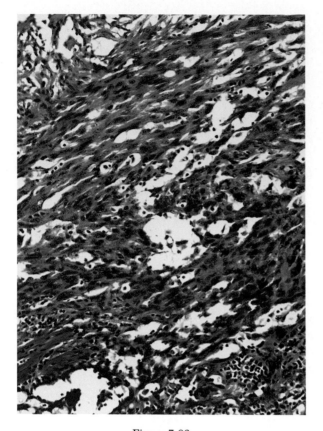

Figure 7-86
ANGIOSARCOMA
This poorly differentiated scalp mass has a predominant spindle cell pattern.

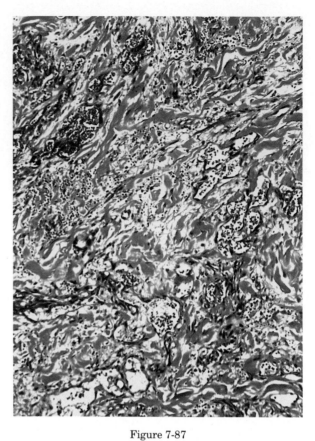

Figure 7-87
ANGIOSARCOMA
Notice the irregular, subtle but extensive dissection of collagen by delicate vascular channels. This comes from the resection margin of an amputation for Stewart-Treves syndrome.

Figure 7-88
EPITHELIOID
ANGIOSARCOMA
Epithelioid lesions most often have a diffuse, sheet-like architecture.

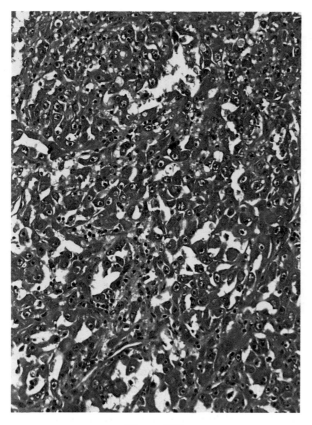

Figure 7-89
EPITHELIOID ANGIOSARCOMA
Tumor cells are large and eosinophilic, with vesicular nuclei and prominent nucleoli.

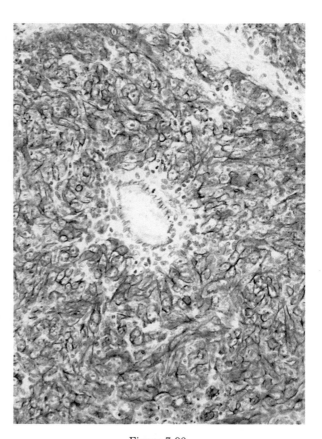

Figure 7-90
ANGIOSARCOMA
Note the strong CD31 positivity in both neoplastic and normal endothelial cells (ABC method).

Special Studies. Reticulin staining can be helpful in outlining a tubular vasoformative architecture, especially in epithelioid lesions. Most angiosarcomas are immunopositive for CD31 (fig. 7-90), which is very specific, and less often for CD34, which is much less specific. Staining for VWF is variable but is much more often positive in epithelioid, rather than conventional, cases. The relative nonspecificity of *Ulex europaeus* I means that this lectin has been largely superceded by CD31 as an endothelial marker. In addition, up to 50 percent of epithelioid angiosarcomas are keratin positive (fig. 7-91) and a small proportion stain for epithelial membrane antigen. Electron microscopic demonstration of endothelial differentiation (Weibel-Palade bodies, pinocytosis, and prominent external lamina) is more easily obtained in epithelioid rather than conventional lesions and therefore is only infrequently useful in routine diagnosis.

Differential Diagnosis. Distinction of conventional-type angiosarcoma from a variety of benign hemangiomas is achieved principally on finding endothelial multilayering as well as endothelial atypia. However, a complex anastomosing growth pattern also favors angiosarcoma. Atypia in the absence of multilayering should be treated with caution since this may represent a reactive pseudosarcomatous feature, especially in ulcerated or otherwise traumatized lesions. Poorly differentiated angiosarcomas are best distinguished from other spindle cell malignant neoplasms by immunohistochemistry, especially using CD31, the most sensitive endothelial marker. Epithelioid angiosarcoma is distinguished from epithelioid hemangioendothelioma by its sheet-like growth pattern and generally larger cell size, although cases exist with overlapping features (see above). Overtly vasoformative foci may also be present in epithelioid angiosarcoma.

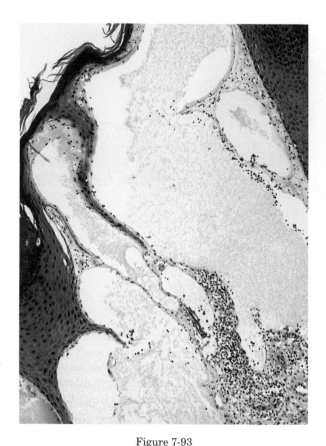

Figure 7-93
LYMPHANGIOMA CIRCUMSCRIPTUM
The lymphatic spaces have a flattened, attenuated endothelial lining. Note the stromal lymphocytes.

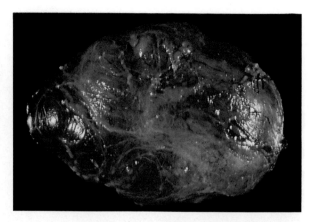

Figure 7-94
CAVERNOUS LYMPHANGIOMA
A typically lobulated cystic example from the neck of a young child.

spongy masses of variable size (fig. 7-94) and are uncommon in the limbs. Among stillborn fetuses with cystic hygroma there is a high incidence of the XO (Turner's) karyotype (159). A significant, but uncommon, subset of cavernous lymphangiomas arise in the abdominal cavity, especially the mesentery, where they often reach a large size and clinically can be confused with a multicystic mesothelioma or, less often, a pancreatic cystic lesion.

Pathologic Findings. Cavernous lymphangioma consists of large, dilated lymphatic spaces with an attenuated endothelial lining (fig. 7-95) that contain variable amounts of lymph, as well as lymphocytes and sometimes red blood cells. The walls of the larger lymphatic spaces often contain discontinuous bundles of smooth muscle and lymphoid aggregates (fig. 7-96), sometimes, especially in larger cystic lesions, forming lymphoid follicles. Large or longstanding lesions often show marked interstitial fibrosis and may

show more diffuse stromal inflammatory changes due to prior infection.

Special Studies. Special stains play no real role in this diagnosis, except for keratin to distinguish cystic mesothelioma from cavernous lymphangioma.

Differential Diagnosis. Some cases may resemble cavernous hemangioma but the latter generally lacks both lymphoid aggregates and mural bundles of smooth muscle. Multicystic mesothelioma, at least focally, shows a greater number of epithelioid or hobnail mesothelial lining cells. If these are hard to find, immunostaining for keratin, which highlights the attenuated lining of each cystic space, readily makes the distinction.

Treatment and Prognosis. Large lesions, particularly those in the abdomen, are prone to become secondarily infected, often repeatedly, for reasons that are not clear. Both cavernous and cystically dilated lesions recur locally, usually as a result of incomplete excision, especially in difficult locations such as the oral cavity.

Progressive Lymphangioma

Definition. Progressive lymphangioma (*benign lymphangioendothelioma*) is a rare, benign, localized lymphatic proliferation occurring in the skin and characterized by dissecting vascular channels.

Clinical Features. Progressive lymphangioma occurs mainly in adults, is more common on

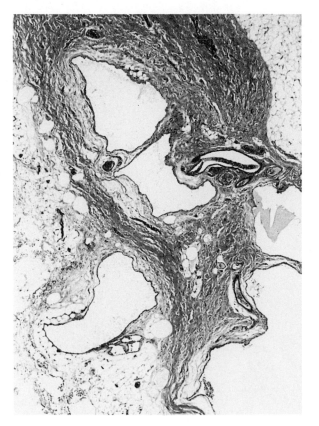

Figure 7-95
CAVERNOUS LYMPHANGIOMA
The dilated lymphatic spaces have thin walls and an irregular outline.

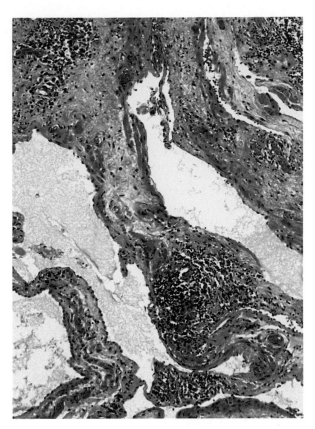

Figure 7-96
CAVERNOUS LYMPHANGIOMA
Note the irregular bundles of smooth muscle in the vessel walls and the stromal aggregates of lymphocytes.

a limb than the trunk, and is characterized clinically by a reasonably circumscribed, pinkish red cutaneous macule which progressively enlarges over a period of years and which may reach a considerable size (greater than 10 cm) (167,172,174a,175). Cutaneous vesicles are not a feature. Among reported cases there is a slight preponderance in males and children are affected occasionally. Exceptional patients with multiple lesions have been described (172).

Pathologic Findings. Progressive lymphangioma consists of thin-walled lymphatic channels located in the dermis which ramify or dissect between dermal collagen, most often in the form of horizontally oriented clefts (fig. 7-97). The lining endothelial cells tend to have somewhat hyperchromatic nuclei but there is no multilayering, atypia, or mitotic activity (fig. 7-98). Occasional lesions extend in a similar fashion into the underlying subcutis.

Special Studies. Special stains play no role in this diagnosis.

Differential Diagnosis. Proper clinical correlation usually allows no differential diagnosis. In the absence of such data, these lesions may be confused histologically with angiosarcoma. However, the latter shows greater endothelial hyperchromasia and pleomorphism, a more complex growth pattern, greater variability in vessel size, and at least focal endothelial multilayering. Hobnail hemangioma differs clinically (see under that entity), tends to have vessels that are more dilated (at least superficially), and has more protuberant endothelial nuclei. Patch stage Kaposi's sarcoma has smaller, more irregular vascular channels, usually associated with stromal plasma cells, erythrocytes, and hemosiderin.

Treatment and Prognosis. Following complete excision, progressive lymphangioma shows no tendency to recur locally.

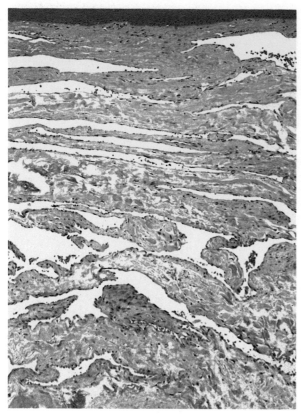

Figure 7-97
PROGRESSIVE LYMPHANGIOMA
Thin-walled lymphatic spaces ramify through the dermis.

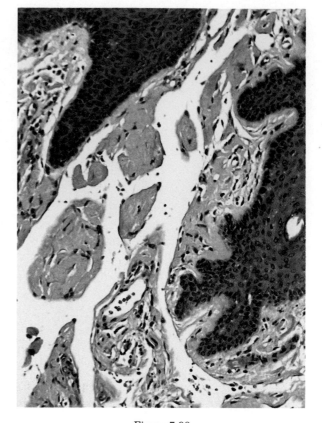

Figure 7-98
PROGRESSIVE LYMPHANGIOMA
The lymphatic channels are generally empty and the lining cells have hyperchromatic nuclei.

Lymphangiomatosis

Definition. Lymphangiomatosis is a diffuse, benign lymphatic proliferation typically affecting multiple tissue planes over a large area.

Clinical Features. This lesion is rare and is best known in its visceral form, which tends to affect multiple parenchymal organs, particularly the lung, as well as bone and skin; usually presents with chylothorax during childhood; and has a poor prognosis (158,163,170,176). The visceral form is described in the Fascicle, Tumors of the Lower Respiratory Tract (161a). However lymphangiomatosis also occurs, possibly more commonly, in a form confined largely to somatic soft tissue (171). Infants and children (with a male predilection) are affected, although the condition persists into adulthood. Patients present with diffuse, boggy swelling of a large part, or all, of a limb. The swelling is fluctuant and compressible and some patients have associated cutaneous vesicles.

Lymphangiography reveals innumerable interconnecting lymphatic spaces throughout all tissue planes, often connected to normal lymphatic channels. Radiologic skeletal survey reveals lytic bone involvement, usually in the same anatomic region, in approximately 50 percent of patients.

Pathologic Findings. Lymphangiomatosis affecting skin and soft tissue has a distinctive morphology (171): countless variably dilated lymphatic channels which ramify throughout skin and subcutis, dissecting between all normal structures (fig. 7-99) and leaving islands of normal tissue apparently "hanging in mid air." All of these spaces are lined by a very attenuated monolayer of endothelial cells (fig. 7-100); the lumina are most often empty or may contain small amounts of lymph. In the adjacent stroma there may be patchy lymphocytic aggregates. Hemosiderin deposition is common, for reasons which are not clear. Overlying epidermal hyperplasia is an occasional feature.

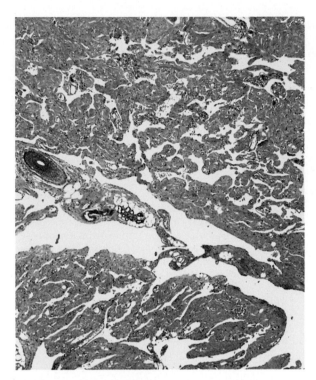

Figure 7-99
LYMPHANGIOMATOSIS
The dermis is diffusely and irregularly dissected by thin-walled lymphatic channels.

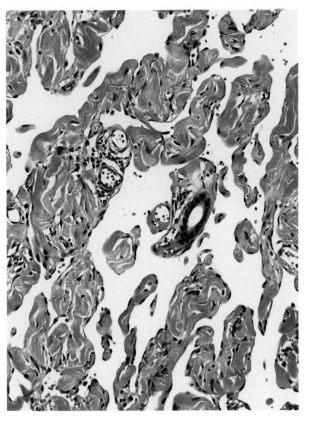

Figure 7-100
LYMPHANGIOMATOSIS
The degree to which normal structures are dissected apart, and thus appear disconnected, is striking. Note the stromal hemosiderin deposition.

Similar, but less extensive, features of lymphangiomatosis may be seen in association with kaposiform hemangioendothelioma.

Special Studies. The appearance may be so striking as to simulate an artefact of tissue disaggregation, hence immunostains for endothelial markers are occasionally helpful to verify the presence of the attenuated lining cells (fig. 7-101).

Differential Diagnosis. In a small biopsy distinction from progressive lymphangioma may be impossible. Angiomatosis is distinguished by its more conventional, nondissecting but diffuse, growth pattern and composition of usual capillary and cavernous-type vessels. Clinical correlation is always advisable.

Treatment and Prognosis. In contrast to cases with visceral involvement, lymphangiomatosis of somatic soft tissue is mainly a cosmetic and symptomatic problem. Growth of the affected tissue usually ceases when patient growth ceases and the lesion is nondestructive. Treatment consists of surgical reduction in a manner comparable to that used in lymphedema.

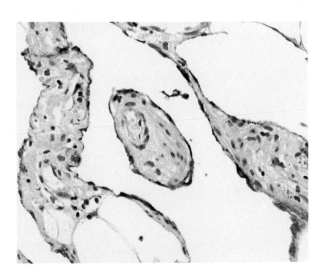

Figure 7-101
LYMPHANGIOMATOSIS
The attenuated endothelial lining is highlighted by VWF immunopositivity (ABC method).

REFERENCES

Introduction

1. Burke A, Virmani R. Tumors of the heart and great vessels. Atlas of Tumor Pathology, 3rd Series, Fascicle 16. Washington, D.C.: Armed Forces Institute of Pathology, 1996.
1a. De Young BR, Wick MR, Figzgibbon JF, Sirgi KE, Swanson PE. CD31. An immunospecific marker for endothelial differentiation in human neoplasms. Appl Immunohistochem 1993;1:97–100.
1b. Lymboussaki A, Partanen TA, Olofsson B, et al. Expression of the vascular endothelial growth C and receptor VEGFR-3 in lymphatic endothelium of the skin and in vascular tumors. Am J Pathol 1998;153:395–403.

Papillary Endothelial Hyperplasia

1c. Clearkin KP, Enzinger FM. Intravascular papillary endothelial hyperplasia. Arch Pathol Lab Med 1976;100:441–4.
2. Hashimoto H, Daimaru Y, Enjoji M. Intravascular papillary endothelial hyperplasia. A clinicopathologic study of 91 cases. Am J Dermatopathol 1983;5:539–45.
3. Kuo TT, Sayers CP, Rosai J. Masson's "vegetant intravascular hemangioendothelioma": a lesion often mistaken for angiosarcoma. Study of seventeen cases located in the skin and soft tissues. Cancer 1976;38:1227–36.
4. Pins MR, Rosenthal DI, Springfield DS, Rosenberg AE. Florid extravascular papillary endothelial hyperplasia (Masson's pseudoangiosarcoma) presenting as a soft tissue sarcoma. Arch Pathol Lab Med 1993;117:259–63.
5. Reed CN, Cooper PH, Swerlick RA. Intravascular papillary endothelial hyperplasia. Multiple lesions simulating Kaposi's sarcoma. J Am Acad Dermatol 1984;10:110–3.

Reactive Angioendotheliomatosis

6. Krell JM, Sanchez RL, Solomon AR. Diffuse dermal angiomatosis: a variant of reactive cutaneous angioendotheliomatosis. J Cutan Pathol 1994;21:363–70.
7. Le Boit PE, Solomon AR, Santa Cruz DJ, Wick MR. Angiomatosis with luminal cryoprotein deposition. J Am Acad Dermatol 1992;27:969–73.
8. Wick MR, Rocamora A. Reactive and malignant "angioendotheliomatosis": a discriminant clinicopathological study. J Cutan Pathol 1988;15:260–71.

Glomeruloid Hemangioma

9. Chan JK, Fletcher CD, Hicklin GA, Rosai J. Glomeruloid hemangioma. A distinctive cutaneous lesion of multicentric Castleman's disease associated with POEMS syndrome. Am J Surg Pathol 1990;14:1036–46.

Bacillary Angiomatosis

9a. Murphy GF, Elder DE. Non-melanocytic tumors of the skin. Atlas of Tumor Pathology. 3rd Series, Fascicle 1. Washington, D.C.: Armed Forces Institute of Pathology, 1991.

Vascular Ectasias

10. Bean WB, Walsh JR. Venous lakes. Arch Dermatol 1956;74:459–63.
11. Edgerton MT, Hiebert JM. Vascular and lymphatic tumors in infancy, childhood and adulthood: challenge of diagnosis and treatment. Curr Probl Cancer 1978;2:41–4.
12. Finley JL, Noe JM, Arndt KA, Rosen S. Portwine stains. Morphologic variations and developmental lesions. Arch Dermatol 1984;120:1453–5.
13. Frain Bell W. Angioma serpiginosum. Br J Dermatol 1957;69:251–68.
14. MacCollum DW, Martin LW. Hemangiomas in infancy and childhood. A report based on 6470 cases. Surg Clin North Am 1956;36:1647–63.
14a. Murphy GF, Elder DE. Non-melanocytic tumors of the skin. Atlas of Tumor Pathology. 3rd Series, Fascicle 1. Washington, D.C.: Armed Forces Institute of Pathology, 1991.
15. Stevenson JR, Lincoln CS. Angioma serpiginosum. Arch Dermatol 1967;95:16–22.
16. Watson WL, McCarthy WB. Blood and lymph vessel tumors. A report of 1056 cases. Surg Gynecol Obstet 1940;71:569–88.

Capillary Hemangioma

17. Bhaskar SM, Jacoway JR. Pyogenic granuloma. Clinical features, incidence, histology and result of treatment: report of 242 cases. J Oral Surg 1961;24:391–8.
18. Calonje E, Mentzel T, Fletcher CD. Pseudomalignant perineurial invasion in cellular ('infantile') capillary haemangiomas. Histopathology 1995;26:159–64.
19. Chan JK, Tsang WY, Calonje E, Fletcher CD. Verrucous hemangioma. A distinctive but neglected variant of cutaneous hemangioma. Int J Surg Pathol 1994;2:171–6.
20. Cho KH, Kim SH, Park KC, et al. Angioblastoma (Nakagawa)–is it the same as tufted angioma? Clin Exp Dermatol 1991;16:110–3.

21. Coffin CM, Dehner LP. Vascular tumors in children and adolescents: a clinicopathologic study of 228 tumors in 222 patients. Pathol Annu 1993;28:97–120.
22. Cooper PH, McAllister HA, Helwig EB. Intravenous pyogenic granuloma. A study of 18 cases. Am J Surg Pathol 1979;3:221–8.
23. Cooper PH, Mills SE. Subcutaneous granuloma pyogenicum. Lobular capillary hemangioma. Arch Dermatol 1982;118:30–3.
23a. Edgerton MT, Hiebert JM. Vascular and lymphatic tumors in infancy, childhood and adulthood: challenge of diagnosis and treatment. Curr Probl Cancer 1978;2:41–4.
24. Imperial R, Helwig E. Verrucous hemangioma. A clinicopathologic study of 21 cases. Arch Dermatol 1967; 96:247–53.
25. Johnson WC. Pathology of cutaneous vascular tumors. Int J Dermatol 1976;15:239–70.
26. Kumakiri M, Muramoto F, Tsukinaga I, et al. Crystalline lamellae in the endothelial cells of a type of hemangioma characterised by the proliferation of immature endothelial cells and pericytes–angioblastoma (Nakagawa). J Am Acad Dermatol 1983;8:68–75.
27. Lister WA. The natural history of strawberry naevi. Lancet 1938;1:1429–34.
27a. MacCollum DW, Martin LW. Hemangiomas in infancy and childhood. A report based on 6470 cases. Surg Clin North Am 1956;36:1647–63.
28. Mancini AJ, Smoller BR. Proliferation and apoptosis within juvenile capillary hemangiomas. Am J Dermatopathol 1996;18:505–14.
29. McGeoch AH. Pyogenic granuloma. Aust J Dermatol 1961;VOL:633–40.
30. Mills SE, Cooper PH, Fechner RE. Lobular capillary hemangioma: the underlying lesion of pyogenic granuloma. A study of 73 cases from the oral and nasal mucous membranes. Am J Surg Pathol 1980;4:471–9.
31. Miyamoto T, Mihara M, Mishima E, Hagari Y, Shimao S. Acquired tufted angioma showing spontaneous regression. Br J Dermatol 1992;127:645–8.
32. Nappi O, Wick MR. Disseminated lobular capillary hemangioma (pyogenic granuloma). A clinicopathologic study of two cases. Am J Dermatopathol 1986;8:379–85.
33. Padilla RS, Orkin M, Rosai J. Acquired "tufted" angioma (progressive capillary hemangioma). A distinctive clinicopathologic entity related to lobular capillary hemangioma. Am J Dermatopathol 1987;9:292–300.
34. Patrice SJ, Wiss K, Mulliken JB. Pyogenic granuloma (lobular capillary hemangioma): a clinicopathologic study of 178 cases. Pediatr Dermatol 1991;8:267–76.
35. Perrone T. Vessel nerve intermingling in benign infantile hemangioendothelioma. Hum Pathol 1985;16:198–200.
36. Renshaw AA, Rosai J. Benign atypical vascular lesions of the lip. A study of 12 cases. Am J Surg Pathol 1993;17:557–65.
37. Warner J, Wilson Jones E. Pyogenic granuloma recurring with multiple satellites. A report of 11 cases. Br J Dermatol 1968;80:218–27.
38. Wilson BB, Greer KE, Cooper PH. Eruptive disseminated lobular capillary hemangioma (pyogenic granuloma). J Am Acad Dermatol 1989;21:391–4.
39. Wilson Jones E, Orkin M. Tufted angioma (angioblastoma). A benign progressive angioma, not to be confused with Kaposi's sarcoma or low-grade angiosarcoma. J Am Acad Dermatol 1989;20:214–25.

Cavernous Hemangioma

40. Calonje E, Fletcher CD. Sinusoidal hemangioma. A distinctive benign vascular neoplasm within the group of cavernous hemangiomas. Am J Surg Pathol 1991;15:1130–5.
41. Coffin CM, Dehner LP. Vascular tumors in children and adolescents: a clinicopathologic study of 228 tumors in 222 patients. Pathol Annu 1993;28:97–120.
42. Edgerton MT, Hiebert JM. Vascular and lymphatic tumors in infancy, childhood and adulthood: challenge of diagnosis and treatment. Curr Probl Cancer 1978;2:41–4.
43. Fine RM, Derbes VJ, Clark WH Jr. Blue rubber bleb nevus. Arch Dermatol 1961;84:802–5.
44. Kasabach HH, Meritt KK. Capillary hemangioma with extensive purpura. Report of a case. Am J Dis Child 1961;59:1063–70.
45. MacCollum DW, Martin LW. Hemangiomas in infancy and childhood. A report based on 6470 cases. Surg Clin North Am 1956;36:1647–63.
46. Rice SJ, Fischer DS. Blue rubber bleb nevus syndrome. Arch Dermatol 1962;86:502–11.
47. Watson WL, McCarthy WB. Blood and lymph vessel tumors. A report of 1056 cases. Surg Gynecol Obstet 1940;71:569–88.

Arteriovenous Hemangioma

48. Angervall L, Nielsen JM, Stener B, Svendsen P. Concomitant arteriovenous vascular malformation in skeletal muscle: a clinical, angiographic and histologic study. Cancer 1979;44:232–8.
49. Connelly MG, Winkelmann RK. Acral arteriovenous tumor. a clinicopathologic review. Am J Surg Pathol 1985;9:15–21.
50. Girard C, Graham JH, Johnson WC. Arteriovenous hemangioma (arteriovenous shunt). A clinicopathologic and histochemical study. J Cutan Pathol 1974;1:73–87.
51. Rusin LJ, Harrell E. Arteriovenous fistula. Cutaneous manifestations. Arch Dermatol 1976;112:1135–8.

Epithelioid Hemangioma

52. Castro C, Winkelmann RK. Angiolymphoid hyperplasia with eosinophilia in the skin. Cancer 1974;34:1696–705.
53. Chan JK, Hui PK, Ng CS, Yuen NW, Kung IT, Gwi E. Epithelioid haemangioma (angiolymphoid hyperplasia with eosinophilia) and Kimura's disease in Chinese. Histopathology 1989;15:557–74.
54. Fawcett HA, Smith NP. Injection-site granuloma due to aluminum. Arch Dermatol 1984;120:1318–22.

55. Fetsch JF, Weiss SW. Observations concerning the pathogenesis of epithelioid hemangioma/angiolymphoid hyperplasia. Mod Pathol 1991;4:449–55.

56. Kuo TT, Shih LY, Chan HL. Kimura's disease, involvement of regional lymph nodes and distinction from angiolymphyoid hyperplasia with eosinophilia. Am J Surg Pathol 1988;12:843–54.

57. Miliauskas JR, Mukherjee T, Dixon B. Postimmunization (vaccination) injection site reactions. A report of four cases and review of the literature. Am J Surg Pathol 1993;17:516–24.

58. Morton K, Robertson AJ, Hadden W. Angiolymphoid hyperplasia with eosinophilia: report of a case arising from the radial artery. Histopathology 1987;11:963–9.

59. Olsen TG, Helwig EB. Angiolymphoid hyperplasia with eosinophilia. A clinicopathologic study of 116 patients. J Am Acad Dermatol 1985;12:781–96.

60. Reed RJ, Terazakis N. Subcutaneous angiolymphoid hyperplasia with eosinophilia (Kimura's disease). Cancer 1972;29:489–97.

61. Rosai J. Angiolymphoid hyperplasia with eosinophilia of the skin. Its nosological position in the spectrum of histocytoid hemangioma. Am J Dermatopathol 1982;4:175–84.

62. Rosai J, Ackerman LR. Intravenous atypical vascular proliferation. A cutaneous lesion simulating a malignant blood vessel tumor. Arch Dermatol 1974;109:714–7.

63. Rosai J, Gold J, Landy R. The histiocytoid hemangiomas. A unifying concept embracing several previously described entities of skin, soft tissue, large vessels, bone and heart. Hum Pathol 1979;10:707–30.

64. Tsang WY, Chan JK. The family of epithelioid vascular tumors. Histol Histopathol 1993;8:187–212.

65. Urabe A, Tsuneyoshi M, Enjoji M. Epithelioid hemangioma versus Kimura's disease. A comparative clinicopathologic study. Am J Surg Pathol 1987;10:758–66.

66. Wells GC, Whimster IW. Subcutaneous angiolymphoid hyperplasia with eosinophilia. Br J Dermatol 1969;81:1–15.

67. Wilson Jones E, Bleehen SS. Inflammatory angiomatous nodules with abnormal blood vessels occurring about the ears and scalp (pseudo or atypical pyogenic granuloma). Br J Dermatol 1969;81:804–16.

Microvenular Hemangioma

68. Aloi F, Tomasini C, Pippione M. Microvenular hemangioma. Am J Dermatopathol 1993;15:534–8.

69. Hunt SJ, Santa Cruz DJ, Barr RJ. Microvenular hemangioma. J Cutan Pathol 1991;18:235–40.

Hobnail Hemangioma

70. Calonje E, Fletcher CD, Wilson Jones E, Rosai J. Retiform hemangioendothelioma. A distinctive form of low-grade angiosarcoma delineated in a series of 15 cases. Am J Surg Pathol 1994;18:115–25.

70a. Guillou L, Calonje E, Speight P, Rosai J, Fletcher CD. Hobnail hemangioma: a pseudomalignant vascular lesion with a reappraisal of targetoid hemosiderotic hemangioma. Am J Surg Pathol 1999;23:97–105.

70b. Mentzel T, Partanen TA, Kutzner H. Hobnail hemangioma ("targetoid hemosiderotic hemangioma"): clinicopathologic and immunohistochemical analysis of 62 cases. J Cutan Pathol 1999;26:279–86.

71. Santa Cruz DJ, Aronberg J. Targetoid hemosiderotic hemangioma. J Am Acad Dermatol 1988;19:550–8.

72. Santonja C, Torrelo A. Hobnail hemangioma. Dermatology 1995;191:154–6.

Spindle Cell Hemangioma

73. Ding J, Hashimoto H, Imayama S, Tsuneyoshi M, Enjoji M. Spindle cell hemangioendothelioma: probably a benign vascular lesion not a low-grade angiosarcoma. A clinicopathological, ultrastructural and immunohistochemical study. Virchows Arch [A] 1992;420:77–85.

74. Fanburg JC, Meis Kindblom JM, Rosenberg AE. Multiple enchondromas associated with spindle cell hemangioendotheliomas. An overlooked variant of Maffucci's syndrome. Am J Surg Pathol 1995;19:1029–38.

75. Fletcher CD, Beham A, Schmid C. Spindle cell haemangioendothelioma: a clinicopathological and immunohistochemical study indicative of a nonneoplastic lesion. Histopathology 1991;18:291–301.

76. Imayama S, Murakamai Y, Hashimoto H, Hori Y. Spindle cell hemangioendothelioma exhibits the ultrastructural features of reactive vascular proliferation rather than of angiosarcoma. Am J Clin Pathol 1992;97:279–87.

77. Perkins P, Weiss SW. Spindle cell hemangioendothelioma. An analysis of 78 cases with reassessment of its pathogenesis and biologic behavior. Am J Surg Pathol 1996;20:1196–204.

78. Scott GA, Rosai J. Spindle cell hemangioendothelioma. Report of seven additional cases of a recently described vascular neoplasm. Am J Dermatopathol 1988;10:281–8.

79. Weiss SW, Enzinger FM. Spindle cell hemangioendothelioma, a low grade angiosarcoma resembling a cavernous hemangioma and Kaposi's sarcoma. Am J Surg Pathol 1986;10:521–30.

80. Zoltie N, Roberts PF. Spindle cell haemangioendothelioma in association with epithelioid haemangioendothelioma. Histopathology 1989;15:544–6.

Intramuscular Angioma

81. Allen PW, Enzinger FM. Hemangioma of skeletal muscle. An analysis of 89 cases. Cancer 1972;29:8–22.

82. Beham A, Fletcher CD. Intramuscular angioma: a clinicopathological analysis of 74 cases. Histopathology 1991;18:53–9.

83. Fergusson IL. Haemangiomata of skeletal muscle. Br J Surg 1972;9:634–7.

84. Lin JJ, Lin F. Two entities in angiolipoma. A study of 459 cases of lipoma with review of the literature on infiltrating angiolipoma. Cancer 1974;34:720–7.

Synovial Hemangioma

85. Devaney K, Vinh TZ, Sweet DE. Synovial hemangioma: a report of 20 cases with differential diagnostic considerations. Hum Pathol 1993;24:737–45.

Angiomatosis

86. Howat AJ, Campbell PE. Angiomatosis: a vascular malformation of infancy and childhood. Report of 17 cases. Pathology 1987;19:377–82.

87. Rao VK, Weiss SW. Angiomatosis of soft tissue. An analysis of the histologic features and clinical outcome in 51 cases. Am J Surg Pathol 1992;16:764–71.

Retiform Hemangioendothelioma

88. Calonje E, Fletcher CD, Wilson Jones E, Rosai J. Retiform hemangioendothelioma: a distinctive form of lowgrade angiosarcoma delineated in a series of 15 cases. Am J Surg Pathol 1994;18:115–25.

89. Dufau JP, Pierre C, De SaintMaur PP, Bellavoir A, Gros P. Hémangioendothélioma rétiforme. Ann Pathol 1997;17:47–51.

90. Duke D, Dvorak AM, Harrist TJ, Cohen LM. Multiple retiform hemangioendotheliomas. A low grade angiosarcoma. Am J Dermatopathol 1996;18:606–10.

91. Fukunaga M, Endo Y, Masui F, et al. Retiform haemangioendothelioma. Virchows Arch 1996;428:301–4.

Malignant Endovascular Papillary Angioendothelioma

91a. Calonje E, Fletcher CD, Wilson Jones E, Rosai J. Retiform hemangioendothelioma: a distinctive form of low grade angiosarcoma delineated in a series of 15 cases. Am J Surg Pathol 1994;18:115–25.

92. Dabska M. Malignant endovascular papillary angioendothelioma of the skin in childhood. Clinicopathologic study of 6 cases. Cancer 1969;24:503–10.

92a. Fanburg-Smith JC, Michal M, Partanen TA, Alitalo K, Miettinen M. Papillary intralymphatic angioendothelioma (PILA). A report of twelve cases of a distinctive vascular tumor with phenotypic features of lymphatic vessels. Am J Surg Pathol 1999;23:1004–10.

93. Fukunaga M, Ushigome S, Shishikura Y, Yokoi K, Ishikawa E. Endovascular papillary angioendotheliomalike tumour associated with lymphoedema. Histopathology 1995;27:243–59.

94. Manivel JC, Wick MR, Swanson PE, Patterson K, Dehner LP. Endovascular papillary angioendothelioma of childhood: a vascular lesion possibly characterized by "high" endothelial cell differentiation. Hum Pathol 1986;17:1240–4.

Kaposiform Hemangioendothelioma

95. Fukunaga M, Ushigome S, Ishikawa E. Kaposiform haemangioendothelioma associated with Kasabach-Merritt syndrome. Histopathology 1996;28:281–4.

96. Lai MF, Allen PW, Yuen PM, Leung PC. Locally metastasizing vascular tumor. Spindle cell, epithelioid or unclassified hemangioendothelioma? Am J Clin Pathol 1991;96:660–3.

97. Mentzel T, Mazzoleni G, Dei Tos AP, Fletcher CD. Kaposiform hemangioendothelioma in adults: clinicopathologic and immunohistochemical analysis of three cases. Am J Clin Pathol 1997;108:450–5.

98. Niedt GW, Alba Greco M, Wieczorek R, Blanc WA, Knowles DM. Hemangioma with Kaposi's sarcomalike features: report of two cases. Pediatr Pathol 1989;9:567–75.

99. Tsang WY, Chan JK. Kaposi-like infantile hemangioendothelioma. A distinctive vascular neoplasm of the retroperitoneum. Am J Surg Pathol 1991;15:982–9.

100. Zukerberg LR, Nickoloff BJ, Weiss SW. Kaposiform hemangioendothelioma of infancy and childhood. An aggressive neoplasm associated with Kasabach-Merritt syndrome and lymphangiomatosis. Am J Surg Pathol 1993;17:321–8.

Polymorphous Hemangioendothelioma

101. Chan JK, Frizzera G, Fletcher CD, Rosai J. Primary vascular tumors of lymph node other than Kaposi's sarcoma. Analysis of 39 cases and delineation of two new entities. Am J Surg Pathol 1992;16:335–50.

102. Nascimento AG, Keeney GL, Sciot R, Fletcher CD. Polymorphous hemangioendothelioma: a report of two cases, one affecting extranodal soft tissues, and review of the literature. Am J Surg Pathol 1997;21:1083–9.

102a. Warnke RA, Weis LM, Chan JK, Cleary ML, Dorfman RF. Tumor of the lymph nodes and spleen. Atlas of Tumor Pathology. 3rd Series, Fascicle 14. Washington, D.C.: Armed Forces Institute of Pathology, 1995.

Giant Cell Angioblastoma

103. Gonzalez Crussi F, Choud P, Crawford SE. Congenital infiltrating giant cell angioblastoma, a new entity? Am J Surg Pathol 1991;15:175–83.

Kaposi's Sarcoma

104. Bayley AC, Lucas SB. Kaposi's sarcoma or Kaposi's disease? A personal reappraisal. In: Fletcher CD, McKee PH, eds. Pathobiology of soft tissue tumours. Edinburgh: Churchill Livingstone 1990:141–63.

105. Bencini PL, Marchesi L, Cainelli T, Crosti C. Kaposi's sarcoma in kidney transplant recipients treated with cyclosporin. Br J Dermatol 1988;118:709–14.

106. Chor PJ, Santa Cruz DJ. Kaposi's sarcoma. A clinicopathologic review and differential diagnosis. J Cutan Pathol 1992;19:6–20.

107. Cossu S, Satta R, Cottoni F, Massarelli G. Lymphangioma-like variant of Kaposi's sarcoma: clinicopathologic study of seven cases with review of the literature. Am J Dermatopathol 1997;19:16–22.

108. Dorfman RF. Kaposi's sarcoma revisited. Hum Pathol 1984;15:1013–7.

109. Dorfman RF. Kaposi's sarcoma. With special reference to its manifestations in infants and children and to the concepts of Arthur Purdy Stout. Am J Surg Pathol 1986;10:68–77.

110. Dutz W, Stout AP. Kaposi's sarcoma in infants and children. Cancer 1960;13:684–93.

111. Gange RW, Wilson Jones E. Kaposi's sarcoma and immunosuppressive therapy: an appraisal. Clin Exp Dermatol 1978;3:135–46.

112. Gange RW, Wilson Jones E. Lymphangioma-like Kaposi's sarcoma. A report of three cases. Br J Dermatol 1979;100:327–34.

113. Gottlieb GJ, Ackerman AB. Kaposi's sarcoma: an extensively disseminated form in young homosexual men. Hum Pathol 1982;13:882–92.

114. Ioachim HL, Adsay V, Giancotti FR, Dorsett B, Melamed J. Kaposi's sarcoma of internal organs. A multiparameter study of 86 cases. Cancer 1995;75:1376–85.

115. Kao GF, Johnson FB, Sulica VI. The nature of hyaline (eosinophilic) globules and vascular slits of Kaposi's sarcoma. Am J Dermatopathol 1990;12:256–67.

116. Krigel RL, Friedman Kien AE. Epidemic Kaposi's sarcoma. Semin Oncol 1990;17:350–60.

117. Lemlich G, Schwam L, Lebwohl M. Kaposi's sarcoma and acquired immunodeficiency syndrome: postmortem findings in twenty-four cases. J Am Acad Dermatol 1987;16:319–25.

118. Moskowitz LB, Hensley GT, Gould EW, Weiss SD. Frequency and anatomic distribution of lymphadenopathic Kaposi's sarcoma in the acquired immunodeficiency syndrome: an autopsy series. Hum Pathol 1985;16:447–56.

119. Nickoloff BJ, Foreman KE. Charting a new course through the chaos of KS (Kaposi's sarcoma). Am J Pathol 1996;148:1323–9.

120. O'Leary JJ, Kennedy MM, McGee JO. Kaposi's sarcoma associated herpes virus (KSHV/HHV8): epidemiology, molecular biology and tissue distribution. Molec Pathol 1997;5:4–8.

121. Rabkin CS, Janz S, Lash A, et al. Monoclonal origin of multicentric Kaposi's sarcoma lesions. N Engl J Med 1997;336:988–93.

122. Stribling J, Weitzner S, Smith GV. Kaposi's sarcoma in renal allograft recipients. Cancer 1978;42:442–6.

123. Tappero JW, Connant MA, Wolfe SF, Berger TG. Kaposi's sarcoma. Epidemiology, pathogenesis, histology, clinical spectrum, staging criteria and therapy. J Am Acad Dermatol 1993;28:371–95.

124. Templeton AC. Kaposi's sarcoma. Pathol Annu 1981;16(2);315–36.

Epithelioid Hemangioendothelioma

125. Ellis GL, Kratochvil FJ. Epithelioid hemangioendothelioma of the head and neck: a clinicopathologic report of twelve cases. Oral Surg Oral Med Oral Pathol 1986;61:61–8.

126. Gray MH, Rosenberg AE, Dickersin GR, Bhan AK. Cytokeratin expression in epithelioid vascular neoplasms. Hum Pathol 1990;21:212–7.

127. Lamovec J, Sobel HJ, Zidar A, Jerman J. Epithelioid hemangioendothelioma of the anterior mediastinum with osteoclastlike giant cells. Light microscopic, immunohistochemical, and electron microscopic study. Am J Clin Pathol 1990;93:813–7.

128. Mentzel T, Beham A, Calonje E, Katenkamp D, Fletcher CD. Epithelioid hemangioendothelioma of skin and soft tissues: clinicopathologic and immunohistochemical study of 30 cases. Am J Surg Pathol 1997;21:363–74.

129. Suster S, Moran CA, Koss MN. Epithelioid hemangioendothelioma of the anterior mediastinum. Clinicopathologic, immunohistochemical and ultrastructural analysis of 12 cases. Am J Surg Pathol 1994;18:871–81.

130. Van Haelst UJ, Pruszczynski M, Ten Cate LN, Mravunac M. Ultrastructural and immunohistochemical study of epithelioid hemangioendothelioma of bone: coexpression of epithelial and endothelial markers. Ultrastruct Pathol 1990;14:141–9.

131. Weiss SW, Enzinger FM. Epithelioid hemangioendothelioma: a vascular tumor often mistaken for a carcinoma. Cancer 1982;50:970–81.

132. Weiss SW, Ishak KG, Dail DH, Sweet DE, Enzinger FM. Epithelioid hemangioendothelioma and related lesions. Semin Diagn Pathol 1986;3:259–87.

133. Williams SB, Butler BC, Gilkey GW, Kapadia SB, Burton DM. Epithelioid hemangioendothelioma with osteoclast like giant cells. Arch Pathol Lab Med 1993;117:315–8.

Angiosarcoma

134. Abratt RP, Williams M, Raff M, Dodd NF, Uys CJ. Angiosarcoma of the superior vena cava. Cancer 1983;52:740–3.
135. Alessi E, Sala F, Berti E. Angiosarcomas in lymphedematous limbs. Am J Dermatopathol 1986;8:371–8.
136. Byers RJ, McMahon RF, Freemont AJ, et al. Epithelioid angiosarcoma arising in an arteriovenous fistula. Histopathology 1992;21:87–9.
137. Capo V, Ozzello L, Fenoglio CM, et al. Angiosarcomas arising in edematous extremities: immunostaining for factor VIII related antigen and ultrastructural features. Hum Pathol 1985;16:144–50.
138. Cooper PH. Angiosarcomas of the skin. Semin Diagn Pathol 1987;4:2–17.
139. Fineberg S, Rosen PP. Cutaneous angiosarcoma and atypical vascular lesions of the skin and breast after radiation therapy for breast carcinoma. Am J Clin Pathol 1994;102:757–63.
140. Fletcher CD, Beham A, Bekir S, Clarke AM, Marley NJ. Epithelioid angiosarcoma of deep soft tissue: a distinctive tumor readily mistaken for an epithelial neoplasm. Am J Surg Pathol 1991;15:915–24.
141. Girard C, Johnson WC, Graham JH. Cutaneous angiosarcoma. Cancer 1970;26:868–83.
142. Goette DK, Detlefs RL. Postirradiation angiosarcoma. J Am Acad Dermatol 1985;12:922–6.
143. Holden CA, Spittle MF, Wilson Jones E. Angiosarcoma of the face and scalp, prognosis and treatment. Cancer 1987;59:1046–57.
144. Jennings TA, Peterson L, Axiotis CA, Friedlander GE, Cooke RA, Rosai J. Angiosarcoma associated with foreign body material. A report of three cases. Cancer 1988;62:2436–44.
145. Kauffman SL, Stout AP. Malignant hemangioendothelioma in infants and children. Cancer 1961;14:1186–96.
146. Leake J, Sheehan MP, Rampling D, Ramani P, Atherton DJ. Angiosarcoma complicating xeroderma pigmentosum. Histopathology 1992;21:179–81.
147. Maddox JC, Evans HL. Angiosarcoma of skin and soft tissues: a study of forty-four cases. Cancer 1981;8:1907–21.
148. Mark RJ, Poen JC, Tran LM, Fu YS, Juillard GF. Angiosarcoma. A report of 67 patients and a review of the literature. Cancer 1996;77:2400–6.
149. Marrogi AJ, Hunt SJ, Santa Cruz DJ. Cutaneous epithelioid angiosarcoma. Am J Dermatopathol 1990;12:350–6.
150. McWilliam LJ, Harris M. Granular cell angiosarcoma of the skin: histology, electron microscopy and immunohistochemistry of a newly recognized tumour. Histopathology 1985;9:1205–16.
150a. Meis-Kindblom JM, Kindblom LG. Angiosarcoma of soft tissue: a study of 80 cases. Am J Surg Pathol 1998;22:683–97.
151. Prescott RJ, Banerjee SS, Eyden BP, Haboubi NY. Cutaneous epithelioid angiosarcoma: a clinicopathological study of four cases. Histopathology 1994;25:421–9.
152. Rosai J, Sumner HW, Kostianovsky M, PerezMesa C. Angiosarcoma of the skin. A clinicopathologic and fine structural study. Hum Pathol 1976;7:83–109.
153. Stewart FW, Treves N. Lymphangiosarcoma in postmastectomy lymphedema. A report of six cases in elephantiasis chirurgica. Cancer 1948;1:64–81.
154. Trassard M, LeDoussal V, Bui BN, Coindre JM. Angiosarcoma arising in a solitary schwannoma (neurilemoma) of the sciatic nerve. Am J Surg Pathol 1996;20:1412–7.
155. Wilson Jones E. Malignant angioendothelioma of skin. Br J Dermatol 1964;76:21–39.
156. Wilson Jones E. Malignant vascular tumours. Clin Exp Dermatol 1976;1:287–312.
157. Woodward AH, Ivins JC, Soule EH. Lymphangiosarcoma arising in chronic lymphedematous extremities. Cancer 1972;30:562–72.

Lymphatic Lesions

158. Asch MJ, Cohen AH, Moore TC. Hepatic and splenic lymphangiomatosis with skeletal involvement: report of a case and review of the literature. Surgery 1974;76:334–9.
159. Bill AH, Sumner DS. A unified concept of lymphangioma and cystic hygroma. Surg Gynecol Obstet 1965;120:79–86.
160. Byrne J, Blanc WA, Warburton D, Wigger J. The significance of cystic hygroma in fetuses. Hum Pathol 1984;15:61–7.
161. Chervenak FA, Issacson G, Blakemore KJ, et al. Fetal cystic hygroma: cause and natural history. N Engl J Med 1983;309:822–5.
161a. Colby TV, Koss MN, Travis WD. Tumors of the lower respiratory tract. Atlas of Tumor Pathology. 3rd Series, Fascicle 13. Washington, D.C.: Armed Forces Institute of Pathology, 1995.
162. Flanagan BP, Helwig EB. Cutaneous lymphangioma. Arch Dermatol 1977;113:24–30.
163. Frack MD, Simon S, Dawson BH. The lymphangiomatosis syndrome. Cancer 1968;22:428–37.
164. Gross RE, Goeringer CF. Cystic hygroma of the neck. Report of twenty-seven cases. Surg Gynecol Obstet 1939;69:48–60.
165. Harkins GA, Sabiston DC. Lymphangioma in infancy and childhood. Surgery 1960;47:811–22.
166. Mallett RB, Curley GK, Mortimer PS. Acquired lymphangioma: report of four cases and a discussion of the pathogenesis. Br J Dermatol 1992;126:380–2.
167. Mehregan DR, Mehregan AH, Mehregan DA. Benign lymphangioendothelioma: report of 2 cases. J Cutan Pathol 1992;19:502–5.
168. Peachey RD, Lim CC, Whimster IW. Lymphangioma of the skin. A review of 65 cases. Br J Dermatol 1970;83:519–27.
169. Prioleau PG, Santa Cruz DJ. Lymphangioma circumscriptum following radical mastectomy and radiation therapy. Cancer 1978;42:1989–91.

170. Ramani P, Shah A. Lymphangiomatosis. Histological and immunohistochemical analysis of four cases. Am J Surg Pathol 1992;16:764–71.

171. Singh Gomez C, Calonje E, Browse NL, Ferrar DW, Fletcher CD. Lymphangiomatosis of the limbs. Clinicopathologic analysis of a series with good prognosis. Am J Surg Pathol 1995;19:125–33.

171a. Warnke RA, Weis LM, Chan JK, Cleary ML, Dorfman RF. Tumors of the lymph nodes and spleen. Atlas of Tumor Pathology. 3rd Series, Fascicle 14. Washington, D.C.: Armed Forces Institute of Pathology, 1995.

172. Watanabe M, Kishiyama K, Ohkawara A. Acquired progressive lymphangioma. J Am Acad Dermatol 1983;8:663–7.

173. Watson WL, McCarthy WB. Blood and lymph vessel tumors. A report of 1056 cases. Surg Gynecol Obstet 1940;71:569–88.

174. Whimster IW. The pathology of lymphangioma circumscriptum. Br J Dermatol 1976;94:473–86.

174a. Wilson Jones E. Malignant vascular tumours. Clin Exp Dermatol 1976;1:287–312.

175. Wilson Jones E, Winklemann RK, Zacharay CB, Reda AM. Benign lymphangioendothelioma. J Am Acad Dermatol 1990;23:229–35.

176. Wolff M. Lymphangiomatosis: clinicopathologic study and ultrastructural confirmation of its histogenesis. Cancer 1973;31:988–1007.

❖❖❖

8

PERIVASCULAR TUMORS

INTRODUCTION

The neoplasms generally considered to constitute the category of perivascular tumors are glomus tumor and hemangiopericytoma (Table 8-1). The former is composed of cells which histologically, ultrastructurally, and immunohistochemically closely resemble normal glomus cells. However, the situation with hemangiopericytoma is quite different. As is discussed in the section devoted to hemangiopericytoma immediately below, several different entities have been included in this category, the evidence that cells of adult hemangiopericytomas are differentiating as pericytes is less than compelling, and several other types of tumors often feature areas histologically indistinguishable from hemangiopericytoma. However, in order not to cause unnecessary confusion, we have continued the custom of placing adult hemangiopericytoma within the perivascular category.

Recently, Fletcher and colleagues have described 24 tumors whose constituent cells demonstrate myoid differentiation but whose histologic features overlap with those of hemangiopericytoma. Based on the morphologic features they have labeled these tumors glomangiopericytoma and myopericytoma, and they have also included adult myofibroma (see chapter 2) within the overlap group (8a). The first two are briefly discussed at the end of this chapter and the third in the myofibroma section of chapter 2. It is possible these tumors may be composed of cells that are differentiated as pericytes and thus represent the "true" hemangiopericytoma.

HEMANGIOPERICYTOMA

Definition. Hemangiopericytoma is a tumor composed of spindled to oval undifferentiated cells which proliferate around and are intimately associated with prominent, thin-walled, often branching ("staghorn") vessels.

General Considerations. Hemangiopericytoma has caused pathologists both conceptual and diagnostic difficulties from the time it was first given its name by Stout in 1942. Diagnostic difficulties occur because the tumor cells are undifferentiated by light microscopy and resemble those in several other tumors. Conceptual difficulties arise because the position of the tumor cells around thin-walled, often "staghorn" vessels suggests they could be demonstrating pericytic differentiation, yet other evidence to support this theory is largely absent (17). Normal pericytes are rather nondescript elongate cells by light microscopy and are similar to the cells found in hemangiopericytoma, but ultrastructurally, normal pericytes usually have elongate cell processes covered at least partially by basal lamina and cytoplasmic filaments with focal dense bodies (5,12). These features are also seen in smooth muscle cells, and indeed in most reports normal pericytes express an actin recognized by the smooth muscle antigen antibody (15). However, in the literature more than half of the adult hemangiopericytomas that have been examined ultrastructurally were composed of cells that failed to demonstrate the myoid features that characterize normal pericytes, and the cells of adult hemangiopericytoma are actin negative (4,5,8,13,15,16). Thus, there is weak, and in some

Table 8-1

PERIVASCULAR TUMORS

Benign
(Managerial Group Ia, Table 1-10)

Glomus tumor

Sinonasal hemangiopericytoma

Intermediate
(Managerial Groups IIa and IIc, Table 1-10)

Hemangiopericytoma*

Malignant
(Managerial Group III, Table 1-10)

Glomangiosarcoma**

Malignant hemangiopericytoma

---

*This implies morphologically benign hemangiopericytoma. Rare examples will recur or metastasize. See text.
**These extraordinarily rare tumors are morphologically malignant but practically never metastasize.

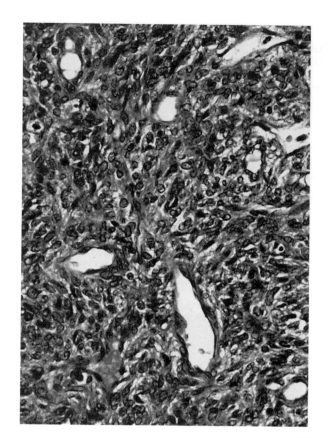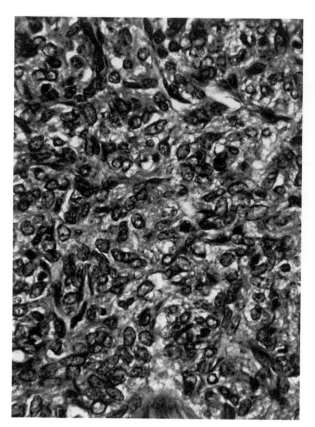

Figure 8-2
HEMANGIOPERICYTOMA

The cells that compose hemangiopericytoma are randomly arranged and have uniform nuclei and indistinct cell margins. A disorganized appearance is characteristic.

Figure 8-3
HEMANGIOPERICYTOMA
The cells may be arranged in short bundles or in a poorly formed storiform pattern in some hemangiopericytomas.

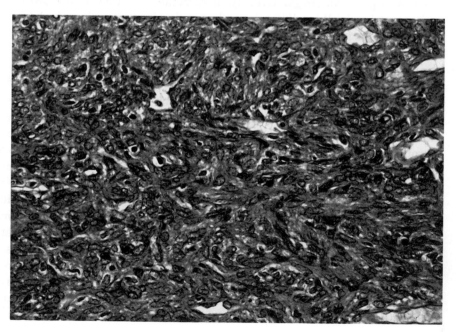

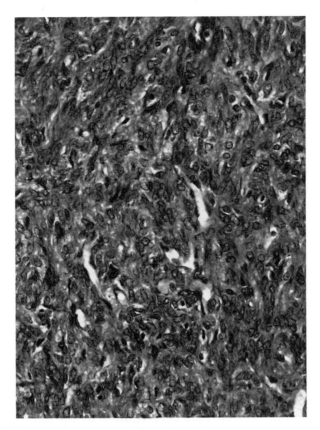

Figure 8-4
HEMANGIOPERICYTOMA
There is considerable overlap between hemangiopericytoma and solitary fibrous tumor and this photomicrograph has features that could be seen in either.

Occasional tumor cell necrosis is an ominous
finding because it is associated with an increased
risk for metastasis. In fact, the combination of
size over 5 cm, mitotic rate over 4 mitoses per 10
high-power fields, and tumor cell necrosis should
elicit a diagnosis of malignant hemangiopericytoma, particularly if the cells are pleomorphic and
have abnormal chromatin patterns (7). On the
other hand, cytologically bland, mitotically inactive hemangiopericytomas should never be diagnosed as "benign" because occasional tumors with
these features will metastasize. The proper designation for these is simply hemangiopericytoma or
a term such as "of uncertain malignant potential"
can be used (1). Uncertain malignant potential
is a useful label for tumors between these ex-
tremes, e.g., tumors with brisk mitotic activity
but no necrosis or those with tumor cell necrosis
in the absence of significant mitotic activity. In
any case, the comments section of the report

should contain information about the expected
behavior of the tumor.

Hemorrhage occurs in some hemangiopericytomas but is not, in itself, an adverse prognostic feature. However, hemorrhage is often associated with tumor cell necrosis which is an
indicator of malignant potential so careful inspection of hemorrhagic areas is worthwhile.
Scattered lymphocytes and mast cells are commonly present and fatty differentiation has been
reported in rare hemangiopericytomas, as has
metaplastic cartilage (14). Nodules of tumor occasionally develop outside the main tumor mass
or in its capsule. This is not known to increase
the risk for recurrence.

Special Studies. Reticulin is abundant
around individual cells in hemangiopericytoma
but this stain is seldom used diagnostically any-
more because so many tumors in the differential
diagnosis have a similar staining pattern. About
50 percent of the hemangiopericytomas so far
tested contain CD34-positive cells (12). Because
most of the tumors that are included among the
main differential diagnostic considerations for
hemangiopericytoma do not contain such cells this
is a useful adjunct to diagnosis. Care must be taken
to be sure it is the tumor cells that are CD34
positive because the endothelial cells lining the
vessels in the tumor are also CD34 positive. CD31
can be useful in this regard because it marks the
endothelial cells lining the vessels but not the
tumor cells. About a third of hemangiopericytomas are CD57 positive and a considerable
number contain factor XIIIa-positive cells, but
antigens recognized by these antibodies are
present in many different types of tumors so
these two immunohistochemical stains are less
helpful in differential diagnosis (4,13,15). Actin,
desmin, and CD99 stains are negative. A few
putative hemangiopericytomas have been reported to be focally positive for factor VIII, S-100
protein, and myelin-associated proteins (13,15).

As noted in the General Considerations section,
over 50 percent of the hemangiopericytomas that
have been examined ultrastructurally lack
myoid features. Rather the cells have the ultrastructural features of fibroblasts or primitive
mesenchymal cells.

Chromosomal studies in a few tumors have
demonstrated various anomalies but there
seems to be a fairly consistent abnormality of the

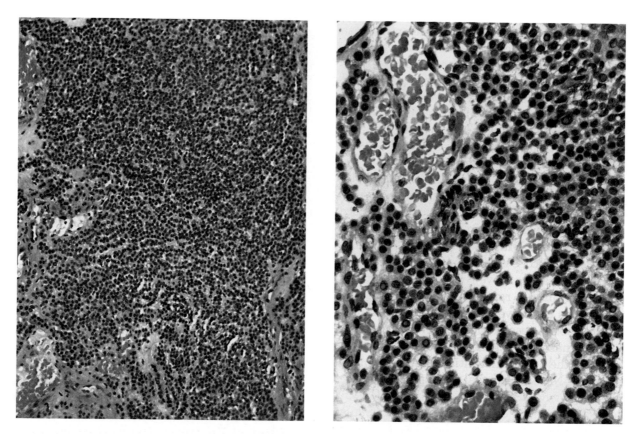

Figure 8-6
GLOMUS TUMOR
Glomus tumors are composed of sheets or packets of cells with round regular nuclei and inconspicuous nucleoli.

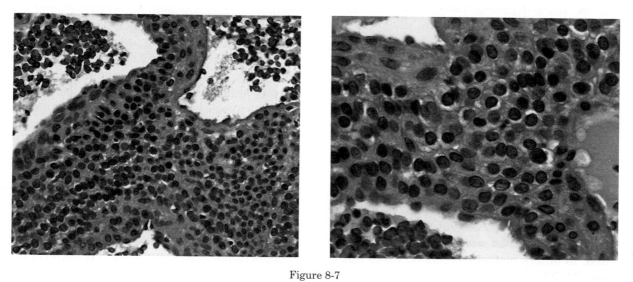

Figure 8-7
GLOMUS TUMOR
The characteristic round regular nuclei and perivascular location of the cells of a glomus tumor are seen here.

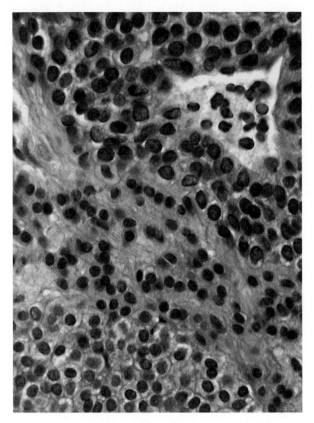

Figure 8-8
GLOMUS TUMOR

In occasional tumors there will be some variation in the size of the tumor cell nuclei, with larger nuclei in areas, as seen on the upper right.

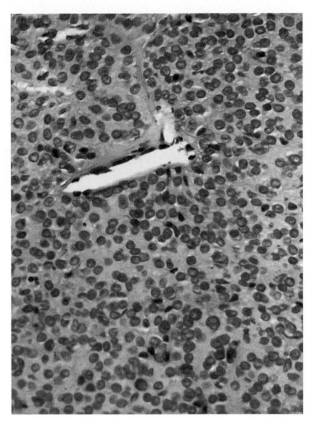

Figure 8-9
GLOMUS TUMOR

The tumor cells grow around vessels and in many instances appear to be in the wall of the vessel, a useful finding.

eosinophilic or amphophilic cytoplasm and hard to see nucleoli, and are devoid of division figures (fig. 8-7). The only deviation from this pattern of monotonous nuclear uniformity is the occasional tumor that contains cells with enlarged nuclei, some of which may resemble the large cells seen in ancient schwannoma (fig. 8-8). Rare glomus tumors are composed of cells with abundant eosinophilic cytoplasm; these have been classified as *oncocytic glomus tumor* (40).

The cells of a glomus tumor are almost always in close proximity to numerous small blood vessels and classically they appear to be in the walls of the vessels (fig. 8-9) (41). Usually, clusters of tumor cells are arranged around numerous vessels set within a hyalinized or myxoid stroma. Even when the tumor cells grow in sheets simulating epithelium, which they often do, or are arranged in packets mimicking the appearance of a paraganglioma, blood vessels are still nu-

merous although they may be slit-like and inconspicuous. Commonly, glomus tumors are surrounded by a rim of thick collagen; tumor cells may be present within this capsule or in the surrounding soft tissue. Indeed, the tumor cells may infiltrate locally.

The pattern of the usual glomus tumor—round regular cells growing around and into the walls of vessels—is one that needs to be kept in mind because of the large number of locations in which these tumors can develop.

Glomangioma. This tumor grossly and microscopically resembles cavernous hemangioma because it contains large, dilated, often thick-walled vascular spaces but it is distinguished from hemangioma on the basis of the nests of glomus cells in the walls of the cavernous vessels and from glomus tumor by the size of the vessels (fig. 8-10). Thrombosis is not uncommon and calcification may be present.

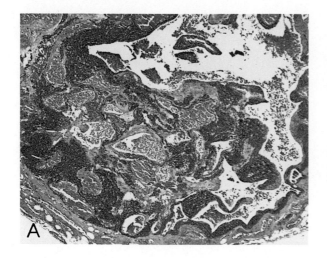

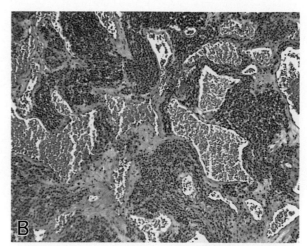

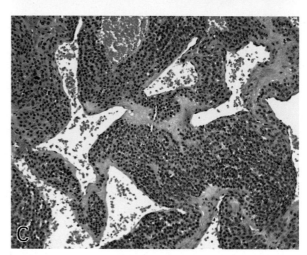

Figure 8-10
GLOMANGIOMA
Glomangiomas are glomus tumors in which the tumor cells grow around cavernous vessels. The cells in glomangioma are identical to those in the usual glomus tumor.

Glomangiomyoma. This tumor resembles either glomus tumor because of perivascular tumor growth or glomangioma because of cavernous vascular spaces but unlike either of these, focally the tumor cells become elongate and take on the features of ordinary smooth muscle cells (31). This change in differentiation is most prominent around thick-walled vessels where the spindled tumor cells often blend into the muscular wall of the vessel.

Glomangiosarcoma. This very rare neoplasm has been reported to have two forms (26,28,32, 35). In one, an otherwise characteristic glomus tumor composed of uniform cells has focal areas in which the cells become spindled or pleomorphic and their nuclei feature prominent nucleoli and easily found mitotic figures. Care must be taken not to confuse glomus tumors that contain cells with large degenerative nuclei with these areas of

morphologic malignant transformation. Mitotic figures, easily found in glomangiosarcoma and essentially absent in glomus tumors including those with enlarged degenerate-appearing nuclei, are probably the most useful feature in this regard. In the other form, the tumor is completely glomangiosarcoma. This is so rare that its existence can be questioned but from the few reports available it would seem that the cells resemble glomus cells except they have larger nuclei with prominent nucleoli and numerous mitotic figures (32). These cells should surround and be present within vessel walls as is seen in the usual glomus tumor. Better yet, electron microscopy should reveal tumor cells with myoid features and the immunohistochemical profile should be that of glomus tumors as described below. Altogether, if a diagnosis of glomangiosarcoma is contemplated, consultation is probably in order.

Special Studies. The cells of glomus tumor and glomangiosarcoma are reactive for muscle-specific actin and vimentin (28,29,32,35,37,39). Some but not all glomus tumors contain cells that are desmin positive (39). Keratin, epithelial membrane antigen, S-100 protein, and carcinoembryonic antigen are negative. Some investigators have reported that rare glomus tumors are factor VIII positive.

Ultrastructurally, the cells composing a glomus tumor or a glomangiosarcoma have smooth muscle features including basal lamina and large numbers of cytoplasmic filaments that insert into dense bodies and often fill the cytoplasm (32,35,41).

Differential Diagnosis. One of the main problems in recognizing glomus tumor is that it is so uncommon that pathologists often fail to think about it unless the tumor is subungual. Once it is considered, the cytologic features of the usual glomus tumor are so distinctive that the diagnosis is seldom in doubt on the basis of light microscopy. In the subcutaneous tissue and skin, the main differential diagnostic concerns are nodular sweat gland tumors and nevi. When faced with this differential diagnosis, immunohistochemistry is very useful because sweat gland tumors are keratin, epithelial membrane antigen, and often carcinoembryonic antigen positive whereas glomus tumors fail to react with these antibodies (33). S-100 protein is a reliable means of recognizing nevi because the cells that compose glomus tumors are S-100 protein negative (37). Glomus tumors in which the cells are in packets might be confused with paraganglioma; a chromogranin stain should clarify the diagnosis. Hemangiopericytomas are actin negative and do not contain cells that resemble those populating glomus tumors. Vascular neoplasms are excluded by identifying glomus cells in the walls and around vessels. Epithelioid smooth muscle tumors do not usually feature the rich vasculature found in glomus tumors and the tumor cells are not present within vessel walls. Of course, care must be taken not to confuse normal glomus structures, such as the glomus coccygeum, with a neoplasm (27).

Treatment and Prognosis. Glomus tumors, glomangiomas, and glomangiomyomas are benign even if the tumor cells are infiltrating. About 10 percent recur but recurrences are not destructive and are easily controlled with conservative reexcision (34,38). Glomangiosarcoma so rarely metastasizes that exceptions to this rule are reported (28).

GLOMANGIOPERICYTOMA AND MYOPERICYTOMA

Fletcher and colleagues have described 24 tumors with myoid differentiation whose morphologic features overlap those of hemangiopericytoma and glomus tumor (42). These included tumors with histologic features of "infantile-type" myofibromatosis occurring in adults (chapter 2), tumors with features of both glomus tumor and hemangiopericytoma (glomangiopericytoma), and glomus tumors with perivascular spindled myoid cells (myopericytoma). Histologically, the glomangiopericytomas featured prominent branching vessels lined by a single layer of endothelial cells surrounded by epithelioid cells with a glomoid appearance. In other areas the tumors had a typical hemangiopericytomatous appearance. Myopericytomas were characterized by a concentric perivascular proliferation of bland spindled to ovoid myoid cells as well as areas with the appearance of hemangiopericytoma. The recurrence rate for the myofibromatosis group was 3/5, for the glomangiopericytoma group 1/6, and for the myopericytoma group 2/5. No patients developed metastasis and all recurrences have been controlled to date.

REFERENCES

Hemangiopericytoma

1. Angervall L, Kindblom LG, Nielsen JM, Stener B, Svendsen P. Hemangiopericytoma: a clinicopathologic, angiographic and microangiographic study. Cancer 1978;42:2412–27.
2. Compagno J. Hemangiopericytoma-like tumors of the nasal cavity: a comparison with hemangiopericytoma of soft tissues. Laryngoscope 1978;88:460–9.
3. Compagno J, Hyams VJ. Hemangiopericytoma-like intranasal tumors. A clinicopathologic study of 23 cases. Am J Clin Pathol 1976;66:672–83.
4. D'Amore ES, Manivel JC, Sung JH. Soft-tissue and meningeal hemangiopericytomas: an immunohistochemical and ultrastructural study. Hum Pathol 1990;21:414–23.
5. Dardick I, Hammar SP, Scheithauer BW. Ultrastructural spectrum of hemangiopericytoma: a comparative study of fetal, adult, and neoplastic pericytes. Ultrastruct Pathol 1989;13:111–54.
6. Eichhorn JH, Dickersin GR, Bhan AK, Goodman ML. Sinonasal hemangiopericytoma. A reassessment with electron microscopy, immunohistochemistry, and long-term follow-up. Am J Surg Pathol 1990;14:856–66.
7. Enzinger FM, Smith BH. Hemangiopericytoma. An analysis of 106 cases. Hum Pathol 1976;7:61–82.
8. Fletcher CD. Haemangiopericytoma–a dying breed? Reappraisal of an "entity" and its variants: a hypothesis. Curr Diagn Pathol 1994;1:19–25.
8a. Granter S, Badizadegan K, Fletcher CD. Myofibromatosis in adults, glomangiopericytoma, and myopericytoma: a spectrum of tumors showing perivascular myoid differentiation. Am J Surg Pathol 1998;22:513–25.
9. Herath SE, Stalboerger PG, Dahl RJ, Parisi JE, Jenkins RB. Cytogenetic studies of four hemangiopericytomas. Cancer Genet Cytogenet 1994;72:137–40.
10. Mandahl N, Orndal C, Heim S, et al. Aberrations of chromosome segment 12q13-15 characterize a subgroup of hemangiopericytomas. Cancer 1993;71:3009–12.
11. Mentzel T, Calonje E, Nascimento AG, Fletcher CD. Infantile hemangiopericytoma versus infantile myofibromatosis. Study of a series suggesting a continuous spectrum of infantile myofibroblastic lesions. Am J Surg Pathol 1994;18:922–30.
12. Nappi O, Ritter JH, Pettinato G, Wick MR. Hemangiopericytoma: histopathological pattern or clinicopathologic entity? Semin Diagn Pathol 1995;12:221–32.
13. Nemes Z. Differentiation markers in hemangiopericytoma. Cancer 1992;69:133–40.
14. Nielsen GP, Dickersin GR, Provenzal JM, Rosenberg AE. Lipomatous hemangiopericytoma. A histologic, ultrastructural and immunohistochemical study of a unique variant of hemangiopericytoma. Am J Surg Pathol 1995;19:748–56.
15. Porter PL, Bigler SA, McNutt M, Gown AM. The immunophenotype of hemangiopericytomas and glomus tumors, with special reference to muscle protein expression: an immunohistochemical study and review of the literature. Mod Pathol 1991;4:46–52.
16. Schurch W, Skalli O, Lagace R, Seemayer TA, Gabbiani G. Intermediate filament proteins and actin isoforms as markers for soft-tissue tumor differentiation and origin. III. Hemangiopericytomas and glomus tumors. Am J Pathol 1990;136:771–86.
17. Stout AP, Murray MR. Hemangiopericytoma: a vascular tumor featuring Zimmermann's pericytes. Ann Surg 1942;116:26–41.
18. van de Rijn M, Rouse RV. CD34: A review. Appl Immunohistochem 1994;2:71–80.
19. Winek RR, Scheithauer BW, Wick MR. Meningioma, meningeal hemangiopericytoma (angioblastic meningioma), peripheral hemangiopericytoma, and acoustic schwannoma. A comparative immunohistochemical study. Am J Surg Pathol 1989;13:251–61.

Infantile Hemangiopericytoma

20. Mentzel T, Calonje E, Nascimento AG, Fletcher CD. Infantile hemangiopericytoma versus infantile myofibromatosis. Study of a series suggesting a continuous spectrum of infantile myofibroblastic lesions. Am J Surg Pathol 1994;18:922–30.

Sinonasal Hemangiopericytoma (Sinonasal Hemangiopericytoma–like Tumor)

21. Compagno J. Hemangiopericytoma-like tumors of the nasal cavity: a comparison with hemangiopericytoma of soft tissues. Laryngoscope 1978;88:460–9.
22. Compagno J, Hyams VJ. Hemangiopericytoma-like intranasal tumors. A clinicopathologic study of 23 cases. Am J Clin Pathol 1976;66:672–83.
23. Eichhorn JH, Dickersin GR, Bhan AK, Goodman ML. Sinonasal hemangiopericytoma. A reassessment with electron microscopy, immunohistochemistry, and long-term follow-up. Am J Surg Pathol 1990;14:856–66.
24. Fletcher CD. Haemangiopericytoma–a dying breed? Reappraisal of an "entity" and its variants: a hypothesis. Curr Diagn Pathol 1994;1:19–23.
25. Nappi O, Ritter JH, Pettinato G, Wick MR. Hemangiopericytoma: histopathological pattern or clinicopathologic entity? Semin Diagn Pathol 1995;12:221–32.

Glomus Tumor

26. Aiba M, Hirayama A, Kuramochi S. Glomangiosarcoma in a glomus tumor. An immunohistochemical and ultrastructural study. Cancer 1988;61:1467–71.

27. Albrecht S, Zbieranowski I. Incidental glomus coccygeum. When a normal structure looks like a tumor. Am J Surg Pathol 1990;14:922–4.

28. Brathwaite CD, Poppiti RJ Jr. Malignant glomus tumor. A case report of widespread metastases in a patient with multiple glomus body hamartomas. Am J Surg Pathol 1996;20:233–8.

29. Dervan PA, Tobbia IN, Casey M, O'Loughlin J, O'Brien M. Glomus tumours: an immunohistochemical profile of 11 cases. Histopathology 1989;14:483–91.

30. Duncan L, Halverson J, De Schryver KK. Glomus tumor of the coccyx. A curable cause of coccygodynia. Arch Pathol Lab Med 1991;115:78–80.

31. Faggioli GL, Bertoni F, Stella A, Bacchini P, Mirelli M, Gessaroli M. Multifocal diffuse glomus tumor. A case report of glomangiomyoma and review of the literature. Int Angiol 1988;7:281–6.

32. Gould EW, Manivel JC, Albores SJ, Monforte H. Locally infiltrative glomus tumors and glomangiosarcomas. A clinical, ultrastructural, and immunohistochemical study. Cancer 1990;65:310–8.

33. Haupt HM, Stern JB, Berlin SJ. Immunohistochemistry in the differential diagnosis of nodular hidradenoma and glomus tumor. Am J Dermatopathol 1992;14:310–4.

34. Hayes MM, Van der Westhuizen N, Holden GP. Aggressive glomus tumor of the nasal region. Report of a case with multiple local recurrences. Arch Pathol Lab Med 1993;117:649–52.

35. Hiruta N, Kameda N, Tokudome T, et al.. Malignant glomus tumor: a case report and review of the literature. Am J Surg Pathol 1997;21:1096–103.

36. Idy–Peretti I, Cermakova E, Dion E, Reygagne P. Subungual glomus tumor: diagnosis based on high-resolution MR images [Letter]. Am J Roentgenol 1992;159:1351.

37. Kaye VM, Dehner LP. Cutaneous glomus tumor. A comparative immunohistochemical study with pseudoangiomatous intradermal melanocytic nevi. Am J Dermatopathol 1991;13:2–6.

38. Nuovo MA, Grimes MM, Knowles DM. Glomus tumors: clinicopathologic and immunohistochemical analysis of forty cases. Surg Pathol 1990;3:31–4.

39. Porter PL, Bigler SA, McNutt M, Gown AM. The immunophenotype of hemangiopericytomas and glomus tumors, with special reference to muscle protein expression: an immunohistochemical study and review of the literature. Mod Pathol 1991;4:46–52.

40. Slater DN, Cotton DW, Azzopardi JG. Oncocytic glomus tumour: a new variant. Histopathology 1987;11:523–31.

41. Tsuneyoshi M, Enjoji M. Glomus tumor: a clinicopathologic and electron microscopic study. Cancer 1982;50:1601–7.

Glomangiopericytoma and Myopericytoma

42. Badizadadegan K, Granter S, Fletcher CD. Myofibromatosis in adults, glomangiopericytoma, and myopericytoma: a spectrum of tumors showing perivascular myoid differentiation. Am J Surg Pathol 1998;22:513–25.

9

SYNOVIAL TUMORS

INTRODUCTION

There is reasonable doubt whether any soft tissue tumors are composed of cells differentiating as synovial cells. Many, but not all, synovial sarcomas contain cells with an epithelial phenotype, at least focally, and there is no evidence that the cells are differentiating as synoviocytes. Consequently, we have moved synovial sarcoma to the miscellaneous category although its name is not changed (also see the introductory comments in the section on synovial sarcoma in chapter 11). This leaves only the localized and diffuse types of tenosynovial giant cell tumors in the synovial tumor category. The immunologic and enzymatic profiles of the most common tenosynovial tumor, localized tenosynovial giant cell tumor (giant cell tumor of tendon sheath), suggest that the constituent cells are of monocyte/macrophage and myofibroblastic lineage and that the giant cells most closely resemble osteoclasts (6,8,9). This does not exclude synovial differentiation because type A synovial cells also express antigens suggesting monocyte/macrophage lineage (7). One could also argue that the lineage of its constituent cells makes localized tenosynovial giant cell tumor a fibrohistiocytic tumor. To further complicate matters, the localized form of tenosynovial giant cell tumor shares clinical, morphologic, and immunologic features with fibroma of tendon sheath which is included among the fibrous tumors. This has led some investigators to maintain that the two lesions represent different parts of the spectrum of the same tumor, while others consider them to be different entities (5,6). The end result is uncertainty about the nosologic position of localized tenosynovial giant cell tumor (giant cell tumor of tendon sheath). Until things become more certain and to avoid confusion, we have elected to leave this tumor in the synovial tumor category while acknowledging its close relationship to fibroma of tendon sheath (Table 9-1).

The issue of a malignant form of tenosynovial giant cell tumor has been raised periodically through the years (2–4). Excluding the giant cell type of malignant fibrous histiocytoma, giant cell osteosarcoma, clear cell sarcoma (it may contain giant cells and typically arises from tendons and fascia), epithelioid sarcoma, and fibrosarcoma, few malignant neoplasms limited to the soft tissues with features of tenosynovial giant cell tumor are left. We concur with the definitional stance taken by Enzinger and Weiss (5) who restrict the term "malignant tenosynovial giant cell tumor" to lesions in which the histologic features of the usual giant cell tumor alternate with areas in which the cells are large and pleomorphic with prominent nucleoli. Tumor cell necrosis is usually prominent and abnormal mitotic figures are almost always present in malignant giant cell tumors, as is infiltration. Tumors that begin as the usual benign giant cell tumor but recur as a cytologically malignant neoplasm would also be classified as malignant giant cell tumor. All other sarcomas containing osteoclast-like giant cells not classifiable as a specific type of sarcoma are labeled as the giant cell variant of malignant fibrous histiocytoma. When these definitions are used, malignant tenosynovial giant cell tumors are very rare indeed, and the only acceptable ones we are aware of have begun in the synovium and extended into the soft tissues. Bertoni and associates (1) have recently presented eight cases from the Mayo Clinic and reviewed seven others presented in the literature.

Tenosynovial giant cell tumors of the localized type are common and most often are referred to

Table 9-1

TUMORS USUALLY CLASSIFIED AS SYNOVIAL

Benign
(Managerial Group Ib, Table 1-10)
Localized tenosynovial tumor
(giant cell tumor of tendon sheath)
Diffuse tenosynovial tumor
(soft tissue pigmented villonodular synovitis)
Malignant
(Managerial Group III, Table 1-10)
Malignant tenosynovial tumor*

---

*The requirements for this diagnosis are presented in the Introduction.

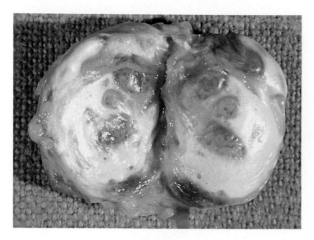

Figure 9-1
LOCALIZED TENOSYNOVIAL GIANT CELL TUMOR
This example of a localized form of tenosynovial tumor has the characteristic gross appearance of white fibrous tissue dissecting the tumor into nodules, which are stained brown by hemosiderin.

as giant cell tumors of tendon sheath. Those of the diffuse type, identical to pigmented villonodular synovitis except for their extra-articular location, are rare.

BENIGN SYNOVIAL TUMORS (MANAGERIAL GROUP Ib, TABLE 1-10)

Tenosynovial Giant Cell Tumor, Localized Type

Definition. Tenosynovial giant cell tumor, localized type, also known as *giant cell tumor of tendon sheath* and *nodular tenosynovitis,* is a circumscribed tumor essentially limited to the hands, feet, ankles, and knees that is composed of both mononuclear cells with round to oblong nuclei and almost always variable numbers of multinuclear giant cells with the same nuclear features.

Clinical Features. The localized type of tenosynovial giant cell tumor develops only in the hands, feet, ankles, and knees, or extremely rarely in the hip (12,13). About 85 percent are in the fingers, usually near an interphalangeal joint. Most patients are between 30 and 50 years of age and the tumor is slightly more common in women (13). The tumors usually are in the soft tissues near tendons but they can develop elsewhere and rarely may erode nearby bone. Skin involvement is rare.

Pathologic Findings. Grossly, localized tenosynovial giant cell tumors are usually under 4

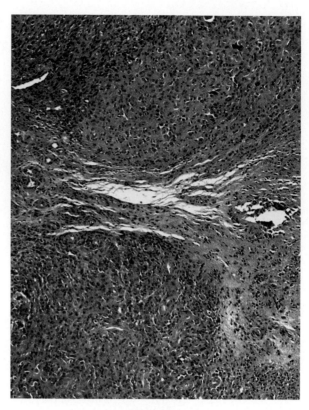

Figure 9-2
LOCALIZED TENOSYNOVIAL GIANT CELL TUMOR
The nodular pattern can also be appreciated microscopically at low magnification.

cm although rare examples can be larger, especially if they arise in the foot or around the ankle. The localized form is circumscribed and often lobulated although rarely it may erode bone and lose its apparent circumscription. On cut section, it is usually white to gray but yellow and brown areas due to xanthoma cells and hemosiderin, respectively, are common (fig. 9-1).

Microscopically, dense fibrous tissue divides the tumor giving it a nodular appearance (fig. 9-2). Localized tenosynovial giant cell tumor is composed of cells with small, round to oblong, often reniform or clefted, uniform nuclei, sometimes with prominent nucleoli. These oblong cells frequently blend with spindled forms. Scattered among these mononuclear cells are variable numbers of multinucleated giant cells with similar nuclei (fig. 9-3) (13). Giant cells are usually readily apparent at low magnification and sometimes are numerous, but in occasional tumors they can be difficult to find or, rarely, are even absent (fig. 9-4).

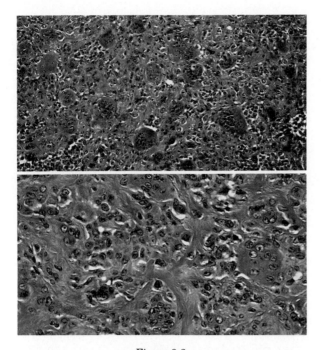

Figure 9-3
LOCALIZED TENOSYNOVIAL GIANT CELL TUMOR
Localized tenosynovial tumor is composed of small, uniform, mononuclear cells which closely resemble histiocytes mixed with variable numbers of multinucleated giant cells.

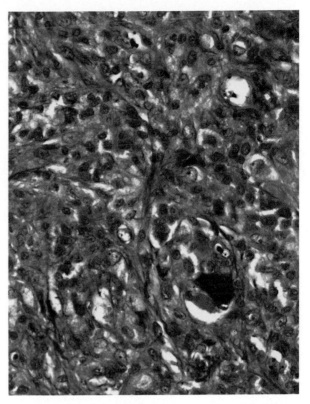

Figure 9-4
LOCALIZED TENOSYNOVIAL GIANT CELL TUMOR
In some instances giant cells are sparse or even absent. Multiple sections may reveal giant cells or uncommonly the diagnosis is based on the appearance of the mononuclear cells.

The giant cells usually contain 8 to 10 nuclei but can have as many as 50 or 60. In some tumors the giant cell nuclei have smudged chromatin. Other low-power features that may be seen include xanthoma cells, hemosiderin outside and inside macrophages, metaplastic bone or cartilage, focally or diffusely hyalinized stroma and, particularly in lesions near large joints, alveolar-like spaces (see fig. 9-6). Mitotic figures are usually sparse but can be numerous and groups of tumor cells can occasionally be found in vascular spaces. Neither elevated mitotic activity nor vascular involvement predicts a more aggressive course.

Special Studies. Many ultrastructural studies suggest that the constituent cells of localized tenosynovial giant cell tumor resemble fibroblasts or histiocytes (13). Enzymatic and immunologic studies provide evidence that the cells may be true histiocytes of monocyte/macrophage lineage although there are cells of such lineage lining the normal synovium. The constituent mononuclear cells are usually CD68 and leukocyte common antigen positive (11). In addition to the cells a subpopulation of desmin-positive,

actin-negative dendritic cells is found in about half the tumors (10a).

Chromosomal analysis reveals cytogenetic heterogeneity, with most of the chromosomal changes clustered in 1p11 and 16q24 (10).

Differential Diagnosis. The localized form of tenosynovial giant cell tumor should be distinguished from the much less common diffuse type. The diffuse form is the soft tissue equivalent of pigmented villonodular synovitis; in fact, most cases are extensions into the soft tissues from an intra-articular primary. Diffuse tenosynovial giant cell tumor, as its name implies, is not circumscribed as is the localized form and occurs mainly around the knee; less commonly, it involves the distal extremity. Microscopically, the tumor cells grow in sheets and resemble those of the localized form except that they are commonly pigmented with hemosiderin. Alveolar-like spaces in the stroma and foam cells are the rule.

If the tumor in question is around the knee and the joint is involved, it is surely the diffuse rather than the localized form of tenosynovial tumor.

Fibroma of tendon sheath occurs in the same location as most localized tenosynovial tumors but is typically paucicellular. It is composed of cells ranging from fibroblasts with vesicular nuclei that resemble those in nodular fasciitis to mature fibrocytes, whereas the cells in localized tenosynovial giant cell tumors tend to have histiocytic features. Giant cells are unusual in fibroma of tendon sheath and paucicellular collagen is usually more extensive than in localized tenosynovial giant cell tumor. However, when giant cells become sparse in localized tenosynovial tumor and fibroma of tendon sheath becomes cellular the two can resemble each other closely, and indeed some investigators think they are morphologic variants of the same tumor (11). Fortunately, both lesions have the same 30 percent incidence of recurrence so there is no penalty for misclassification. Necrobiotic granulomas feature palisaded histiocytes that can resemble the constituent cells of tenosynovial giant cells, but these surround necrotic areas, and necrosis is unusual in localized tenosynovial giant cell tumor. Moreover, giant cells are usually absent or at most sparse in necrobiotic granulomas. Foreign body and infectious granulomas contain chronic inflammatory cells in addition to histiocytes, and sometimes there is necrosis. Epithelioid sarcoma can occasionally contain giant cells but tumor cells of larger size, brightly eosinophilic cytoplasm, and keratin positivity distinguish epithelioid sarcoma from tenosynovial giant cell tumor.

Treatment and Prognosis. About 30 percent of localized tenosynovial giant cell tumors recur but rarely aggressively and recurrences are almost always controlled by reexcision. Rarely, extension into bone does occur but this can be controlled by removal of the tumor. Some studies suggest that high cellularity and easily found mitotic figures are predictive of recurrence.

Tenosynovial Giant Cell Tumor, Diffuse Type (Soft Tissue Pigmented Villonodular Synovitis)

Definition and Clinical Features. This very rare lesion is histologically identical to intra-articular pigmented villonodular synovitis which is described in the Fascicle, Tumors of the Bones and Joints (14a). As it turns out, many but by no means all of the soft tissue cases reported are extensions of intra-articular pigmented villonodular synovitis (16,18). Consequently, most diffuse tenosynovial giant cell tumors develop around the knee with a smaller subset occurring around the ankle and foot. Rarely toes, fingers, elbows, the sacroiliac area, and the temporomandibular soft tissues can be the site of involvement.

Pathologic Findings. Grossly, most diffuse tenosynovial giant cell tumors are large and bulky. They are usually white to brown but may be yellow when large numbers of xanthoma cells are present (14,15). Unlike their juxta-articular counterparts, diffuse tenosynovial giant cell tumors are not villous, however, they frequently are nodular (fig. 9-5, left). They are highly cellular and the constituent cells most frequently grow in sheets within the nodules. Hemosiderin pigment is usually prominent (fig. 9-5, right). Numerous cleft-like spaces, often referred to as alveolar spaces, are common (fig. 9-6). The cells vary from small polygonal cells with scant, sometimes pigmented, cytoplasm to spindled cells (figs. 9-7, 9-8). Xanthoma cells are common. Multinucleated giant cells may be present but are usually not numerous while chronic inflammatory cells are usually prominent. Mitotic activity is often brisk.

Special Studies. The constituent cells are usually CD68 positive and iron stains can identify hemosiderin. A subpopulation of desmin-positive, actin-negative dendritic cells is found in about half the tumors (10a). Cytogenetically, diffuse lesions often show clonal rearrangements of 1p11-13 as well as trisomy 5 and 7 (17).

Differential Diagnosis. Because of their size and high cellularity, concern for a malignant process is often foremost in the observer's mind when a diffuse tenosynovial giant cell tumor is encountered. This concern is heightened when the often destructive growth pattern of these lesions is revealed by imaging studies. However, the constituent histiocytic cells are uniform and often pigmented (an iron stain is helpful) and they do not demonstrate the chromatin abnormalities, nucleomegaly, or abnormal mitotic figures expected in a sarcoma. Inflammatory malignant fibrous histiocytoma may come to mind because of the large numbers of foam cells and lymphocytes but this tumor hardly ever occurs around a joint and is associated with neutrophils rather than chronic

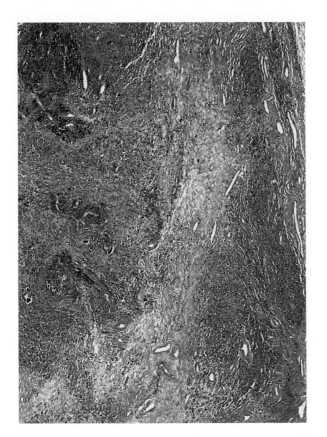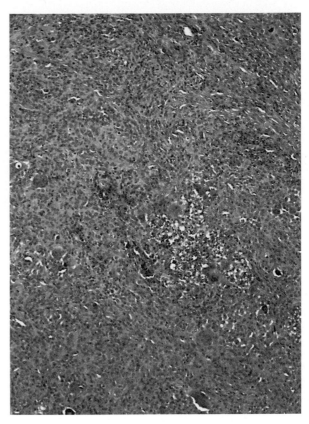

Figure 9-5
DIFFUSE TENOSYNOVIAL GIANT CELL TUMOR
Left: Giant cells are usually sparse or absent and the uniform cells tend to grow in large nodules separated by fibrous tissue.
Right: Hemosiderin is commonly present.

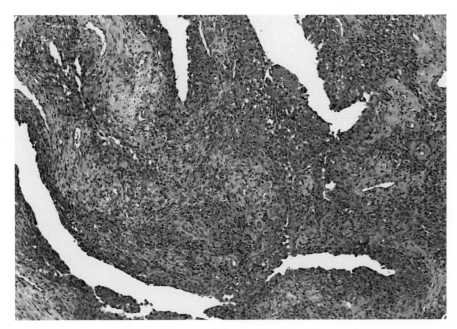

Figure 9-6
DIFFUSE TENOSYNOVIAL
GIANT CELL TUMOR
Pseudosynovial clefts, also labeled alveolar-like spaces, are commonly present throughout.

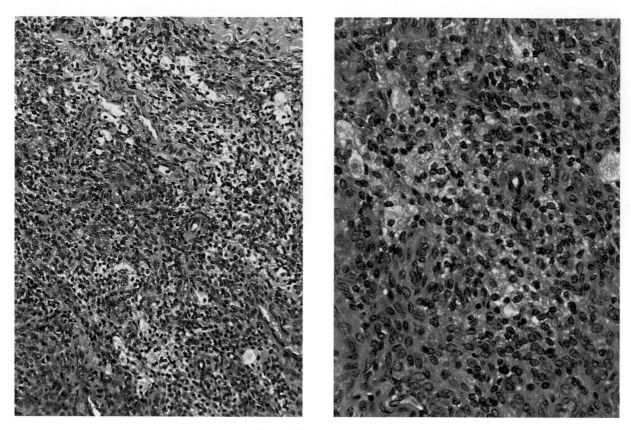

Figure 9-7
DIFFUSE TENOSYNOVIAL GIANT CELL TUMOR
The constituent cells resemble those found in the localized form of giant cell tumor and have uniform nuclei. Foam cells and chronic inflammation are common.

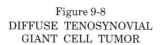

Figure 9-8
DIFFUSE TENOSYNOVIAL
GIANT CELL TUMOR
The cells in the diffuse type can be spindled but retain their uniform appearance. It is the bland appearance of the nuclei that help distinguish this tumor from sarcoma.

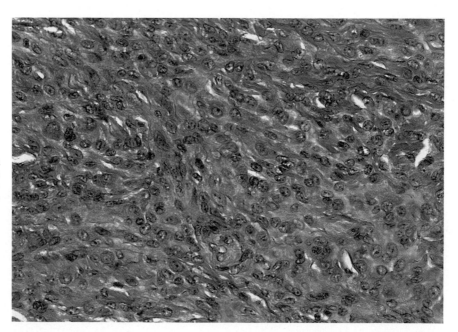

inflammation. The alveolar-like spaces might raise a question of alveolar rhabdomyosarcoma or synovial sarcoma but the elongate spindle cell component of synovial sarcoma, with its stubby nuclei, and the rhabdomyoblastic cells of alveolar rhabdomyosarcoma are not present in diffuse tenosynovial giant cell tumor. Desmin stains are positive in rhabdomyosarcoma; keratin and epithelial membrane antigen are positive in synovial sarcomas containing glands that mimic the alveolar spaces of diffuse tenosynovial giant cell tumor; these stains are negative in diffuse tenosynovial giant cell tumor. Most importantly, imaging studies frequently reveal intra-articular involvement as well as a soft tissue tumor, which is very rare in synovial sarcoma and unheard of in rhabdomyosarcoma. In cases where chronic inflammation and alveolar spaces are prominent angiomatoid fibrous histiocytoma enters the differential diagnosis. However, the alveolar spaces of diffuse tenosynovial giant cell tumor are not filled with blood as are the spaces in angiomatoid fibrous histiocytoma and giant cells are usually more numerous.

Treatment and Prognosis. The diffuse form of tenosynovial giant cell tumor may recur, in fact 30 to 50 percent do so (15,18). A small minority of these lesions metastasize (see below) and, exceptionally, such cases may be morphologically bland (18). Treatment is surgical removal.

MALIGNANT TENOSYNOVIAL GIANT CELL TUMOR (MANAGERIAL GROUP III, TABLE 1-10)

The definitional requirements for this rare tumor have been provided in the introduction. A recent review of eight cases from the Mayo Clinic and seven from the literature which presumably arose in joints has been provided by Bertoni and associates (1). Similar cases have also been described recently in extra-articular locations (18). Malignant lesions most often show transition from conventional giant cell tumor to nondistinctive sarcoma. Such lesions are associated with a significant risk of metastasis to lymph nodes and lung.

REFERENCES

Introduction

1. Bertoni F, Krishnan KU, Beabout JW, Sim FH. Malignant giant cell tumor of the tendon sheaths and joints (malignant pigmented villonodular synovitis). Am J Surg Pathol 1997;21:153–63.
2. Bliss BO, Reed RJ. Large cell sarcomas of tendon sheath. Malignant giant cell tumors of tendon sheath. Am J Clin Pathol 1968;49:776–81.
3. Carstens PH, Howell RS. Malignant giant cell tumor of tendon sheath. Virchows Arch [A] 1979;382:237–9.
4. Dal Cin P, Sciot R, Samson I, et al. Cytogenetic characterization of tenosynovial giant cell tumors (nodular tenosynovitis). Cancer Res 1994;54:3986–7.
5. Enzinger FM, Weiss SW. Soft tissue tumors, 3rd ed. St. Louis: Mosby, 1995:749.
6. Maluf HM, De YB, Swanson PE, Wick MR. Fibroma and giant cell tumor of tendon sheath: a comparative histological and immunohistological study. Mod Pathol 1995;8:155–9.
7. Palmer DG, Sclvendran Y, Allen C, Revell PA, Hogg N. Features of synovial membrane identified with monoclonal antibodies. Clin Exp Immunol 1985;59:529–38.
8. Ushijima M, Hashimoto H, Tsuneyoshi M, Enjoji M. Giant cell tumor of the tendon sheath (nodular tenosynovitis). A study of 207 cases to compare the large joint group with the common digit group. Cancer 1986;57:875–84.
9. Wood GS, Beckstead JH, Medeiros LJ, Kempson RL, Warnke RA. The cells of giant cell tumor of tendon sheath resemble osteoclasts. Am J Surg Pathol 1988;12:444–52.

Tenosynovial Giant Cell Tumor, Localized Type

10. Dal Cin P, Sciot R, Samson I, et al. Cytogenetic characterization of tenosynovial giant cell tumors (nodular tenosynovitis). Cancer Res 1994;54:3986–7.
10a. Folpe AL, Weiss SW, Fletcher CD. Tenosynovial giant cell tumors: evidence for a desmin-positive dendritic cell subpopulation. Mod Pathol 1998;11:939–44.
11. Maluf HM, De YB, Swanson PE, Wick MR. Fibroma and giant cell tumor of tendon sheath: a comparative histological and immunohistological study. Mod Pathol 1995;8:155–9.
12. Rao AS, Vigorita VJ. Pigmented villonodular synovitis (giant-cell tumor of the tendon sheath and synovial

membrane). A review of eighty-one cases. J Bone Joint Surg 1984;66:76–94.

13. Ushijima M, Hashimoto H, Tsuneyoshi M, Enjoji M. Giant cell tumor of the tendon sheath (nodular tenosynovitis). A

study of 207 cases to compare the large joint group with the common digit group. Cancer 1986;57:875–84.

Tenosynovial Giant Cell Tumor, Diffuse Type

14. Arthaud JB. Pigmented nodular synovitis: report of 11 lesions in non-articular locations. Am J Clin Pathol 1972;58:511–7.

14a. Fechner RE, Mills SE. Tumors of the bones and joints. Atlas of Tumor Pathology. Fascicle 8, 3rd Series. Washington, D.C.: Armed Forces Institute of Pathology, 1993.

15. Rao AS, Vigorita VJ. Pigmented villonodular synovitis (giant-cell tumor of the tendon sheath and synovial membrane). A review of eighty-one cases. J Bone Joint Surg 1984;66:76–94.

16. Schwartz HS, Unni KK, Pritchard DJ. Pigmented villonodular synovitis: a retrospective review of large affected joints. Clin Orthop 1989;247:243–55.

17. Sciot R, Rosai J, Dal Cin P, et al. Analysis of 35 cases of localized and diffuse tenosynovial giant cell tumor: a report from the Chromosomes and Morphology (CHAMP) Study Group. Mod Pathol 1999;12:576–9.

18. Somerhausen NS, Fletcher CD. Diffuse-type giant cell tumor: clinicopathologic and immunohistochemical analysis of 50 cases with extra-articular disease. Am J Surg Pathol 2000;24:479–92.

10

CARTILAGINOUS AND OSSEOUS TUMORS

INTRODUCTION

Cartilaginous tumors of the soft tissues are defined as those in which the lesional cells produce cartilage, while osseous tumors are those in which lesional cells lay down osteoid or bone in the absence of any other line of differentiation other than fibrous or fibrohistiocytic. These definitions raise several problems: 1) How is tumor osteoid distinguished from collagen and neoplastic cartilage from chondroid?; 2) Given the presence of convincing bone or cartilage in a soft tissue neoplasm, how does one determine whether this matrix is metaplastic or neoplastic?; and 3) What is the best way to classify sarcomas that sometimes but not always contain tumor cartilage or bone? Osteoid is dense collagen which if mineralized becomes bone. Because osteoid laid down by tumor cells, whether benign or malignant, is considered to be evidence of osseous differentiation and because osteoid is morphologically indistinguishable from collagen except for its configuration, it is important to know the features that count as tumor osteoid. Unfortunately, a crisp description of the minimal histologic features that should be present before a matrix is accepted as tumor osteoid is generally lacking in both the orthopedic and soft tissue pathology literature.

Faced with this vacuum, different investigators employ different definitions. Our convention for classifying a soft tissue tumor as of osseous type based solely on tumor osteoid is to require the putative osteoid to be abundant, densely eosinophilic, and rimmed by tumor cells. In addition, it is most often laid down in long narrow trabeculae with irregular margins and cross branches, an arrangement that has been likened to lace; less often, acceptable tumor osteoid is produced in sheets or broad trabeculae with irregular margins. In benign osseous lesions, the osteoid trabeculae tend to have a smoother contour and are often broader than the typically more narrow trabeculae seen in osteosarcoma. Moreover, the osteoid-producing cells in benign osseous lesions are uniform and have bland nuclei. Even in benign lesions, we still require osteoid to be abundant and dense. When tumor osteoid mineralizes it often takes on a purplish hue when stained with hematoxylin and eosin (H&E) and this tinctorial quality, combined with its irregular thin trabecular arrangement, almost always allows easy recognition of mineralized tumor bone. We exclude from the osseous tumor group soft tissue lesions that have a dense collagenous stroma which does not fulfill the requirements set out above for tumor osteoid. If the tumor with "suggestive osteoid" is malignant, we place it into the pleomorphic malignant fibrous histiocytoma (MFH) group if histiocyte-like cells are present and the constituent cells do not demonstrate any other line of differentiation, or the undifferentiated sarcoma category if neither histiocyte-like cells or differentiated cells are present. Of course, nothing much is at stake except classificatory nicety because the management and prognosis for pleomorphic MFH, undifferentiated sarcoma, and soft tissue osteosarcoma are the same.

While tumor osteoid is accepted as evidence of osseous differentiation, we do not accept "chondroid" as evidence of cartilaginous differentiation. Chondroid is essentially acid mucopolysaccharide and morphologically nonspecific so with the exception of myxoid chondrosarcoma, as described below, we require cartilaginous tumors to produce at least focally differentiated cartilage featuring cells in lacunae surrounded by a uniform, dense, basophilic matrix. When both neoplastic cartilage and neoplastic bone or osteoid are present in the same soft tissue sarcoma, the rule that applies to malignant skeletal tumors also applies in the soft tissue: tumor bone takes precedence and the tumor is classified as an osteosarcoma. Benign tumors composed of bone and cartilage are very rare in the soft tissue but as in bone they are classified as osteochondromas.

The second problem that arises is distinguishing metaplastic bone and cartilage, which can be found in a wide variety of soft tissue tumors, both benign and malignant, from tumor bone and cartilage. If the bone or cartilage is of the latter type, the tumor is classified as an osseous or cartilaginous one; tumors containing metaplastic bone or cartilage are not so classified. This problem is particularly acute in malignant soft tissue tumors because a considerable number of sarcomas, such as synovial sarcoma, epithelioid sarcoma, MFH, and liposarcoma, contain metaplastic bone or cartilage. Metaplastic bone usually does not have the irregular, fine, lace-like trabecular pattern of tumor bone formed by malignant cells as seen in osteosarcoma, nor does it have its lavender hue; rather, metaplastic bone is usually deposited as regular fragments of well-formed, most often eosinophilic bone, which has smooth outlines and sometimes a lamellar pattern. Characteristically, metaplastic bone is located at the periphery of the tumor and is sparse in contrast to tumor bone, which is typically more widely distributed throughout the lesion. Definitionally, the cells forming metaplastic bone must be cytologically benign. Even with these guidelines, it may be impossible in some cases to determine whether bone is neoplastic or metaplastic. The important decision is not about the type of bone but the malignant potential of the tumor, and almost all tumors that are acceptable as osteosarcoma except for uncertainty about the type of bone are composed of cells that are obviously malignant on cytologic grounds. For malignant neoplasms containing cartilage the situation can be equally problematic and one is usually reduced to trying to decide whether the cartilage-forming cells are benign (metaplasia) or malignant; the latter would allow classification of the tumor as chondrosarcoma. Care should be taken not to interpret infiltrated normal bone or cartilage as evidence of a soft tissue osteosarcoma or chondrosarcoma. Imaging studies, which should always be done to be sure an apparent soft tissue bone- or cartilage-forming tumor is not actually primary in bone, are usually helpful in this regard.

For benign bone- and cartilage-containing tumors, taxonomic practice as reported in the literature can only be judged inconsistent. Since bone and cartilage in benign tumors are cytologically bland, they could be considered metaplastic as they are in those benign bone- and cartilage-forming lesions classified as other than of osseous or cartilaginous type, e.g., calcifying aponeurotic fibroma and ossifying fibromyxoid tumor. On the other hand, some benign tumors with an osseous or cartilaginous stroma are placed in the osseous or cartilaginous category, e.g., myositis ossificans and chondroma. This latter classificatory maneuver is used most often when the bone or cartilage in the lesion is abundant. When differentiated tissue other than a fibrous stroma is present, a dual label is sometimes used, e.g., chondrolipoma, or the bone and cartilage is considered metaplastic and the label of the other differentiated tissue is used, e.g., leiomyoma with osseous metaplasia. The term benign mesenchymoma has been suggested for benign tumors whose constituent cells demonstrate more than one line of cellular differentiation but we do not use this term and it is seldom used in the literature. Our convention is to list the differentiated tissue present in the diagnostic label unless the lesion in question already has an assigned name.

The third problem is how to classify sarcomas that sometimes (but not always) possess an osseous or cartilaginous matrix elaborated by tumor cells but contain no other differentiated cells except fibroblasts or cells that would warrant classifying the tumor as a fibrous histiocytoma. The best known examples of these problematic tumors are giant cell sarcoma of the soft tissues (which is usually included among the malignant fibrous histiocytomas even though about half of them produce neoplastic bone or cartilage) and myxoid chondrosarcoma (only rare examples of which contain neoplastic cartilage). Presumably, investigators have not included the bone- and cartilage-forming type of giant cell sarcoma among the osseous and cartilaginous tumors because bone and cartilage formation is inconstant and often focal. Going against this trend, we think sarcomas containing neoplastic osteoid or bone and a fibrous or fibrohistiocytic stroma should be classified as osteosarcoma. If the tumor otherwise meets the criteria for giant cell sarcoma or another type of MFH and does not contain neoplastic bone or cartilage, it is classified as MFH. Rare soft tissue sarcomas containing malignant cartilage or bone plus an additional differentiated cell type (other than fibrous or fibrohistiocytic) or sarcomas that contain two or more differentiated cell types other than bone or cartilage have been classified by some as malignant mesenchymomas. We think it better to classify such tumors based on the predominant differentiated cell type and specify that other differentiated tissues are also present. For example, liposarcomas and leiomyosarcomas containing malignant bone or cartilage would be classified as such rather than as malignant mesenchymoma, e.g., leiomyosarcoma with chondrosarcoma. An equally acceptable alternative is to label such sarcomas as mixed and specify the differentiated components present, e.g., mixed sarcoma, leiomyosarcoma and chondrosarcoma.

Less than 10 percent of the tumors classified as myxoid chondrosarcoma contain recognizable tumor cartilage but all tumors with the characteristic histologic pattern of this neoplasm are classified as chondrosarcoma. Classificatory common sense would suppose that only the cartilage-containing tumors be classified as chondrosarcoma and the others be provided with another label, but this is not the case. The reasons for making this widely recognized exception are the ultrastructural resemblance of soft tissue myxoid chondrosarcoma cells to chondroblasts, and the fact that the stroma of myxoid chondrosarcoma may contain some of the same acid mucopolysaccharides that are found in hyaline cartilage.

It is thus apparent that classificatory consistency is not widely practiced when it comes to soft tissue tumors containing bone and cartilage. For the sake of reproducibility, we think the only exception to the conventions provided above for the sarcomas should be myxoid chondrosarcoma. The situation with the benign bone- and cartilage-containing tumors is too ingrained to change and one simply has to learn the labels that have been applied to the various morphologic patterns.

There is one benign soft tissue tumor in the cartilaginous category, chondroma, and two soft tissue tumors that are classified as chondrosarcoma, myxoid chondrosarcoma, and mesenchymal chondrosarcoma. We are unconvinced of the existence of clinically malignant cartilaginous neoplasms arising in the soft tissues that are composed of cells differentiating as hyaline cartilage with the histologic features of grade I chondrosarcoma of bone. Benign lesions in the extraskeletal osseous category include myositis ossificans and related lesions such as fibro-osseous pseudotumor of the digits, ossifying fasciitis, and ossifying panniculitis as well as a distinctly different lesion, progressive fibrodysplasia ossificans, a rare inherited disorder. Osteosarcoma is the only malignant soft tissue neoplasm in the osseous category. We

Table 10-1

EXTRAOSSEOUS CARTILAGINOUS AND OSSEOUS TUMORS

Benign
(Managerial Groups Ia and Ib, Table 1-10)

Chondroma (and osteochondroma)

Myositis ossificans and related lesions, including fibro-osseous pseudotumor of the digits and panniculitis ossificans

Fibrodysplasia ossificans progressiva (Managerial Group IV, Table 1-10)

Malignant
(Managerial Group III, Table 1-10)

Myxoid chondrosarcoma

Mesenchymal chondrosarcoma

Extraskeletal osteosarcoma

consider soft tissue osteomas to be a form of osseous metaplasia and the rare, purely soft tissue osteochondroma is discussed with chondroma. Synovial chondromatosis is discussed in the Fascicle, Tumors of the Bones and Joints (4a). There are no "intermediate" cartilaginous or osseous tumors so all tumors in this category are classified as either benign (mostly reactive) or malignant (Table 10-1).

BENIGN EXTRASKELETAL CARTILAGINOUS TUMORS (MANAGERIAL GROUPS Ia AND Ib, TABLE 1-10)

Chondroma

Definition. Soft tissue chondroma is an extraskeletal, extrasynovial, benign soft tissue tumor composed, at least in part, of hyaline cartilage and no other differentiated tissue except a fibrous or myxoid stroma.

General Considerations. Definitionally, soft tissue chondromas must have, at least focally, a dense basophilic matrix that contains cells within lacunae, i.e., differentiated hyaline cartilage must be identified. When chondromas are attached to either bone or synovium, they are considered to have arisen in those sites even though they may protrude into the soft tissues. In about two thirds

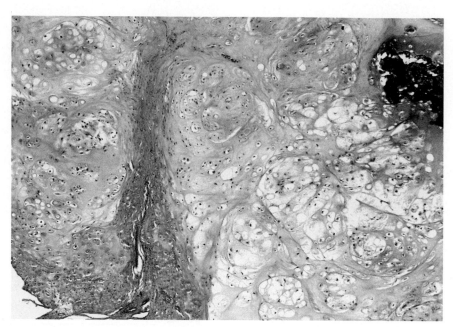

Figure 10-1
EXTRAOSSEOUS
CHONDROMA
Extraosseous chondromas are lobulated tumors composed of hyaline cartilage. Most occur on the hands and feet.

of soft tissue chondromas, cartilage is abundant and obvious, but in the remainder, variable amounts of fibrous tissue, myxoid stroma, and calcium replace or obscure the cartilage and multiple sections may be required to find diagnostic areas. Extraskeletal chondromas with extensive fibrous tissue are sometimes labeled as *fibrochondroma* while those with a prominent myxoid stroma may be classified as *myxochondroma*.

Clinical Features. Extraskeletal chondromas are unusual neoplasms. Most occur in the hands and feet, and about half develop in the fingers. They are rare in the head and neck and on the trunk. They often grow in the vicinity of tendons and joints, but by definition they must be extraosseous and not attached to synovium or periosteum. Most patients are middle-aged, although the reported range is from 9 to 79 years. The usual symptom is a painless lump and almost all chondromas are single. The tumor is slightly more common in men than women. Imaging techniques may aid in the diagnosis (5,6).

Pathologic Findings. Grossly, extraskeletal chondromas are usually lobulated and often have sharply demarcated edges. They may appear cartilaginous on cut section and cysts are sometimes present. Almost all are under 2 cm and rarely are larger than 5 to 6 cm.

Microscopically, the typical chondroma is lobulated and composed predominantly or exclusively of differentiated hyaline cartilage with cells in lacunae (fig. 10-1) (2,3). Variable amounts of fibrous tissue and myxoid stroma are usually present and in some tumors can be so abundant that the required cartilage is focal and inconspicuous. Calcification is present in many chondromas and can be so extensive as to obscure the cartilage (2). The center of the tumor is most commonly calcified and the calcified chondrocytes may exhibit degenerative changes or be outlined by flecks of calcium. Multinucleated giant cells are common and some tumors contain collections of epithelioid and giant cells which mimic a granulomatous reaction or giant cell tumor of tendon sheath.

As in enchondromas of bone, the cells of extraskeletal chondroma can exhibit a considerable range of appearances. Most are small with smooth dense chromatin but not infrequently the cells display variation in size and shape and there can be considerable nuclear enlargement as well as hyperchromatism (fig. 10-2) (3). However, they never have cytologically malignant features. The cells tend to grow in clusters and individual cells may be retracted from the edges of the lacunar spaces. Cells with eosinophilic cytoplasm and round to spindled nuclei embedded in a myxoid matrix are sometimes scattered throughout the tumor. These are thought to be chondroblasts and vessels may be prominent in

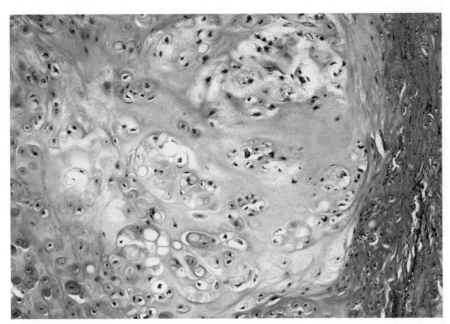

Figure 10-2
EXTRAOSSEOUS
CHONDROMA
The cells composing chondromas are usually small with dense smooth chromatin, but they can vary considerably in size and shape.

such areas. When chondroblasts are numerous and hyaline cartilage sparse the label *chondroblastic chondroma* may be used.

Mitotic figures may be seen in some tumors, but they are usually sparse and never abnormal. Myxoid areas composed of small cells with elongate nuclei and scant cytoplasm are a feature of some chondromas. Chondromas are usually surrounded by dense connective tissue or tendon. As would be expected, the cells within the differentiated areas of chondroma are S-100 protein positive, but immunohistochemistry is seldom needed to make the diagnosis.

Differential Diagnosis. A major concern is distinguishing chondroma from chondrosarcoma. Chondrosarcomas of the hands and feet, the most common site of chondroma, are vanishingly rare. Moreover, chondrosarcomas composed solely of differentiated hyaline cartilage identical to grade I chondrosarcoma of the skeleton have not been reported in the soft tissues, so this is not a diagnostic consideration if a primary in the skeleton has been excluded, something that should always be done before assuming a cartilaginous lesion is primary in the soft tissues. As a result, chondromas in the soft tissues can be as cellular and as atypical as grade I chondrosarcoma of bone. The latter, while it practically never metastasizes, can dedifferentiate to higher grade sarcoma, an occurrence not reported for soft tissue chondromas.

Myxoid chondrosarcoma, discussed in detail below, is a major differential diagnostic consideration when chondromas have a prominent myxoid stroma. Differentiated hyaline cartilage, a required component of chondroma and prominent in the vast majority, is absent in about two thirds of myxoid chondrosarcomas and hard to find in almost all the remainder. The chain-like arrangement of the cells which touch one another, a requirement for myxoid chondrosarcoma, is uncommon in chondroma; chondromas occur mainly in the hands and feet, which are rare sites for myxoid chondrosarcomas; and myxoid chondrosarcomas are usually larger than 3 cm, a size rarely attained by chondromas. Mesenchymal chondrosarcoma features small round blue cells with focal islands of differentiated cartilage and often a pericytic type of vascular pattern, so it is not a serious differential diagnostic consideration for chondroma.

Another major differential diagnostic concern when contemplating a diagnosis of chondroma is excluding lesions primary in nearby bone, periosteum, or synovium, or a metastasis. By definition, soft tissue chondromas do not arise in nor are they attached to these structures. Cartilaginous tumors arising in bone or periosteum should be classified as primary in bone and their malignant potential evaluated as such even if they extend into the soft tissues (1). The same applies to cartilaginous lesions arising in the synovium (4). Imaging studies are the best method to determine the primary site of a cartilaginous neoplasm. Synovial chondromatosis is histologically identical to soft tissue chondroma but it is localized to the synovium (4). Moreover, it usually develops around large joints and consists of multiple tumor nodules whereas chondromas are almost always single and mainly occur in the hands and feet. However, synovial chondromatosis has been reported in the hands (4). As would be expected, on rare occasions, multiple nodules of bland hyaline cartilage may be present away from the synovium in the soft tissues. This occurs almost exclusively around large joints, is benign, and has been labeled extra-articular synovial chondromatosis.

As noted in the Introduction to this chapter, bland hyaline cartilage may be found in a number of other types of benign soft tissue tumors. By convention, the cartilage is either considered to be metaplastic and the lesion is classified on the basis of morphologic features other than the cartilage, or the tumor is given a dual name such as chondrolipoma. Two such lesions that figure prominently in the differential diagnosis of chondroma because of their frequent location in the hand are giant cell tumor of tendon sheath with cartilaginous metaplasia and calcifying aponeurotic fibroma (CAF). CAF has a dense fibrous stroma that surrounds nodules which may have a center composed of cartilage. A distinct feature of CAF not present in chondroma is the circular, parallel rows of cells that form the nodules. Chondroma occurs mainly in adults while CAF is mainly a lesion of childhood. Both can recur but are otherwise nonaggressive, so distinction between the two is not critical. Multinucleated giant cells are occasionally a feature of chondroma and rarely, tenosynovial giant cell tumor (giant cell tumor of tendon sheath) can feature metaplastic cartilage. However, metaplastic cartilage is almost always focal in the latter and the characteristic plump histiocytic tumor cells are always found. The cells in the differentiated areas of chondroma are almost always S-100 protein positive, while the cells in giant cell tumor are often CD68 and CD15 positive, but S-100 protein negative.

Bland cartilage within a sarcoma is generally considered to be metaplastic and the sarcoma is classified on the basis of the noncartilaginous areas. Soft tissue tumors containing cytologically malignant cartilage with atypia beyond that allowed in chondroma practically always have other components and are classified according to the guidelines presented in the Introduction.

Treatment and Prognosis. Extraskeletal chondromas are classified as benign, but about 15 to 20 percent recur (2). However, they do not recur aggressively and they do not dedifferentiate to sarcoma. Recurrences are successfully managed by local excision.

MALIGNANT EXTRASKELETAL CARTILAGINOUS TUMORS (MANAGERIAL GROUP III, TABLE 1-10)

Myxoid Chondrosarcoma

Definition. Myxoid chondrosarcoma is a neoplasm with a myxoid stroma and a lobular configuration in which the constituent cells generally form long rows and interconnecting strands that extend from the periphery of the lobules toward the center, and are usually attached to each other. About one third of the tumors contain differentiated cartilage.

General Considerations. Only rare extraskeletal myxoid chondrosarcomas contain cartilage, and even then cartilaginous differentiation is usually immature, focal, and inconspicuous. Why then are all of these tumors classified as of cartilaginous type whether they contain cartilage or not? The decision to place them all in this category is based on the ultrastructural resemblance of extraskeletal myxoid chondrosarcoma cells to chondroblasts, a matrix that displays many of the histochemical reactions of cartilage, the S-100 protein–positive cells in a minority of extracellular myxoid chondrosarcomas and, of course, the observation that some of the tumors contain cartilage (see Introduction). The important message is that not all myxoid chondrosarcomas will contain differentiated cartilage by light microscopy and in that circumstance the tumor is recognized on the basis of its other histologic features. In the past, myxoid chondrosarcomas without differentiated cartilage were classified by some as chordoid sarcoma (12).

Clinical Features. Myxoid chondrosarcoma is almost exclusively a tumor of adults, with a median age of about 50 years (9,13). The tumor

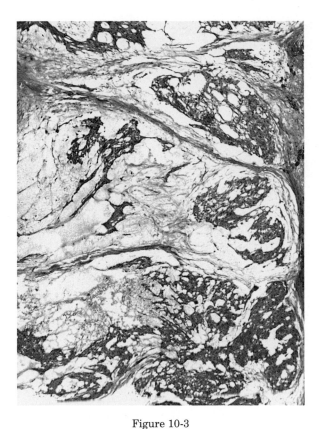

Figure 10-3
MYXOID CHONDROSARCOMA
Myxoid chondrosarcoma almost always has a lobular pattern of growth, a feature that helps in its recognition.

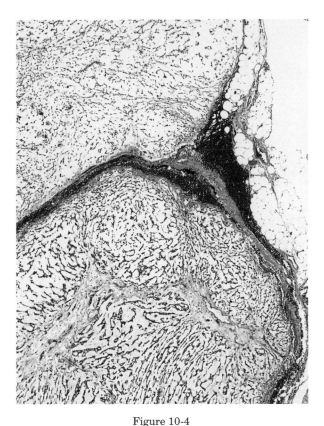

Figure 10-4
MYXOID CHONDROSARCOMA
The lobular pattern of myxoid chondrosarcoma is apparent, as is the chain-like arrangement of the tumor cells.

is so rare in children and adolescents that consultation is probably in order when a possible example is encountered in a patient this young. The extremities are the favored site and more than two thirds develop in the legs, most commonly around the knee and in the thigh. These tumors practically never occur in the hands and feet. Although most are in the deep soft tissues, myxoid chondrosarcoma has been reported to arise in the subcutaneous tissue. Because most are deep, the median size at the time of diagnosis is around 7 cm. As would be expected, patients most often come to the attention of a physician because a mass has been detected. It is twice as common in men as in women.

Pathologic Findings. The lobulation or nodularity of extraskeletal myxoid chondrosarcoma that is a definitional feature microscopically can often be appreciated grossly. On cut surface, the tumor typically appears gelatinous or slimy and areas of hemorrhage are common (9). Low-

power microscopic examination reveals the characteristic division of the tumor into lobules surrounded by fibrous tissue (figs. 10-3, 10-4) (15). The lobules are of variable cellularity and their matrix is myxoid. They tend to be more cellular near the periphery and the constituent cells most often arrange themselves in rows or chains that extend from the periphery toward the center (fig. 10-5) (9,10). Unlike the cells in most other myxoid lesions, the cells in this tumor have discernible cytoplasm and usually are attached to one another, a phenomenon that is important in recognizing this tumor and one we refer to as "cells reaching out to touch one another" (fig. 10-6). Sometimes the tumor cells are arranged in whorls or clusters rather than chains. The constituent cells are usually small, round to stellate, relatively uniform, and have dense chromatin but in a few tumors they are distinctly spindled (fig. 10-7). Intranuclear inclusions are sometimes noted and in about 10 percent of tumors cytoplasmic hyaline

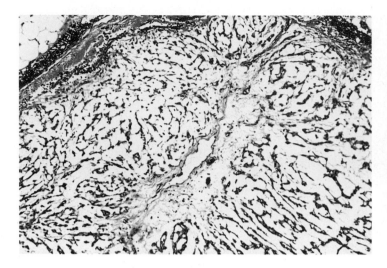

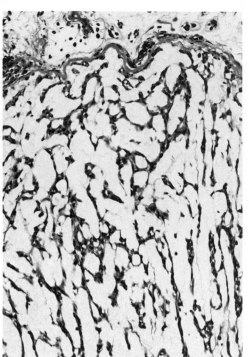

Figure 10-5
MYXOID CHONDROSARCOMA
Characteristically, the tumor cells grow in a linear fashion and seem to hang from the edge of the tumor lobule toward the center.

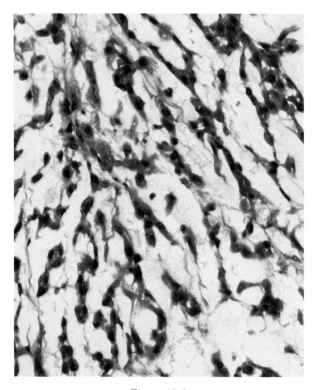

Figure 10-6
MYXOID CHONDROSARCOMA
Unlike most myxoid neoplasms, the cells in myxoid chondrosarcoma often have easily seen eosinophilic cytoplasm and most are in contact with each other.

inclusions, resembling those seen in the cells of rhabdoid tumors, are present (15). Characteristically, the tumor cells have a small amount of easily visible eosinophilic cytoplasm which may be vacuolated. Mitotic figures are usually sparse but can be numerous, particularly in more cellular areas. Some tumors are more cellular and some of these are composed focally of uniform round cells that resemble those of PPNET/Ewing's sarcoma while others contain areas resembling monophasic synovial sarcoma (13). Stainable glycogen is usually present in the tumor cells. Hemorrhage is common while necrosis is usually absent. Hyaline cartilage is rarely present.

The keys to recognizing myxoid chondrosarcoma are: 1) the lobularity; 2) the myxoid stroma; and 3) cells with easily seen cytoplasm that often are arranged in rows and touch each other. A myxoid tumor around the knee or in the thigh should always alert the observer to the possibility of myxoid chondrosarcoma.

Special Studies. A number of investigators have reported acid mucopolysaccharides of the type found in cartilage to be present in the stroma of extraskeletal myxoid chondrosarcoma. For diagnostic purposes, the most useful demonstration of these mucopolysaccharides is their

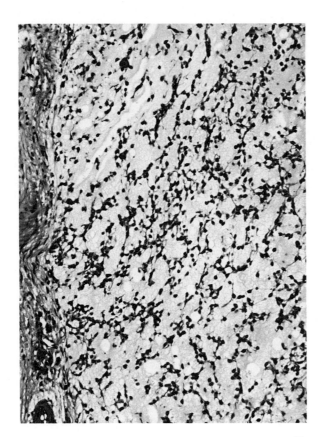 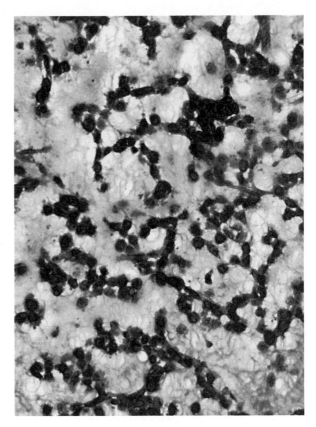

Figure 10-7
MYXOID CHONDROSARCOMA
Characteristically, the small uniform tumor cells, most often with round nuclei, are embedded in a myxoid matrix. Cartilage is rarely found.

staining with Alcian blue or colloidal iron after hyaluronidase predigestion. Although this procedure is advocated by some investigators, we have not found it entirely reliable and usually it is not necessary to make the diagnosis. The critical electrolyte concentration technique to detect cartilaginous acid mucins is seldom if ever used diagnostically.

Wick and associates (20) reported 4 of 5 myxoid chondrosarcomas to be S-100 protein and Leu-7 positive and 3 of 5 to be epithelial membrane antigen (EMA) positive. Meis-Kindblom and associates found that the cells in 38 percent of 48 myxoid chondrosarcomas were S-100 protein positive but the staining was focal and weak while EMA was positive in 3 of the 48 (13). Of the 39 tumors studied by Dei Tos and associates (8) S-100 protein was negative in more than 80 percent (7 of 39 were positive); 6 of 34 were EMA positive, 1 of 37 keratin positive,

and 1 of 30 glial fibrillary acidic protein positive. Thus, S-100 protein staining often is not helpful in diagnosing myxoid chondrosarcoma and the cells may be EMA and keratin positive.

Ultrastructurally, the constituent cells of extraskeletal myxoid are small and embedded in a granular matrix that resembles that of cartilage (18,19). The cells demonstrate features, while not specific, that are characteristic of chondroblasts: abundant rough endoplasmic reticulum often containing granular material, glycogen, intermediate filaments, and lipid droplets (14). Moreover, about a third of myxoid chondrosarcomas are composed of cells with parallel arrays of microtubules within rough endoplasmic reticulum (7,17). These structures, while not absolutely specific, are rarely found in other neoplasms and constitute a very helpful diagnostic feature when the histologic features are consistent with myxoid chondrosarcoma. However, electron microscopy is seldom needed to make the diagnosis. Cytogenetic studies have revealed nonrandom reciprocal translocations involving chromosomes 9 and 22: t(9:22)(q22-31;q11-12)(7, 11,14a,16).

Differential Diagnosis. Myxoid chondrosarcoma figures prominently in the differential diagnosis of soft tissue tumors with a myxoid stroma. A useful first step when faced with a myxoid neoplasm is to determine whether the tumor is one of the three most common malignant myxoid neoplasms, namely, myxoid liposarcoma, myxoid MFH (myxofibrosarcoma), or myxoid chondrosarcoma. Myxoid liposarcomas have a predilection for the same sites on the extremities as myxoid chondrosarcoma, except that only on the rarest occasions do they arise in the subcutaneous tissue. Also, myxoid liposarcoma has a prominent plexiform vascular pattern missing in myxoid chondrosarcoma; the cells, at least in the paucicellular areas are usually not discernibly attached to each other as the cells are in myxoid chondrosarcoma; it typically contains fibrous as well as myxoid areas; and it contains lipoblasts or lipocytes. Myxoid MFH at least focally features larger and more pleomorphic cells than are allowed in the definition of myxoid chondrosarcoma and a lobular pattern is not characteristic. Low-grade fibromyxoid sarcoma lacks the lobularity and characteristic chain-like arrangement of the cells with easily seen cytoplasm that are the hallmark of myxoid chondrosarcoma. Neural lesions often possess a myxoid stroma and all neurofibromas, schwannomas, and about half of malignant peripheral nerve sheath tumors (MPNSTs) are S-100 protein positive. Moreover, neural tumors except for epithelioid MPNST lack the other features of myxoid chondrosarcoma.

Myxoid areas in rhabdomyosarcoma, mixed salivary gland tumors, and sweat gland tumors, particularly chondroid syringoma, can all mimic myxoid chondrosarcoma. In fact, cutaneous mixed tumors may be very similar to myxoid chondrosarcoma by light microscopy when the epithelial component is inconspicuous because the myoepithelial component may be lobulated and the cells may resemble those of myxoid chondrosarcoma. To further confuse matters some myxoid chondrosarcomas contain keratin- and EMA-positive cells, stains that are positive in the epithelial and myoepithelial elements of a mixed tumor. The usually superficial location of mixed tumors should clarify the situation and carcinoembryonic antigen and BRST-2 immunostains may be positive in sweat gland tumors. Essentially all embryonal rhabdomyosarcomas contain desmin-positive cells, while the cells of myxoid chondrosarcoma are desmin negative. Myxomas of the soft tissues, including intramuscular myxoma and juxtacortical myxoma, are even more paucicellular than myxoid chondrosarcoma, have cells that do not touch each other, and do not have a well-formed lobular pattern.

Soft tissue chondromas may have an extensive myxoid stroma and sparse amounts of differentiated cartilage. This differential diagnosis is discussed in the Chondroma section above. Chordomas are uniformly keratin and S-100 protein positive while only a small subset of extraskeletal myxoid chondrosarcomas contain cells that express these markers. The usual locations of chordomas and myxoid chondrosarcomas are quite different and physaliphorous cells are not a feature of myxoid chondrosarcoma. Physaliphorous cells typically contain intracytoplasmic epithelial mucin which can be detected with periodic acid–Schiff (PAS) or mucicarmine stains while the cells of myxoid chondrosarcoma are PAS negative. Parachordoma may contain keratin-positive cells not found in myxoid chondrosarcoma; the stroma is a combination of myxoid and hyaline while that of chondrosarcoma is uniformly myxoid; and the cells are not arranged in a chair-like fashion as they often are in myxoid chondrosarcoma.

Ossifying fibromyxoid tumor often features bone in its capsule and has more vessels than does myxoid chondrosarcoma. Both lesions may contain S-100 protein–positive cells.

Treatment and Prognosis. Extraskeletal myxoid chondrosarcoma is a malignant neoplasm which often follows a prolonged course. Although most patients do well over the short term, about three quarters of the tumors eventually recur locally and metastasize (9,13,15). Recurrences and metastases 10 to 20 years after the tumor has been excised are not unusual. About 75 percent of the patients are alive at 10 years, but some of these will have already experienced recurrence or metastasis. The most common sites of metastasis are the lungs, soft tissues, bone, and lymph nodes. Although high cellularity and a high mitotic index have been found by some to be high risk features, they were not accurate predictors of outcome in the series from M.D. Anderson (15). We are not convinced that histologic features reliably stratify patients into groups with a differing prognosis.

Extraskeletal Mesenchymal Chondrosarcoma

Definition. This rare neoplasm has a biphasic pattern: one population of cells is undifferentiated and reminiscent of the cells that comprise small round blue cell tumors while the other is differentiated as hyaline cartilage.

General Considerations. Although generally considered to be a cartilaginous neoplasm, recent studies have shown that the small noncartilaginous cells in mesenchymal chondrosarcomas are CD99 positive and that at least some have a t(11;22) translocation identical to that found in peripheral primitive neuroendocrine tumor (PPNET)/Ewing's sarcoma (24,27). These findings plus the histologic appearance suggest that mesenchymal chondrosarcoma may be a PPNET/Ewing's sarcoma with focal cartilaginous differentiation but further studies are needed before this concept is accepted.

Clinical Features. Mesenchymal chondrosarcoma has a predilection for the meninges, orbit, neck, spine, and the lower extremities, although it has been reported in a wide variety of other sites (21,22,25,28,29). It occurs at all ages, but the majority develop in individuals in the third and fourth decades (23). Mesenchymal chondrosarcomas in the head and neck often produce symptoms early in their course because of their location, meningeal lesions can cause symptoms of an intracranial mass, and orbital lesions can interfere with vision or produce exophthalmos.

Pathologic Findings. Macroscopically, mesenchymal chondrosarcomas are soft masses which may contain visible or palpable areas of calcium or cartilage. Areas of hemorrhage and necrosis are unusual. Tumors within the cranium and within the head and neck area are usually small when diagnosed because their location causes early symptoms, whereas those in the deep soft tissues frequently grow to large size.

Microscopically, the visual image of the typical mesenchymal chondrosarcoma is that of a sea of

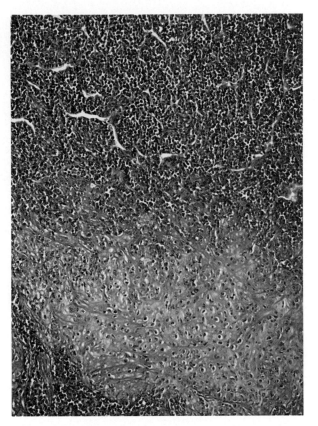

Figure 10-8
MESENCHYMAL CHONDROSARCOMA
Three features that can be discerned at low magnification in most mesenchymal chondrosarcomas are illustrated here: small round basophilic tumor cells, a pericytic vascular pattern, and the presence of cartilage.

small round blue cells dotted by islands of cartilage (fig. 10-8) (23,25,26,28). Often there is a vascular pattern similar to that found in hemangiopericytoma. The undifferentiated small blue cells have round to elongate or even spindled nuclei, with coarse granular chromatin and scant, indistinct cytoplasm (fig. 10-9). Glycogen is variably present. The undifferentiated cells may grow in sheets or nodules surrounded by fibrous tissue, but often they proliferate around narrow, slit-like vessels as well as staghorn-shaped ("pericytic") sinusoidal vessels (figs. 10-8, 10-9C). In some tumors the required cartilage is abundant, but in others it is sparse and many sections may be needed to find it. We do not accept a "chondroid" matrix as evidence of cartilaginous differentiation unless it has the appearance of hyaline cartilage and the cells lie within lacunae (fig. 10-10). The cartilage may become

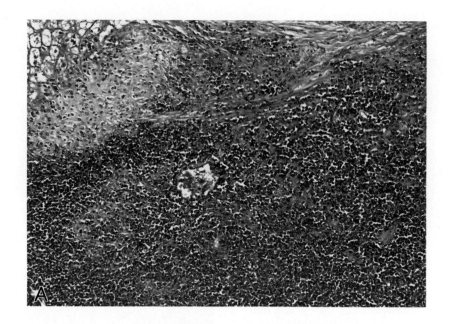

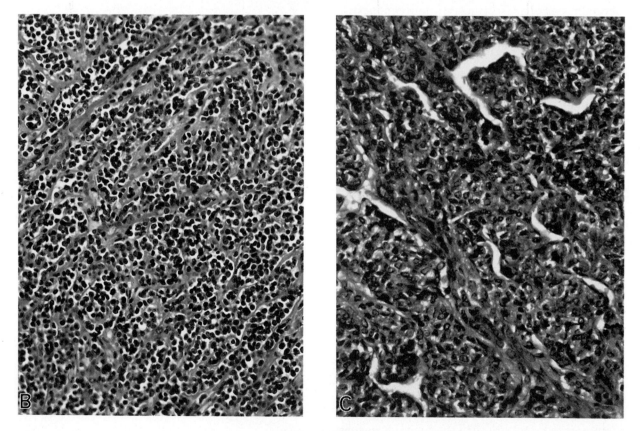

Figure 10-9
MESENCHYMAL CHONDROSARCOMA

The small round blue cells that compose mesenchymal chondrosarcoma blend into cartilage (A) and resemble cells of other small round blue cell tumors (B). They are often associated with a pericytic vascular pattern (C).

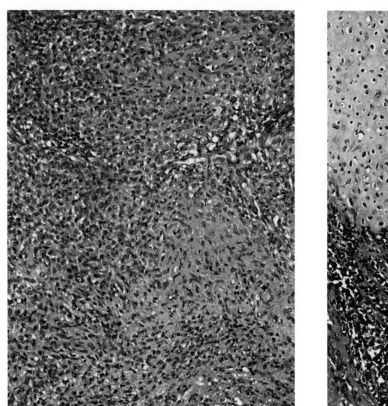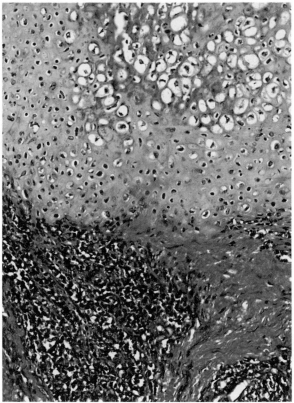

Figure 10-10

MESENCHYMAL CHONDROSARCOMA

Left: "Chondroid" areas are common in mesenchymal chondrosarcomas but also in other small round blue cell tumors.
Right: The presence of well-differentiated cartilage identifies mesenchymal chondrosarcoma.

calcified or ossified. Mitotic figures can usually be found but are not usually numerous or abnormal. Necrosis and hemorrhage are usually absent or inconspicuous.

Special Studies. The cartilaginous cells usually stain for S-100 protein (6 of 9 cases in one study [30]) and both the small undifferentiated cells and the cartilaginous cells are positive for CD57 in about two thirds of the cases (30). We have found that small cells in almost all mesenchymal chondrosarcomas are also positive for CD99 (24). Most importantly for differential diagnostic purposes, the tumor cells are almost always negative for desmin, CD45, chromogranin, keratin, EMA, and actin (see Differential Diagnosis below). Electron microscopy confirms what can be seen by light microscopy, that the tumor is composed of cartilaginous and undifferentiated cells. A mesenchymal chondrosarcoma in a child has been reported to have a t(11;22)

translocation identical to that found in PPNET/Ewing's sarcoma (see General Considerations above) (27).

Differential Diagnosis. Because the undifferentiated cells in mesenchymal chondrosarcoma resemble those found in small round blue cell tumors, all of the latter enter into the differential diagnosis. When cartilage is encountered, the diagnosis should be straightforward, but in situations where a biopsy does not contain cartilage, immunohistochemistry can be useful. Desmin is absent in mesenchymal chondrosarcoma and but present in practically all embryonal rhabdomyosarcomas. Essentially all of the tumors in the PPNET/Ewing's category are CD99 positive, as are mesenchymal chondrosarcomas. Thus, the only distinguishing features between the two by light microscopy are cartilaginous differentiation and a hemangiopericytoma-like vascular pattern in mesenchymal chondrosarcoma. Neuroblastoma usually occurs at a younger age and is associated with catecholamine production; lymphomas are positive for CD15 or other lymphoid markers.

The staghorn vascular pattern found in most mesenchymal chondrosarcomas should raise concern about other tumors that feature such vessels. These include hemangiopericytoma, synovial sarcoma, and fibrous histiocytoma. The presence of cartilage should clarify the situation, except that cartilaginous metaplasia can occur in synovial sarcoma. In doubtful cases, keratin and EMA stains may help identify synovial sarcoma and the cells in monophasic synovial sarcoma tend to be more elongate and organized into fascicles compared to those in mesenchymal chondrosarcoma. Both synovial sarcoma and mesenchymal chondrosarcoma may contain CD99-positive cells. About half of hemangiopericytomas are CD34 positive, a stain not reported to be positive in mesenchymal chondrosarcoma, and the cells are much more fibroblastic. Fibrous histiocytomas are not composed of small round blue cells. Care must be taken to be sure that an apparent soft tissue mesenchymal chondrosarcoma does not in fact represent either a soft tissue extension from a primary bone tumor or a metastasis. Extraskeletal myxoid chondrosarcoma has morphologic features that are quite different from mesenchymal chondrosarcoma (see above).

A difficult diagnostic dilemma is posed by the small round blue cell tumor that does not fit any of the known classifiable categories but could be mesenchymal chondrosarcoma except for the absence of cartilage. We think cartilage should be present before a definitive diagnosis of mesenchymal chondrosarcoma is made, so this implies that a tumor suspected of being mesenchymal chondrosarcoma in which cartilage is not found has been thoroughly and extensively sectioned. In our view it is better to interpret tumors that are otherwise mesenchymal chondrosarcoma but do not have cartilage as malignant undifferentiated small round blue cell tumors unless the CD99 stain is positive, in which case PPNET/Ewing's sarcoma may be considered if the histologic features support that diagnosis.

Treatment and Prognosis. About half of mesenchymal chondrosarcomas metastasize, most often to the lung, from a few months after initial excision up to 20 or more years. The median time to metastasis is about 5 years. The overall survival rate is about 50 percent at 5 years and 25 percent at 10 years (23,25,28). Histologic features and grading do not seem to correlate with outcome.

EXTRASKELETAL OSSEOUS TUMORS

As discussed in the Introduction to this chapter, tumors in this category are required to have, at least focally, a matrix of tumor bone or neoplastic osteoid of the type found in skeletal osseous tumors. Recognizing bone (mineralized collagen) is usually straightforward, but distinguishing lesional bone from metaplastic bone and deciding whether a collagenous matrix qualifies as "tumor osteoid" is subjective, with definitional variation. Our conventions are presented in the Introduction.

BENIGN EXTRASKELETAL OSSEOUS TUMORS (MANAGERIAL GROUPS Ia AND Ib, TABLE 1-10)

This section deals with two benign osseous lesions, myositis ossificans and progressive fibrodysplasia ossificans, a rare familial disorder. The latter has sometimes been referred to as progressive myositis ossificans, a term which can cause confusion with myositis ossificans, a quite different lesion. As a result, we think the term myositis ossificans should be reserved for the reactive process which, in contrast to progressive fibrodysplasia, is a harmless, solitary, nonprogressive lesion. Although myositis ossificans is by definition limited to skeletal muscle, identical or nearly identical reactive processes occur in the periosteum, subcutis, tendons, and fingers. Depending on location, these have been designated as panniculitis ossificans, fasciitis ossificans, parosteal fasciitis, and fibro-osseous pseudotumor of the digits (florid reactive periostitis) (33,38). All of these share the histologic features of myositis ossificans except that a zonal arrangement of osteoid and bone is usually limited to myositis ossificans, and all, including myositis ossificans, are basically forms of nodular fasciitis with an osteoid or bony matrix. Because myositis ossificans is by far the most common and best known of these reactive processes and because the clinical and histologic features of panniculitis ossificans, fasciitis ossificans, and fibro-osseous pseudotumor are essentially similar, all will be discussed in the following section under the heading of myositis ossificans. Parosteal fasciitis is not discussed because it is a skeletal lesion but the discussion also applies to it. Foci of metaplastic bone in the soft tissues, often in areas of inflammation, sometimes referred to as osteomas, are not discussed.

Myositis Ossificans (Including Panniculitis Ossificans, Fasciitis Ossificans, and Fibro-osseous Pseudotumor of the Digits [Florid Reactive Periostitis])

Definition. Myositis ossificans is an intramuscular reactive condition associated with an osseous or osteoid matrix, at least focally. The constituent cells resemble those found in nodular fasciitis and granulation tissue or they resemble osteoblasts in a healing fracture. Similar reactive bone-containing lesions outside muscle have received different names: panniculitis ossificans when the lesion occurs in the subcutaneous tissue, fibro-osseous pseudotumor of the digits when it is in the fingers, and fasciitis ossificans for those developing elsewhere in the soft tissues (32,33,38).

Clinical Features. About half the patients with myositis ossificans present with pain and a rapidly growing intramuscular mass following a known episode of trauma; the other half have no history of trauma and sometimes no pain, only a mass (31). Myositis ossificans affects all ages, but the majority develop in individuals under the age of 35. It is very rare in children. Over three fourths of the lesions occur in the muscles of the arms and legs. Panniculitis ossificans definitionally presents as a mass in the subcutaneous tissue, sometimes with a history of trauma; the same lesion is labeled as fasciitis ossificans elsewhere in the soft tissues. Patients with fibro-osseous pseudotumor of the digits come to a physician because they detect a rapidly enlarging nodule, sometimes painful, in a digit, most commonly the index finger, less commonly the other fingers or the toes. The lesions may be attached to the periosteum or free in the soft tissue.

Radiographically, fully developed myositis ossificans is usually distinctive on plain films, and radiologists are frequently able to make the correct diagnosis and avoid biopsy. Therefore, radiographic consultation is a key part of the diagnostic process and if preoperative films were taken, pathologists should not make a diagnosis of myositis ossificans until they are aware of the radiographic findings. The pattern of calcification that makes myositis ossificans radiographically distinctive occurs 3 to 6 weeks after the trauma; X rays taken before that time are usually nonspecific (34). Imaging studies reveal soft tissue masses that almost always are calcified (35).

Pathologic Findings. Like most reactive lesions, myositis ossificans is rarely larger than 6 cm and most lesions are in the 3 to 5 cm range. On cut section, calcified examples are gritty. The center of the lesion is often red and myxoid or cystic, and it becomes more yellow to white toward the periphery. Microscopically, myositis ossificans is famous for its "zonation" phenomenon, in which the center of the lesion lacks bone and has an appearance essentially of nodular fasciitis, while in the middle zone the cells form trabecular osteoid which in the outer zone calcifies and becomes bone (fig. 10-11) (31). In actuality, we have found the zonation phenomenon to be of limited diagnostic use because not infrequently the zones are poorly demarcated and the specimens may be fragmented and difficult to orient. However, when present and identifiable, it can be useful because sarcomas associated with bone formation, the most important consideration in the differential diagnosis, may not display a zonal phenomenon, or if they do, bone tends to be in the center of the mass rather than at the periphery ("reverse zonation").

The constituent cells of myositis ossificans are the most important key to the diagnosis. In areas away from osteoid and bone formation, they are essentially the same cells that populate nodular fasciitis (fig. 10-12). While their nuclei may be larger than those of the usual fibroblasts, their chromatin is usually fine and evenly distributed, nucleoli are small and regular, and pleomorphism if present is not marked. Cells rimming the osteoid and bone take on the features of the osteoblasts seen in healing fractures and thus can have denser chromatin and more prominent nucleoli, but are essentially uniform (fig. 10-13). Mitotic figures may be numerous but are not abnormal. Arborizing vessels, inflammatory cells, fibrin, and

409

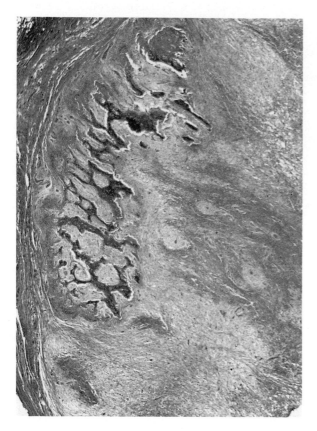 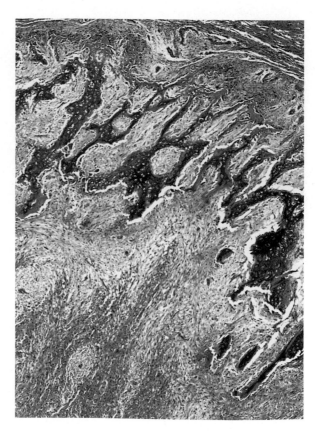

Figure 10-11
MYOSITIS OSSIFICANS

The famous zonation phenomenon, whereby mature bone is at the periphery of the lesion, fibrous tissue resembling nodular fasciitis is in the center, and osteoid is in between, is illustrated.

multinucleated giant cells, usually of the osteo-clastic type, are all common and there may be damaged skeletal muscle at the periphery.

The osteoid and bone are very similar to those seen in a fracture callus. Areas where early osteoid is present are marked by hypercellularity, eosino-philic matrix with the features of osteoid (see Introduction), and eventually, rimming of oste-oid trabeculae by lesional cells (fig. 10-13). The osteoid tends to be laid down in broad trabeculae. Variable numbers of the osteoid trabeculae un-dergo mineralization, usually most prominently at the periphery, and lamellar bone may be seen in some lesions. Early lesions contain little bone, but as the lesion matures more and more bone is formed, and when the lesion is mainly osseous the center may have a dense collagenous stroma containing mature fibrocytes (fig. 10-14). In some longstanding lesions the center may un-dergo cystic degeneration resulting in an appear-ance that sometimes mimics aneurysmal bone cyst (37). Cartilage is present in some lesions.

The features, then, that best help identify myositis ossificans are: 1) a cellular pattern in the non–bone-forming areas that resembles nod-ular fasciitis or granulation tissue, 2) cellular uniformity although the nuclei may be enlarged, 3) normal mitotic figures, and 4) zonal layers of osteoid and bone rimmed by osteoblasts. In ad-dition, the radiographic features are usually dis-tinctive and the patients are most often younger than those with soft tissue osteosarcoma (34). Immunohistochemistry and electron microscopy are not needed to make the diagnosis.

Panniculitis ossificans, fasciitis ossificans, and fibro-osseous pseudotumor of the digits are histo-logically identical to myositis ossificans except that a zonation phenomenon is usually absent and bone and osteoid are laid down at random in these lesions (32,33,38).

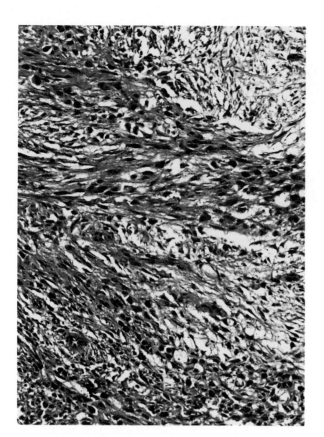 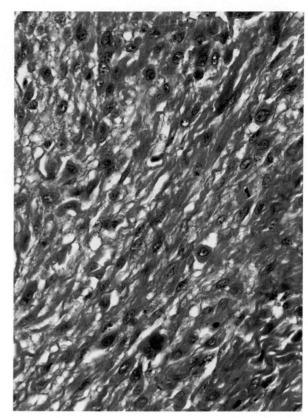

Figure 10-12
MYOSITIS OSSIFICANS
The fibroblastic and myofibroblastic portions of myositis ossificans are composed of cells that closely resemble those that populate nodular fasciitis. Note the nuclear uniformity.

Differential Diagnosis. The most important consideration is distinguishing myositis ossificans and other reactive bone-forming lesions (i.e., panniculitis ossificans, fasciitis ossificans, and fibro-osseous pseudotumor of the digits) from osteosarcoma, either primary in the soft tissue or a skeletal primary extending from the bone or metastatic from another site (36). Soft tissue osteosarcoma is a very rare neoplasm, and it occurs almost exclusively in individuals over 40 to 45 years, an age when these reactive conditions are unusual. Moreover, radiographs of myositis ossificans are often distinctive and help determine that the bone-forming soft tissue lesion being evaluated is not extending from a nearby bone. Armed with information about the age of the patient and the radiographic findings, the pathologist should have a good idea whether a bone-forming intramuscular lesion is likely to be osteosarcoma or not. Histologically, the cells

in osteosarcoma are more pleomorphic than those of myositis ossificans, and typically have nuclei with increased, often grainy chromatin and prominent nucleoli. Abnormal mitotic figures, not present in myositis ossificans and the other bone-forming reactive conditions under discussion, are not unusual and osteosarcoma is usually more cellular than most examples of myositis ossificans. The osteoid and bone in osteosarcoma are usually thinner and more irregular than that seen in reactive processes, and osteosarcoma may demonstrate a "reverse" zonation phenomenon with bone at the center of the mass and infiltrating malignant cells at the periphery, in contrast to myositis ossificans in which bland bone often forms a sharp margin at the periphery. The osteoid, typically broad, and bone in fasciitis ossificans, panniculitis ossificans, and fibro-osseous pseudotumor of the digits are almost always laid down randomly rather

411

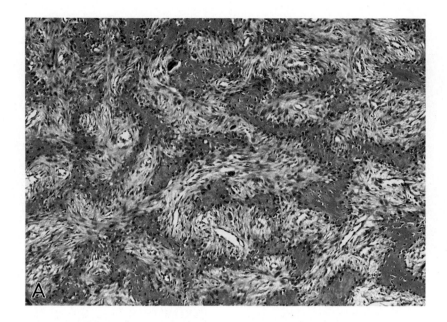

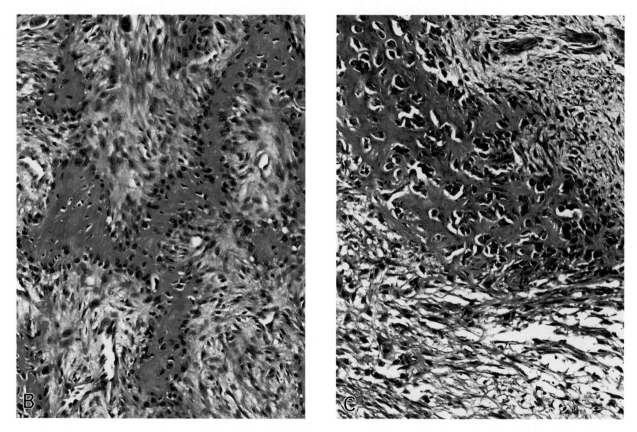

Figure 10-13

MYOSITIS OSSIFICANS

The osteoid in myositis ossificans tends to be broader than that in osteosarcoma (A). The osteoblasts can have large nuclei with prominent nucleoli, but clues to the benign nature of the process are the reactive fibrous areas (B), the relatively uniform pattern of osteoid deposition, and the uniform but often enlarged nuclei (C).

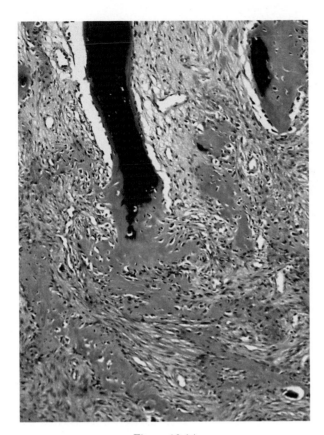

Figure 10-14
MYOSITIS OSSIFICANS
Osteoid undergoing mineralization in myositis ossificans.

than in "zones" but the cells are essentially those found in myositis ossificans and nodular fasciitis. Specifically, significant pleomorphism, abnormal mitotic figures, and cytologically malignant nuclei are absent in these reactive processes (33,38).

Proliferative myositis and proliferative fasciitis rarely may feature foci of bone. Such lesions are identified by the ganglion-like cells that define them. There may be momentary concern whether to label an intramuscular reactive process proliferative myositis or myositis ossificans. This concern is immediately dissipated when it is realized that the distinction makes no difference as long as the process is recognized as reactive. Osteomas consist entirely of mature bone and there may be fat or bone marrow present.

Treatment and Prognosis. Myositis ossificans is benign, and although it may continue to grow if incompletely removed it does not do so aggressively. Because it is benign, because the radiographic features are so distinctive, and because it usually spontaneously regresses over time there is probably no need to remove it if radiographic follow-up is available to be sure destructive growth does not occur. Myositis ossificans does not dedifferentiate to sarcoma.

Fibrodysplasia Ossificans Progressiva

Definition. This is a progressive multifocal disease characterized first by fibrous replacement of tissue and then calcification of the fibrous foci. Bone is often present. The lesion most commonly involves subcutaneous tissue, fat, muscle, and tendons.

General Considerations. This very rare familial disease has also been referred to as *myositis ossificans progressiva,* a label that is to be discouraged because of possible confusion with the reactive, harmless, localized more common lesion, myositis ossificans.

Clinical Findings. Fibrodysplasia ossificans progressiva almost always manifests by age 5 or 6, although rarely, it may first become apparent in older children and even young adults (39,40, 42a). It is transmitted as an autosomal dominant trait (40,41). The first symptoms are the presence of a mass or masses, usually in the upper trunk or head and neck area. As the disease progresses, more and more masses appear, proceeding cranial to caudal and proximal to distal, resulting in distortion of the extremities which causes ambulatory problems, and malformation of the trunk which leads to respiratory difficulties. Commonly, some of the digits are missing, and not infrequently, some of the remaining ones are distorted. This is a useful clue to the diagnosis.

Pathologic Findings. Fibrodysplasia ossificans begins as a fibroblastic proliferation in which a collagenous matrix replaces skeletal muscle and the subcutaneous tissue. This is followed by calcification of the fibrous masses (42). Calcification begins most often in the center of the nodules and is usually followed by bone formation in the calcified areas. The masses become confluent and as they do so they become larger and larger and eventually replace muscle, subcutaneous tissue, and tendons. The initial fibroblastic proliferation is composed of uniform fibroblasts of the type seen in nodular fasciitis set in an edematous stroma. This is followed by

413

the formation of mature collagen upon which calcium is deposited and bone forms.

Differential Diagnosis. Myositis ossificans is a single, intramuscular reactive process and is described above. The age of the patient, the digital abnormalities, and the multiplicity of lesions of fibrodysplasia ossificans serves to distinguish the two and the zonation phenomenon seen in many examples of myositis ossificans is absent in fibrodysplasia ossificans. Abnormal mitotic figures and significant pleomorphism, features of sarcoma, are absent in fibrodysplasia ossificans. During the early stages of fibrodysplasia, distinction from fibromatosis may be difficult, but the multiple lesions, digital involvement, and eventual calcification should clarify the diagnosis. Other conditions in which soft tissue calcification can occur causing them to be in the differential diagnosis include dermatomyositis, multiple areas of trauma, and pseudohypoparathyroidism.

Treatment and Prognosis. Most patients die of this poorly understood disorder within 10 to 20 years of diagnosis, usually as a result of compromise of respiratory function secondary to thoracic immobilization. There is no known effective therapy (42a).

MALIGNANT EXTRASKELETAL OSSEOUS LESIONS (MANAGERIAL GROUP III, TABLE 1-10)

Osteosarcoma of the Soft Tissues

Definition. Osteosarcoma is a malignant soft tissue tumor in which the constituent cells form osteoid or bone (and sometimes cartilage) but no other differentiated tissue except fibrous tissue or a fibrohistiocytic stroma.

General Considerations. Osteosarcoma of the soft tissues is distinctly rare and hardly ever occurs in individuals under the age of 40 to 45 years. An osteosarcoma in the soft tissue of a young patient is much more likely to be an extension from a nearby bone or a metastasis than a primary in the soft tissue. Even in older individuals, a sarcoma containing bone may well represent another type of neoplasm with metaplastic bone. "Tumor" or "malignant" osteoid is accepted as evidence of bony differentiation in soft tissue sarcomas as it is for intraosseous ones, so the problem of distinguishing tumor osteoid from

collagen is as difficult for soft tissue tumors as it is for skeletal tumors. Our conventions for accepting a matrix as tumor osteoid or tumor bone are presented in the Introduction to this chapter. Preliminary studies suggest that antibodies raised against two bone proteins, osteocalcin and osteonectin, may identify tumor cells differentiated as osteocytes or osteoblasts (47,48). Further studies are needed to confirm the initial observations and to determine sensitivity and specificity based on a larger number of cases.

Clinical Features. As noted above, osteosarcoma of the soft tissue is mainly a tumor of middle-aged and older individuals and is very rare in children and young adults (43,44,46,49, 51). Patients usually present with a mass, which may be painful, most often in the lower extremity, particularly the thigh (51). The retroperitoneum, the upper extremities, and the pelvis are the next most frequently involved sites and many other sites have been the subject of a small number of case reports. Most soft tissue osteosarcomas are deep-seated, but the neoplasm can develop in the subcutaneous tissue. Osteosarcoma may arise in radiated sites (50). Imaging studies usually reveal a mass with variable amounts of calcification.

Pathologic Findings. On cut section, soft tissue osteosarcomas may be gritty and areas of bone or cartilage can be apparent. Areas of hemorrhage and necrosis are common. Microscopically, the required feature is a sarcoma in which tumor cells produce tumor osteoid or bone as defined in the Introduction (figs. 10-15, 10-16). Almost all soft tissue osteosarcomas have obviously malignant cytologic features and are easy to recognize as high-grade sarcoma, that is, most are composed of cells that display significant pleomorphism, striking increases in the amount and granularity of chromatin, and abnormal mitotic figures (51) In other words, almost all are identical to pleomorphic MFH except for tumor bone formation (44). However, we are aware of a single report of a tumor considered to be an osteosarcoma that was as well differentiated as parosteal osteosarcoma, although the tumor did not recur or metastasize (52).

The amount of tumor osteoid and bone in soft tissue osteosarcoma varies considerably from tumor to tumor and cartilage may be present as well (46). As is the case for osteosarcoma of bone, tumors with both tumor cartilage and tumor

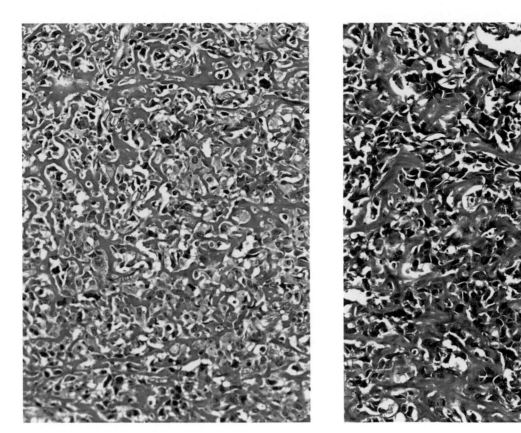

Figure 10-15
OSTEOSARCOMA

As is the case in bone, osteosarcoma arising in the soft tissues is a sarcoma in which some of the tumor cells produce osteoid or bone. Osteoid formed by malignant cells ("malignant osteoid") is most often narrow and laid down in a pattern in which the rows of osteoid are connected as in lace (left and right). It is this pattern of osteoid deposition plus the cytologic features of the cells that allows recognition of osteosarcoma.

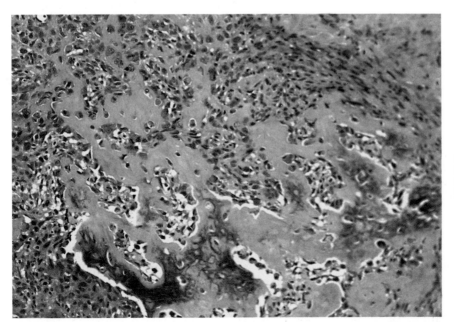

Figure 10-16
OSTEOSARCOMA

In this example of osteosarcoma, the osteoid is thicker but still connected. Mineralization of osteoid often gives bone a purplish hue, as seen at the bottom.

bone are classified as osteosarcoma. Osteosarcomas containing neoplastic cartilage are sometimes classified as *chondroblastic osteosarcoma,* while those composed predominantly of spindled cells resembling the cells in fibrosarcoma may be classified as *fibroblastic osteosarcoma* (43). Giant cells are present in many osteosarcomas, and when they are numerous the term *giant cell–rich osteosarcoma* is sometimes used (46). Telangiectatic osteosarcomas are very rare in the soft tissues, as are small cell types (44). None of these subtypes has therapeutic or prognostic significance, so it is not critical to identify them but it is important to recognize that osteosarcomas may have these variable histologic patterns.

Tumor osteoid and bone, most often laid down in long thin trabeculae with irregular edges, tend to be localized towards the center of the tumor in contrast to the predominance of bone at the periphery of many examples of myositis ossificans. This has been referred to as "reverse" zonation and is sometimes used to help distinguish myositis ossificans from osteosarcoma. This is further discussed in the Differential Diagnosis section of myositis ossificans.

Immunohistochemistry may be useful to exclude mimics of soft tissue osteosarcoma and, as noted in the introductory remarks at the beginning of this chapter and this section, antiosteocalcin and antiosteonectin antibodies may be useful markers for bone cells. Further studies are needed to confirm initial observations (47,48).

Differential Diagnosis. The only benign lesions that are likely in the differential diagnosis are myositis ossificans and its variants: fasciitis ossificans, panniculitis ossificans, parosteal fasciitis, and fibro-osseous pseudotumors of the digits. The features that allow distinction of these lesions and rare examples of proliferative myositis and proliferative fasciitis that contain bone from osteosarcoma are discussed in the Myositis Ossificans section above. Soft tissue osteosarcoma is almost always a tumor of older individuals and an apparent osteosarcoma in a younger individual may well be another lesion, osteosarcoma extending from bone, or a metastatic osteosarcoma.

One diagnostic dilemma that arises is whether an obvious high-grade sarcoma is osteosarcoma or another type of sarcoma with metaplastic bone. Metaplastic bone is usually focal, at the periphery of the tumor, and must be formed by bland cells. It frequently lacks the trabecular or lacelike pattern typical of tumor osteoid and tumor bone. Another situation that may be encountered is a pleomorphic high-grade sarcoma that is undifferentiated or qualifies as a pleomorphic MFH except that focally the tumor cells form a substance that is suspicious for tumor osteoid. Our convention is to require unequivocal evidence of tumor osteoid, as defined in the Introduction, before classifying the tumor as osteosarcoma. Even if unequivocal tumor osteoid or bone is present some investigators have based classification on whether tumor osteoid or bone is focal and sparse (not osteosarcoma) or abundant and diffuse (osteosarcoma), while others have decided that any amount of matrix they accept as tumor osteoid qualifies the tumor as an osteosarcoma (43,46). Dorfman and associates (45) have taken the position that if the tumor bone and osteoid are in fibrous septa, they define the tumor as MFH and if diffuse, osteosarcoma. Obviously, all of these are conventions and it makes no practical difference whether such tumors are interpreted as undifferentiated sarcoma, pleomorphic MFH, or osteosarcoma. For the sake of uniformity, we suggest that if the tumor cells are producing unequivocal osteoid or bone, irrespective of amount or location, it should be classified as osteosarcoma, and if the osteoid is doubtful, it should be diagnosed as pleomorphic MFH or undifferentiated sarcoma.

A more important decision, however, is whether an osteosarcoma apparently primary in the soft tissues is in fact extending from a bone or is a metastasis. This is particularly important when the lesion has features that would qualify it as one of the types of skeletal osteosarcoma that arise on the surface of bone. Imaging studies should always be performed before accepting any bone-forming sarcoma as primary in the soft tissues. The dedifferentiated component of dedifferentiated liposarcoma occasionally has the histologic features of osteosarcoma.

Treatment and Prognosis. The short-term outlook at 2 to 3 years for patients with soft tissue osteosarcoma is similar to that for any high-grade sarcoma, that is, about 50 percent of the tumors recur and 50 percent metastasize, often after recurrence (44,46,51). At 5 years less than 30 percent of the patients are alive. The most common sites of metastasis are lungs, lymph nodes, bone, and soft tissue. In the M.D. Anderson series (44), all survivors had tumors less than 5 cm in diameter, and histologic features, including the subtype of the osteosarcoma, did not affect outcome. In the Mayo Clinic series (51) size was not a significant predictor of outcome.

REFERENCES

Chondroma

1. Bauer TW, Dorfman HD, Latham J. Periosteal chondroma. A clinicopathologic study of 23 cases. Am J Surg Pathol 1982;6:631–7.
2. Chung EB, Enzinger FM. Chondroma of soft parts. Cancer 1978;41:1414–24.
3. Dahlin DC, Salvador AH. Cartilaginous tumors of the soft tissues of the hands and feet. Mayo Clin Proc 1974;49:721–6.
4. De Benedetti MJ, Schwinn CP. Tenosynovial chondromatosis in the hand. J Bone Joint Surg [Am] 1979;61:898–903.
4a. Fechner RE, Mills SE. Tumors of the bones and joints. Atlas of Tumor Pathology. Fascicle 8, 3rd Series. Washington, D.C.: Armed Forces Insitute of Pathology, 1993.
5. Wong L, Dellon AL. Soft tissue chondroma presenting as a painful finger: diagnosis by magnetic resonance imaging. Ann Plast Surg 1992;28:304–6.
6. Zlatkin MB, Lander PH, Begin LR, Hadjipavlou A. Soft-tissue chondromas. Am J Roentgenol 1985;144:1263–7.

Myxoid Chondrosarcoma

7. Antonescu CR, Argani P, Erlandson RA, Healey JH, Ladanyi M, Huvos AG. Skeletal and extraskeletal myxoid chondrosarcoma: a comparative clinicopathologic, ultrastructural, and molecular study. Cancer 1998;83:1504–21.
8. Dei Tos AP, Wadden C, Fletcher CD. Extraskeletal myxoid chondrosarcoma: an immunohistochemical reappraisal of 39 cases. App Immuno 1997;5:73–7.
9. Enzinger FM, Shiraki M. Extraskeletal myxoid chondrosarcoma. An analysis of 34 cases. Hum Pathol 1972;3:421–35.
10. Fletcher CD, Powell G, McKee PH. Extraskeletal myxoid chondrosarcoma: a histochemical and immunohistochemical study. Histopathology 1986;10:489–99.
11. Hinrichs SH, Jaramillo MA, Gumerlock PH, Gardner MB, Lewis JP, Freeman AE. Myxoid chondrosarcoma with a translocation involving chromosomes 9 and 22. Cancer Genet Cytogenet 1985;14:219–26.
12. Martin RF, Melnick PJ, Warner NE, Terry R, Bullock WK, Schwinn CP. Chordoid sarcoma. Am J Clin Pathol 1973;59:623–35.
13. Meis-Kindblom JM, Bergh P, Gunterberg B, Kindblom LG. Extraskeletal myxoid chondrosarcoma: a reappraisal of its morphologic spectrum and prognostic factors based on 117 cases. Am Surg Pathol 1999;23:636–50.
14. Povysil C, Matejovsky Z. A comparative ultrastructural study of chondrosarcoma, chordoid sarcoma, chordoma and chordoma perifericum. Pathol Res Pract 1985;179:546–59.
14a. Rao UN, Surti U, Hoffner L, et al. Extraskeletal and skeletal myxoid chondrosarcoma: a multiparameter analysis of three cases including cytogenetic analysis and fluorescence in situ hybridization. Mol Diagn 1996;1:99–107.
15. Saleh G, Evans HL, Ro JY, Ayala AG. Extraskeletal myxoid chondrosarcoma. A clinicopathologic study of ten patients with long-term follow-up. Cancer 1992;70:2827–30.
16. Sciot R, Dal Cin P, Fletcher C, et al. t(9; 22)(q22–31; q11–12) is a consistent marker of extraskeletal myxoid chondrosarcoma: evaluation of three cases. Mod Pathol 1995;8:765–8.
17. Suzuki T, Kaneko H, Kojima K, Takatoh M, Hasebe K. Extraskeletal myxoid chondrosarcoma characterized by microtubular aggregates in the rough endoplasmic reticulum and tubulin immunoreactivity. J Pathol 1988;156:51–7.
18. Tsuneyoshi M, Enjoji M, Iwasaki H, Shinohara N. Extraskeletal myxoid chondrosarcoma–a clinicopathologic and electron microscopic study. Acta Pathol Jpn 1981;31:439–47.
19. Weiss SW. Ultrastructure of the so-called "chordoid sarcoma". Evidence supporting cartilaginous differentiation. Cancer 1976;37:300–6.
20. Wick MR, Burgess JH, Manivel JC. A reassessment of "chordoid sarcoma". Ultrastructural and immunohistochemical comparison with chordoma and skeletal myxoid chondrosarcoma. Mod Pathol 1988;1:433–43.

Extraskeletal Mesenchymal Chondrosarcoma

21. Bagchi M, Husain N, Goel MM, Agrawal PK, Bhatt S. Extraskeletal mesenchymal chondrosarcoma of the orbit. Cancer 1993;72:2224–6.
22. Bloch DM, Bragoli AJ, Collins DN, Batsakis JG. Mesenchymal chondrosarcomas of the head and neck. J Laryngol Otol 1979;93:405–12.
23. Dabska M, Huvos AG. Mesenchymal chondrosarcoma in the young. Virchows Arch [A] 1983;399:89–104.
24. Granter SR, Renshaw AA, Fletcher CD, Bhan AK, Rosenberg AE. CD99 reactivity in mesenchymal chondrosarcoma. Hum Pathol 1996;27:1273–6.

cellularity; limited or absent cytologic atypia; and a variable tendency to recur locally but not to metastasize. In many of these lesions it remains unknown whether they are neoplastic or whether they represent localized reactive or metabolic abnormalities. The best known tumor in this category is intramuscular myxoma. For convenience, angiomyxomas are also included since they differ from the other group members only by their prominent vascularity. Lesions in this group definitionally show only fibroblastic or myofibroblastic differentiation, thus excluding myxoid variants of other mesenchymal neoplasms showing specific differentiation (e.g., myxoid smooth muscle tumors or nerve sheath neoplasms). Myxoid MFH (myxofibrosarcoma) is excluded from this category by its nuclear atypia and cytologic pleomorphism (even if mild) and it is accepted generally that none of the true soft tissue myxomas has metastatic potential. For this reason it is not uncommon for large or somewhat cellular but cytologically bland myxomatous lesions of unclassified type to be termed cellular myxoma or "low-grade myxoid neoplasm with recurrent potential" and some also use the latter designation for myxoid MFH (myxofibrosarcoma) of the lowest grade. We believe that this managerial term, if used carefully, is of practical value in designating the infrequent lesions that fall into this gray area, but we would not encourage its use as an alternative to low-grade myxofibrosarcoma or as a "catch-all" diagnosis. Dermal nerve sheath myxoma is discussed in the Fascicles devoted to non-melanocytic skin tumors and nerve sheath tumors. It is our opinion that the term myxoma should not used in unqualified form (i.e., myxoma, not otherwise specified [NOS]) since this provides no clinically useful information and might conceal a variety of differing biologic potentials. For this reason these lesions should be subclassified when possible.

Intramuscular Myxoma

Definition. Intramuscular myxoma is a hypocellular lesion with a sparse or inconspicuous vasculature, is composed of bland spindle to stellate fibroblasts, and arises in skeletal (voluntary) muscle.

Clinical Features. Intramuscular myxoma is relatively uncommon, with a reported annual incidence of 1 case per million people (7). It affects principally adults, especially those in the fifth to seventh decades, and shows a moderate predilection for females (1–4,6–8). Cases in childhood are exceptionally rare (1). It presents usually as a solitary, slowly growing, painless intramuscular mass; most occur in the thigh or gluteal region, with a much smaller number arising around the upper limb girdle. Average maximum diameter of these tumors is 5 cm and examples which exceed 10 cm are distinctly rare. A small subset of patients (less than 5 percent) may develop multiple lesions; in these cases and in perhaps 5 percent of patients with a solitary lesion, there is associated fibrous dysplasia of the underlying or adjacent bone, most often the femur (4,10). Patients with multiple myxomas generally have polyostotic disease (10). The basis for this interesting association is not understood.

Pathologic Findings. Grossly, intramuscular myxoma is usually round to ovoid, appears deceptively well-circumscribed, and has a pale mucoid or gelatinous cut surface (fig. 11-1) from which thick translucent material may drip. Cystic spaces and fibrous trabeculae are often noted. Necrosis and hemorrhage are absent unless as a result of preceding biopsy.

Microscopically, these are poorly circumscribed, seemingly infiltrative lesions which merge with surrounding skeletal muscle and fascial tissue (fig. 11-2). At low-power magnification they are generally so hypocellular as to appear completely banal. Another notable, diagnostically important feature is the virtual absence (or only very small number) of intralesional blood vessels (fig. 11-3). In addition to this classic pattern, types that are focally more cellular have been recently described (7a). Tumor cells are small, spindle to stellate shaped, with pale indistinct cytoplasm and small somewhat hyperchromatic nuclei in which mitoses are rare (fig. 11-4). Small muciphages with bubbly cytoplasm are usually present. Nuclear atypia or pleomorphism and multinucleate cells are not seen. Especially towards the periphery of the lesion, the hypocellular myxoid tissue may contain strands of fibrocollagenous tissue (fig. 11-5), which appear disrupted or infiltrated; at the margin, the same pattern of infiltration is seen between longitudinally arranged muscle fibers (fig. 11-6).

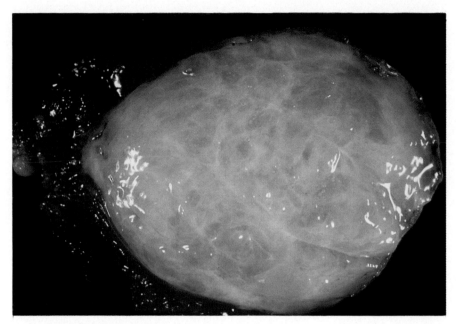

Figure 11-1
INTRAMUSCULAR MYXOMA
A typically well-circumscribed example with a myxoid and trabeculated cut surface.

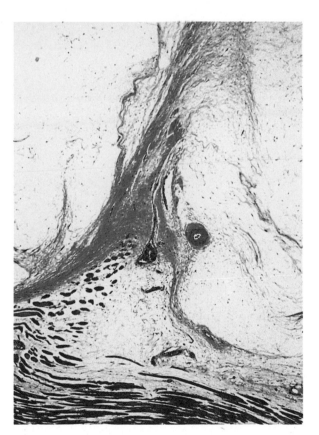

Figure 11-2
INTRAMUSCULAR MYXOMA
Note the poorly defined margin.

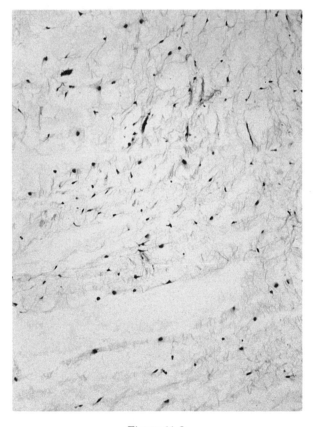

Figure 11-3
INTRAMUSCULAR MYXOMA
Medium-power examination shows the usual bland hypocellularity.

421

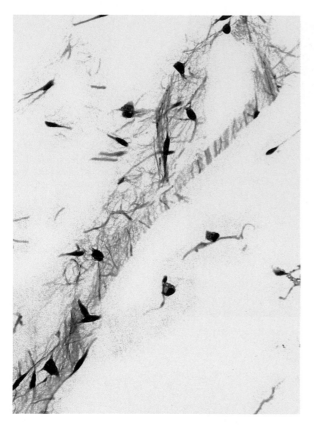

Figure 11-4
INTRAMUSCULAR MYXOMA
Note the uniform small fibroblasts and muciphages.

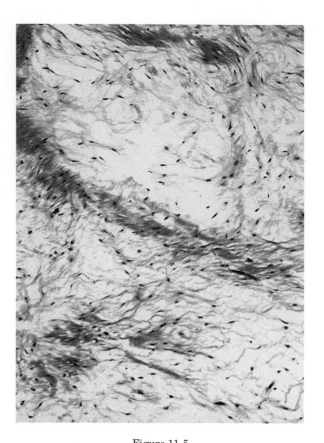

Figure 11-5
INTRAMUSCULAR MYXOMA
Areas, especially toward the periphery, may be somewhat more collagenous.

Figure 11-6
INTRAMUSCULAR MYXOMA
Although the margin appears infiltrative, recurrence is rare.

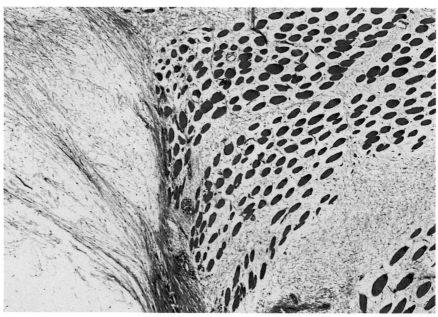

Special Studies. Mucin histochemical stains, including the formerly popular critical electrolyte concentration technique of Alcian blue staining, show, as in most benign myxomas, that the matrix consists of hyaluronic acid (5,9). Immunostaining shows only vimentin positivity, although very rare cells may be weakly actin positive in some cases, in keeping with the nature of myofibroblasts. As one would anticipate, the muciphages stain with histiocyte markers such as CD68. Importantly, staining for S-100 protein is consistently negative. Electron microscopy shows that the lesional cells have fibroblastic or myofibroblastic features.

Differential Diagnosis. Because local recurrence is rare in intramuscular myxomas, careful consideration should be given to the differential diagnosis. Classic examples are so hypocellular that they are easy to recognize. However, more cellular intramuscular myxomas have been reported, and these must be carefully distinguished from myxoid lesions with a greater risk of recurrence, particularly low-grade myxoid MFH. Whenever there is nuclear pleomorphism, and more than a rare mitotic figure, the lesion should be classified as low-grade MFH (myxofibrosarcoma). If hypocellular areas cannot be found, the lesion should not be considered to be an intramuscular myxoma (see Unclassified Bland Myxoid Lesions below). Low-grade myxoid MFH (myxofibrosarcoma) is also more cellular, and the vessels are more numerous, tend to be curvilinear, and are slightly thicker walled; importantly, there is nuclear and cytologic atypia and pleomorphism, even in the lowest grade lesions and these features are not allowed in myxomas, including "cellular" myxomas. Obviously, if the myxoid lesion in question is not within a muscle it is not intramuscular myxoma. Juxta-articular myxoma (see below) is morphologically similar but tends to be somewhat more cellular and is definitionally located outside muscle. Myxoid neurofibroma is usually somewhat more cellular, contains intralesional nerve fibers, and is S-100 protein positive. Myxoid liposarcoma is more cellular and far more vascular, the delicate vessels typically being arranged in an arborizing or arching pattern; small univacuolated or multivacuolated lipoblasts should be evident, especially close to vessels. Myxoid malignant peripheral nerve sheath tumor and myxoid leiomyosarcoma are more cellular, nearly always have at least some fascicular foci, and show immunohistochemical or ultrastructural evidence of specific differentiation.

Treatment and Prognosis. If carefully defined, the local recurrence rate of intramuscular myxoma is very low, probably less than 5 percent. This holds true even for lesions which have been shelled-out or in which there is residual microscopic disease. In one study, none of 38 cases of "cellular" intramuscular myxoma recurred, however, the follow-up time was short (an average of 30 months) (7a). For this reason, simple local excision is adequate treatment. The rare examples which recur are nondestructive.

Juxta-Articular Myxoma

Definition. Juxta-articular myxoma is similar morphologically to intramuscular myxoma (see above) but occurs immediately adjacent to a large joint, often in association with cystic degeneration of the adjacent articular cartilage.

Clinical Features. As implied by the name, juxta-articular myxoma generally arises adjacent to a large joint, with an overwhelming predilection for the knee (11,13). Rare cases affect the shoulder, elbow, or hip. Almost invariably, adults are affected, with a striking male predominance and a peak incidence in the fourth to sixth decades. Most examples measure less than 5 cm and the majority are associated with degenerative changes in the adjacent joint, especially meniscal cysts; probably for this reason, pain is a common symptom (12). Although these features are very suggestive of a reactive process, the tendency for recurrence (see below) suggests otherwise.

Pathologic Findings. In most cases these lesions are morphologically indistinguishable from intramuscular myxoma (see above) other than by their anatomic location (figs. 11-7, 11-8). However, a small proportion of cases show somewhat increased cellularity in the absence of atypia (fig. 11-9). Probably as a consequence of their more exposed and more mobile location, as well as the proximity of an often damaged joint, juxta-articular myxomas more often show foci of inflammation, hemorrhage, or fibrosis than their intramuscular counterparts.

Special Studies. Findings are the same as in intramuscular myxoma (see above).

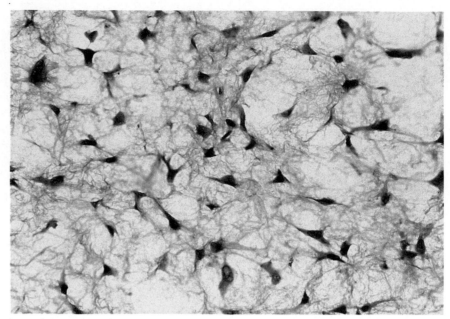

Figure 11-7
JUXTA-ARTICULAR MYXOMA
Pleomorphism is absent in lesional fibroblasts.

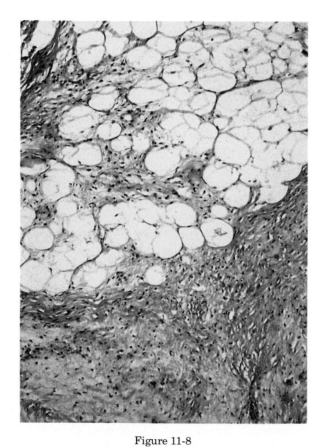

Figure 11-8
JUXTA-ARTICULAR MYXOMA
These lesions often have a poorly defined or infiltrative margin, similar to that in intramuscular myxoma.

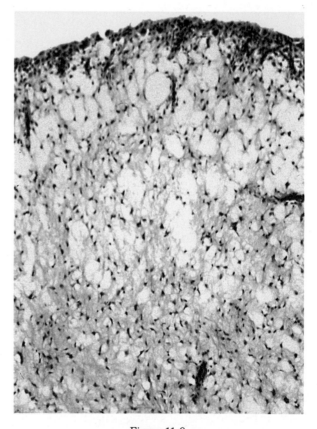

Figure 11-9
JUXTA-ARTICULAR MYXOMA
This lesion, which abuts on synovium (top), shows higher cellularity than is usual in the more common intramuscular lesions.

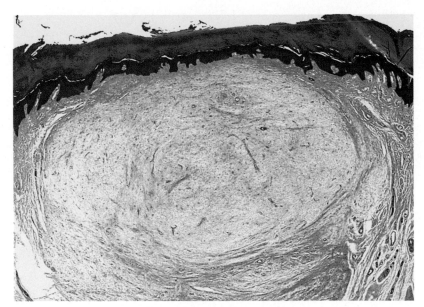

Figure 11-10
DIGITAL MYXOMA
Typical low-power appearance of the dermal nodule.

Differential Diagnosis. The principal lesions which require distinction are discussed under intramuscular myxoma (see above). In more cellular cases, the tumor must be distinguished from a low-grade myxoid MFH (myxofibrosarcoma). The most reliable diagnostic features of the latter are cellular pleomorphism (albeit often mild in low-grade lesions) and more prominent vessels. A ganglion or bursa is distinguished by its more typical clinical location, its usually thick-walled cystic architecture, and its generally lower cellularity.

Treatment and Prognosis. In contrast to intramuscular myxomas, juxta-articular myxomas are reported to have a 30 percent local recurrence rate (13). Recurrences may repeat and appear to infiltrate adjacent tissues. While this published data perhaps may reflect inadvertent inclusion of a small number of low-grade myxofibrosarcomas, it is also possible that the tendency to recur results from the persistence of the putative etiologic factor, i.e., the adjacent degenerative arthropathy. This entity highlights perfectly the difficulty in distinguishing between a reactive or neoplastic pathogenesis.

Digital Myxoma

Definition. Digital myxoma (also known as *digital mucous cyst*) is a dermal lesion usually occurring on the finger, and composed of fibroblasts which elaborate a copious myxoid matrix.

Clinical Features. Digital myxoma affects adults, principally females, and almost exclusively arises as a solitary, often painful nodule, less than 1 cm in diameter, on a finger (14,15). There is no anatomic association with interphalangeal joints. Histologically comparable lesions very rarely affect the skin elsewhere. It has been postulated that digital myxoma may represent a localized counterpart of focal cutaneous mucinosis, but this is unproven and seems unlikely given the predilection of the latter for the head and neck region (15).

Pathologic Findings. Digital myxoma generally forms a deep dermal nodule which, by extending superficially, gives rise to an elevated cutaneous lump (fig. 11-10). The cut surface is gelatinous and may be cystic. Histologic features are similar to those of intramuscular myxoma (see above) (fig. 11-11) but hypercellularity is more common, such that some cases could descriptively be termed digital fibromyxoma (fig. 11-12). The overlying epidermis may be either hyperplastic or atrophic. Infiltration into deeper tissues is not a feature and, superficially, the lesion merges imperceptibly with dermal connective tissue (fig. 11-13). Mitoses are scarce and necrosis is not seen.

Special Studies. Tumor cells show vimentin and variable actin or CD34 positivity by immunohistochemistry. Importantly, S-100 protein is consistently negative.

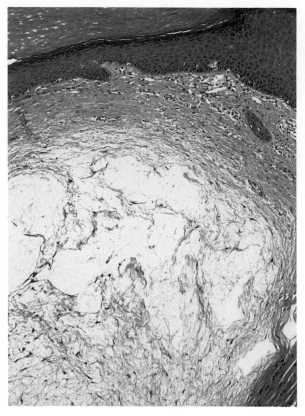

Figure 11-11
DIGITAL MYXOMA
This hypocellular, somewhat cystic lesion resembles intramuscular myxoma.

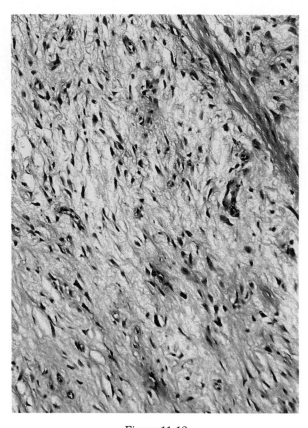

Figure 11-12
DIGITAL MYXOMA
This is a somewhat more cellular and collagenous example. It has also been termed "fibromyxoma."

Differential Diagnosis. The principal differential diagnoses are myxoid neurofibroma, dermal nerve sheath myxoma (neurothekeoma), and low-grade myxoid MFH (myxofibrosarcoma). Myxoid neurofibroma has wavy or buckled nuclei, contains small nerve fibers, and is S-100 protein positive. Dermal nerve sheath myxoma has a lobulated growth pattern, commonly contains scattered epithelioid or multinucleate cells, and is S-100 protein positive. Low-grade myxoid MFH (myxofibrosarcoma) shows cellular pleomorphism and nuclear hyperchromasia and is more vascular.

Treatment and Prognosis. Digital myxomas commonly recur locally, perhaps in more than 30 percent of cases, unless the lesion is excised completely with a narrow margin of normal tissue. Recurrence is neither infiltrative nor destructive.

Aggressive Angiomyxoma

Definition. Aggressive angiomyxoma is a locally infiltrative tumor, usually arising in the pelviperineal soft tissue. It is composed of fibroblasts and myofibroblasts, and numerous, often thick-walled blood vessels in a copious myxoid matrix.

General Considerations. Aggressive angiomyxoma differs from any of the other lesions in this section on myxomas by its propensity for infiltrative growth and recurrence. Although covered in the Fascicle, Tumors of the Cervix, Vagina, and Vulva (21a), it is included here also since it may occur in extragenital tissues and affect males. It seems increasingly likely that aggressive angiomyxoma, at least in most cases, differentiates towards specialized (perhaps unique) genital stroma.

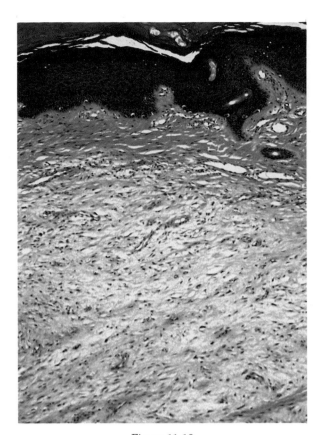

Figure 11-13
DIGITAL MYXOMA
The lesional margin is not sharply defined.

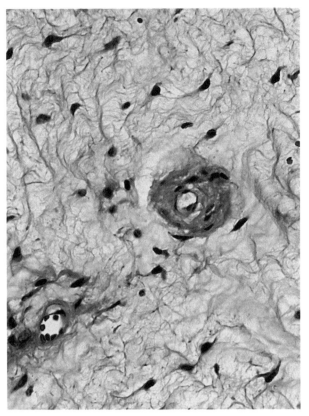

Figure 11-14
AGGRESSIVE ANGIOMYXOMA
The presence of bland spindle to stellate cells with delicate eosinophilic cytoplasm associated with thick-walled vessels is characteristic of aggressive angiomyxoma.

Clinical Features. Aggressive angiomyxoma affects almost exclusively adults in the third to fifth decades, with a very marked predilection for females (16,18,19,23). Perhaps 5 percent of cases occur in males (17,20,24) and examples occurring in prepubertal girls are very rare (25); lesions in postmenopausal women are also uncommon. Most patients present with a relatively large (often greater than 10 cm), slowly growing, painless mass in the pelviperineal region, which may give rise to pressure effects on the adjacent urogenital or anorectal tracts. Exophytic, polypoid growth is rare. In females the mass most often presents in the vulva or perineum, less frequently in the vagina or pelvis, and in males the scrotum or perineum is usually affected. Inguinal lesions occur in either sex. Imaging studies often reveal that the mass is substantially larger, due to deep-seated extension, than is evident by clinical examination alone.

Pathologic Findings. Grossly, aggressive angiomyxoma usually but not always exceeds 10 cm in maximum diameter; occasional cases measure more than 20 cm. Lesions under 5 cm are unusual. Most lesions have a lobulated appearance, often with finger-like extensions into the surrounding tissue, and are composed of gray-pink or tan, rubbery or gelatinous tissue. Precise delineation of macroscopic margins is usually impossible.

Microscopically, tumor cells are small, uniform, spindle to stellate shaped, with poorly defined, palely eosinophilic cytoplasm and bland, often vesicular nuclei (fig. 11-14). These cells are set in a copious myxoid matrix which contains variable numbers of usually rounded, medium-sized to large vessels, the walls of which are often thickened or hyalinized, at least focally (fig. 11-15). Commonly also present in the stroma and often

427

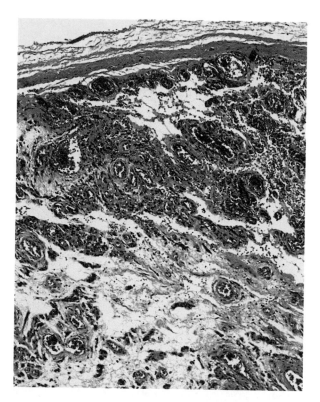

Figure 11-27
ANGIOMYOFIBROBLASTOMA
A fibrous pseudocapsule is characteristic.

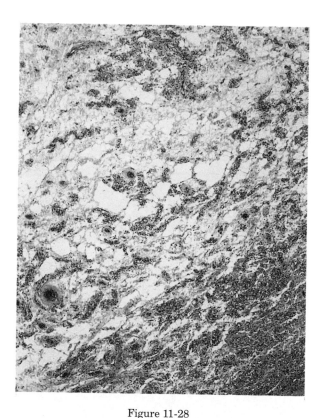

Figure 11-28
ANGIOMYOFIBROBLASTOMA
This photomicrograph demonstrates the typical variation in cellularity.

(see page 427), with which it may be confused. Recognition of this "entity" prompted the discovery of the commonly desmin-positive nature of many vulvovaginal stromal lesions.

Clinical Features. Angiomyofibroblastoma (38,39,41–45,47) affects mainly females between the menarche and menopause, although occasional cases occur in older patients (45,46) and rare examples have been recognized in adult males (38,47). Scrotal tumors with hybrid features of angiomyofibroblastoma and spindle cell lipoma have been reported (44). Most cases present as a slowly growing, painless vulvar mass, with perhaps 10 to 15 percent occurring in the vagina; rare tumors in males have arisen in the scrotum. Most examples are subcutaneous and measure less than 5 cm; although tumors around 10 cm have been described, lesions larger than 5 cm should always prompt very careful diagnostic appraisal. The most common preoperative diagnosis is of a Bartholin's gland cyst.

Pathologic Findings. Grossly, angiomyofibroblastoma is well-circumscribed but not obviously

encapsulated. The cut surface is usually tan to pink, with a soft, homogeneous consistency.

Microscopically, these tumors are well delineated, being bounded by a narrow fibrous pseudocapsule (fig. 11-27). At low-power magnification, angiomyofibroblastoma shows variably hypercellular and hypocellular areas with a prominent vascular pattern throughout (fig. 11-28). The vessels are generally thin-walled and often ectatic, although some may show sclerosis of their walls, and, along with the tumor cells, are set in an abundant, edematous, hypocellular matrix (fig. 11-29). Tumor cells are spindled to round or epithelioid and often appear to be concentrated around vessels. The cells have small amounts of eosinophilic cytoplasm and uniform ovoid nuclei with a variable chromatin pattern and inconspicuous nucleoli (fig. 11-30). Binucleate or multinucleate tumor cells are common (fig. 11-31) and some cells have denser cytoplasm with more hyaline, producing a plasmacytoid appearance. Mitoses are very scarce.

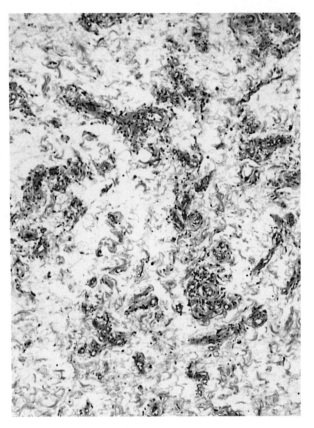

Figure 11-29
ANGIOMYOFIBROBLASTOMA
Vessels typically cuffed by rounded tumor cells are distributed in a loose edematous matrix. This pattern is very common in angiomyofibroblastoma and helps identify it.

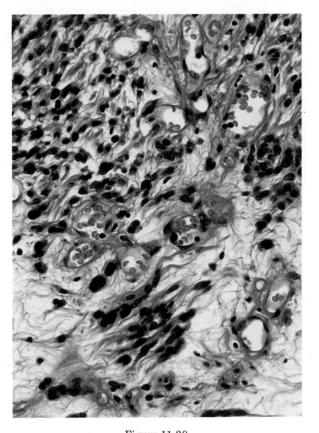

Figure 11-30
ANGIOMYOFIBROBLASTOMA
Tumor cells are round or spindle shaped and have eosinophilic cytoplasm.

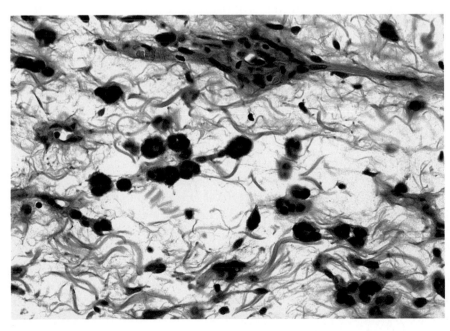

Figure 11-31
ANGIOMYOFIBROBLASTOMA
Multinucleate giant cells are commonly present.

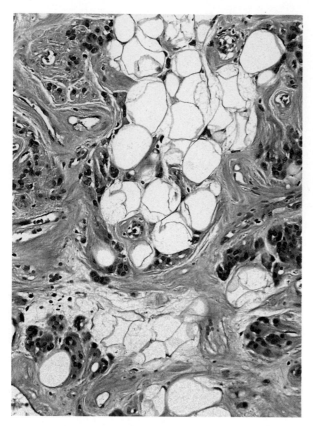

Figure 11-32
ANGIOMYOFIBROBLASTOMA
Some cases contain mature adipocytes.

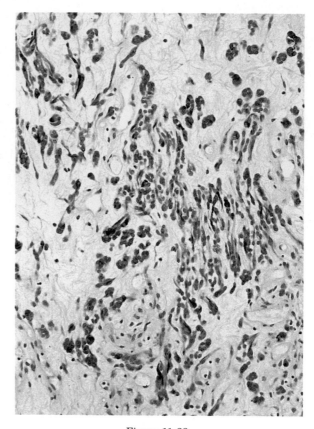

Figure 11-33
ANGIOMYOFIBROBLASTOMA
Desmin immunopositivity is a consistent finding.

Infrequent features include a great number of spindle cell areas (reminiscent of leiomyoma), degenerative nuclear hyperchromasia and atypia (comparable to ancient schwannoma), or looser, hypocellular areas with stellate cells (reminiscent of aggressive angiomyxoma) (40). Entrapment of nerves or glandular tissue is not seen but approximately 10 percent of cases contain intralesional mature adipocytes (fig. 11-32); whether these are truly lesional or entrapped is uncertain (45). Stromal mast cells and perivascular lymphocytes are commonly seen. Thus, angiomyofibroblastoma should be considered whenever a variably cellular mesenchymal lesion with prominent vessels and edematous matrix is encountered in the genital area, especially if plasmacytoid or epithelioid cells are clustered around the vessels.

Special Studies. Tumor cells usually do not contain glycogen nor are they obviously fuchsinophilic on trichrome stains. The hypocellular

matrix contains little or no mucin. Immunohistochemical staining reveals that the majority of tumor cells are strongly desmin positive in effectively all cases (fig. 11-33), while only a minority of cells in occasional cases show positivity for either smooth muscle actin or pan-muscle actin (HHF35) (38,42,45,47). Tumor cells are negative for S-100 protein, keratin, fast myosin, and myoglobin. The few cases examined ultrastructurally have shown fibroblastic features in most cells, with a minority showing myofibroblastic differentiation (38,42,45).

Differential Diagnosis. Differential diagnosis is limited largely to those mesenchymal lesions which occur in vulvovaginal tissue. Aggressive angiomyxoma is poorly circumscribed and infiltrative, is both less cellular and less vascular, and has vessels that tend to have thicker walls, around which smooth muscle bundles may be oriented. It is almost always larger than 5 cm. It should be

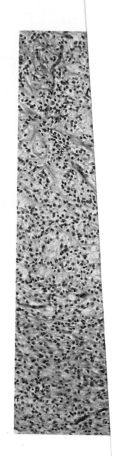

OSSIFYIN

Most lesions are
are numerous.

A small proport
percent, show atyp
tures (50); such cas
if metastatic, *mal*
often takes the for
ripherally, located I
laid down by plum
thus raising the pos
(see Differential Di
ical form is charact
tion but increased
activity in the lobul
11-40). Cytologic ple
be a feature of atypi
notable that recurre
may be morphologic

Special Studies.
glycogen and are ge
(PAS) negative. Immu
veals positivity for S-

acknowledged, however, that rare lesions show hybrid features of angiomyofibroblastoma and angiomyxoma (40). Fibroepithelial stromal polyp is an exophytic, poorly marginated, submucosal lesion which generally has spindle cells and often bizarre stellate or multinucleate cells in the immediately subepithelial zone of the vagina and cervix. Immunohistochemistry does not distinguish angiomyofibroblastoma from either of these entities as all are commonly desmin positive.

Other diagnostic considerations include epithelioid leiomyoma, which is more cellular, generally lacks prominent vessels, and usually is also actin positive; cellular angiofibroma (46), which is much more cellular and is desmin negative; and glomus tumor, which has more uniformly rounded cells, sharp cell membranes, and is rarely as hypocellular.

Treatment and Prognosis. To date, angiomyofibroblastoma has never been recorded to recur locally, even after marginal excision or a shell-out procedure, thus underlining the importance of its distinction from aggressive angiomyxoma. The authors are aware of perhaps one example of a clinically malignant counterpart (40a), although reliable distinction from an epithelioid leiomyosarcoma seems problematic. With regard to those rare cases that overlap morphologically with aggressive angiomyxoma, follow-up data is limited but individual cases have recurred, suggesting that such hybrid lesions are better regarded, and treated, as angiomyxomas.

Ossifying Fibromyxoid Tumor

Definition. Ossifying fibromyxoid tumor (OFMT) is a neoplasm of uncertain differentiation characterized by lobules of monomorphic rounded cells with pale cytoplasm. The lesion is bounded by a fibrous capsule which usually but not always contains metaplastic bone.

General Considerations. OFMT is a recently characterized neoplasm whose direction of differentiation is as yet uncertain, despite fairly reproducible immunohistochemical and ultrastructural features (49). At the present time, the balance of evidence tends somewhat to favor neural crest lineage. Although the majority of cases are entirely benign, a small subset of lesions demonstrate worrisome histologic features

which appear to correlate with increased risk of recurrence and potential for rare metastasis.

Clinical Features. OFMT affects mainly adults, with a peak incidence in the fifth to seventh decades and a slight predominance in males (49, 51–53). Cases before age 20 are uncommon (54a). The usual presentation is as a solitary, slowly growing, subcutaneous painless mass, but up to 20 percent of lesions are subfascial and very rare multicentric examples have been reported (54). Most measure less than 5 cm but tumors greater than 10 cm have been described. Anatomic location is variable and while 60 percent occur the limbs, the remainder are equally divided between the head and neck region and trunk. Some head and neck lesions are submucosal. If preoperative radiographs are available, a peripheral rim of calcification may be evident.

Pathologic Findings. Grossly, OFMT is well circumscribed and encapsulated, and therefore often able to be shelled out. The outer and cut surfaces may be bony hard; the cut surface is generally ovoid and lobulated.

Microscopically, almost all tumors have a relatively thick, hypocellular fibrous capsule, which may extend into the lesion to a variable degree as fibrous septa. Within the capsule and fibrous septa, areas of metaplastic ossification characteristically are present in most cases (fig. 11-34). Inevitably, this is susceptible to sampling error and therefore the absolute reality of nonossifying examples of OFMT is hard to confirm (fig. 11-35). The bone is most often lamellar in type and osteoblastic rimming is absent or inconspicuous. Lobules of tumor may extend beyond the capsule (in a manner reminiscent of salivary mixed tumors) and this may account for recurrence in some cases. Tumor cells are round, ovoid or, less often, spindled and have pale or eosinophilic cytoplasm (fig. 11-36). They have a uniform appearance and vesicular nuclei, sometimes with a small nucleolus. Cellularity is usually moderate (fig. 11-37) and the tumor cells are commonly arranged in intersecting cords and strands within a fibromyxoid matrix (fig. 11-38). This matrix also usually contains prominent thin-walled blood vessels, some of which are often thrombosed. In almost all cases pleomorphism is absent, necrosis is not seen, and mitoses are scarce, averaging less than 1 per 10 high-power fields.

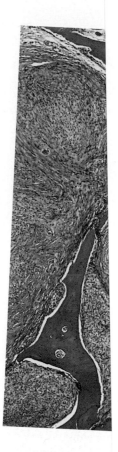

OSSIFYING
Note the lobulated
plastic bone in capsule

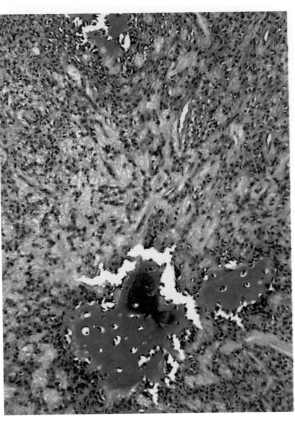

Figure 11-39
ATYPICAL OSSIFYING FIBROMYXOID TUMOR
Note that the osteoid is centrally located and is rimmed by plump tumor cells.

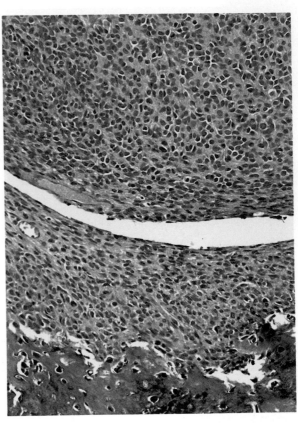

Figure 11-40
ATYPICAL OSSIFYING FIBROMYXOID TUMOR
In this case cellularity is markedly increased.

Figure 11-36
OSSIFYING
FIBROMYXOID TU
These uniform cells wi
vesicular nuclei are a consis
ture of ossifying fibromyxoi

Figure 11-41
OSSIFYING
FIBROMYXOID TUMOR
Most cases show clear-cut S-100 protein immunopositivity.

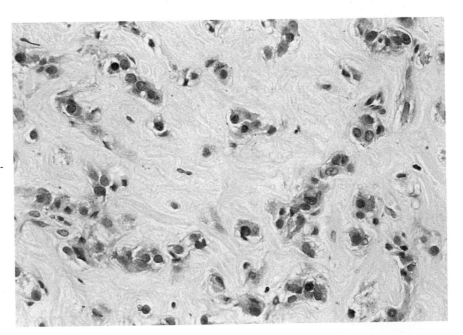

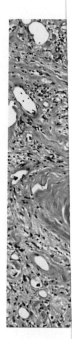

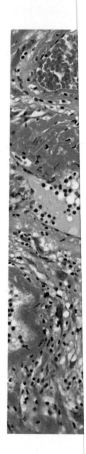

The vessels i
characteristically

with PAS-positive cytoplasm, has generally fewer vessels, and lacks the peripheral rim of ossification. A glomus tumor is excluded by the lack of lobularity, absence of ossification, and negativity of S-100 protein. Atypical OFMTs with central active bone formation are distinguished from osteosarcoma by their otherwise characteristic uniform cytomorphology and lobular growth pattern, S-100 protein positivity and, if needed, ultrastructural findings which are identical to those in benign OFMT.

Treatment and Prognosis. Histologically typical cases have a local recurrence rate of 10 percent, which usually is a consequence of marginal or incomplete excision (49). Such recurrence is occasionally repeated but is nondestructive. The risk of recurrence in atypical OFMT (see above) seems higher, although reported case numbers are limited (50,54a). Two published cases metastasized to lung (50,54a). In most cases complete excision with a narrow margin of normal tissue is adequate treatment.

Parachordoma

Definition. Parachordoma is a benign neoplasm composed of often vacuolated cells of uncertain differentiation, set in a myxoid or eosinophilic hyaline matrix that resembles the notochord.

General Considerations and Clinical Features. This tumor, first described in English by Dabska, occurs in teenagers and adults, usually in the deep soft tissues but occasionally in the subcutis (55). Eleven new cases have recently been reported bringing the total in the literature to less than 50 (56,56a). They are slowly growing tumors and patients often notice a mass years before they seek medical attention. Morphologically, they may resemble mixed tumors of sweat gland type which occasionally occur in the subcutaneous tissue and rarely, even in the deep soft tissues but arguably they lack evidence of myoepithelial differentiation by immunohistochemistry (56a,58).

Pathologic Findings. Grossly and microscopically, the tumor is lobulated and almost always under 5 cm (60). Microscopically, parachordoma features nodules of cells separated by bands of fibrous tissue (fig. 11-42). Most of the cells have vesicular to pyknotic nuclei, often with abundant, often vacuolated cytoplasm, and grow in small clusters or cords set in a prominent

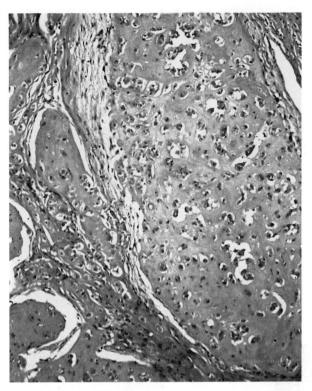

Figure 11-42
PARACHORDOMA
The tumor cells in parachordoma characteristically form lobules surrounded by fibrous tissue.

myxoid or hyaline matrix that can appear "chondroid" (fig. 11-43) (55,57). Spindle cells are seen in some cases. The cytoplasmic margins of the tumor cells are usually sharp and distinct. The overall appearance mimics the notochord and if vacuolated cells resembling physalipherous cells are present parachordoma can appear identical to chordoma (59). Compact nests of spindled cells are also often present. The stroma is Alcian blue positive, a reaction that is abolished by hyaluronidase digestion.

The reported immunohistochemical profile of parachordoma is somewhat inconsistent: all tumors subjected to immunohistochemistry have contained S-100 protein–positive cells and in some, cells are also keratin and EMA positive (56a). Positive staining for S-100 protein and keratin is characteristic of chordoma, suggesting parachordoma is related to chordoma; however, parachordoma occurs in areas where chordoma does not develop and the cytokeratin types are reported to be different in each (56,56a). Cytogenetically, the

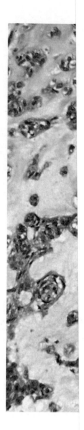

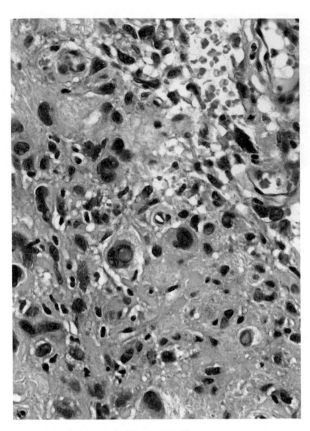

Figure 11-46
PLEOMORPHIC HYALINIZING
ANGIECTATIC TUMOR OF SOFT PARTS (PHAT)
Higher power view shows the pleomorphic cells within a
hyalinized stroma. Intranuclear inclusions are present.

In this tumor th

tumors stud
of chromoso:

Differen
ular pattern
grow in cord
portant con:
drosarcoma
lacks the eos
istic of parac
ent cells. Th
in chains th;
the center (
staining of th
tion. Both le
EMA-, and
myxoid chon
negative. Ch
parachordon
wise these tv
collagen stai
doma but r
syringoma of

Differential Diagnosis. This tumor, with its
hyalinized stroma, ectatic vessels, and pleomorphic cells, most resembles "ancient" schwannoma
but the negative S-100 protein stain eliminates
that consideration. Moreover, Antoni A and B
areas are not present. The pleomorphism suggests MFH but the low cellularity and paucity of
mitotic figures discourage that diagnosis, and
some PHATs are CD34 positive, a result which
is essentially never found in pleomorphic MFH.

Treatment and Prognosis. Four of the eight
patients on whom Weiss and associates (61) were
able to obtain follow-up had recurrences. One
recurrence was uncontrolled and required amputation and another was repeated over many
years. No metastases have been reported.

MALIGNANT NEOPLASMS (MANAGERIAL GROUPS III AND IV, TABLE 1-10)

Peripheral Primitive Neuroectodermal Tumor/Ewing's Sarcoma Family of Tumors

Definition. Tumors of the peripheral primitive neuroectodermal tumor/Ewing's sarcoma
(PPNET/ES) group are malignant neoplasms in
which the constituent cells vary from those with
uniform, small, round, pale, lightly stippled nuclei
and glycogen-rich cytoplasm growing in no specific
pattern to larger cells with more irregular nuclei,
some of which may be arranged in Homer-Wright
rosettes and pseudorosettes. The tumor cells express the *MIC*2 gene recognized by CD99, and
demonstrate several novel reciprocal chromosomal translocations and fusion gene transcripts.

General Considerations. Ewing's sarcoma
of bone and its soft tissue counterpart, extraskeletal Ewing's sarcoma, and peripheral
primitive neuroectodermal tumor of bone and
soft tissue (*peripheral neuroepithelioma; Askin's
tumor*) have until recently been thought to represent separate neoplasms. In the past, bone and
soft tissue tumors featuring sheets of uniform
primitive cells with sparse cytoplasm and
cytoplasmic glycogen were usually classified as
Ewing's sarcoma and extraskeletal Ewing's sarcoma, whereas tumors featuring cells with more
nuclear variability in shape and size, more abundant cytoplasm, variable glycogen content, and
Homer-Wright rosettes and pseudorosettes were
usually classified as peripheral primitive neuroectodermal tumor (PPNET), or if located in the
chest wall as Askin's tumor. However, there is
enough overlap in the light microscopic features
of bony Ewing's sarcoma, bony PPNET, atypical
Ewing's sarcoma of bone, extraskeletal Ewing's
sarcoma, the small cell tumor of thoracopulmonary origin or Askin tumor, and soft tissue PPNET
to suggest that these may not be different neoplasms. These overlapping light microscopic features include cell size and shape, patterns of
growth, the presence of Homer-Wright rosettes
and pseudorosettes, and the presence of cytoplasmic glycogen.

Recent studies also demonstrate overlapping
immunohistologic features and common genetic
abnormalities among these tumors, further supporting the contention they are in fact a single

entity. Among these are the observations that monoclonal antibody CD99 decorates the cells of all these neoplasms whether they have morphologic features which in the past would have caused them to be classified as Ewing's sarcoma or as PPNET (62) and that both of these tumors demonstrate identical chromosomal translocations and fusion gene transcripts. Thus the evidence supports the conclusion that PPNET/ES represents a single morphologic spectrum in which tumors display variable degrees of neuroectodermal differentiation, i.e., tumors designated in the past as PPNET are the most differentiated while those designated as Ewing's sarcoma represent the undifferentiated or most primitive part of the spectrum. Consequently, neural markers such as intermediate neurofilament, S-100 protein, neuron-specific enolase, CD57, synaptophysin, and chromogranin are more commonly positive in tumors featuring Homer-Wright rosettes and demonstrating fine structural evidence of neural differentiation (PPNET), as compared to tumors lacking these light and electron microscopic features (Ewing's sarcoma). A standard label has yet to be agreed upon but we prefer peripheral primitive neuroectodermal tumor/ Ewing's sarcoma (PPNET/ES).

There is another small cell soft tissue sarcoma, the *primitive malignant ectomesenchymoma* or *biphenotypic sarcoma* with myogenic and neural differentiation, which resembles PPNET/ES except that it contains cells demonstrating skeletal muscle differentiation (93). This tumor appears to be a variant of PPNET/ES and so it is discussed in this chapter.

Clinical Features. PPNET/ES occurs at any age but 80 percent are discovered in the second and third decades of life; it is rare after the age of 40 years, and is unusual in patients less than 5 years old. The mean age for patients to develop the tumor is about 14 to 20 years, and there is a slight male predilection. Essentially, the age of the patients and the distribution of lesions is the same for tumors diagnosed in the past as bony or soft tissue Ewing's sarcoma as for those diagnosed as PPNET. PPNET/ES has a predilection for bone and the soft tissues of the lower extremities and thorax but it can develop in any bone or soft tissue site. It also may develop in organs.

Pathologic Findings. Soft tissue PPNET/ ES has a variegated macroscopic appearance (63). It may be lobulated or multinodular, well circumscribed or infiltrative, and tan, yellow, or gray-white. Most are soft and friable with areas of hemorrhagic necrosis. Some lesions are partially cystic. The soft tissue lesions measure between 2 to 40 cm when first recognized, with a mean near 10 cm. An occasional tumor is attached to a peripheral nerve.

As would be expected when a tumor receives several different designations, there is a morphologic continuum that extends from what was formerly classified as Ewing's sarcoma to tumors that were designated as PPNET. Some neoplasms have features of one or the other end of the continuum while others have features of both. This continuum is the same whether the tumor arises in bone, soft tissue, or another organ. At the Ewing's sarcoma end of the spectrum, the tumor cells are arranged in diffuse or lobulated sheets and alveolar, angiomatoid, and fascicular patterns (fig. 11-47). They have uniform compact, round to oval nuclei and a modest amount of pale amphophilic or eosinophilic, sometimes vacuolated cytoplasm (fig. 11-48) (63,88). The nuclei not only are uniform and small but also have smooth outlines; pale, finely stippled chromatin; and small round nucleoli (fig. 11-48). A few tumors contain variable numbers of spindled or polygonal cells. There is little or no intervening intercellular stroma, but the lobules or masses of cells may be separated by fibrovascular septa (fig. 11-47B). Eighty-five to 90 percent of the tumors are composed of cells with abundant cytoplasmic glycogen (79). Mitotic figures are almost always present and vary from 5 to 50 per 10 high-power fields. On rare occasions, metaplastic cartilage or bone is formed.

Those cases reported in the past as "atypical" Ewing's sarcoma of bone and soft tissue contain cells in which the nuclei feature indented outlines, prominent heterochromatin, and small to medium-sized nucleoli (fig. 11-49). The cells are arranged in sheets or lobules as in the classic case, but they form alveolar, angiomatoid (fig. 11-47), and fascicular patterns more often than the cells in classic Ewing's sarcoma (72,89,96). The tumor cells in these atypical tumors less frequently contain glycogen but more frequently form Homer-Wright rosettes and pseudorosettes. The histologic features of atypical Ewing's tumors are essentially those that have been reported for PPNET.

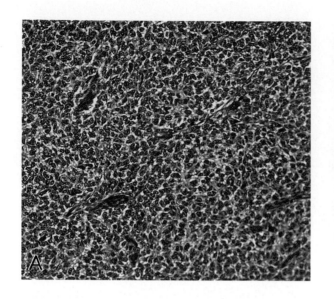

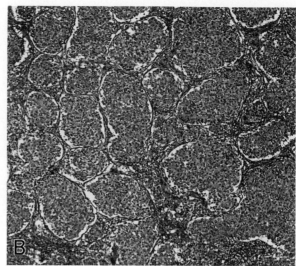

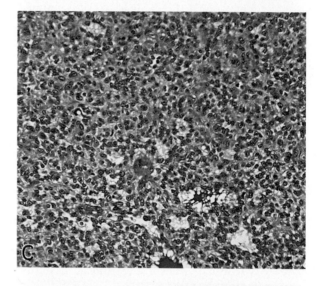

Figure 11-47
PERIPHERAL PRIMITIVE NEUROECTODERMAL
TUMOR/EWING'S SARCOMA
The cells in PPNET/Ewing's sarcoma may be arranged
in diffuse nondescript sheets (A), lobulated masses (B),
alveolar patterns (C), angiomatoid formations (D), or organoid pseudoglandular structures (E).

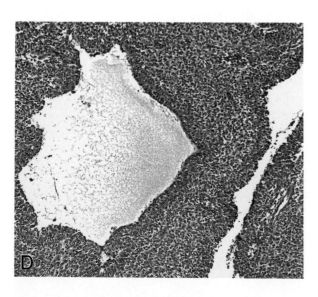

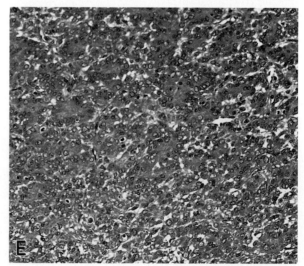

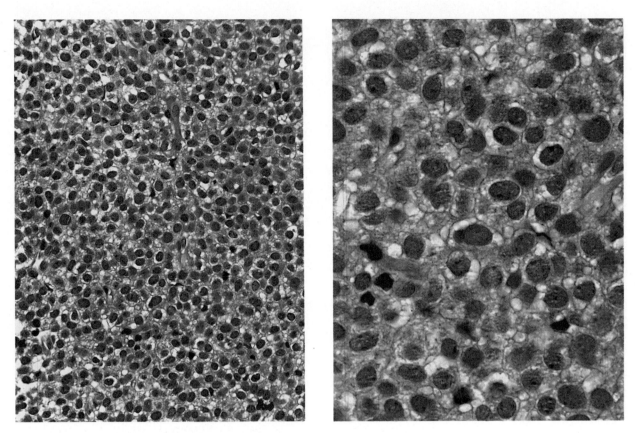

Figure 11-48
PERIPHERAL PRIMITIVE NEUROECTODERMAL TUMOR/EWING'S SARCOMA
At the undifferentiated (Ewing's) end of the PPNET/Ewing's sarcoma spectrum, the cells are compact and have round to oval nuclei and small amounts of amphophilic and sometimes eosinophilic cytoplasm. Nuclear chromatin is finely granular and nucleoli are absent or inconspicuous.

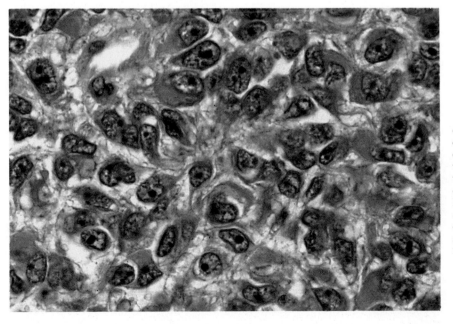

Figure 11-49
PERIPHERAL PRIMITIVE
NEUROECTODERMAL
TUMOR/EWING'S SARCOMA

At the differentiating (PPNET) end of the PPNET/Ewing's sarcoma spectrum, the nuclei are often larger and more atypical than at the less differentiated end; the cells have irregular nuclear outlines and prominent nucleoli. In some cases, there is considerable eosinophilic or amphophilic cytoplasm. The latter findings can suggest the possibility of skeletal muscle or neural differentiation.

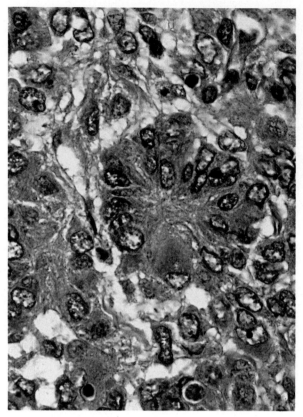

Figure 11-50

PERIPHERAL PRIMITIVE NEUROECTODERMAL
TUMOR/EWING'S SARCOMA

PPNET/Ewing's sarcoma at the differentiated end of the spectrum demonstrates evidence of neural differentiation, including the Homer-Wright rosettes seen here.

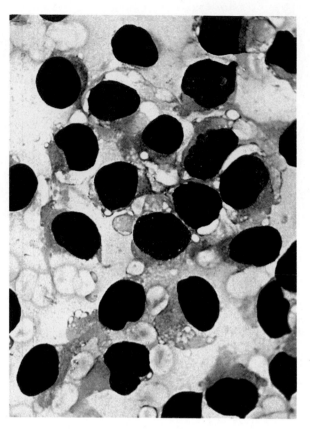

Figure 11-51

PERIPHERAL PRIMITIVE NEUROECTODERMAL
TUMOR/EWING'S SARCOMA

Fine needle aspiration biopsies of PPNET/Ewing's sarcoma at the less differentiated end of the spectrum consist of single and discohesive clusters of very uniform cells having dense fine chromatin and no nucleoli. The cytoplasm is delicate, vacuolated, and amphophilic. These cytologic features are not specific for PPNET/Ewing's sarcoma but immunohistochemical staining may allow diagnosis.

The morphologic feature that marks the PPNET end of this morphologic continuum is neural differentiation, usually in the form of Homer-Wright rosettes and pseudorosettes (figs. 11-47E, 11-50). The tumor cells are small to medium-sized; round, oval, polygonal, and sometimes focally spindled; and grow in formless sheets, interlacing nests, lobules, or alveoli identical to the patterns reported in the atypical Ewing's sarcoma noted above (fig. 11-47) (64,67,68,81,90). They may be densely packed or noncohesive and may contain a considerable amount of eosinophilic cytoplasm, giving them a neural or rhabdoid appearance (fig. 11-49). The Homer-Wright rosette, the cardinal feature of the PPNET part of the continuum, is characterized by a focus of sparse to abundant eosinophilic fibrillary material surrounded by tumor cells (figs. 11-47E, 11-50). Rosettes may be well formed but most

often are ill-defined. In many cases the fibrillary material is attached to a centrally placed blood vessel, and in this case the structure is labeled a pseudorosette. The tumor cell nuclei are usually irregular in size and shape, and have a prominent heterochromatin pattern and small nucleoli; they thus are identical to those described in atypical Ewing's sarcoma (figs. 11-49–11-51). Nearly 80 percent of bony and 50 percent of soft tissue PPNETs contain cytoplasmic glycogen, although the Askin tumor chest wall cases as originally reported were all glycogen negative (64). A brisk mitotic rate, which varies from 2 to 20 or more mitoses per 10 high-power fields, is typical of these lesions. Metaplastic cartilage or bone may be found in the soft tissue PPNET.

PPNET/ES with divergent skeletal muscle differentiation, also known as *primitive malignant ectomesenchymoma,* demonstrates light microscopic, immunohistologic, and molecular features of typical PPNET/ES, but, in addition, there is immunohistologic and sometimes light microscopic evidence of skeletal muscle differentiation. As described by Triche (95), the light microscopic features are suggestive of alveolar rhabdomyosarcoma and consist of poorly differentiated small round cells and clearly identifiable rhabdomyoblasts arranged in solid alveolar nests separated by fibrous septa (93).

Immunohistochemical and Electron Microscopic Findings. The most useful immunohistologic reagent for the diagnosis of PPNET/ES is the monoclonal antibody CD99 (HBA/1, 12E7 and 013) which recognizes a cell surface protein, MIC2, located on the pseudoautosomal region of the X and Y chromosomes. The CD99 antibody is strongly positive in more than 90 percent of cases reported as PPNET (62,86) and in nearly 100 percent of cases reported as Ewing's sarcoma (62, 74,84,86). Whether the negative cases represent other tumors is unknown since most were not examined for either the characteristic translocations or for the fusion gene products found in PPNET/ES. The CD99 antibody typically decorates the cell membrane of each tumor cell (fig. 11-52). However, CD99 is not specific for PPNET/ES and the list of other tumors that may contain CD99-positive cells is growing. Immunohistochemical staining for FLI1 protein is positive in about 70 percent of PPNET/ES but is not specific. It may prove to be a useful adjunct for diagnosis (75a).

The intermediate filament, vimentin, is found in 80 to 90 percent of PPNET/ES (67,69,72,89) but is so ubiquitous as to be of no diagnostic significance. The finding of cytokeratin, recognized by CAM 5.2, in 6 percent of PPNETs and 3 percent of Ewing's sarcomas, may be confusing diagnostically, but only scattered positive cells are found and this finding in conjunction with a positive CD99 should not lead to an erroneous diagnosis. Desmin-positive cells (83,95) have been reported in a few tumors but it is probable that some of these lesions represent PPNET/ES with divergent skeletal muscle differentiation (93,95).

Neural markers show variable results depending upon the degree of neuroectodermal differentiation by light microscopy; tumors classified in the

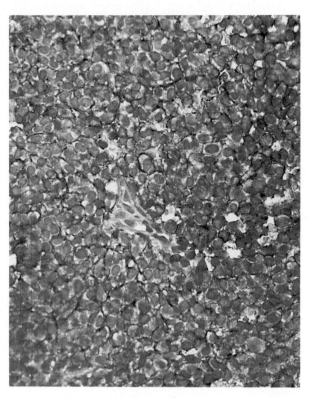

Figure 11-52
PERIPHERAL PRIMITIVE NEUROECTODERMAL TUMOR/EWING'S SARCOMA
Immunohistochemical staining for CD99 demonstrates diffuse membranous staining of the cell surface in PPNET/Ewing's sarcoma.

past as PPNET are more commonly positive than the less differentiated Ewing's sarcoma. Neuron-specific enolase is reported in up to 80 to 90 percent of PPNETs, synaptophysin in 50 percent, CD57 in 40 percent, S-100 protein and chromogranin in 25 percent, and when frozen tissue is available, neurofilament has also been found in nearly 50 percent (67,68,89,90). On the other hand, neuron-specific enolase is reported in 40 to 50 percent of Ewing's sarcomas, synaptophysin in 40 percent, CD57 in 15 percent, S-100 protein in only 2 percent, and chromogranin in 0 percent, and when frozen tissue is available, neurofilament was found in only 5 percent (67–69,89,90).

Because CD99 is positive, by our definition of PPNET/ES, in nearly 100 percent of cases, the other antibodies listed above, as well as the fine structural features listed below, are of limited diagnostic utility and can be viewed as ancillary tests if one is interested in estimating the degree of neuroectodermal differentiation.

Fine structural study also shows a spectrum of features from the less differentiated Ewing's sarcoma to differentiating lesions which were formerly interpreted as PPNET. The less differentiated tumors consist of uniformly round or oval small cells, 8 to 14 μm in diameter (82). The nuclei are round or oval as well, have sparse chromatin, and small to medium-sized nucleoli. Cytoplasmic organelles are scant but glycogen is abundant in more than 90 percent of cases. A few primitive intercellular junctions are evident in most cases. By definition, dense core neurosecretory granules are not present, but a few microtubules and a few blunt dendritic processes may be found, and are perhaps the earliest morphologic sign of differentiation.

The most differentiated tumors containing Homer-Wright rosettes or pseudorosettes usually contain cells with dense core neurosecretory granules and microtubules in the main part of the cell or within dendritic processes. The dense core granules measure between 50 and 200 nm but are usually 100 to 150 nm (81). Interdigitating dendritic processes of varying numbers are found: these may be short and blunt or quite long, extending between adjacent cells (67,81). The cells and nuclei of these more differentiated tumors have irregular shapes, the chromatin is more clumped, and small to medium-sized nucleoli are apparent.

Cytogenetics, Molecular Genetic, and Flow Cytometry Findings. Five unique chromosomal translocations, all involving the *EWS* (Ewing's sarcoma) gene located at band q12 on chromosome 22, have been found in cells composing the PPNET/ES family of tumors. The translocation t(11;22)(q24;q12) occurs in 80 to 90 percent of cases (97), and the translocation t(21;22)(q22;q12) in the majority of the remaining cases (75,92,99). Less frequent translocations are t(7;22)(p22;q12) (73), t(17;22)(q12;q12) (78), and t(2;22)(q33;q12) (85). These rearrangements may be associated with other complex translocations. Southern blot and reverse transcription polymerase chain reaction analyses to detect hybrid transcripts are sensitive and easier to perform than cytogenetic analysis from cell culture which is technically difficult and fails to provide suitable chromosomes for analysis in up to 50 percent of cases (70,80). The chromosomal translocations can also be detected by fluorescence in situ hybridization (FISH) using frozen sections (81a) or formalin-fixed paraffin-imbedded tissue (79a).

The translocations t(11;22) and t(21;22) fuse the *EWS* gene on chromosome 22q12 to the FLI 1 gene (Friend leukemia virus integration 1) on 11q24 (67), or the *ERG* gene on 21q22 (75,92,99). The translocation, t(7;22), fuses *EWS* to the *ETV1* gene (ETS translocation variant) (73) located on chromosome 7 at band p22 (76). The translocation t(17;22), fuses *EWS* to the *E1AF* gene (adenovirus E1A enhancer binding protein) at band q12 on chromosome 17 (78), while the translocation t(2;22) fuses the *EWS* gene to the *FEV* (fifth Ewing's variant) gene at band q33 on chromosome 2 (85). These fusion genes are heterogeneous since several different breakpoints have been described (75). This heterogeneity may prove to be of therapeutic and prognostic importance (98). The "type 1" *EWS-FKI*1 fusion gene appears to be associated with a significantly better prognosis as compared to other *EWS-FLI*1 fusion types (69a,80a). The *EWS/FLI1/ERG/ETV1/E1AF/FEV* fusion genes likely play a role in PPNET/ES oncogenesis since there is evidence that the gene products alter transcriptional activation properties (65).

Less than 5 percent of tumors interpreted as PPNET/ES by light microscopic, electron microscopic, or immunohistologic analysis lack the translocations or fusion genes described above, suggesting that they are not PPNET/ES. However, it is also possible that there are still other undiscovered fusion genes.

The finding of the *EWS/FLI*1 fusion gene product in biphenotypic sarcomas with neural and skeletal muscle differentiation supports the concept that these small cell neoplasms with skeletal muscle differentiation are another variant of the PPNET/ES family (93).

The oncogene c-*myc,* but not n-*myc,* is upregulated in PPNET/ES (62). *EWS-FLI*1 is a transactivator of the c-*myc* promotor which suggests the upregulation is controlled by *EWS-FLI*1 (65).

No difference in outcome has been found between cases differing in the fraction of cells in cell cycle, in combinations of S+G2/M, or between aneuploid and diploid tumors (94).

To summarize, five distinct translocations and fusion genes are found in over 95 percent of cases of PPNET/ES. These findings support the concept of the PPNET/ES family and point to a common progenitor.

Differential Diagnosis. First and foremost in the differential diagnosis of PPNET/ES are the other round blue cell tumors: lymphoma, embryonal and alveolar rhabdomyosarcoma, undifferentiated small round cell sarcoma, and neuroblastoma. All of these tumors, except lymphoblastic lymphoma, are CD99 negative or at most weakly and focally CD99 positive, and they all lack the *EWS-FL1*1 or *EWS-ERG* fission gene product and t(11:22)(q24:q12) translocation. Moreover, there are immunohistologic differences between these tumors that can be exposed by a panel of monoclonal antibodies.

Malignant lymphoma/leukemia may be difficult to separate from a less differentiated PPNET/ES on the basis of hematoxylin and eosin–stained sections, and prominent staining of cell surfaces with CD99 occurs in 50 to 80 percent of cases T-cell leukemias and T-cell lymphoblastic lymphomas (81). However, lymphomas usually lack glycogen and are decorated by common leukocyte antigen (CD45) or other lymphoid/leukemia cell markers which are negative in PPNET/ES.

Sometimes PPNET/ES resembles embryonal rhabdomyosarcoma since the nuclear features can be similar and both contain abundant cytoplasmic glycogen. However, in most embryonal rhabdomyosarcomas the nuclei contain dense smooth chromatin and inconspicuous nucleoli, while the nuclei in tumors in the Ewing's end of the spectrum are paler and more lightly stippled, and small nucleoli are easily seen. When there is doubt, a panel of antibodies is very helpful because desmin and muscle-specific actin are expressed by the cells of essentially all rhabdomyosarcomas, while CD99 is negative or only weakly and focally positive in no more than 10 percent (81,95). Unless there is divergent muscle differentiation, the cells in PPNET/ES are desmin negative.

PPNET/ES with divergent skeletal muscle differentiation (primitive malignant ectomesenchymoma) may be mistaken for alveolar rhabdomyosarcoma because the former not only may feature an alveolar growth pattern, but some cells are desmin and muscle-specific actin positive, and skeletal muscle differentiation is evident at the fine structural level (93,95). However, PPNET/ES with divergent skeletal muscle differ-

entiation is also CD99 positive while the cells in alveolar rhabdomyosarcoma are CD99 negative. Moreover, PPNET/ES with divergent skeletal muscle differentiation demonstrates the translocation t(11;22) or t(21;22) of the PPNET/ES family and lacks the translocation t(1;13) and t(2;13) of alveolar rhabdomyosarcoma.

There is a small number of small round and spindle cell sarcomas, estimated at about 5 percent by the Intergroup Rhabdomyosarcoma Study, that cannot presently be further subclassified (83a). The cells of these tumors are similar to those of PPNET/ES but show no discernible differentiation when examined with current diagnostic modalities.

Neuroblastoma can mimic PPNET/ES histologically; however, neuroblastoma cells do not stain with CD99 (62,84) and the anatomic site and elevated serum catecholamine levels are helpful in identifying neuroblastoma. The nuclei of most neuroblastoma cells are dense and hyperchromatic unlike the more finely stippled nuclei of most PPNET/ES, especially at the Ewing's end of the spectrum.

Depending on the age of the patient and the location of the tumor, Wilms' tumor, desmoplastic small cell tumor, esthesioneuroblastoma, small cell undifferentiated carcinoma, small cell osteosarcoma, and mesenchymal chondrosarcoma enter the differential diagnosis. Metastatic oat cell carcinomas can also mimic PPNET/ES, but the older age of the patient, the presence of nuclear molding, the lack of cytoplasm, the Azzopardi effect, and the diffuse cytokeratin staining, often with a dot-like pattern, allows accurate separation of these two lesions. On the other hand, the cells of 5 to 10 percent of oat cell carcinomas react with CD99. Small cell osteosarcoma, by definition, contains malignant osteoid or bone, but evidence of such differentiation may be focal and if the bone is missed these lesions can easily be mistaken for PPNET/ES. Although the constituent cells of small cell osteosarcoma contain cytoplasmic glycogen they are CD99 negative (62,71). Mesenchymal chondrosarcoma consists of diffuse or lobular collections of small round cells similar at those of PPNET/ES but can be differentiated by the islands of hyaline cartilage which are required for its diagnosis. The cartilaginous cells in mesenchymal chondrosarcoma but not the undifferentiated cells are S-100 protein positive while the undifferentiated cells, in our experience, are CD99 positive. The finding of CD99-positive cells could lead to an erroneous diagnosis if only a small biopsy is available for examination. Wilms' tumor can usually be excluded by location and its constituent cells are usually CD99 negative. However, weak CD99 staining has been reported in about 10 percent of Wilms' tumors. The cells of esthesioneuroblastoma and sinonasal undifferentiated carcinoma are CD99 negative. The cells composing desmoplastic small cell tumor are desmin, cytokeratin, and EMA positive and CD99 negative. Just the opposite profile is found in PPNET/ES, which also lacks a desmoplastic stroma.

Other tumors which may contain CD99-positive cells but which do not have histologic features that would be easily confused with PPNET/ES include islet cell and carcinoid tumors, thymoma and thymic carcinoma, ependymoma, glioblastoma multiforme, leiomyosarcoma, fibrosarcoma, malignant peripheral nerve sheath tumor, synovial sarcoma, and malignant fibrous histiocytoma.

Treatment and Prognosis. The treatment and prognosis for patients with PPNET/ES has dramatically changed over the past 30 years. The combination of surgical excision, irradiation, and multidrug chemotherapy has resulted in a significant improvement in disease-free survival rates for patients without metastasis, although those with metastatic disease still have a dismal prognosis and most such patients are dead of disease within 2 years of presentation (66,67,77,87). The disease-free survival rates for patients with localized disease has improved: 56 to 68 percent 5-year rate for PPNET (66,73,91), 50 to 64 percent for bony Ewing's sarcoma (73,89), and 50 percent for soft tissue Ewing's sarcoma (87).

Desmoplastic Small Cell Tumor

Definition. Desmoplastic small cell tumor (DSCT) is composed of well-defined nests and islands of small cells with scant cytoplasm situated in a prominent desmoplastic stroma. These cells demonstrate multidirectional epithelial, mesenchymal, and neural differentiation, which is reflected by positive desmin, epithelial membrane antigen, keratin, and CD57 staining. They also have a characteristic translocation, t(11;22)(p13;q12), and the fusion gene product *EWS-WT1*.

General Considerations. DSCT is a recently described, highly aggressive malignant neoplasm of young adults. This unusual neoplasm appears to arise from subserosal cells of the peritoneum or pleura which have the capacity for multipotential cellular differentiation. The primary lesions line the peritoneal and, less commonly, the pleural cavities and infiltrate nearby soft tissues and adjacent organs. By light microscopy, the tumor cells have an epithelial appearance which in the past has caused pathologists to diagnose these tumors as malignant mesothelioma, metastatic poorly differentiated carcinoma, neuroendocrine carcinoma, or PPNET. The possibility of this neoplasm is suggested by its light microscopic appearance and clinical presentation, and is confirmed by demonstrating that the tumor cells are desmin, cytokeratin, epithelial membrane antigen, and CD57 positive and CD99 negative.

Clinical Features. Nearly all patients with DSCT present with symptoms related to an abdominal tumor, usually abdominal distention, pain, and a palpable mass. Nausea, vomiting, or constipation due to gastrointestinal obstruction; hematuria, frequency, and dysuria due to bladder or ureteral involvement; ascites; an acute abdomen; and back pain are other symptoms (103,104,108). In several patients the primary site appeared to be the tunica vaginalis (102, 108). Several patients with a pleural primary have presented with shortness of breath, chest pain, and pleural effusion (100,109), and one patient presented with both pleural and peritoneal tumors. The age range is 3 to 48 years with a mean of 22 years. There is a marked preference for males of 5 to 1.

Unfortunately, by the time of laparotomy, most patients have extensive studding of the pelvic and abdominal peritoneal surfaces, and often massive omental, mesenteric, and retroperitoneal involvement. Invasion of the organs comprising the genitourinary and gastrointestinal tracts as well as liver and lymph node metastases may be found at this time or, even more frequently, develop later.

Pathologic Findings. The tumors consist of hard, gray-white, multinodular, bosselated masses attached to the peritoneal or rarely the

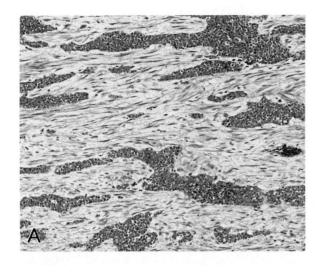

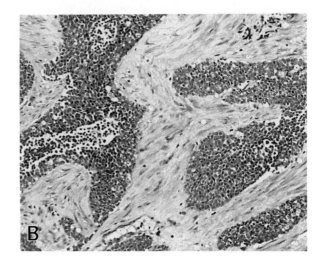

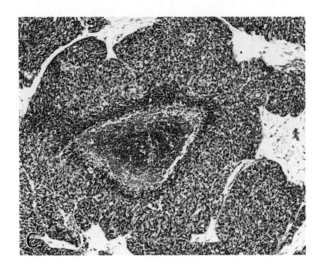

Figure 11-53
DESMOPLASTIC SMALL CELL TUMOR
At low-power magnification, small cell tumor with desmoplastic stroma consists of sharply outlined, large, solid, round to oval and elongate nests and islands or clusters and cords of cells set within a highly desmoplastic stroma. Centrally desquamated cells (B) and coagulative tumor cell necrosis (C) are found in some cases.

pleural surfaces. They often are so extensive that they replace the omentum and mesentery, and often the tumor involves the retroperitoneal soft tissues. Most DSCTs are entirely solid but some are multicystic and have soft, pale yellow areas of necrosis and red-brown areas of hemorrhage. The lesions usually measure from 2 to 15 cm in aggregate. The ovaries measured 38 cm in one case in which they were involved by the DSCT. Some tumors are so massive that debulking procedures produce lesions weighing up to 5 kg.

As seen with low-power microscopy, the tumor characteristically grows as sharply outlined, large, solid, round to elongate nests and islands, or tiny clusters and slender cords of small to medium-sized cells distributed in a highly desmoplastic stroma (fig. 11-53) (104,108). In

some tumors the cells at the periphery of the nests take on a basaloid appearance and grow in a palisading fashion. Loss of cell cohesion or necrosis (fig. 11-53C) may be seen in the center of the nests and islands, imparting an alveolar appearance (fig. 11-53B). Irregular spaces, rarely large enough to be considered cysts (fig. 11-54, left), are found in some tumors and sometimes the tumor cells form tubules with lumens (fig. 11-54, right) which may contain PAS-positive diastase-resistant and mucicarmine-positive substances. The constituent cells are uniform, measuring 15 to 20 µm, and round, oval, or spindled (fig. 11-55). The cytoplasm is scant and may contain glycogen, while cell borders are indistinct. Conforming to the shape of the cells, the nuclei are round or oval and their chromatin

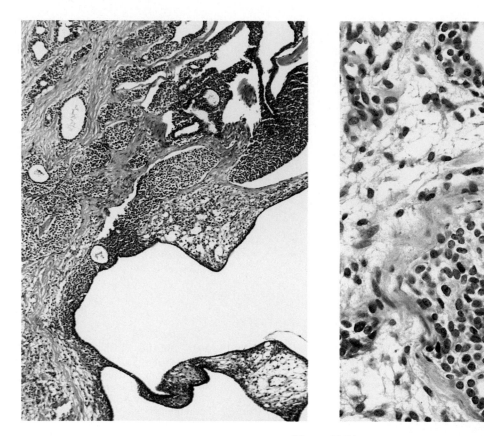

Figure 11-54
DESMOPLASTIC SMALL CELL TUMOR
Irregular cystic spaces are found in some cases of small cell tumor with desmoplastic stroma (left) but, perhaps more commonly, small tubules with lumens are encountered, suggesting the possibility of an epithelial neoplasm (right).

is darkly staining and granular, with inconspicuous nucleoli (fig. 11-55). In some tumors the nuclear contours are irregular and have deep invaginations. Mitotic figures are frequent with up to 30 per 10 high-power fields (103). Focal Homer-Wright rosettes and pseudorosettes; eosinophilic, round cytoplasmic inclusions similar to those seen in rhabdoid cells (fig. 11-55D); prominent spindling (fig. 11-55C); and scattered cells with optically clear cytoplasm and pleomorphic nuclei are additional features which may be encountered (fig. 11-56). Some of these features apparently are induced by chemotherapy.

The abundant desmoplastic stroma, populated by widely spaced spindled cells reminiscent of those found in nodular fasciitis, is the eye-catching feature at low magnification, but the stroma is also often edematous or myxomatous (fig. 11-53A,B). In some cases the stroma is not as abundant (fig. 11-55B). Metastatic lesions are usually recogniz-

able as DSCT because the metastatic deposits retain the prominent desmoplastic stroma.

Immunohistochemical and Electron Microscopic Findings. The immunohistologic profile of this unusual tumor is so consistent that it has become definitional (104,108). Cytokeratin (90 percent) (fig. 11-57, left), desmin (90 percent) (fig. 11-57, right), and EMA (88 percent) are found in the cells of nearly all tumors, and if these stains are not positive, we think the diagnosis of DSCT is in doubt and should not be made without consultation (108). Vimentin is positive in 85 percent of DSCTs, CD15 in 75 percent, and neuron-specific enolase in about 80 percent. Chromogranin-, S-100 protein-, alpha-smooth muscle antigen-, and synaptophysin-positive cells are reported in 10 to 15 percent of the cases and another neural marker, CD57, is found in about half the cases (108). Stains for glial fibrillary acidic protein, neurofilaments, carcinoembryonic

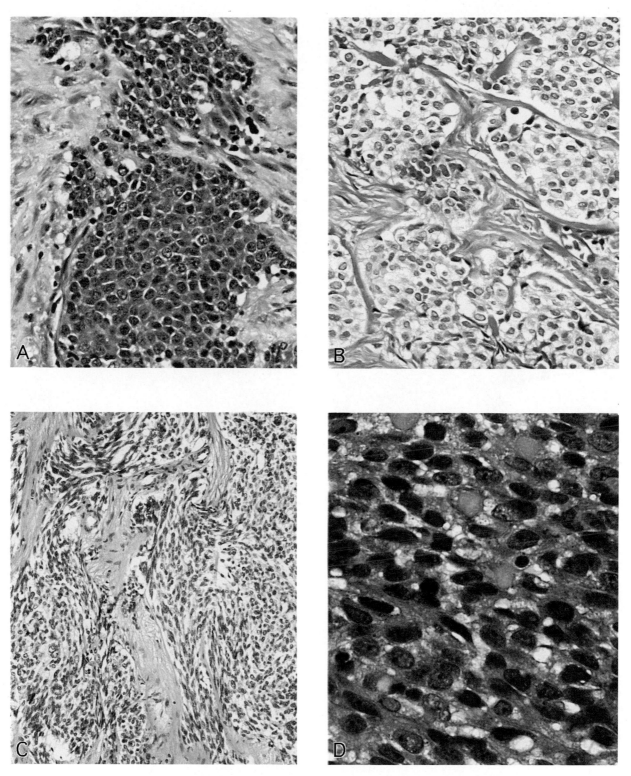

Figure 11-55
DESMOPLASTIC SMALL CELL TUMOR
The cells in small cell tumor with desmoplastic stroma are typically medium sized and round (A,B), spindled (C), or oval (D). The cytoplasm is usually scant, cell borders are indistinct, and nucleoli are inconspicuous. In some cases, the cells have a rhabdoid appearance (D).

Figure 11-56
DESMOPLASTIC
SMALL CELL TUMOR
A few small cell tumors with desmoplastic stroma contain cells with pleomorphic nuclei and more abundant cytoplasm, as illustrated here.

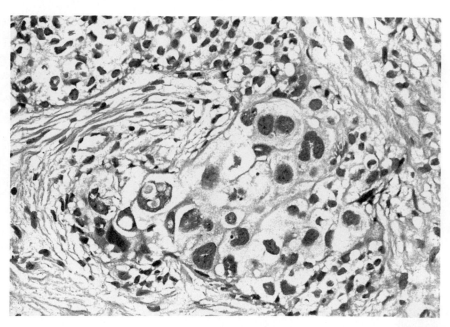

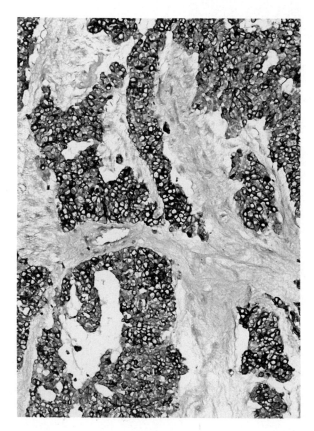
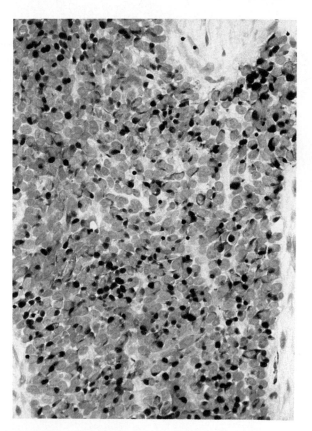

Figure 11-57
DESMOPLASTIC SMALL CELL TUMOR

Small cell tumor with desmoplastic stroma has a characteristic immunohistochemical profile, including strong cytoplasmic staining for cytokeratin (left) and variable, often dot-like cytoplasmic staining for desmin (right). The cells also usually stain for EMA, CD15, and CD57.

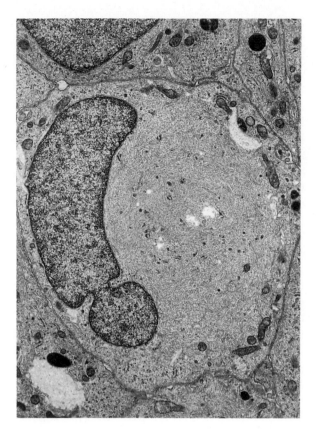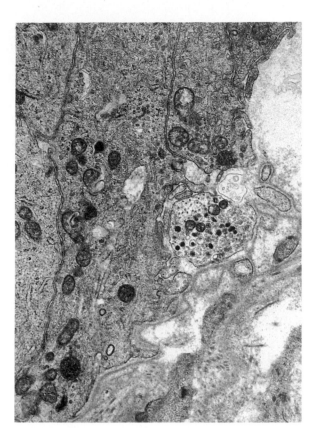

Figure 11-58
DESMOPLASTIC SMALL CELL TUMOR
The ultrastructural features include rhabdoid cells with abundant intermediate filaments (left) and dendritic cytoplasmic processes which may contain dense core secretory granules (right).

antigen, HMB45, alpha-fetoprotein, CD99, and myoglobin are almost always negative (108). Muscle-specific actin is rarely identified.

The minimal histologic and immunohistochemical findings that must be present, then, before diagnosing DSCT include solid nests of small cells which stain for desmin, cytokeratin, and EMA, embedded in a prominent desmoplastic stroma.

Although electron microscopy is not necessary to establish the diagnosis, examination of the fine structure has confirmed the epithelial, mesenchymal, and neural differentiation suggested by light microscopic and immunohistologic techniques. The most prominent ultrastructural feature, which most cases demonstrate, is paranuclear bundles and whorls of intermediate filaments (fig. 11-58, left) (104,108). These correspond to the cytokeratin-, desmin-, or vimentin-positive dot-like structures and the eosinophilic hyaline inclusions seen by optical microscopy. These intermediate filaments often displace the nucleus to an eccentric location in the cell. In a few tumors the intermediate filaments have the configuration of tonofilaments and some tumors contain cells with evidence of neural differentiation (104,108). Such cells may have dendritic processes, sometimes they form Homer-Wright rosettes, and occasionally dense core secretory granules and microtubules are present (fig. 11-58, right). Less frequent are tumor cells arranged in acinar formations with central lumens lined by microvilli (108).

Cytogenetic and Flow Cytometry Findings. A novel reciprocal translocation, t(11;22)(p13;q12)(101,110,111,113), has been reported in DSCT. As in the PPNET/ ES family of tumors and soft tissue clear cell sarcoma, a *EWS* rearrangement located at 22q12 has been found (106). However, unlike in PPNET/ES, the *EWS* gene product is fused to the *WT*1 gene located at 11p13 to form a chimeric *EWS-WT*1 fusion protein (106.) The introduction of the *EWS-WT*1 fusion gene into osteosarcoma cell lines induces expression of endogenous platelet-derived growth factor-alpha (PDGF), a potent fibroblast growth factor (107). PDGF has also been demonstrated in tumor cells of DSCT, which may explain the florid desmoplastic stroma so characteristic of this tumor (107).

The DNA ploidy and proliferative fraction do not correlate with any histologic feature or the length of patient survival (112).

Differential Diagnosis. By light microscopy, DSCT is not easily confused with other small cell tumors such as PPNET/ES, neuroblastoma, or embryonal rhabdomyosarcoma, because of its prominent desmoplastic stroma which these other tumors lack. The immunohistologic staining pattern of DSCT overlaps that of several of the above neoplasms as well as malignant rhabdoid tumor, but attention to the light microscopic appearance and the location and presentation of the primary tumor should prevent interpretative errors. Poorly differentiated carcinoma or a neuroendocrine carcinoma might be confused with DSCT by light microscopy but the former are desmin negative and only DSCT consistently occurs in young patients. Malignant mesotheliomas can be desmin, EMA, and cytokeratin positive, but mesotheliomas are CD15 and CD57 negative, whereas most DSCT are positive for antigens recognized by these antibodies. Furthermore, mesothelioma usually does not resemble DSCT cytologically.

Treatment and Prognosis. This neoplasm has been associated with a very poor outcome and has been generally unresponsive to therapeutic intervention. Despite multidrug chemotherapy, 75 percent of the patients are dead 4 to 72 months (average, 26 months) after presentation (103,104, 108) and only about 5 percent live beyond 5 years without evidence of tumor. The short-term prognosis, however, may not be so grim. Intensive alkylator-based therapy with aggressive surgery and radiotherapy to high-risk sites has resulted in prolonged progression-free survival (105).

Malignant Extrarenal Rhabdoid Tumor

Definition. Malignant extrarenal rhabdoid tumor is a highly malignant neoplasm which entirely consists of discohesive cells with vesicular nuclei and large eosinophilic nucleoli. At least some of the cells must contain eosinophilic keratin-positive paranuclear inclusions, show EMA positivity, or demonstrate abnormalities of chromosome 22q11.

General Considerations. The nosologic position of renal rhabdoid tumors is well established but there is some uncertainty about whether extrarenal rhabdoid tumors occur in the soft tissues and in organs other than the kidneys. This uncertainty results from the observation that many different types of malignant neoplasms focally contain cells which are cytologically identical to those that compose malignant rhabdoid tumor. These include malignant melanoma, poorly differentiated carcinomas of the kidney and gastrointestinal tract, malignant mesothelioma, epithelioid sarcoma, Wilms' tumor, neuroendocrine carcinoma, transitional cell carcinoma of the bladder, malignant lymphoma, central and peripheral nerve sheath tumors, desmoplastic small cell tumor, and embryonal and alveolar rhabdomyosarcomas. When rhabdoid features are focal in an otherwise characteristic, nonrhabdoid neoplasm there is general agreement that the nonrhabdoid features take precedence in classifying the tumor, although some would also add "with rhabdoid features" to the diagnosis. The problem becomes more difficult for extrarenal tumors that are entirely rhabdoid in appearance. There is fairly wide acceptance of extrarenal malignant rhabdoid tumors as distinct neoplasms in pediatric patients but many feel that such tumors in adults are other types of neoplasms, whether primary or metastatic, in which differentiating features cannot be discerned or have been missed. Our position is that the diagnosis of extrarenal malignant rhabdoid tumor should only be made when the tumor is composed exclusively or at least predominantly of cells with rhabdoid features by light microscopy, and light microscopy, immunohistology, and other studies do not reveal another line of differentiation. That is, the diagnosis of extrarenal malignant rhabdoid tumor is one of exclusion. The following discussion includes only tumors that meet this definition.

Clinical Features. Malignant rhabdoid tumors, whether of renal or extrarenal origin, occur predominately in the infant and child (121,125, 128,129). The mean age at presentation is 8 to 9 years, but this tumor occurs in the newborn and

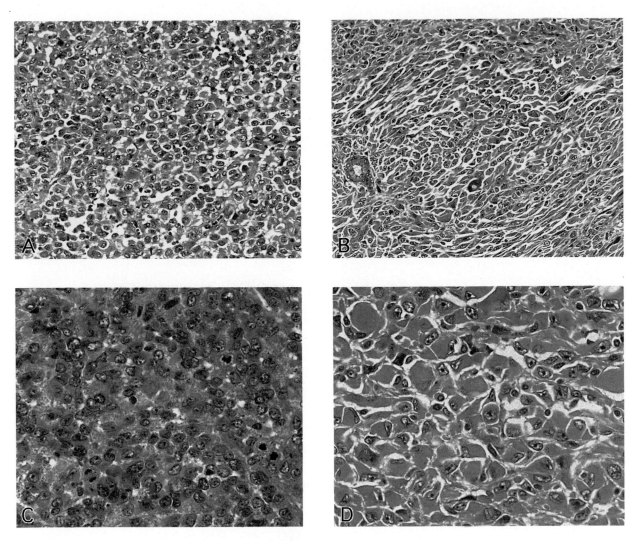

Figure 11-59
MALIGNANT RHABDOID TUMOR

The cells in malignant rhabdoid tumor are arranged in patternless sheets or irregular fascicles (A,B). The cells are discohesive, round with poorly defined cytoplasmic borders (C), or polygonal and spindle shaped with well-defined cytoplasmic borders (D). These nondescript cytologic features are typical of many types of poorly differentiated carcinomas and sarcomas.

middle-aged adults. For comparison, the mean age of patients with renal malignant rhabdoid tumor is only 11 months (129). Approximately 30 percent of malignant rhabdoid tumors occur in extrarenal sites, the most common of which are the soft tissues of the trunk (29 percent), the extremities (25 percent), head and neck (15 percent), abdomen, pelvis and retroperitoneum (20 percent), and solid organs other than the kidney (13 percent). Most patients present with a rapidly growing painful mass.

Pathologic Findings. Grossly, rhabdoid tumors appear as irregularly shaped, nonencapsu-

lated, gray-white to tan, multinodular solid masses that measure from 1 to 18 cm when discovered. The tumor is soft to moderately firm and may have a variegated appearance due to areas of yellow necrosis and red hemorrhage.

Almost all renal and extrarenal malignant rhabdoid tumors consist of sheets of discohesive, large, polygonal and sometimes spindled cells, with round to kidney bean-shaped vesicular nuclei that almost always contain a large, central eosinophilic nucleolus and abundant amphophilic or eosinophilic cytoplasm (fig. 11-59). The cardinal histologic feature is the paranuclear,

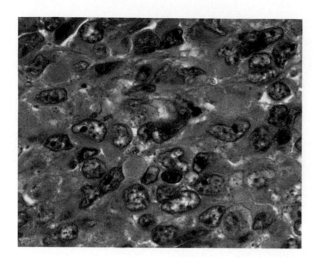

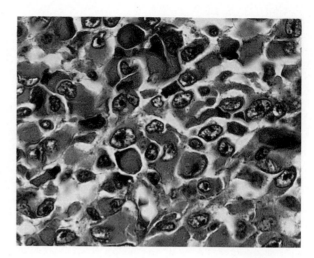

Figure 11-60
MALIGNANT RHABDOID TUMOR

The tumor is composed of large rounded cells (left). The cardinal feature is the paranuclear cytoplasmic eosinophilic or glassy inclusion seen best on the right. These cytoplasmic inclusions are typically vimentin and cytokeratin positive.

cytoplasmic, eosinophilic hyaline or glassy inclusion (fig. 11-60). These inclusions have a globular configuration and may be inconspicuous and present in only a few cells or they may be present in many cells and occasionally in every neoplastic cell (121,123). The cytoplasmic inclusions may be slightly PAS positive and often displace the nucleus, but cross-striations are not present. In fine needle aspiration biopsies the discohesive cells have round and oval nuclei, fine chromatin, and multiple medium-sized nucleoli. The cytoplasm contains eosinophilic inclusions which may displace the nucleus (fig. 11-61). The mitotic rate is typically high, with up to 2 or more per high-power field (121). There is little interstitial tissue in most tumors but some have an edematous to focally myxoid stroma.

In addition to the patterns described above, renal rhabdoid tumors can have hyalinizing or chondroid stroma and pseudoglandular, epithelioid, and histiocytoid cellular patterns (129). The latter two may be associated with multinucleated giant cells. The cells of an extrarenal malignant rhabdoid tumor may also be disposed in patterns other than the diffuse sheets described above, including alveolar, nesting, and trabecular arrangements (121).

The light microscopic features, then, which must be present before a diagnosis of extrarenal malignant rhabdoid tumor is made are large

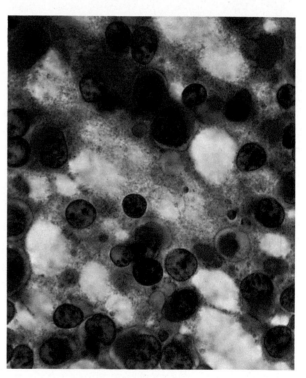

Figure 11-61
MALIGNANT RHABDOID TUMOR

Fine needle aspiration biopsies demonstrate rounded cells containing eosinophilic cytoplasmic inclusions which may displace the nucleus. Similar features can be found in differentiating PPNET/Ewing's sarcoma, rhabdomyosarcoma, small cell tumors with desmoplastic stroma, malignant melanoma, and numerous poorly differentiated carcinomas. Immunohistochemical staining with a panel approach may be useful in suggesting the diagnosis.

The "rl
olar rhal
malignan
inclusions
with desr
Muscle-sp
rhabdomy
reverse is
Furthermc
tiation in
hyperchror
points to r
doid tumor
renal tume
desmin, mi
itive and cy
be classifiec
less cytoger
abnormaliti
tumor or se
keratin stai
tumor shou
myosarcoma
convincingly

A diagnos
tumor migh
metastatic m
ferentiated c
tain cells wi
sions, large n
In the older a
be especially
logic profile of
mas and malig
tical; however
of consequenc
having a prir
tumor is a met

Malignant r
dren; it present
lesion rather tl
papillary or acir
acteristic ultras
cal features whi

Extensive se
identifies evide
tema, and tubu
in those Wilms
doid tumors.

An occasiona
PPNET/ES cont

polygonal or spindle-shaped discohesive tumor cells with vesicular nuclei, a large eosinophilic nucleolus, and abundant eosinophilic cytoplasm. Paranuclear eosinophilic inclusions must be identified in at least a few tumor cells. In addition, the diagnosis requires the characteristic immunohistochemical profile described in the next section, so the diagnosis must be confirmed by utilizing immunohistology to exclude other neoplasms.

Immunohistochemical and Electron Microscopic Findings. Both renal and nonrenal rhabdoid tumors have similar immunohistologic features, suggesting they are differentiating along the same lines. The paranuclear inclusions usually stain in a dot-like pattern for keratin and vimentin, but in occasional tumors, some cells display diffuse cytoplasmic staining for one or both of these intermediate filaments. Cytoplasmic cytokeratin was found in 70 percent of renal tumors reported as malignant rhabdoid tumors, vimentin in 100 percent, desmin in 35 percent, and neurofilament in 10 percent (125,129,129a), while 80 to 85 percent of tumors interpreted as nonrenal malignant rhabdoid tumors have been reported to stain for cytokeratin, 90 percent for vimentin, and 10 percent for desmin (117a,121,123,125,129a). Glial fibrillary acidic protein has not been reported in either renal or nonrenal tumors. Nearly 60 percent of renal and 70 percent of nonrenal cases reported as malignant rhabdoid tumors stain for EMA (117a,121,125). Myoglobin and S-100 protein have been reported in 3 of 11 and 1 of 11 renal cases, respectively, and in 10 to 15 percent of nonrenal cases (125,129). Neuron-specific enolase, a marker on which we place little weight, has been reported in one third of both renal and nonrenal cases.

It is these variable staining results that has lead many to consider extrarenal malignant rhabdoid tumor a nonentity. For a diagnosis of extrarenal malignant rhabdoid tumor, the minimal histologic and clinical features as described in the Pathologic Findings section must be met and the paranuclear inclusions should be cytokeratin positive. Usually the cells are also EMA positive. In our opinion, tumors that contain desmin-, monoclonal myoglobin-, neuron-specific enolase-, neurofilament-, or S-100 protein-positive cells, as reported in several series, should not be included among the extrarenal malignant rhabdoid tumors.

Fine structural examination is useful in confirming the presence of paranuclear whorled aggregates or bundles of intermediate filaments in both renal (129) and extrarenal (121,123,130) rhabdoid tumors (fig. 11-62). In some cases some of the intermediate filaments take on the appearance of tonofilaments. Arrays of rough endoplasmic reticulum, mitochondria, and lipid droplets are often trapped in the whorls of filaments. Cytoplasmic glycogen, primitive or complex intercellular junctions, and focal basal lamina occur in about 25 percent of cases.

Cytogenetic and Flow Cytometry Findings. The cytogenetic and molecular findings of only a small number of extrarenal malignant rhabdoid tumors have been reported. These have demonstrated monosomy or deletion of the long arm of chromosome 22 (116,117,129a) and translocations involving chromosome 22 at band q11 (114,115,122, 123a,124) or band p11 (119). Similar translocations and deletions involving chromosome 22 band q11 have been reported (126) in malignant rhabdoid tumors of the kidney (120,122,127). Schofield et al. (126) in a study of 30 primary renal rhabdoid tumors, showed loss of heterogeneity at chromosome 22q11-12 in 80 percent of the cases. These findings suggest that there is a tumor suppressor gene located on chromosome 22q11, and although the number of renal and extrarenal malignant rhabdoid tumors that have been examined for cytogenetic and molecular abnormalities is small, the chromosomal abnormalities described so far suggest that there may be a common progenitor for both. This may prove to be of diagnostic usefulness in the future if further studies identify a rhabdoid tumor gene.

Differential Diagnosis. Epithelioid sarcoma, embryonal and alveolar rhabdomyosarcoma, malignant melanoma, poorly differentiated carcinomas of the kidney, urinary bladder, and gastrointestinal tract, malignant mesothelioma, Wilms' tumors, neuroendocrine carcinomas, primitive neuroepithelial tumors, small round cell tumor with desmoplastic stroma, and rare malignant lymphomas are the main considerations in the extensive differential diagnosis of neoplasms with the histologic features of extrarenal rhabdoid tumors.

Epithelioid sarcoma usually involves the distal upper and, less frequently, the lower extremity; it has a peak age incidence in the third decade, a time when rhabdoid tumors are uncommon; and it has a characteristic nodular growth pattern, often

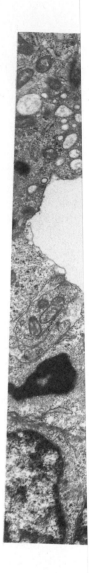

Fine structur
filaments in most

with central r
phoid infiltrate
ded in abunda
which is not a
the case for ma
composing epit
vimentin, and e
itive, and ultra
ate filaments
About 50 percen
CD34-positive c
tive in maligna
neoplasms feat

tumor cells characteristically contain abundant glycogen which is often not present or sparse in melanoma cells; the histologic features are almost always the same from tumor to tumor, unlike melanomas which show considerable histologic variation; and clear cell sarcoma has a more indolent course than many melanomas. Chromosomal analysis has revealed that about 75 percent of clear cell sarcomas display a nonrandom translocation involving chromosomes 12 and 22, namely t(12;22)(q13-14;q12-13), never reported in malignant melanoma (131,138–140). Interestingly, chromosome 22 participates in the t(11;22) (q24;q12) translocation that is characteristic of PPNET/ES; in fact, the same gene is involved in both tumors, the *EWS* gene on chromosome 22 (143). However, preferential rearrangements of chromosomes frequently found in malignant melanoma also have been reported in clear cell sarcoma (131,142).

Because of these clinical, histologic, and chromosomal differences, we think clear cell sarcoma should be classified separately from malignant melanoma. We have included this tumor among the miscellaneous soft tissue neoplasms rather than the neural neoplasms because it does not display nerve or nerve sheath differentiation, rather it is closer to malignant melanoma than any other differentiated tumor type. Malignant melanoma of soft parts is an acceptable alternative designation so long as the differences from cutaneous malignant melanoma are clearly understood.

Clinical Features. Clear cell sarcoma develops most frequently on the extremities, mostly on the lower extremity (75 percent of cases) (132,136). The foot, including the ankle and heel, is by far the most common site, followed by the knee and thigh. About 25 percent of the tumors arise in the upper extremity, particularly the hand and wrist, while involvement of the head and neck and trunk is distinctly rare. Most patients are young, with a median age of 30 years, although these tumors have been reported in patients from age 7 to 85. Females are more frequently affected than males. The tumor typically grows slowly, causes pain in about half the patients, and is usually deep-seated around tendons and fascia.

Pathologic Findings. Grossly, clear cell sarcomas are usually lobulated and gray-white on cut section, although foci of brown or black pigment are visible in some tumors. Areas of hemorrhage

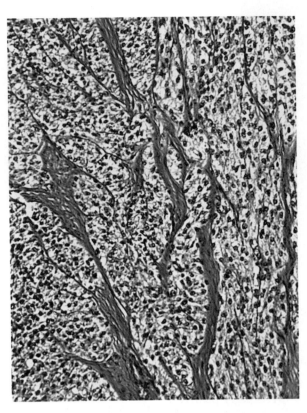

Figure 11-63
CLEAR CELL SARCOMA
In many clear cell sarcomas, fibrous tissue bands dissect the tumor cells into groups.

and necrosis are often found and a few tumors contain cysts. Most tumors are about 3 to 4 cm when discovered although they can be quite large and bulky (136). This unusually small size for a malignant soft tissue tumor is probably the result of the slow progression that is characteristic of clear cell sarcoma and the frequent location around the foot and ankle, a site where a tumor often becomes apparent when it is small.

Microscopically, the usual clear cell sarcoma is distinctive at low-power magnification because the tumor cells are most often arranged in packets or nests surrounded by delicate to thick fibrous bands (fig. 11-63) (132,134,135). In many tumors, the cells arrange themselves in short fascicles or rows, while in others they are in whorls. The constituent cells are medium-sized to large, vary from round to polygonal to spindled, and have vesicular nuclei with prominent nucleoli (figs. 11-64, 11-65)(136). Nuclear pleomorphism is not significant except in rare examples and in some recurrences and

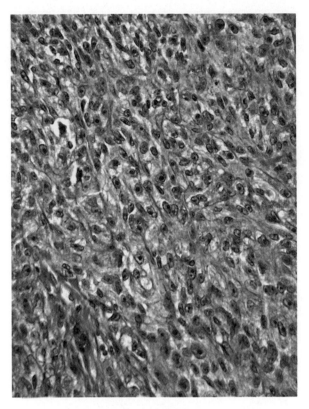

Figure 11-64
CLEAR CELL SARCOMA
Cells with large uniform nuclei and prominent nucleoli
are a constant feature of clear cell sarcoma.

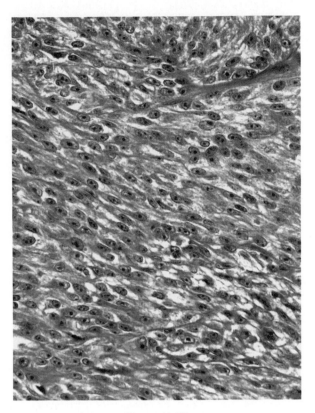

Figure 11-65
CLEAR CELL SARCOMA
The cytoplasm may be clear or lightly eosinophilic.

metastases (figs. 11-66, 11-67). The name of the tumor suggests that the cytoplasm of the constituent cells should be clear and indeed it is in many tumor cells, but in most tumors the majority of the cells have lightly to deeply eosinophilic cytoplasm (fig. 11-67). Multinucleated tumor giant cells with a wreath-like arrangement of the nuclei are found in a significant number of clear cell sarcomas and these have the same vesicular nuclei and large nucleoli as do the other tumor cells.

PAS stains, with and without diastase digestion, reveal abundant intracytoplasmic glycogen in about two thirds of the tumors but no intracellular mucin. Melanin, both intracellular and extracellular, can be seen in the hematoxylin and eosin-stained sections in some cases, but when a melanin stain is used about half to three fourths of the cases have demonstrable melanin. Hemosiderin is commonly present and can be confused with melanin, so iron stains are sometimes useful. Mitotic figures are distinctly sparse. Rarely,

large areas of the stroma may be hyalinized, and tumor cell necrosis is present in about a third of clear cell sarcomas. Often, clear cell sarcoma extends from the soft tissue around the fascia and tendons to the deep dermis or into muscle, but involvement of the epidermis is rare.

The key histologic features then of clear cell sarcoma are: 1) packets or groups of medium-sized to large polygonal to fusiform cells surrounded by fibrous tissue, 2) uniform polygonal to spindled tumor cells with large nucleoli and clear to eosinophilic cytoplasm, 3) intracytoplasmic glycogen, 4) presence of melanin, 5) multinucleated tumor giant cells with a wreath-like arrangement of the nuclei, and 6) usually sparse mitotic figures (figs. 11-63–11-67) (132,136).

Special Studies. About 80 percent of clear cell sarcomas contain cells that express S-100 protein and more than three quarters are HMB45 positive (132,135,136,141). Cytokeratin, EMA, desmin, actin, and leukocyte common antigen stains are negative. Ultrastructurally,

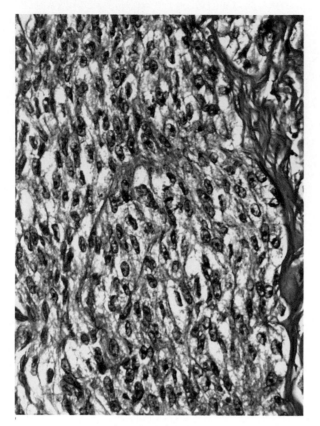

Figure 11-66
CLEAR CELL SARCOMA
In many clear cell sarcomas the nuclei are round but they can also be elongate.

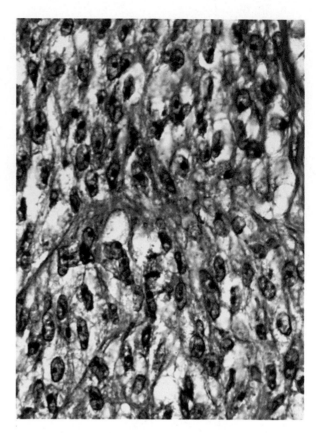

Figure 11-67
CLEAR CELL SARCOMA
Note the nuclear uniformity and large prominent nucleoli in this high-power view of clear cell sarcoma. These are almost constant features of clear cell sarcoma.

most tumors contain cells with melanosomes in varying degrees of development and occasionally long cell processes which interdigitate among one another. The distinctive chromosomal abnormalities found in clear cell sarcomas are discussed in General Considerations above.

Differential Diagnosis. Distinction of clear cell sarcoma from primary malignant melanoma is largely based on location. The diagnosis of primary malignant melanoma, except for desmoplastic melanoma, requires neoplastic transformation of melanocytes at the dermal-epidermal or the mucosal-submucosal junction. This area is rarely involved by clear cell sarcoma and only when the tumor is very large and erodes through the dermis. Desmoplastic melanoma, which unlike clear cell sarcoma usually arises in the skin of the head and neck in an older individual, may or may not be associated with lentigo maligna or lentigo maligna melanoma, but its constituent

cells are not arranged in packets as is characteristic of clear cell sarcoma, its stroma is collagenous, and most of the tumor cells have features of fibroblasts. The cells of spindle cell melanoma may have large nucleoli and may form groups surrounded by fibrous tissue, but this tumor is associated with junctional proliferation of melanocytes. Glycogen may be present in the tumor cells of cutaneous melanoma, but is usually more abundant in clear cell sarcoma. Of course, S-100 protein and HMB45 are of little value in making this distinction.

The most common and difficult differential diagnostic problem is distinguishing clear cell sarcoma from metastatic malignant melanoma. Features that favor melanoma are significant cellular pleomorphism, a high mitotic index, tumor cell necrosis and, of course, a history of a primary melanoma. The latter is most important, and when it is absent and the tumor cells are uniform and mitotically inactive it may be impossible to be sure whether the tumor is clear cell sarcoma or metastatic malignant melanoma.

Cellular blue nevi may feature packets of cells separated by fibrous stroma and intracytoplasmic glycogen, but they occur primarily on the trunk, a site not often involved by clear cell sarcoma. Melanin is usually more abundant in cellular blue nevi than in clear cell sarcomas, and cellular blue nevi are usually superficial and rarely involve the tendons, fascial structures, or aponeuroses. Malignant blue nevus is also generally superficial, most commonly occurs on the scalp, and may be associated with benign blue nevus. In rare circumstances, it may be impossible to distinguish malignant blue nevus and clear cell sarcoma, but this is not a serious problem because both tumors are treated alike and essentially behave alike, although clear cell sarcoma usually is slower to metastasize.

The spindled cells in synovial sarcoma superficially resemble the elongate cells in some clear cell sarcomas but they lack prominent nucleoli. About half of monophasic synovial sarcomas and 100 percent of biphasic synovial sarcomas are keratin positive, a stain that is negative in clear cell sarcoma. Only about 30 percent of synovial sarcomas are S-100 protein positive. Essentially, synovial sarcoma is HMB45 negative while at least three fourths of the cases of clear cell sarcoma are HMB45 positive. Calcification is common in synovial sarcoma and almost always absent in clear cell sarcoma. Finally, melanin is often present in clear cell sarcoma, but not in synovial sarcoma, while mucin may be present in biphasic synovial sarcoma, but not in clear cell sarcoma. Fibrosarcomas lack the packet-like arrangement of the cells found in the usual clear cell sarcoma and the tumor cells are negative for S-100 protein, HMB45, and glycogen. Leiomyosarcomas may be epithelioid but the cells are not divided into packets and actin and desmin stains may be positive.

Malignant peripheral nerve sheath tumor (MPNST) and clear cell sarcoma can have overlapping histologic features and both can be S-100 protein positive. However, most MPNSTs arise from a nerve, from a neurofibroma, or in a patient with von Recklinghausen's disease, patterns of origin not usually observed in clear cell sarcoma. Moreover, they rarely contain glycogen or melanin pigment, they are usually HMB45 negative, and mitotic figures are usually numerous, in contrast to clear cell sarcoma. In occasional cases, distinction between clear cell sarcoma and MPNST may be unclear but this is not of great concern since both tumors have a similar prognosis. Most carcinomas, including renal cell carcinoma, can be distinguished from clear cell sarcoma by a keratin stain.

Because the cells of clear cell sarcoma are often separated into clusters by fibrous bands, neuroendocrine tumors, particularly paraganglioma, enter into the differential diagnosis. However, the nuclei of the cells that compose clear cell sarcoma are not stippled and large prominent nucleoli are not a feature of paragangliomas. A chromogranin or synaptophysin stain usually clarifies the situation because one or both should be positive in paraganglioma and negative in clear cell carcinoma.

Treatment and Prognosis. In the short term, clear cell sarcomas behave in a manner similar to most other adult sarcomas in that about 50 percent metastasize within 5 years; however, in some cases the pace of tumor progression is decidedly slower than for most other sarcomas, resulting in a significant number of metastases appearing after 5 years (132–134,136,137). Most often metastasis follows local recurrence, which can occur on multiple occasions. Tumor size appears to be the only variable that predicts metastatic potential: tumors over 5 cm have a significantly higher incidence of metastasis than do tumors under 5 cm. The most common sites of metastatic tumor are the regional lymph nodes, lungs, and bone. Patient survival is determined mainly by metastasis, and thus continues to decline with more extended follow-up.

Alveolar Soft Part Sarcoma

Definition. Alveolar soft part sarcoma is composed of large uniform cells with abundant granular to vacuolated eosinophilic cytoplasm divided into packets by thin-walled, often sinusoidal vessels.

General Considerations. This morphologically distinctive neoplasm is composed of cells whose direction of differentiation has been the object of speculation ever since its description in 1952 by Christopherson, Foote, and Stewart (146). Based on its appearance some have postulated it is a paraganglioma or a neural tumor but ultrastructural and immunohistochemical studies do not support this contention (144,147). Most recent studies support myogenic differentiation, specifically primitive or myoblastic skeletal muscle differentiation, because both desmin and MyoD1 stains are positive in many alveolar soft part sarcomas (150,156,157,162,166,168). However, Wang and associates (172) in a recent study failed to find nuclear staining by MyoD1 and Western blot analysis did not reveal a protein band that would correspond to MyoD1. Desmin was positive in the cells in 6 of the 12 tumors studied. Even though some of the tumor cells contained desmin, the lack of MyoD1 expression must raise serious doubts about the hypothesis that the tumor cells in alveolar soft part sarcoma are differentiated as skeletal muscle cells. Cytoplasmic staining by MyoD1 most likely represents a nonspecific cross reaction with another antigen or diffusion from nearby skeletal muscle cells. Altogether, it seems the direction of differentiation of the tumor cells remains a mystery. In any event, this rare tumor has morphologic features that make recognition easy, it has no benign counterpart, metastases not infrequently occur a decade or more after the primary has been excised and, contrarily, a significant number of patients initially present with symptoms caused by metastasis rather than the primary tumor.

Clinical Features. Much of what is known about the clinical presentation and outcome of patients with alveolar soft part sarcoma has been provided by two large series, one from Memorial Sloan-Kettering (153a), the other from the Armed Forces Institute of Pathology (AFIP) (148). Most patients are adolescents and young adults between 15 and 35 years of age, although all ages may be affected. However, alveolar soft part sarcoma is distinctly rare in individuals over 50 and under 5. There is a female predilection, particularly if the patient is under 20. About half the tumors arise in the anterior thigh and buttock while most of the remainder are discovered in the distal lower extremity, upper extremity, and trunk. However, this neoplasm has been reported in almost every location; in children, the head and neck is a common site (163,164). Unusual sites to keep in mind are retroperitoneum, uterine cervix and corpus, tongue, and orbit (155,160,167).

Alveolar soft part sarcoma is almost unique among sarcomas because of its unusual propensity to present initially as a metastasis, particularly to brain and lung (154,165). The primary tumor grows slowly and often is asymptomatic, and this plus the proclivity of the tumor for vascular invasion and the frequency of brain metastases which are symptomatic when small probably explains this phenomenon. Even patients who present because of the discovery of the primary tumor have a significant chance of synchronous metastases. As a consequence, imaging studies of all possible sites of metastasis are usually performed whenever a patient is diagnosed with alveolar soft part sarcoma (159,170). The prominent vascularity of the tumor often causes the radiologist to think of this tumor when computerized tomography (CT) scans are reviewed.

Pathologic Findings. Grossly, on cut section, alveolar soft part sarcomas usually demonstrate focal areas of hemorrhage and necrosis, while the viable tumor varies from yellow to gray. Microscopically, fibrous bands of varying width divide the tumor into nodules but it is the small packets of cells within the nodules that catch the attention of the viewer (fig. 11-68). Initially, at low magnification, one has the impression that thin, delicate fibrous tissue is dividing small groups of around 25 to 50 cells into the packets, but closer inspection reveals it is dilated sinusoidal thin-walled veins and delicate hard-to-see reticulin fibers that separate the clusters of tumor cells (fig. 11-69). Within the packets, central necrosis and cell loss are common and the remaining centrally located tumor cells are often discohesive, while viable cohesive cells line the outside perimeter of the packets. It is this combination of partially empty central areas and peripheral viable tumor cells, mimicking the alveolar lining cells of the lung, that gives the tumor its alveolar appearance (fig. 11-70). Often, clusters of tumor cells protrude into the vascular channels giving rise to a "glomeruloid" appearance (fig. 11-69, right). Occasionally, particularly in children and infants, the organoid pattern of the tumor is lost and the uniform cells grow in sheets.

The tumor cells are large but uniform, with abundant granular to vacuolated cytoplasm and large, round to polygonal, vesicular nuclei, often with prominent nucleoli (fig. 11-71). Cell margins are characteristically sharp and easily seen.

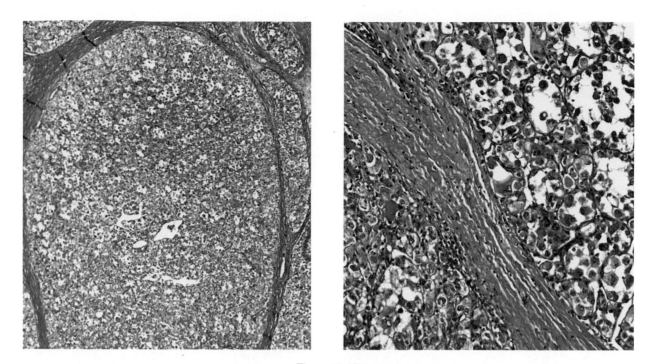

Figure 11-68
ALVEOLAR SOFT PART SARCOMA
Left: Typically, nodules of tumor cells are surrounded by fibrous tissue septa.
Right: Within the nodules the tumor cells are further subdivided into packets.

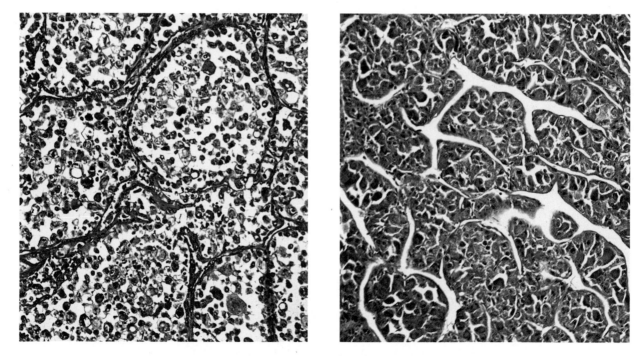

Figure 11-69
ALVEOLAR SOFT PART SARCOMA
At low magnification, it may appear that the packets of tumor cells are separated by fibrous tissue (left) but it is actually sinusoidal vessels that divide the tumor cells into packets (right).

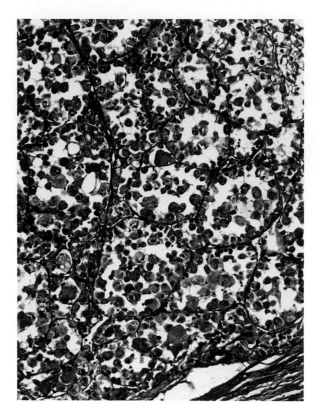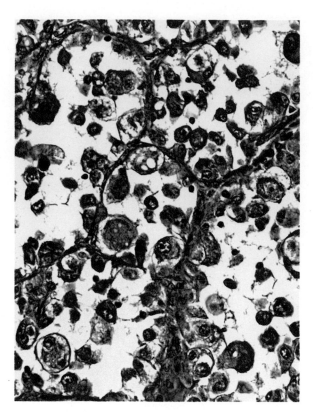

Figure 11-70
ALVEOLAR SOFT PART SARCOMA
It is the relatively empty centers of the packets (left) and the cells resting on vascular basement membranes (right) that give this tumor its lung-like appearance.

Although occasional examples feature focal areas where the cells are pleomorphic, pleomorphism is not a feature of most alveolar soft part sarcomas and even if it is present it is focal (149). Diffuse pleomorphism is so rare that it should cause the observer to think about another type of neoplasm. Some tumor cells contain two nuclei, and sometimes 5 to 10 nuclei are present in a single cell. Mitotic figures, if present, are rare. The cytoplasm is characteristically eosinophilic and granular but may be vacuolated. PAS stains reveal glycogen, at least focally, in the cytoplasm of the cells of most tumors as well as PAS-positive diastase-resistant material. Sometimes the latter is in the form of crystals: in fact, about 80 percent of tumors contain cells with rod-like to rhomboid crystals so these are a useful marker (fig. 11-72). However, crystals may be difficult to find or, as noted, absent. Vascular invasion is commonly present and often multifocal. Psammoma bodies have been reported (145).

Special Studies. Reported immunohistochemical studies of alveolar soft part sarcoma record inconsistent results. More specifically, some investigators have reported the tumor cells to be desmin, muscle-specific actin, smooth muscle actin, MyoD1, and S-100 protein positive while others have reported these to be negative, or positive only focally, or positive in some but not all tumors (150,152,156,157,162,166,168). Stains for cytokeratins, EMA, myoglobin, chromogranin, and neurofilaments are negative in almost all reports. Thus, immunohistochemistry is most important diagnostically in excluding other neoplasms with an immunologic profile not reported for alveolar soft part sarcoma. The variable immunohistochemical results do not resolve the longstanding question about the direction of differentiation of the constituent cells (see General Considerations above) (157).

Ultrastructurally, there are few filaments, no thick and thin filaments, and no mature skeletal

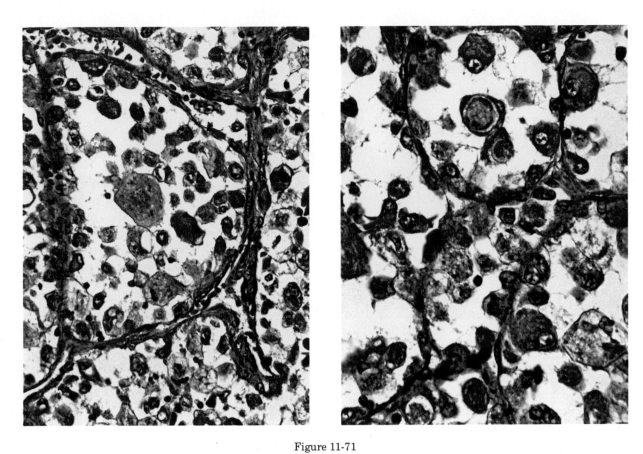

Figure 11-71
ALVEOLAR SOFT PART SARCOMA
The cells composing alveolar soft part sarcoma have abundant granular to vacuolated cytoplasm and nuclei with prominent nucleoli.

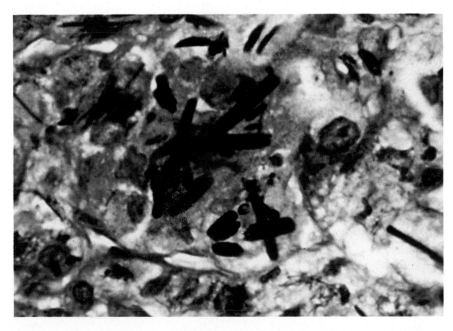

Figure 11-72
ALVEOLAR
SOFT PART SARCOMA
A PAS stain will often aid in identifying the crystals present in many tumors.

471

muscle features (158,159,161,162,171). The Golgi is typically extensive and contains granules and dense structures which often merge with crystals with a linear periodicity. Chromosomal analysis of a few tumors has revealed a consistent abnormality of 17q25 as well as other multiple and complex abnormalities (151,168,169).

Differential Diagnosis. The clusters of uniform large cells, some of which may contain crystals, surrounded by thin-walled sinusoidal vessels, are so distinctive that the diagnosis of alveolar soft part sarcoma is seldom in doubt. This pattern may raise a question of metastatic renal cell carcinoma but a keratin stain will resolve the issue because 99 percent or more of renal cell carcinomas contain keratin-positive cells while this stain is negative in alveolar soft part sarcoma. Moreover, renal cell carcinoma is very rare in the age group in which alveolar soft part sarcoma is most common. The nests of cells could raise concern for paraganglioma but the cells are too large, their vesicular nuclei and prominent nucleoli are unusual for paraganglioma, and chromogranin stains are negative in alveolar soft part sarcoma. Moreover, paragangliomas do not occur in the extremities. Alveolar rhabdomyosarcoma features clusters of cells surrounded by fibrous tissue, not sinusoidal veins, and has cells that are smaller and more pleomorphic than the cells of alveolar soft part sarcoma. Moreover, the nuclei of the constituent cells of rhabdomyosarcoma are dense while they are vesicular in alveolar soft part sarcoma and prominent nucleoli are not a feature in most rhabdomyosarcomas. Immunohistochemical stains may be of limited value in this situation because both may contain desmin-positive cells, but if the desmin stain is negative the tumor is almost certainly not alveolar rhabdomyosarcoma. Granular cell tumors are composed of cells with more densely eosinophilic cytoplasm and the cells are S-100 protein positive. Only rare alveolar soft part sarcomas contain S-100 protein-positive cells and granular cell tumors do not feature dilated sinusoidal vessels around clusters of cells. In women, ovarian clear cell carcinoma may be considered but this tumor lacks sinusoidal vessels surrounding groups of cells and the keratin stain should be positive.

When alveolar soft part sarcomas feature sheet-like growth or significantly large areas with pleomorphic cells the diagnosis becomes more difficult.

Cutting many sections to find more characteristic areas is often fruitful and immunohistochemical stains help rule out other tumors such as carcinoma or melanoma. Because some alveolar soft part sarcomas contain desmin-positive cells, this stain can also be considered.

Treatment and Prognosis. The patterns of behavior exhibited by alveolar soft part sarcoma are distinctly different from those of most other adult sarcomas (148,153). First, local recurrence is unusual whereas it is common with most other sarcomas. Second, the metastatic rate is higher than it is for most other adult sarcomas and metastasis commonly occurs in the absence of local recurrence. Third, not infrequently patients initially present because of a metastasis, particularly in the brain or lungs. Fourth, metastases may develop decades after the primary tumor has been excised. Because of the latter, survival figures continue to decline over long periods of time. In the large Memorial Hospital series (153), survival was 77 percent at 2 years, 60 percent at 5 years, 38 percent at 10 years, and 15 percent at 20 years. Tumor size has been reported to be an important predictor of patient survival (149).

This is a slowly growing neoplasm which seldom causes symptoms until it is very large but which metastasizes so early in its course that it is wise to consider it a systemic disease at the onset. Unfortunately, there is no known effective therapy unless the initial excision cures the patient.

Synovial Sarcoma

Definition. Synovial sarcoma is a biphasic soft tissue sarcoma with epithelial and spindle cell components, or a monophasic sarcoma having the same histologic features as the spindle cell component of biphasic synovial sarcoma.

General Considerations. Because many synovial sarcomas arise not far from joints, areas of epithelial differentiation in biphasic tumors were, on the basis of light microscopic observation, originally thought to represent synovial differentiation and hence the name. However, it is now known that the epithelial cells and some of the spindle cells in synovial sarcoma express cytokeratins and EMA, antigens not expressed by synovial cells. Moreover, the epithelial cells in synovial sarcoma have ultrastructural features identical to those found in normal epithelial cells, including desmosomes, microvilli on luminal surfaces, tight junctions, and basal lamina. None of these features has ever been described in normal or reactive synovium. Thus, the epithelial cells in synovial sarcoma are indeed epithelial and not synovial. The idea that a soft tissue neoplasm could demonstrate epithelial differentiation has been difficult to accept, and has caused some investigators to suggest renaming biphasic synovial sarcoma as carcinosarcoma (193,215). We think it unwise to change the names of tumors to fit the latest scientific revelations unless a useful clinical purpose is served by such label changes. In our opinion, changing the name to carcinosarcoma does not meet this criterion and in fact could cause confusion, and, moreover, future investigations may well suggest a better name. The epithelial cells in biphasic synovial sarcoma have long been referred to as "epithelioid" because they were originally thought to be synovial cells with an epithelial appearance. Because it is now clear they are epithelial cells, we think their lineage can be respected by application of the term "epithelial."

The concept of monophasic spindle cell synovial sarcoma arose from the observation that there were purely spindle cell tumors whose constituent cells morphologically resembled the spindled component of biphasic synovial sarcoma. Following these observations, a period of uncertainty about how to distinguish monophasic synovial sarcoma from fibrosarcoma ensued. This ended when it became apparent that monophasic synovial sarcomas often have morphologic features not seen in fibrosarcomas, such as calcification, thick ropy collagen, and a hemangiopericytoma-like vascular pattern. Further evidence that monophasic synovial sarcoma existed was provided by immunohistochemical demonstration of keratin or EMA expression by some of the spindled cells in synovial sarcoma and finding that a balanced chromosomal translocation between chromosomes X and 18 is present in both the monophasic and biphasic variants (see Special Studies below).

Recently, a third variant of synovial sarcoma, the poorly differentiated type, has been recognized. Poorly differentiated areas occur in about 20 percent of otherwise characteristic synovial sarcomas but rarely is an entire synovial sarcoma poorly differentiated. The latter have the same t(x;18) translocation as ordinary synovial sarcoma and are described below (238a).

A purely epithelial synovial sarcoma has been postulated (187). However, a glandular neoplasm in the soft tissues that is a candidate for an epithelial synovial sarcoma without spindle cells must be distinguished from metastatic adenocarcinoma, adenocarcinoma locally extending from a nearby organ such as the skin, and deep-seated mixed tumors including myoepitheliomas before it is considered to be an epithelial synovial sarcoma. This can only be accomplished by imaging techniques and clinical findings in addition to morphology because pure epithelial synovial sarcoma cannot be recognized on morphologic grounds. We have never seen a convincing example of purely epithelial synovial sarcoma. Pure epithelial synovial sarcomas are so rare, if they exist at all, that the term monophasic synovial sarcoma refers only to the spindle cell type of synovial sarcoma.

Clinical Features. Synovial sarcoma occurs chiefly in young adults and teenagers, although these tumors do occur in older adults and preteen children (174,176,178,184–186,194,197,208,219, 223,230,242,243,245). There is a slight male predominance in most studies. The majority develop in the extremities and limb girdles, and synovial sarcoma is one of the rare sarcomas that occurs with some frequency in the distal extremities, including the hands and feet. Although often located near a large joint, synovial sarcoma only rarely involves intra-articular tissues. Less common locations include the head and neck (more often the latter) (177,222,226,228,233) and the abdominal wall (188); even more unusual sites are the retroperitoneum (232), the pleura and lung (192,244), and the thoracic area, most often the mediastinum (240). Very rarely, synovial sarcoma arises in the heart (175,198) or the interior of a major vein (214,231). Within the soft tissues, the neoplasm is typically situated in deeper structures such as tendon or muscle rather than in the subcutis. Synovial sarcomas vary from small to large at discovery; as might be expected, smaller examples are more often located distally where they become apparent sooner. Imaging studies may reveal areas of calcification in some tumors.

Pathologic Findings. Synovial sarcomas are typically yellow-tan to gray on cut section and vary from soft to firm. Occasionally, there is grossly apparent calcification and areas of necrosis are

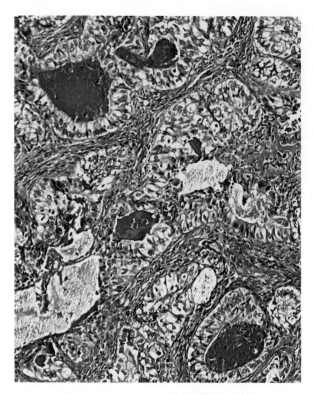

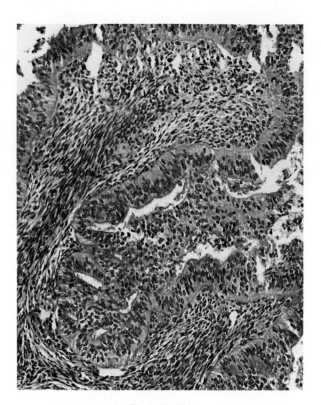

Figure 11-73
BIPHASIC SYNOVIAL SARCOMA
There are two distinct, intermingled but sharply marginated components. The epithelial component is composed of larger and paler cells that form glandular spaces while the spindle cell component between the glands is made up of small, uniform spindle cells with a high nuclear-cytoplasmic ratio. The material in the glandular lumens has the staining characteristics of epithelial mucin.

Figure 11-74
BIPHASIC SYNOVIAL SARCOMA
Here the epithelial component demonstrates a combination of glandular and solid growth. The tall columnar character of the cells of the gland-forming portion is striking.

common. Some synovial sarcomas demonstrate obvious infiltration of adjacent tissues, whereas others appear more circumscribed. Cyst formation may be present.

Microscopically, there are two main forms: biphasic and monophasic. Biphasic synovial sarcomas contain distinct but intermingled epithelial and spindle cell components which are characteristically sharply demarcated from each other, but which may merge gradually in some areas (figs. 11-73–11-77). The epithelial component forms solid nests and, frequently, glandular or tubular structures (figs. 11-73–11-75). Less common is a papillary pattern in which the papillae are lined by epithelial cells and have cores composed of the spindle cell component (fig. 11-76). The epithelial cells in synovial sarcomas are characteristically larger and paler, and have more cytoplasm than

the cells in the spindle cell component; they vary from flattened to cuboidal to tall columnar around glandular spaces and are usually cuboidal or polygonal, although occasionally somewhat spindled, in solid nests (fig. 11-77). Their nuclei are typically round and vesicular, and the cytoplasmic margins are usually clearly seen. Hyalinized collagen is occasionally present among the epithelial cells. The glandular lumens often contain epithelial mucin which is more commonly eosinophilic and granular or clumped but which may be basophilic and colloid-like (fig. 11-73). This material stains with PAS after diastase digestion and thus has the character of epithelial mucin. The epithelial compartment in biphasic synovial sarcoma varies from very focal and difficult to find to so greatly predominant that the spindle cell component is hard to identify, although a relatively even mix is most frequent. Rarely, focal squamous differentiation has been reported (185,217,225).

474

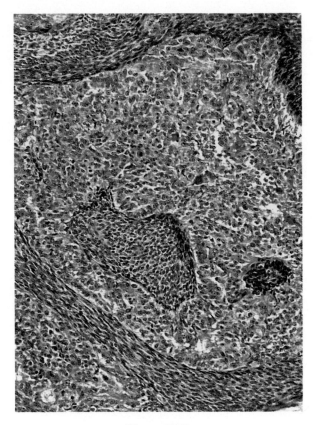

Figure 11-75
BIPHASIC SYNOVIAL SARCOMA
In this example, the epithelial component is mostly solid.
Note the difference between the more vesicular epithelial
cell nuclei and the darker spindle cell nuclei.

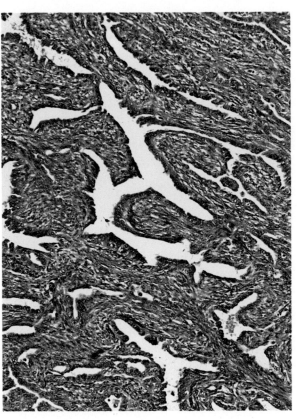

Figure 11-76
BIPHASIC SYNOVIAL SARCOMA
WITH PAPILLARY PATTERN
Cuboidal epithelial cells line the surfaces of the papillae,
while the cores are composed of spindle cells.

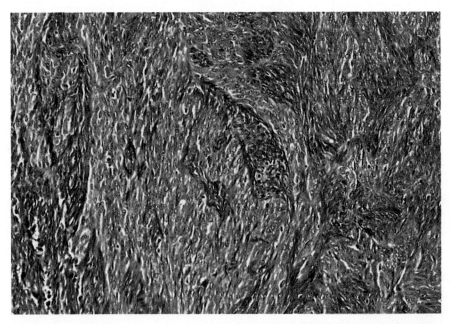

Figure 11-77
BIPHASIC
SYNOVIAL SARCOMA
Occasionally the cells of the
epithelial component are spindle
shaped; however, their open nuclei
contrast sharply with the darker
nuclei of the spindle cells and they
have more abundant cytoplasm.

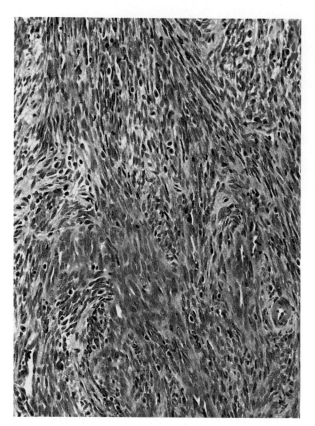 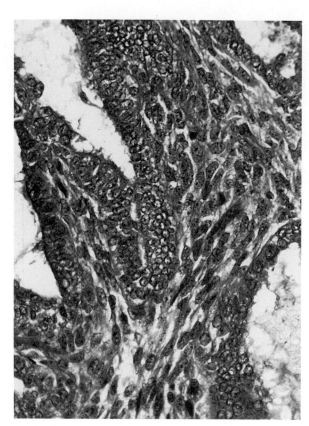

Figure 11-78
BIPHASIC SYNOVIAL SARCOMA
The spindle cells are small, uniform, and closely packed and have a high nuclear-cytoplasmic ratio. The chromatin is often finely stippled.

The spindle cell component of biphasic synovial sarcomas is made up of small, uniform spindled cells with a high nuclear-cytoplasmic ratio, growing in solid sheets or fascicles (fig. 11-78, left). Occasionally, the cells are more rounded than spindled, but when this occurs they maintain their small size and scant cytoplasm (fig. 11-79). The spindle cell nuclei stain darkly and usually have evenly distributed, finely stippled chromatin (fig. 11-78, right). The tapered cytoplasm is often hard to discern and cell margins are usually indistinct. Areas of nodularity, a swirling pattern, and foci of myxoid change or fine fibrosis with decreased cellularity may be observed. There are three characteristic findings in the spindle cell component which, although not always present, are very distinctive when they are: 1) thick, ropy collagen bundles that contrast with the thin adjacent cells and may be almost osteoid-like (fig. 11-80); 2) calcification (figs. 11-81, 11-82);

and 3) a rich, hemangiopericytoma-like vascular network (fig. 11-83). The extent of calcification is variable but may be massive and often is detected by imaging studies.

Monophasic synovial sarcoma is recognized by its resemblance to the spindle cell component of biphasic synovial sarcomas. Our basic histologic criteria for this diagnosis require the cells to be of the appropriate small, uniform type, as described above, and, since the cytologic features while characteristic are not entirely specific by themselves, it is very helpful if at least one of the three other distinctive findings enumerated just above is present (figs. 11-78, 11-80, 11-81, 11-83, 11-84) (181,186). Other features observed in the spindle cell component of both biphasic and monophasic synovial sarcomas include, rather frequently, numerous mast cells and, less frequently and focally, nuclear palisading, pseudorosette formation, a myxoid stroma, a herring-bone pattern,

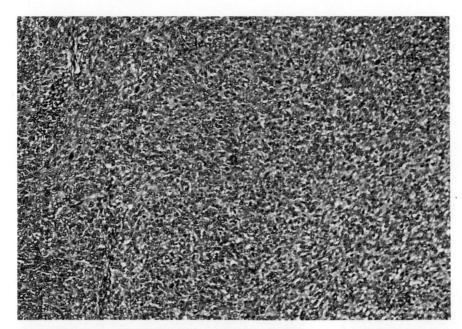

Figure 11-79
BIPHASIC SYNOVIAL
SARCOMA: SPINDLE
CELL COMPONENT
In this area of the spindle cell component, the cells are more rounded than spindled and their nuclei are vesicular. However, the paucity of cytoplasm indicates they are spindle cells rather than epithelial cells.

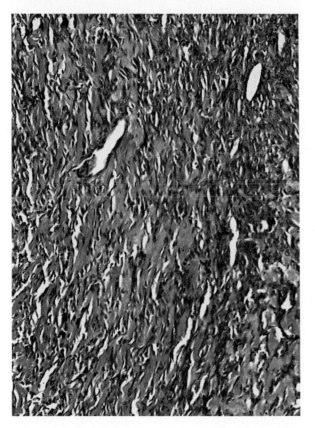
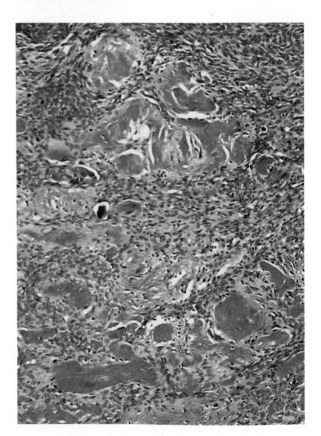

Figure 11-80
MONOPHASIC SYNOVIAL SARCOMA
Thick collagen bundles are characteristic of synovial sarcoma and their presence in a spindle cell tumor should cause the observer to think of synovial sarcoma. The cells demonstrate the typical small size, uniformity, and high nuclear-cytoplasmic ratio of monophasic synovial sarcoma and the spindle cell component of biphasic synovial sarcoma. There is no epithelial component. The collagen can be almost osteoid-like (right).

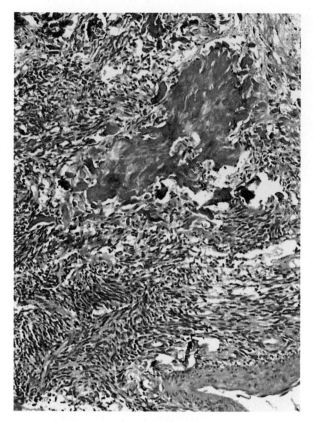

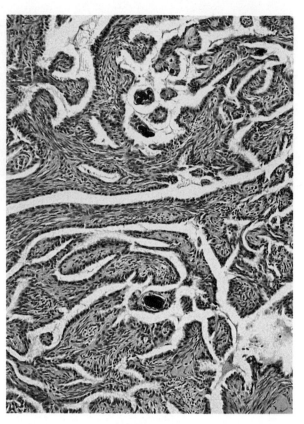

Figure 11-81
MONOPHASIC SYNOVIAL SARCOMA
An area of calcification is present. The cells are of the appropriate small, uniform type. Calcification is common in synovial sarcomas and always should cause the observer to think of this possibility.

Figure 11-82
BIPHASIC SYNOVIAL SARCOMA
An unusual form of calcification is the presence of psammomatous formations in the cores of papillae in the papillary variant of biphasic synovial sarcoma.

and a retiform microcystic arrangement of the tumor cells (figs. 11-85, 11-86). Areas of slightly larger cells that blend into adjacent areas composed of the usual small cells may be present and are not generally considered to be evidence of a biphasic pattern (fig. 11-87). Occasionally, zones of moderately large, rounded, somewhat epithelioid cells growing in solid sheets and lacking lumens are found along with areas of small spindle cells, although not intermingled in a biphasic pattern (fig. 11-88) (186). These cells are identical to those composing the epithelioid variant of poorly differentiated synovial sarcoma (see below). More than mild nuclear pleomorphism is not allowed in the definition of synovial sarcoma and the only tumors we have accepted as monophasic synovial sarcoma with significant pleomorphism are ones excised after irradiation or recurrences in elderly patients. Another un-

usual occurrence is metaplastic bone or cartilage formation (216).

The mitotic rate is variable, and in biphasic examples division figures may be found in both the epithelial and spindle cell components. Tumor cell necrosis is not infrequent, especially in larger neoplasms, and large areas of cystic change are occasionally observed. Local recurrences typically resemble the original tumor, although in biphasic examples the proportion of epithelial and spindle cell elements may vary (the spindle cell component is more often increased). Regional lymph node metastases from biphasic synovial sarcomas that are predominantly epithelial often maintain the dominance of the epithelial component, or even increase it. Distant metastases of biphasic synovial sarcoma may contain both components or either alone; in the latter event it is more frequently the spindle

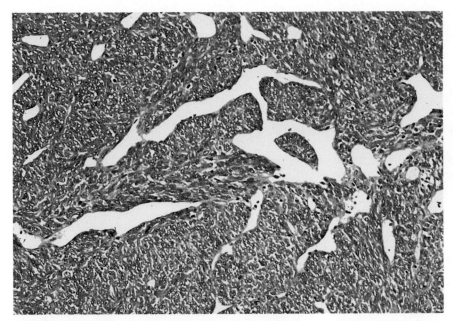

Figure 11-83
MONOPHASIC
SYNOVIAL SARCOMA

A hemangiopericytoma-like vascular pattern in monophasic synovial sarcoma is shown here. Thick collagen bundles, calcification, and hemangiopericytoma-like vascularity, as illustrated in figures 11-80, 11-81, 11-83, and 11-84, are commonly seen in the spindle cell component of biphasic synovial sarcoma and are very helpful in the diagnosis of monophasic synovial sarcoma (see text). Whenever a diagnosis of hemangiopericytoma is contemplated, synovial sarcoma should be considered also.

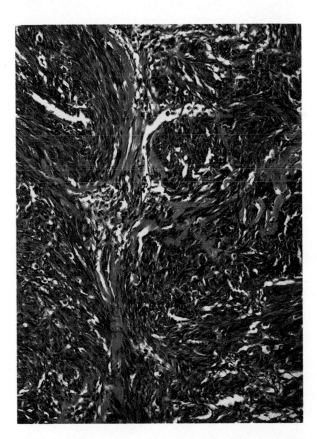
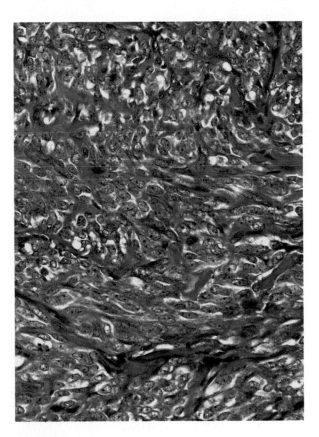

Figure 11-84
MONOPHASIC SYNOVIAL SARCOMA

The nuclei of the spindle cells often but not always appear quite dense at low magnification (note the osteoid-like collagen) (left) and often have stippled chromatin (right).

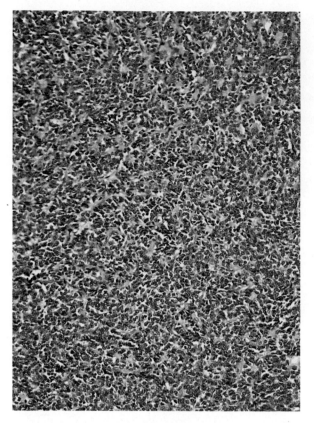

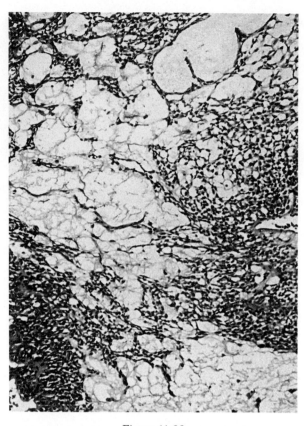

Figure 11-85
MONOPHASIC SYNOVIAL SARCOMA
Pseudorosette formation is a rare occurrence in synovial sarcoma. When glands are not present, distinction from peripheral neuroectodermal tumor is aided by the presence of more typical spindle cell areas elsewhere. CD99 is often positive as it is in PPNET/Ewing's sarcoma.

Figure 11-86
RETIFORM, MICROCYSTIC PATTERN
IN SYNOVIAL SARCOMA
This pattern is occasionally observed in the spindle cell component of biphasic synovial sarcoma and in monophasic synovial sarcoma.

Figure 11-87
MONOPHASIC
SYNOVIAL SARCOMA
Areas with somewhat larger cells and more open nuclei blend with adjacent smaller cells with darker nuclei. Although the cells with more vesicular nuclei resemble those in the epithelial areas of a biphasic tumor, they do not have much cytoplasm. Therefore, we do not consider this to represent a biphasic pattern, although it borders on such.

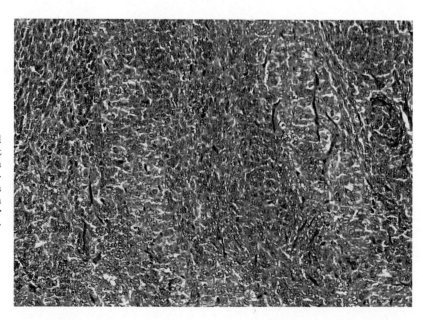

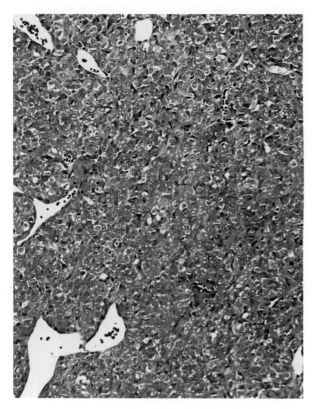

Figure 11-88
SYNOVIAL SARCOMA WITH SOLID ZONES
OF LARGER ROUNDED EPITHELIOID CELLS
There are occasional synovial sarcomas that have discrete areas with a solid (nongland-forming) proliferation of moderately large, rounded epithelioid cells. Other areas of the tumor invariably contain smaller spindle cells typical of monophasic synovial sarcoma.

cell component that is solely present but occasionally a metastatic synovial sarcoma may consist entirely of epithelial elements. Recurrences and metastases of monophasic synovial sarcoma almost always contain only the spindle cell component, i.e., such tumors remain monophasic.

A poorly differentiated form of synovial sarcoma characterized by a solid proliferation of uniform, closely packed, relatively small rounded to spindled cells, resembling those found in small round cell tumors, at most a vague or focal biphasic pattern, and frequently a hemangiopericytoma-like vascular network has been reported (185,188,210,238a). Rarely, structures resembling pseudorosettes may be present. In addition, some investigators have placed tumors composed of epithelioid cells with round irregular nuclei and prominent nucleoli (epithelioid vari-

ant) and those in which the spindle cells grow in fibrosarcoma-like fascicles (fibrosarcoma-like variant) in the poorly differentiated category (238). Poorly differentiated areas may be found in up to 20 percent of otherwise characteristic synovial sarcomas. Identifying typical patterns elsewhere allows proper classification of such tumors as synovial sarcoma (185). Very rarely, synovial sarcomas may be entirely poorly differentiated. The tumor cells in poorly differentiated examples, whether focally present in an otherwise typical synovial sarcoma or composing the entire tumor, contain the characteristic t(x;18) translocation (see below) (238a).

We think tumors with focal areas of poor differentiation should be classified as "synovial sarcoma with focal poorly differentiated areas" and those composed entirely of poorly differentiated cells as "poorly differentiated synovial sarcoma." Poorly differentiated histology, whether focal or diffuse, may have prognostic importance (see Treatment and Prognosis below).

Special Studies. Immunohistochemically, the epithelial component of biphasic synovial sarcoma stains for cytokeratin in almost 100 percent of cases and EMA is also frequently expressed. The spindle cells in some but not all tumors also express cytokeratin or EMA although the staining is usually focal and less intense than that observed in the epithelial cells (179,181,185,189,203,205, 212,213,218,220,229,235). The reported range of tumors that contain cytokeratin-positive spindled cells is wide but roughly half of the monophasic cases and two thirds to three fourths of the biphasic cases contain such cells. In a smaller percentage of cases the spindle cells express EMA; however, spindle cells that express EMA also usually express keratin. Examples of EMA-positive, keratin-negative monophasic synovial sarcomas have been reported (173,238a). Vimentin is expressed by the epithelial elements in about 15 to 30 percent of biphasic tumors. The spindle cells, whether in monophasic or biphasic tumors, express vimentin in 80 to 90 percent of cases. Carcinoembryonic antigen is expressed by the epithelial, and less often, the spindle cells in a few synovial sarcomas and the staining is usually focal. About a third of tumors are S-100 protein positive, usually in a focal distribution, and 60 percent contain CD99-positive cells (182, 185,190,196,221). The latter antibody stains the tumor cells in nearly all PPNET/ES sarcomas. A recent study of poorly differentiated synovial sarcoma found that only about 40 percent are keratin positive but 95 percent were EMA positive (238a). Like the usual synovial sarcoma, a significant number of poorly differentiated examples are CD99 and S-100 protein positive (238a). Another recent study largely confirmed these results and also reported that 9 out of 10 tumors were positive for CD57, 8 of 8 for CD56, and 6 of 10 for neurofilaments (190a).

Ultrastructurally, the epithelial cells of biphasic synovial sarcoma demonstrate features expected in epithelial cells. These include desmosomes, microvilli on luminal surfaces, juxtaluminal tight junctions, and basement membrane at the border with the spindle cell component. The cells of the latter are less distinctive but may display desmosomes and more poorly formed junctions, focal basement membrane material, and cytoplasmic processes, especially adjacent to small intercellular spaces, which clearly distinguishes them from fibroblasts (173,181,183,189,191,211,221).

Cytogenetic evaluation of synovial sarcomas, both biphasic and monophasic, has demonstrated a balanced translocation involving chromosomes X and 18 in up to 90 percent of cases (180,198,200, 204,209,218,224,236). This translocation is probably not specific for synovial sarcoma, but the type of *SYT-SSX* gene fusion transcript may influence the morphologic subtype of synovial sarcoma. Biphasic tumors appear to uniformly contain a *SYT-SSX*1 fusion transcript, whereas equal numbers of monophasic tumors contain the *SYT-SSX*1 and *SYT-SSX*2 fusion transcript (198a,238). Fluorescent in situ hybridization and reverse transcription polymerase chain reaction can be utilized to detect the *SYT-SSX* fusion gene associated with t(x;18). Diagnostically, these techniques may be useful when synovial sarcomas are poorly differentiated or have unusual histologic features.

Differential Diagnosis. Because of its distinctive composition, biphasic synovial sarcoma is unlikely to be confused with other neoplasms. The only other malignant soft tissue tumor that has a biphasic pattern is the glandular variant of malignant peripheral nerve sheath tumor (MPNST)(241). The glands in this tumor, however, unlike those in biphasic synovial sarcoma, usually

are formed by cells that contain cytoplasmic as well as luminal mucin; there is also a second population of basally located chromogranin-positive cells of neuroendocrine type. Also, the spindle cells, which generally comprise the bulk of glandular MPNST, are often larger than those of the spindle cell component of biphasic synovial sarcoma, although not always, and may demonstrate pleomorphism. Thick collagen bundles, calcification, and hemangiopericytoma-like vascularity, common findings in synovial sarcoma, are not usually features of MPNST (whether glandular or not), and MPNSTs usually demonstrably arise from a major nerve, from a neurofibroma, or in a patient with neurofibromatosis (or more than one of these).

Biphasic synovial sarcomas in which the epithelial component greatly outweighs the spindle cell component are occasionally confused with metastatic or skin adnexal adenocarcinoma. This problem can be avoided by careful search for the spindle cell component, which may be quite focal. We have seen rare purely epithelial metastases from a biphasic synovial sarcoma, as indicated previously; the history and imaging studies are critical for making this diagnosis. Skin adnexal (sweat gland) adenocarcinomas would, in general, be expected to be more superficial than synovial sarcoma, as would mixed tumors and myoepitheliomas.

Monophasic synovial sarcoma is most likely to be confused with fibrosarcoma; in fact, it has been argued in the past that monophasic synovial sarcoma cannot be distinguished from fibrosarcoma (207). However, we believe that it is clearly separable and distinguishable on the basis of the criteria given above, namely, small, uniform cells with a high nuclear-cytoplasmic ratio associated with thick collagen bundles, calcification, or hemangiopericytoma-like vascularity. This position is of course further supported by the clinical similarity of monophasic to biphasic synovial sarcoma and by the presence of the same chromosomal translocation in both. On the other hand, fibrosarcoma is a spindle cell sarcoma without specialized differentiation in which the cells are arranged in bundles that intersect at acute angles (see Fibrous Tumors). The rare fibrosarcoma-like variant of poorly differentiated synovial sarcoma can be distinguished from fibrosarcoma by finding characteristic areas of synovial sarcoma elsewhere in the tumor or by immunohistochemistry, chromosomal analysis, or molecular techniques (see Special Studies above).

The cells in leiomyosarcoma have longer nuclei and more abundant cytoplasm than the spindle cells of synovial sarcoma and are often desmin positive. A biphasic pattern is not seen in leiomyosarcoma but smooth muscle tumors may contain keratin-positive or epithelioid cells. Epithelioid sarcoma occurs at roughly the same age as synovial sarcoma but is often superficial rather than deep, and many occur on the distal extremities rather than near a large joint. Epithelioid sarcoma grows with a more pronounced nodular pattern than synovial sarcoma and central necrosis of the nodules is often a prominent feature. The cells in epithelioid sarcoma may superficially resemble the epithelial cells in biphasic synovial sarcoma or the cells in the epithelioid variant of synovial sarcoma. This is particularly a problem when dealing with the proximal variant of epithelioid sarcoma (195). The constituent cells of epithelioid sarcoma consistently express an antigen recognized by keratin, but they have more deeply eosinophilic cytoplasm and do not form the glands found in most biphasic synovial sarcomas. Moreover, the cells in about half of epithelioid sarcomas express CD34, a reaction that is not seen in synovial sarcoma cells.

The cells in clear cell sarcoma have a plump, spindled to epithelioid appearance but are arranged in packets separated by delicate connective tissue, do not form glands, and have large eosinophilic nucleoli. S-100 protein is strongly and diffusely expressed by the tumor cells in almost all clear cell sarcomas and HMB45 is commonly expressed, whereas keratin is negative. S-100 protein expression is found in about a third of synovial sarcomas, but is usually focal. Synovial sarcoma of the neck has some similarity to the tumor known as spindled epithelial tumor with thymus-like differentiation or spindle cell tumor of the thyroid, but the latter contains cysts lined by mucinous epithelium not found in synovial sarcoma and the spindle cells have less dense chromatin.

A monophasic synovial sarcoma with a prominent hemangiopericytoma-like vascular pattern could be confused with hemangiopericytoma. However, monophasic synovial sarcoma would, in general, be expected to have greater cellularity with a higher nuclear-cytoplasmic ratio, more mitotic figures, and at least focal areas without hemangiopericytoma-like vascularity. In addition, the cells of hemangiopericytoma tend to have irregular nuclei and to follow the contours of the vessels in a "tuft and weave" pattern that differs from the straighter cell alignment of synovial sarcoma. We suspect that some cases that have been reported as "malignant hemangiopericytoma" were actually monophasic synovial sarcoma; certainly before a tumor is deemed to be a hemangiopericytoma, synovial sarcoma should be excluded.

The small round cells in poorly differentiated synovial sarcoma can lead to confusion with PPNET/ES. The latter does not feature the spindle cells that are characteristic of synovial sarcoma and PPNET/ES lacks the hemangiopericytoma-like vascular pattern and thick bundles of collagen present in most synovial sarcomas. It should be kept in mind that CD99-positive cells can be found in both. Molecular techniques may be needed in doubtful cases to detect either the t(x;18) translocation in synovial sarcoma or the t(11;22) translocation in PPNET/ES.

Sometimes monophasic synovial sarcomas, especially those of smaller size that have myxoid or fibrous areas of lesser cellularity, are misdiagnosed as a benign neoplasm, particularly schwannoma (neurilemoma). This error is particularly likely if nuclear palisading is present. Schwannoma, however, differs from monophasic synovial sarcoma in that it is encapsulated, may be recognizably related to a nerve, often has wavy-appearing nuclei, sometimes has cellular fascicles separated by hypocellular tissue, may show nuclear pleomorphism ("ancient" changes), demonstrates fibrotic or hyalinized thick-walled vessels, generally lacks the thick collagen bundles and hemangiopericytoma-like vascularity of the type seen in synovial sarcoma (although calcification may be present), and is consistently and diffusely S-100 protein positive and keratin negative.

Treatment and Prognosis. Synovial sarcoma has a reputation for being an aggressive sarcoma both in terms of local recurrence and distant metastasis, but patient survival is about the same as with many other sarcomas. Recurrences and metastases usually become manifest during the first few years after diagnosis but may do so considerably later (185,201,219).

In general, local recurrence is related to inadequate local therapy, with the recurrence rate significantly higher when treatment consists of excision alone rather than excision combined with radiation (186). The major predictor of distant metastasis is tumor size: distant metastasis occurs in a high proportion of cases when a synovial sarcoma measures 5 cm or more in its greatest dimension but is relatively uncommon when the tumor is smaller than this (186). Since patient survival is primarily related to distant metastasis, tumor size is also the primary determinant of survival (174,178,186,202,227,230,234,242,243, 245). No consistent difference in tumor behavior between biphasic and monophasic synovial sarcomas has been observed (174,186,196,201,219,223, 227,234,242,243,245); intervals to recurrence and metastasis and patient survival were somewhat longer with monophasic synovial sarcoma in a study carried out by one of us (186), but the differences were not statistically significant. More recent investigations have suggested that poorly differentiated synovial sarcoma may have a worse prognosis than conventional synovial sarcoma (199). In one study more than 20 percent poorly differentiated areas in a synovial sarcoma significantly worsened the prognosis (206). Favorable prognostic factors other than small tumor size that have been proposed by various investigators include prominent calcification (239), a high proportion of glandular and epithelial elements (176), numerous mast cells (219,237), DNA diploidy (184), low proliferating cell nuclear antigen (PCNA) score (220), and low mitotic rate (176, 184,194,219,227,234,245). However, there has been disagreement about the importance of these findings among different studies, and we suspect that they are all more likely to be present in small synovial sarcomas than in large ones and may not have independent significance. The 82 percent 5-year survival rate reported by Varela-Duran and Enzinger (239) for highly calcified tumors is the best ever recorded.

Another prognostic factor in synovial sarcoma may be related to the type of *SYT-SSX* fusion gene transcript. Patients with *SYT-SSX*2 fusion transcripts and monophasic synovial sarcoma appear to have a lower risk of early metastases and have a better short-term survival rate than patients with *SYT-SSX*1 fusion transcripts and biphasic synovial sarcoma (198a,218a).

Epithelioid Sarcoma

Definition. Epithelioid sarcoma is a histologically distinctive malignant soft tissue tumor which is composed of cells that have the light microscopic appearance, ultrastructural features, and immunohistologic profile of epithelial cells.

General Considerations. In spite of its name, which suggests it is only epithelial-like, the constituent cells of epithelioid sarcoma actually have the immunohistochemical profile of epithelial cells and resemble epithelial cells by light microscopy. Thus, epithelioid sarcoma is, in some sense, a carcinoma arising in the soft tissue although the more generally held concept is that it is a sarcoma with an epithelial phenotype. There are other sarcomas with an epithelial phenotype including synovial sarcoma, epithelioid vascular tumors, and gland-forming neural tumors (however, the cells in epithelioid nerve sheath tumors are keratin negative).

The clinical and pathologic features of the usual or classic epithelioid sarcoma are well known. More recently, it has been suggested that a subset of the tumors, usually classified as nonrenal malignant rhabdoid tumors presenting in adults, has histologic and immunologic features similar enough to epithelioid sarcoma to include it within the latter category (255). However, these tumors demonstrate significant clinical and histologic differences from "classic" epithelioid sarcoma and at least for the present time we think they should be considered to be a separate type of epithelioid sarcoma. In the following discussion the term epithelioid sarcoma refers to classic epithelioid sarcoma and *proximal type epithelioid sarcoma* refers to the tumor formerly classified by some and still classified by others as extrarenal malignant rhabdoid tumor. Proximal epithelioid sarcoma is also known as *large cell epithelioid sarcoma*.

Clinical Features. Classic epithelioid sarcoma most frequently occurs in young adults and teenagers but rarely it can occur in children and older adults (248,265). There is an approximately 2 to 1 ratio of male to female patients. The predominant tumor location by far is the distal upper extremity, especially the fingers, hand, and wrist, but it can arise in other sites, particularly the distal lower extremity (247,249,252,253). It is most rare in the trunk and head and neck. Examples have been reported in the vulva and penis (257,268, 270) but most if not all of these are probably the proximal type of epithelioid sarcoma (see above). Epithelioid sarcoma may arise in the subcutis or in the deeper soft tissues; in the latter instance, there is often involvement of tendons, tendon sheath, or fascial tissue. When it is superficial there can be upward extension of the tumor into the dermis and even ulceration of the epidermis. In this latter circumstance, epithelioid sarcoma is easily mistaken clinically for an inflammatory process with draining sinuses or ulcers. The tumor may be uninodular or multinodular and most often is ill-defined. Classic epithelioid sarcoma varies in size from less than 1 cm to quite large (up to 7.5 cm in a series studied by one of us [253]). Occasional patients with epithelioid sarcoma have multiple tumor nodules extending up the extremity, usually the arm, or enlarged, involved regional lymph nodes at presentation.

The median age of patients with the proximal type of epithelioid sarcoma is around 35 years, which is somewhat older than patients with classic epithelioid sarcoma (255). Patients present with a mass and there is a predilection for the tumor to develop in the genitalia, especially the vulva and penis, the pelvis, and the buttocks although the proximal extremities, trunk, and head and neck also can be involved. As would be expected from their sites of predilection, most proximal epithelioid sarcomas are large and can grow to 20 cm or more.

Pathologic Findings. Grossly, epithelioid sarcoma characteristically forms a mononodular or multinodular mass with irregular, often ill-defined borders (249). The cut surface varies from white to gray to tan and frequently necrosis can be appreciated.

Microscopically at low power most classic epithelioid sarcomas are composed of cells with eosinophilic cytoplasm aggregated into nodules in which brightly eosinophilic collagen is also present (fig. 11-89) (249,252). Usually the tumor nodules, which may undergo central necrosis, are well defined and separated by hyalinized paucicellular collagen, but in some tumors they are inconspicuous or ill-formed or they may fuse together to form irregular larger masses which frequently undergo necrosis (figs. 11-90, 11-91) (252). In many cases, in addition to a nodular pattern, there are areas of more diffuse sheet-like growth

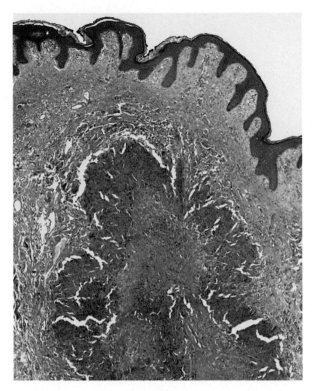

Figure 11-89
EPITHELIOID SARCOMA

A nodular growth pattern with necrotic centers causes epithelioid sarcoma to resemble a granuloma. Consequently, this neoplasm should enter the differential diagnosis of an apparent granuloma of the skin or soft tissue, particularly if an extremity is involved.

of the tumor cells or an irregular growth pattern in which columns of tumor cells stream through the stroma in a serpiginous fashion (fig. 11-92). Chronic inflammatory cells are commonly present, usually at the periphery of the nodules.

The tumor cells that compose classic epithelioid sarcoma range from medium-sized to large and their shape varies from rounded or oval to plump spindled (253). The rounded cells resemble epithelial cells while the spindled forms can resemble fibroblasts. Both have relatively large nuclei and the more rounded cells have abundant, brightly eosinophilic cytoplasm and easily seen cell margins (figs. 11-93, 11-94) (252). Both types of cells blend with one another although the spindle cells tend to predominate at the periphery of the nodules. Rare examples made up entirely of spindle cells (*the fibroma-like variant*) have been reported (261). Nuclear pleomorphism is generally slight but may be moderate in

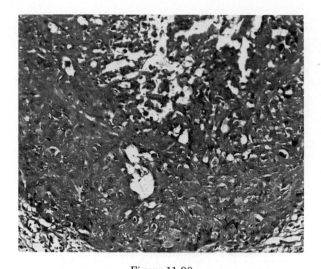

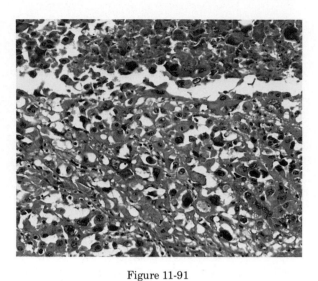

Figure 11-90
EPITHELIOID SARCOMA
A round nodule of tumor with central necrosis resembles a granuloma.

Figure 11-91
EPITHELIOID SARCOMA
Central necrosis in the nodules of epithelioid sarcoma is common.

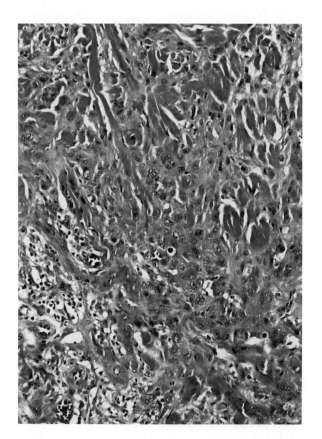

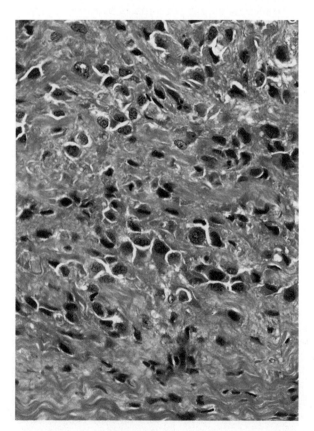

Figure 11-92
EPITHELIOID SARCOMA
The collagen as well as the tumor cell cytoplasm is usually eosinophilic in epithelioid sarcoma. In the left figure, cells are arranged in sheets while in the right they are arranged in columns.

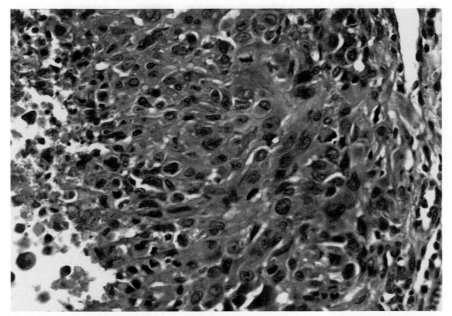

Figure 11-93
EPITHELIOID SARCOMA
Most often, viable tumor cells are at the periphery of the tumor nodule. The cells display their characteristic highly eosinophilic cytoplasm.

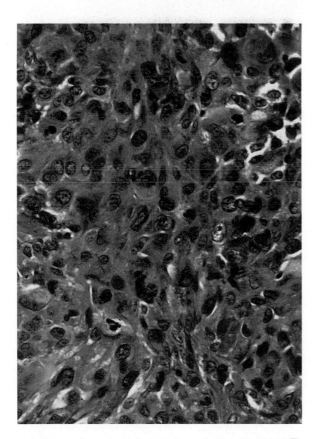
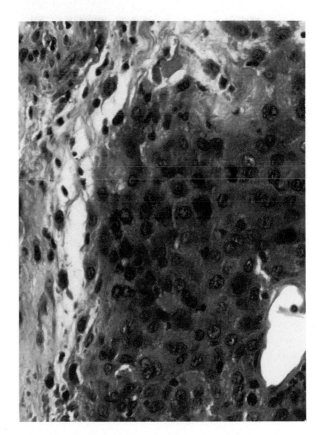

Figure 11-94
EPITHELIOID SARCOMA
The cells in epithelioid sarcoma are generally more atypical than those in a granuloma and their brightly eosinophilic cytoplasm is a helpful clue to the correct diagnosis.

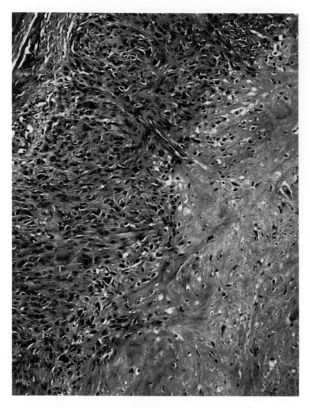

Figure 11-95
EPITHELIOID SARCOMA
Sometimes the centers of tumor nodules are made up of eosinophilic hyalinized collagen or myxoid tissue.

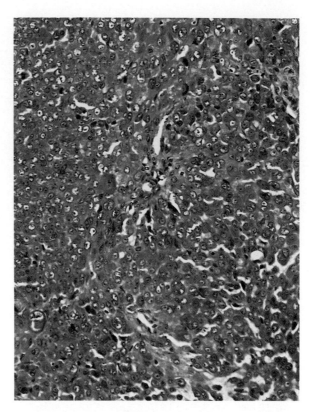

Figure 11-96
EPITHELIOID SARCOMA, PROXIMAL TYPE
The epithelioid tumor cells in the proximal type tumors are arranged in a vaguely nodular pattern but not in the granuloma type pattern seen in classic epithelioid sarcoma. Intranodular collagen is absent or sparse.

areas and mitotic figures are usually sparse but can be numerous (fig. 11-94). Some tumors contain cells with intracytoplasmic vacuoles or rhabdoid type inclusions. Perineural invasion is common but vascular involvement is rare, although vascular invasion is more common in recurrences. It is common for epithelioid sarcoma to grow along tendons and fascia beyond the grossly visible margins of the tumor so complete excision is often difficult. A higher mitotic rate, more prominent necrosis, and perineural invasion appear to be more frequently observed in larger tumors. Metastatic lesions generally resemble the primary neoplasm, although nodular growth may be less prominent microscopically.

Features seen in a minority of cases include extensive hyalinization, focal calcification, metaplastic bone, myxoid areas, hemorrhage, cyst formation or pseudovascular spaces secondary to discohesion of the tumor cells, a focal storiform arrangement of spindle cells, and

smaller tumor cells with inconspicuous cytoplasm (fig. 11-95) (249). Sometimes the latter are arranged linearly in a manner reminiscent of lobular carcinoma (fig. 11-92, right).

The profile that should cause the observer to think of classic epithelioid sarcoma is a teen-aged or young adult patient with a nodular or ulcerated lesion on the distal extremity that has a microscopic pattern reminiscent of a granuloma, rheumatoid nodule, or carcinoma, particularly if the constituent cells have abundant, brightly eosinophilic cytoplasm and sharp cell margins.

The histologic pattern of the proximal type of epithelioid sarcoma is intermediate between that of epithelioid sarcoma and extrarenal malignant rhabdoid tumor (255). Similarities to epithelioid sarcoma include an often nodular growth pattern, although intranodular collagen and granuloma-like tumor growth with central necrosis of nodules is frequently lacking (fig. 11-96). Features that are different from classic epithelioid sarcoma and more like rhabdoid tumor are large cells with copious amphophilic rather than eosinophilic cytoplasm and large nuclei (fig. 11-97). The nuclei are either pleomorphic with inconspicuous nucleoli or vesicular with prominent nucleoli (fig. 11-98). Discohesion may not be as prominent as in the usual extrarenal malignant rhabdoid tumor.

Special Studies. The constituent cells of epithelioid sarcoma are mucin negative, express both high and low weight keratins, and demonstrate membrane staining with EMA (250,258, 259). Keratin staining is usually diffuse and strong although it may be focal in some tumors; it is so universally present in epithelioid sarcoma that it has become definitional for the diagnosis of this tumor. Co-expression of vimentin is also found in nearly all epithelioid sarcomas (246, 259). About 50 percent of epithelioid sarcomas

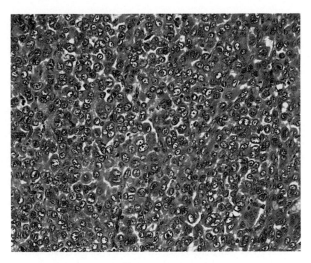

Figure 11-97
EPITHELIOID SARCOMA, PROXIMAL TYPE
Sheet-like growth of cells with malignant rhabdoid-like features is seen in many proximal type tumors.

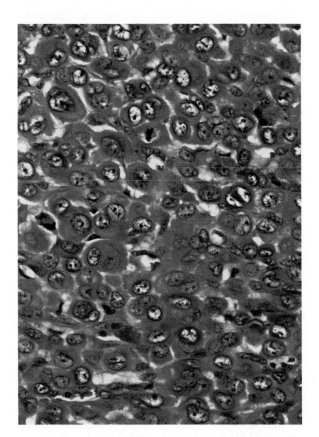 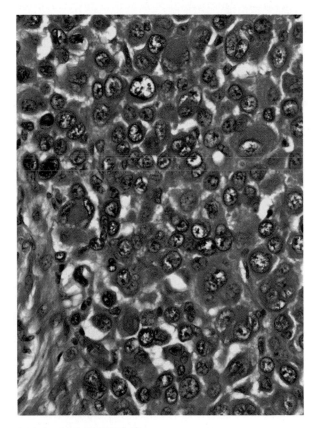

Figure 11-98
EPITHELIOID SARCOMA, PROXIMAL TYPE
The cells in the proximal type more closely resemble the cells in adult malignant rhabdoid tumors with their large nuclei, prominent nucleoli, and amphophilic rather than highly eosinophilic cytoplasm. Cytoplasmic inclusions are prominent on the right.

contain CD34-positive cells (246,269). A positive CD34 stain is very useful because this antibody rarely decorates carcinomas or melanomas, two major considerations in the differential diagnosis of epithelioid sarcoma. We think keratin and CD34 stains should be routinely considered if epithelioid sarcoma is in the differential diagnosis (246). S-100 protein and CD31 are focally positive in rare cases while factor VIII is negative (246, 266). Ultrastructurally, the most notable feature is intracytoplasmic intermediate filaments, which are often aggregated into a mass in a paranuclear location (254,258,260). Occasionally, there are interdigitating cell processes, desmosome-like junctions, and small pseudolumens. Loss of heterozygosity of chromosome 22q in 6 of 10 epithelioid sarcomas suggests that there may be a suppressor gene in this region that may play a role in the pathogenesis of epithelioid sarcoma (264). Reports about the ploidy of the tumor cells are contradictory (251,258,262).

The immunohistochemical profile of the proximal type of epithelioid sarcoma is similar to that of classic epithelioid sarcoma (255). Ultrastructurally, the tumor cells often contain paranuclear, intracytoplasmic, intermediate filament aggregates and some tumor cells demonstrate evidence of epithelial differentiation.

Differential Diagnosis. Because epithelioid sarcoma resembles so many other lesions, both reactive and neoplastic, the differential diagnosis is extensive. However, the immunohistochemical profile of epithelioid sarcoma outlined above is very helpful in identifying this neoplasm. The reactive process most often confused with epithelioid sarcoma, in our experience, is a palisaded granuloma such as rheumatoid nodule or granuloma annulare (particularly deep granuloma annulare). Thinking about the possibility of epithelioid sarcoma whenever a diagnosis of palisaded granuloma is contemplated, particularly if the lesion is on the distal extremity, is important, as is the liberal use of immunohistochemistry (272). Epithelioid sarcoma also resembles granulomatous inflammation and abscesses containing histiocytes, but the cells in these latter lesions are not keratin or CD34 positive. Moreover, the cells in inflammatory and reactive processes are generally smaller and lack the distinct cytoplasmic eosinophilia and sharp cell membranes often displayed by the cells in classic epithelioid sarcoma.

The neoplasms most apt to be confused with epithelioid sarcoma, whether of the classic or proximal type, are squamous cell carcinoma, malignant melanoma, clear cell sarcoma, epithelioid angiosarcoma, epithelioid hemangioendothelioma, sweat gland tumors, metastatic carcinoma, localized tenosynovial giant cell tumor (giant cell tumor of tendon sheath), synovial sarcoma, malignant rhabdoid tumors, epithelioid malignant peripheral nerve sheath tumor (MPNST) and, when the cells of epithelioid sarcoma are predominantly spindled, fibrosarcoma.

Epithelioid sarcomas that have ulcerated the skin are those most likely to engender consideration of squamous cell carcinoma. However, the latter typically occurs in older people, is usually associated with actinic damage, often demonstrates dysplastic changes in adjacent epidermis, and at least focally displays keratinization. Positive keratin staining would obviously not be helpful in this differential but squamous cell carcinomas are CD34 negative and seldom co-express vimentin. Malignant melanoma may occur in young people and the constituent cells commonly are epithelioid. Distinguishing features of melanoma include a junctional component, pigmentation (not always present), lack of intralesional collagen bundles, and a fascicular or nested growth pattern. Deeply invasive and recurrent melanomas are most likely to create problems, and in these instances immunohistochemical positivity for S-100 protein (almost always) and HMB45 (often), together with negativity for keratin and CD34, allows recognition of melanoma. Clear cell sarcoma (malignant melanoma of soft parts) has the same immunohistochemical staining reactions as other malignant melanomas, and in addition, the characteristic histologic pattern is one of small groups of cells with clear to pale cytoplasm outlined by fibrous septa rather than the nodules of cells with eosinophilic cytoplasm and internodular collagen seen in epithelioid sarcoma.

Sweat gland tumors are more superficial than most epithelioid sarcomas and the cells do not express CD34 although they may be BRST-2 positive. However, rarely, mixed tumors and myoepitheliomas may be subfascial and epithelioid sarcoma may ulcerate the skin. These tumors are S-100 protein positive and often actin positive. Metastatic carcinoma is unusual on the distal extremities where epithelioid sarcoma is most common, it usually demonstrates more mitotic activity and pleomorphism, and the cells rarely are CD34 positive.

Epithelioid hemangioendothelioma and epithelioid angiosarcoma may cytologically resemble epithelioid sarcoma. The former usually has a myxoid to collagenous background that can compound the problem, but epithelioid hemangioendothelioma grows predominantly in small nests and cords, is often centered around or within the wall of a large vessel (normally a vein), and is uncommon on the distal extremities. Cytoplasmic vacuoles are found in both epithelioid hemangioendothelioma and epithelioid sarcoma so they are of no help in making a distinction between these two tumors. Immunohistochemical staining for CD31 is typically present in epithelioid hemangioendothelioma and keratin staining is normally absent, although the latter has been noted in a few cases. Epithelioid angiosarcoma is composed at least in part of large epithelioid cells growing in a sheetlike pattern. This is most often associated with vasoformative areas in the usual cutaneous/subcutaneous angiosarcoma, although the rare deep soft tissue angiosarcoma may lack such areas or they may be difficult to identify. Angiosarcoma cells, particularly when epithelioid, may express keratin and CD34 and often stain more weakly and inconsistently for vascular markers, especially factor VIII, than less malignant vascular neoplasms. However, CD31 is usually positive in angiosarcoma and usually negative in epithelioid sarcoma. Differential diagnostic help is provided by the lack of nodular growth and intranodular collagen in angiosarcoma and by the virtual absence of this tumor from the distal extremities except in the setting of chronic lymphedema.

Localized tenosynovial giant cell tumor (giant cell tumor of tendon sheath) is composed of cells whose nuclei can resemble those of epithelioid sarcoma; however, they generally lack the eosinophilic cytoplasm of the cells in epithelioid sarcoma. Moreover, the cells in epithelioid sarcoma are keratin positive and often CD34 positive, stains that are negative in tenosynovial giant cell tumor. Giant cells may be present in epithelioid sarcoma but are usually absent.

Synovial sarcomas may occur on the distal extremities and biphasic examples contain epithelial cells as well as spindled cells; the former are typically keratin positive and the latter may be. However, epithelioid sarcoma lacks a biphasic pattern, and glands, not a feature of epithelioid sarcoma, are often present in biphasic synovial sarcoma. The cells in synovial sarcoma do not express CD34 and ulceration, a not uncommon manifestation of epithelioid sarcoma, is distinctly rare in synovial sarcoma. A few synovial sarcomas contain epithelioid cells but such cells are almost always focal in an otherwise typical synovial sarcoma. Malignant rhabdoid tumors, while commonly keratin positive, are rare in the extremities, and the cells generally lack brightly eosinophilic cytoplasm and are not set within abundant eosinophilic collagen. Instead, they are discohesive and have prominent nucleoli.

The distinction between proximal epithelioid sarcoma and malignant rhabdoid tumor is often arbitrary and probably not of great importance because both tumors pursue an equally aggressive course. Nodular tumor growth would favor epithelioid sarcoma as does a positive CD34 stain. On the other hand, classic epithelioid sarcoma should be carefully distinguished from malignant rhabdoid tumor because of the better prognosis of the former. Epithelioid MPNST is keratin negative and may contain S-100 protein–positive cells; origin from a nerve or a neurofibroma may also help distinguish this tumor from epithelioid sarcoma. Fibrosarcoma, rare on the distal extremities, should only be a consideration when epithelioid sarcomas are predominantly composed of spindled cells, a rare event. Immunohistochemistry helps in this situation.

Treatment and Prognosis. Classic epithelioid sarcoma is prone to both local recurrence and distant metastasis, and is one of the few sarcomas that commonly metastasizes to regional lymph nodes (249). Local recurrence is very frequent when treatment of the primary lesion consists of simple excision alone, but is much less common when the excision is wide or is supplemented with radiation (256,267). If local recurrences become uncontrolled they can often be successfully treated by amputation but amputation as the initial therapy seems to offer little or no advantage over wide excision (271). At times, recurrence takes the form of tumor nodules spreading up the involved extremity (most often the arm) and metastases to the skin are common. This pattern of growth accounts for a significant percentage of uncontrolled local recurrences of epithelioid sarcoma. Regional lymph node metastasis is relatively frequent and is strongly associated with distant metastasis and death due to tumor (249). Distant metastases are most common in the lungs and the skin of the scalp; sites less often involved include other skin locations, bone, and distant lymph nodes. Both local recurrence and metastasis usually occur in the first few years after diagnosis but may become manifest after considerably longer intervals (252). Overall, the long-term survival rate is about 65 to 70 percent (256,249).

Unfavorable prognostic factors identified in different series include older patient age, male sex, more proximal tumor location, larger tumor size, higher mitotic rate, tumor cell necrosis, vascular invasion (rare in our experience), and local recurrence, in addition to regional lymph node metastasis (248,249,256,263). In a study carried out by one of us, tumor size was the major parameter related to outcome: patients with neoplasms

5 cm or larger experienced significantly shorter survival periods primarily as a result of more frequent distant metastasis (253). Regional lymph node metastasis was also more common when the tumor was 5 cm or larger, and this probably was responsible at least partly for the negative prognostic impact of larger size. When tumor size was taken into account, patient age and sex, tumor location, mitotic rate, and tumor necrosis were not significant predictors of survival or metastasis. Local recurrence was unrelated to survival in the group with large tumors, although there was a suggestion it might be an adverse indicator among patients with small tumors.

The proximal type of epithelioid sarcoma is much more aggressive than the classic type; in fact, proximal epithelioid sarcomas have a course identical to extrarenal malignant rhabdoid tumors, with frequent recurrences, a high incidence of metastasis, resistance to chemotherapy, and a high mortality rate. It is thus apparent that the proximal form of epithelioid sarcoma must be distinguished from the classic type.

REFERENCES

Intramuscular Myxoma

1. Dutz W, Stout AP. The myxoma in childhood. Cancer 1961;14:629–35.
2. Enzinger FM. Intramuscular myxoma. A review and follow-up study of 34 cases. Am J Clin Pathol 1965;43:104–13.
3. Hashimoto H, Tsuneyoshi M, Daimaru Y, Enjoji M, Shinohara N. Intramuscular myxoma. A clinicopathologic, immunohistochemical and electron microscopic study. Cancer 1986;58:740–7.
4. Ireland DC, Soule EH, Ivins JC. Myxoma of somatic soft tissues. A report of 58 patients, 3 with multiple tumors and fibrous dysplasia of bone. Mayo Clin Proc 1973;48:401–10.
5. Kindblom LG, Angervall L. Histochemical characterization of mucosubstances in bone and soft tissue tumors. Cancer 1975;38:958–96.
6. Kindblom LG, Stener B, Angervall L. Intramuscular myxoma. Cancer 1974;34:1737–44.
7. Miettinen M, Höckerstedt K, Reitamo J, Tötterman S. Intramuscular myxoma—a clinicopathological study of twenty three cases. Am J Clin Pathol 1985;84:265–72.
7a. Nielsen GP, O'Connell JX, Rosenberg AE. Intramuscular myxoma: a clinicopathologic study of 51 cases with emphasis on hypercellular and hypervascular variants. Am J Surg Pathol 1998;22:1222–7.
8. Rosin RD. Intramuscular myxomas. Br J Surg 1973;60:122–4.
9. Scott JE, Dorling J. Differential staining of acid glycosaminoglycans (mucopolysaccharides) by Alcian blue in salt solutions. Histochemie 1965;5:221–33.
10. Wirth WA, Leavitt D, Enzinger FM. Multiple intramuscular myxomas. Another extraskeletal manifestation of fibrous dysplasia. Cancer 1971;27:1167–73.

Juxta-articular Myxoma

11. Daluiski A, Seeger LL, Doberneck SA, Finerman GA, Eckardt JJ. A case of juxta-articular myxoma of the knee. Skeletal Radiol 1995;24:389–91.
12. Ghormley RK, Dockerty MB. Cystic myxomatous tumors about the knee: their relation to cysts of the menisci. J Bone Jt Surg 1943;25A:306–18.
13. Meis JM, Enzinger FM. Juxtaarticular myxoma. A clinical and pathologic study of 65 cases. Hum Pathol 1992;23:639–46.

Digital Myxoma

14. Hill TL, Jones BE, Park KH. Myxoma of the skin of the finger. J Am Acad Dermatol 1990;22:343–5.

15. Johnson WC, Graham JH, Helwig EB. Cutaneous myxoid cyst. A clinicopathological and histochemical study. JAMA 1965;191:15–20.

Aggressive Angiomyxoma

16. Begin LR, Clement PB, Kirk ME, Jothy S, McCaughey WT, Ferenczy A. Aggressive angiomyxoma of pelvic soft parts: a clinicopathologic study of nine cases. Hum Pathol 1985;16:621–8.

17. Clatch RJ, Drake WK, Gonzalez JG. Aggressive angiomyxoma in men. A report of two cases associated with inguinal hernias. Arch Pathol Lab Med 1993;117:911–3.

18. Fetsch JF, Laskin WB, Lefkowitz M, Kindblom LG, Meis-Kindblom JM. Aggressive angiomyxoma. A clinicopathologic study of 29 female patients. Cancer 1996;78:79–90.

19. Granter SR, Nucci M, Fletcher CD. Aggressive angiomyxoma: reappraisal of its relationship to angiomyofibroblastoma in a series of 16 cases. Histopathology 1997;30:3–10.

20. Iezzoni JC, Fechner RE, Wong LS, Rosai J. Aggressive angiomyxoma in males. A report of four cases. Am J Clin Pathol 1995;104:391–6.

21. Kazmierczak B, Wanschuwa S, Meyer-Bolte K, et al. Cytogenetic and molecular analysis of an aggressive angiomyxoma. Am J Pathol 1995;147:580–5.

21a.Kurman RJ, Norris HJ, Wilkinson E. Tumors of the cervix, vagina, and vulva. Atlas of Tumor Pathology. Fascicle 4, 2nd Series. Washington, D.C.: Armed Forces Institute of Pathology, 1992.

22. Skalova A, Michal M, Husek K, Zamecnik M, Leivo I. Aggressive angiomyxoma of the pelviperineal region. Immunohistochemical and ultrastructural study of seven cases. Am J Dermatopathol 1993;15:446–51.

23. Steeper TA, Rosai J. Aggressive angiomyxoma of the female pelvis and perineum. Report of nine cases of a distinctive type of gynecologic soft tissue neoplasm. Am J Surg Pathol 1983;7:463–75.

24. Tsang WY, Chan JK, Lee KC, Fisher C, Fletcher CD. Aggressive angiomyxoma. A report of four cases occurring in men. Am J Surg Pathol 1992;16:1059–65.

25. White J, Chan YF. Aggressive angiomyxoma of the vulva in an 11-year-old girl. Pediatr Pathol 1994;14:27–37.

26. Wick MR, Ockner DM, Sayadi H, Swanson PE, Ritter JH. Genital angiomyofibroblastoma: comparison with aggressive angiomyxoma and other myxoid neoplasms of skin and soft tissue. Am J Clin Pathol 1997;107:36–44.

Superficial Angiomyxoma

27. Allen PW, Dymock RB, MacCormac WB. Superficial angiomyxomas with or without epithelial components. Report of 30 tumors in 28 patients. Am J Surg Pathol 1988;12:519–30.

28. Carney JA, Headington JT, Wu SP. Cutaneous myxomas. A major component of the complex of myxomas, spotty pigmentation and endocrine overactivity. Arch Dermatol 1986;122:790–8.

29. Ferreiro JA, Carney JA. Myxomas of the external ear and their significance. Am J Surg Pathol 1994;18:274–80.

30. Fetsch JF, Laskin WB, Tavassoli FA. Superficial angiomyxoma (cutaneous myxoma): a study of 15 cases arising in the genital region. Int'l Gynecol Pathol 1997;16:325–34 .

31. Guerin D, Calonje E, McCormick D, Fletcher CD. Superficial angiomyxoma: clinicopathological analysis of a series of distinctive but poorly recognized cutaneous tumors with a tendency for recurrence. Am J Surg Pathol 1999;23:910–17.

Myxoid Lesions with Recurrent Potential

32. Allen PW, Dymock RB, MacCormac LB. Superficial angiomyxomas with and without epithelial components. Report of 30 tumors in 28 patients. Am J Surg Pathol 1988;12:519–30.

33. Meis JM, Enzinger FM. Juxta-articular myxoma: a clinical and pathologic study of 65 cases. Hum Pathol 1992;23:639–46.

34. Mentzel T, Calonje E, Wadden C, et al. Myxofibrosarcoma. Clinicopathologic analysis of 75 cases with emphasis on the low-grade variant. Am J Surg Pathol 1996;20:391–405.

35. Merck C, Angervall L, Kindblom LG, Oden A. Myxofibrosarcoma. A malignant soft tissue tumor of fibroblastic-histiocytic origin. A clinicopathologic and prognostic study of 110 cases using multivariate analysis. Acta Pathol Microbiol Immunol Scand Suppl 1983;282:1–40.

36. Nielsen GP, O'Connell JX, Rosenberg AE. Intramuscular myxoma. A clinicopathologic study of 51 cases with emphasis on the hypercellular variant. Am J Surg Pathol 1998;22:1222–7.

37. Steeper TA, Rosai J. Aggressive angiomyxoma of the female pelvis and perineum. Report of nine cases of a distinctive type of gynecologic soft-tissue neoplasm. Am J Surg Pathol 1983;7:463–75.

Angiomyofibroblastoma

38. Fletcher CD, Tsang WY, Fisher C, Lee KC, Chan JK. Angiomyofibroblastoma of the vulva. A benign neoplasm distinct from aggressive angiomyxoma. Am J Surg Pathol 1992;16:373–82.

39. Fukunaga M, Nomura K, Matsumato K, Doi K, Endo Y, Ushigome S. Vulval angiomyofibroblastoma. Clinicopathologic analysis of six cases. Am J Clin Pathol 1997;107:45–51.

40. Granter SR, Nucci MR, Fletcher CD. Aggressive angiomyxoma: reappraisal of its relationship to angiomyofibroblastoma in a series of 16 cases. Histopathology 1997;30:3–10.

41. Hiruki T, Thomas MJ, Clement PB. Vulvar angiomyofibroblastoma [Letter]. Am J Surg Pathol 1993;17:423–4.

42. Hisaoka M, Kouho H, Aoki T, Daimaru Y, Hashimoto H. Angiomyofibroblastoma of the vulva: a clinicopathologic study of seven cases. Pathol Int 1995;45:487–92.

43. Katenkamp D, Kosmehl H, Mentzel T, Reinke J. Angiomyofibroblastoma of the vulvar and paravaginal region—a new entity. Pathologe 1993;14:131–7.

44. Laskin WB, Fetsch JF, Mostofi KF. Angiomyofibroblastoma-like tumor of the male genital tract: analysis of 11 cases with comparisons to female angiofibroblastoma and spindle cell lipoma. Am J Surg Pathol 1998;22:6–16.

44a. Laskin WB, Fetsch JF, Tavassoli FA. Angiofibroblastoma of the female genital tract: analysis of 17 cases including a lipomatous variant. Hum Pathol 1997;28:1046–55.

45. Nielsen GP, Rosenberg AE, Young RH, Dickersin GR, Clement PB, Scully RE. Angiomyofibroblastoma of the vulva and vagina. Mod Pathol 1996;9:284–91.

45a. Nielsen GP, Young RH, Dickersin GR, Rosenberg AE. Angiomyofibroblastoma of the vulva with sarcomatous transformation ("angiomyofibrosarcoma"). Am J Surg Pathol 1997;28:1046–55.

46. Nucci M, Granter SR, Fletcher CD. Cellular angiofibroma: a benign neoplasm distinct from angiomyofibroblastoma and spindle cell lipoma. Am J Surg Pathol 1997;21:636–44.

47. Ockner DM, Sayadi H, Swanson PE, Ritter JH, Wick MR. Genital angiomyofibroblastoma: comparison with aggressive angiomyxoma and other myxoid neoplasms of skin and soft tissue. Am J Clin Pathol 1997;107:36–44

Ossifying Fibromyxoid Tumor

48. Donner LR. Ossifying fibromyxoid tumor of soft parts: evidence supporting Schwann cell origin. Hum Pathol 1992;23:200–2.

49. Enzinger FM, Weiss SW, Liang CY. Ossifying fibromyxoid tumor of soft parts. A clinicopathologic analysis of 59 cases. Am J Surg Pathol 1989;13:817–27.

50. Kilpatrick SE, Ward MG, Mozes M, Miettinen M, Fukanaga M, Fletcher CD. Atypical and malignant variants of ossifying fibromyxoid tumor: clinicopathologic analysis of six cases. Am J Surg Pathol 1995;19:1039–46.

51. Miettinen M. Ossifying fibromyxoid tumor of soft parts. Additional observations of a distinctive soft tissue tumor. Am J Clin Pathol 1991;95:142–9.

52. Schofield JB, Krausz T, Stamp GW, Fletcher CD, Fisher C, Azzopardi JG. Ossifying fibromyxoid tumor of soft parts: immunohistochemical and ultrastructural analysis. Histopathology 1993;22:101–12.

53. Williams SB, Ellis GL, Meis JM, Heffner DK. Ossifying fibromyxoid tumor (of soft parts) of the head and neck: a clinicopathological and immunohistochemical study of nine cases. J Laryngol Otol 1993;107:75–80.

54. Yoshida H, Minamizaki T, Yumoto T, Furose K, Nakadera T. Ossifying fibromyxoid tumor of soft parts. Acta Pathol Jpn 1991;41:480–6.

54a. Zámecnik M, Michal M, Simpson RH, et al. Ossifying fibromyxoid tumor of soft parts: a report of 17 cases with emphasis on unusual histological features. Ann Diagn Pathol 1997;1:73–81.

Parachordoma

55. Dabska M. Parachordoma: a new clinicopathologic entity. Cancer 1977;40:1586–93.

56. Fisher C, Miettinen M. Parachordoma: a clinicopathologic and immunohistochemical study of four cases of an unusual soft tissue neoplasm. Ann Diag Pathol 1997;1:3–10.

56a. Folpe AL, Agoff SN, Willis J, Weiss SW. Parachordoma is immunohistochemically and cytogenetically distinct from axial chordoma and extraskeletal myxoid chondrosarcoma. Am J Surg Pathol 1999;23:1059–67.

57. Ishida T, Oda H, Oka T, Imamura T, Machinami R. Parachordoma: an ultrastructural and immunohistochemical study. Virchows Arch [A] 1993;422:239–47.

58. Kilpatrick SE, Hitchcock MG, Kraus MD, Calonie E, Fletcher CD. Mixed tumors and myoepitheliomas of soft tissue: a clinicopathologic study of 19 cases with a unifying concept. Am J Surg Pathol 1997;21:13–22.

59. Sangueza OP, White CJ. Parachordoma. Am J Dermatopathol 1994;16:185–8.

60. Shin HJ, Mackay B, Ichinose H, Ayala AG, Romsdahl MM. Parachordoma. Ultrastruct Pathol 1994;18:249–56.

Pleomorphic Hyalinizing Angiectatic Tumor of Soft Parts

61. Smith ME, Fisher C, Weiss SW. Pleomorphic hyalinizing angiectatic tumor of soft parts: a low-grade neoplasm resembling neurilemoma. Am J Surg Pathol 1996;20:21–9.

Peripheral Primitive Neuroectodermal Tumor/Ewing's Sarcoma Family of Tumors (PPNET/ES)

62. Ambros IM, Ambros PF, Strehl S, Kovar H, Gadner H, Salzer KM. MIC2 is a specific marker for Ewing's sarcoma and peripheral primitive neuroectodermal tumors. Evidence for a common histogenesis of Ewing's sarcoma and peripheral primitive neuroectodermal tumors from MIC2 expression and specific chromosome aberration. Cancer 1991;67:1886–93.

63. Angervall L, Enzinger FM. Extraskeletal neoplasm resembling Ewing's sarcoma. Cancer 1975;36:240–51.

64. Askin FB, Rosai J, Sibley RK, Dehner LP, McAlister WH. Malignant small cell tumor of the thoracopulmonary region in childhood: a distinctive clinicopathologic entity of uncertain histogenesis. Cancer 1979;43:2438–51.

65. Bailly RA, Bosselut R, Zucman J, et al. DNA-binding and transcriptional activation properties of the EWS-FLI-1 fusion protein resulting from the t(11; 22) translocation in Ewing sarcoma. Mol Cell Biol 1994;14:3230–41.

66. Beck JD, Bier V, Jurgens H, et al. Maligne periphere neuroepitheliale tumoren im kindesalter. Monatsschr Kinderheilkd 1987;135:214–7.

67. Cavazzana AO, Ninfo V, Roberts J, Triche TJ. Peripheral neuroepithelioma: a light microscopic, immunocytochemical, and ultrastructural study. Mod Pathol 1992;5:71–8.

68. Contesso G, Llombart BA, Terrier P, et al. Does malignant small round cell tumor of the thoracopulmonary region (Askin tumor) constitute a clinicopathologic entity? An analysis of 30 cases with immunohistochemical and electron-microscopic support treated at the Institute Gustave Roussy. Cancer 1992;69:1012–20.

69. Daugaard S, Kamby C, Sunde LM, Myhre JO, Schiodt T. Ewing's sarcoma. A retrospective study of histological and immunohistochemical factors and their relation to prognosis. Virchows Arch [A] 1989;414:243–51.

69a. DeAlava E, Kawai A, Healey JH, et al. EWS-FLI-1 fusion transcript structure is an independent determinant of prognosis in Ewing's sarcoma. J Clin Oncol 1998;16:1248–55.

70. Delattre O, Zucman J, Melot T, et al. The Ewing family of tumors–a subgroup of small-round-cell tumors defined by specific chimeric transcripts. N Engl J Med 1994;331:294–9.

71. Devaney K, Vinh TN, Sweet DE. Small cell osteosarcoma of bone: an immunohistochemical study with differential diagnostic considerations. Hum Pathol 1993;24:1211–25.

72. Dierick AM, Roels H, Langlois M. The immunophenotype of Ewing's sarcoma. An immunohistochemical analysis. Pathol Res Pract 1993;189:26–32.

73. Dunst J, Jurgens H, Sauer R, et al. Radiation therapy in Ewing's sarcoma: an update of the CESS 86 trial. Int J Radiat Oncol Biol Phys 1995;32.919–30.

74. Fellinger EJ, Garin CP, Glasser DB, Huvos AG, Rettig WJ. Comparison of cell surface antigen HBA71 (p30/32MIC2), neuron-specific enolase, and vimentin in the immunohistochemical analysis of Ewing's sarcoma of bone. Am J Surg Pathol 1992;16:746–55.

75. Giovannini M, Biegel JA, Serra M, et al. EWS-erg and EWS-Fli1 fusion transcripts in Ewing's sarcoma and primitive neuroectodermal tumors with variant translocations. J Clin Invest 1994;94:489–96.

75a. Hill C, Weiss SW, Folpe AL. Is FLI-1 protein expression specific for Ewing's sarcoma/primitive neuroectodermal tumor (ES/PNET)? A study of 78 round cell tumors, with emphasis on CD99-positive mimics of ES/PNET. Mod Pathol 2000;13:11A.

76. Jeon IS, Davis JN, Braun BS, et al. A variant Ewing's sarcoma translocation (7;22) fuses the EWS gene to the ETS gene ETV1. Oncogene 1995;10:1229–34.

77. Jurgens H, Bier V, Dunst J, et al. [The German Society of Pediatric Oncology Cooperative Ewing Sarcoma Studies CESS 81/86: report after 6 1/2 years]. Klin Padiatr 1988;200:243–52.

78. Kaneko Y, Yoshida K, Handa M, et al. Fusion of an ETS-family gene, EIAF, to EWS by t(17;22)(q12;q12) chromosome translocation in an undifferentiated sarcoma of infancy. Genes Chromosom Cancer 1996;15:115–21

79. Kissane JM, Askin FB, Foulkes M, Stratton LB, Shirley SF. Ewing's sarcoma of bone: clinicopathologic aspects of 303 cases from the Intergroup Ewing's Sarcoma Study. Hum Pathol 1983;14:773–9.

79a. Kumar S, Pack S, Kumar D, et al. Detection of EWS-FLI-1 fusion in Ewing's sarcoma/peripheral primitive neuroectodermal tumor by fluorescence in situ hybridization using formalin-fixed paraffin-embedded tissue. Hum Pathol 1999;30:324–30.

80. Ladanyi M, Lewis R, Garin CP, et al. EWS rearrangement in Ewing's sarcoma and peripheral neuroectodermal tumor. Molecular detection and correlation with cytogenetic analysis and MIC2 expression. Diagn Mol Pathol 1993;2:141–6.

80a. Lin PP, Brody RI, Hamelin AC, Bradner JE, Healey JH, Ladanyi M. Differential transactivation by alternative EWS-FLI-1 fusion proteins correlates with clinical heterogeneity in Ewing's sarcoma. Cancer Res 1999;59:1428–32.

81. Llombart-Bosch A, Lacombe MJ, Peydro-Olaya A, Perez-Bacete M, Contesso G. Malignant peripheral neuroectodermal tumours of bone other than Askin's neoplasm: characterization of 14 new cases with immunohistochemistry and electron microscopy. Virchows Arch [A] 1988;412:421–30.

81a. Monforte-Munoz H, Lopez-Terrada D, Affendie H, Rowland JM, Triche TJ. Documentation of EWS gene rearrangements by fluorescence in situ hybridization (FISH) in frozen sections of Ewing's sarcoma-peripheral primitive neuroectodermal tumor. Am J Surg Pathol 1999;23:309–15.

82. Navas-Palacios JJ, Aparacio-Duque R, Valdes MD. On the histogenesis of Ewing's sarcoma: an ultrastructural, immunohistochemical, and cytochemical study. Cancer 1984;53:1882–901.

83. Parham DM, Webber B, Holt H, Williams WK, Maurer H. Immunohistochemical study of childhood rhabdomyosarcomas and related neoplasms. Results of an Intergroup Rhabdomyosarcoma Study project. Cancer 1991;67:3072–80.

84. Perlman EJ, Dickman PS, Askin FB, Grier HE, Miser JS, Link MP. Ewing's sarcoma—routine diagnostic utilization of MIC2 analysis: a Pediatric Oncology Group/Children's Cancer Group Intergroup study. Hum Pathol 1994;25:304–7.

85. Peter M, Couturier J, Pacquement H, et al. A new member of the ETS family fused to EWS in Ewing tumors. Oncogene 1997;14:1159–64.

86. Ramani P, Rampling D, Link M. Immunocytochemical study of 12E7 in small round-cell tumours of childhood: an assessment of its sensitivity and specificity. Histopathology 1993;23:557–61.

87. Rud NP, Reiman HM, Pritchard DJ, Frassica FJ, Smithson WA. Extraosseous Ewing's sarcoma. A study of 42 cases. Cancer 1989;64:1548–53.

88. Schmidt D, Harms D. [Cooperative Ewing's Sarcoma Studies 81/86: pathologico-anatomic and immunohistochemical findings and differential diagnosis of Ewing sarcoma]. Klin Padiatr 1988;200:236–42.

89. Schmidt D, Herrmann C, Jurgens H, Harms D. Malignant peripheral neuroectodermal tumor and its necessary distinction from Ewing's sarcoma. A report from the Kiel Pediatric Tumor Registry. Cancer 1991;68:2251–9.

90. Shishikura A, Ushigome S, Shimoda T. Primitive neuroectodermal tumors of bone and soft tissue: histological subclassification and clinicopathologic correlations. Acta Pathol Jpn 1993;43:176–86.

91. Silliman CC, Mierau GW, Strain JD, et al. Peripheral neuroepithelioma of the soft tissues. A retrospective analysis of fifteen pediatric patients. Am J Pediatr Hematol Oncol 1993;15:299–305.

92. Sorensen PH, Lessnick SL, Lopez TD, Liu XF, Triche TJ, Denny CT. A second Ewing's sarcoma translocation, t(21;22), fuses the EWS gene to another ETS-family transcription factor, ERG. Nat Genet 1994;6:146–51.

93. Sorensen PH, Shimada H, Liu XF, Lim JF, Thomas G, Triche TJ. Biphenotypic sarcomas with myogenic and neural differentiation express the Ewing's sarcoma EWS/FLI1 fusion gene. Cancer Res 1995;55:1385–92.

94. Swanson PE, Jaszcz W, Nakhleh RE, Kelly DR, Dehner LP. Peripheral primitive neuroectodermal tumors. A

95. Triche TJ. Pathology of pediatric malignancies. In: Pizzo PA, Poplack DG, eds. Principles and practice of pediatric oncology. Philadelphia: JB Lippincott, 1993:115–52.

96. Tsokos M. Peripheral primitive neuroectodermal tumors. Diagnosis, classification, and prognosis. Perspect Pediatr Pathol 1992;16:27–98.

97. Turc-Carel C, Aurias A, Mugneret F, et al. Chromosomes in Ewing's sarcoma. I. An evaluation of 85 cases and remarkable consistency of t(11;22)(q24;q12). Cancer Genet Cytogenet 1988;32:229–38.

98. Zoubek A, Dockhorn-Dworniczak G, Delattre O, et al. Does expression of different EWS chimeric transcripts define clinically distinct risk groups of Ewing tumor patients? J Clin Oncol 1996;14:1245–51.

99. Zucman J, Melot T, Desmaze C, et al. Combinatorial generation of variable fusion proteins in the Ewing family of tumours. Embo J 1993;12:4481–7.

flow cytometric analysis with immunohistochemical and ultrastructural observations. Arch Pathol Lab Med 1992;116:1202–8.

Small Cell Tumor with Desmoplastic Stroma

100. Bian Y, Jordan AG, Rupp M, Cohn H, McLaughlin CJ, Miettinen M. Effusion cytology of desmoplastic small round cell tumor of the pleura. A case report. Acta Cytol 1993;37:77–82.

101. Biegel JA, Conard K, Brooks JJ. Translocation (11;22)(p13;q12): primary change in intra-abdominal desmoplastic small round cell tumor. Genes Chromosom Cancer 1993;7:119–21.

102. Cummings OW, Ulbright TM, Young RH, Dei Tos AP, Fletcher CD, Hull TT. Desmoplastic small round cell tumors of the paratesticular region. A report of six cases. Am J Surg Pathol 1997;21:219–25.

103. Gerald WL, Landanyi M, de Alava E, et al. Clinical, pathologic, and molecular spectrum of tumors associated with t(11;22)(p13;q12): desmoplastic small round cell tumor and its variants. J Clin Oncol 1998;16:3028–36.

104. Gerald WL, Miller HK, Battifora H, Miettinen M, Silva EG, Rosai J. Intra-abdominal desmoplastic small round-cell tumor. Report of 19 cases of a distinctive type of high-grade polyphenotypic malignancy affecting young individuals. Am J Surg Pathol 1991;15:499–513.

104a. Gerald WL, Rosai J. Desmoplastic small cell tumor with multi-phenotypic differentiation. Zentralbl Pathol 1993;139:141–51.

105. Kushner BH, LaQuaglia MP, Wollner N, et al. Desmoplastic small round-cell tumor: prolonged progression-free survival with aggressive multimodality therapy. J Clin Oncol 1996;14:1526–31.

106. Ladanyi M, Gerald W. Fusion of the EWS and WT1 genes in the desmoplastic small round cell tumor. Cancer Res 1994;54:2837–40.

107. Lee SB, Kolquist KA, Nichols K, et al. The EWS-WT1 translocation product induces PDGFA in desmoplastic small round-cell tumour. Nat Genet 1997;17:309–13.

108. Ordoñez NG. Desmoplastic small round cell tumor. II: An ultrastructural and immunohistochemical study with emphasis on new immunohistochemical markers. Am J Surg Pathol 1998;22:1314–27.

109. Parkash V, Gerald WL, Parma A, Miettinen M, Rosai J. Desmoplastic small round cell tumor of the pleura. Am J Surg Pathol 1995;19:659–65.

110. Rodriguez E, Sreekantaiah C, Gerald W, Reuter VE, Motzer RJ, Chaganti RS. A recurring translocation, t(11;22)(p13;q11.2), characterizes intra-abdominal desmoplastic small round-cell tumors. Cancer Genet Cytogenet 1993;69:17–21.

111. Sawyer JR, Tryka AF, Lewis JM. A novel reciprocal chromosome translocation t(11;22)(p13;q12) in an intraabdominal desmoplastic small round-cell tumor. Am J Surg Pathol 1992;16:411–6.

112. Schmidt D, Köster E, Harms D. Intraabdominal desmoplastic small-cell tumor with divergent differentiation: clinicopathological findings and DNA ploidy. Med Pediatr Oncol 1994;22:97–102.

113. Shen WP, Towne B, Zadeh TM. Cytogenetic abnormalities in an intraabdominal desmoplastic small cell tumor [Letter]. Cancer Genet Cytogenet 1992;64:189–91.

Malignant Rhabdoid Tumor

114. Biegel JA, Allen CS, Kawasaki K, Shimizu N, Budarf ML, Bell CJ. Narrowing the critical region for a rhabdoid tumor locus in 22q11. Genes Chromosomes Cancer 1996;16:94–105.

115. Biegel JA, Burk CD, Parmiter AH, Emanuel BS. Molecular analysis of a partial deletion of 22q in a central

nervous system rhabdoid tumor. Genes Chromosomes Cancer 1992;7:104–8.

116. Biegel JA, Rorke LB, Packer RJ, Emanuel BS. Monosomy 22 in rhabdoid or atypical tumors of the brain. J Neurosurg 1990:73:710–4.

117. Douglass EC, Valentine M, Rowe ST, et al. Malignant rhabdoid tumor: a highly malignant childhood tumor with minimal karyotypic changes. Genes Chromosomes Cancer 1990;2:210–6.

117a.Fanburg-Smith JC, Hengge M, Hengge UR, Smith JS Jr, Miettinen M. Extrarenal rhabdoid tumor of soft tissue: a clinicopathologic and immunohistochemical study of 18 cases. Ann Diagn Pathol 1998;2:351–62.

118. Guillou L, Wadden C, Coindre JM, Krausz T, Fletcher CD. "Proximal-type" epithelioid sarcoma, a distinctive aggressive neoplasm showing rhabdoid features. Clinicopathologic, immunohistochemical, and ultrastructural study of a series. Am J Surg Pathol 1997;21:130–46.

119. Handgretinger R, Kimmig A, Koscielniak E, et al. Establishment and characterization of a cell line (Wa-2) derived from an extrarenal rhabdoid tumor. Cancer Res 1990;50:2177–82.

120. Karnes PS, Tran TN, Cui MY, Bogenmann E, Shimada H, Ying KL. Establishment of a rhabdoid tumor cell line with a specific chromosomal abnormality, 46,XY,t(11;22)(p15.5;q11.23). Cancer Genet Cytogenet 1991;56:31–8.

121. Kodet R, Newton WA Jr, Sachs N, et al. Rhabdoid tumors of soft tissues: a clinicopathologic study of 26 cases enrolled on the Intergroup Rhabdomyosarcoma Study. Hum Pathol 1991;22:674–84.

122. Ota S, Crabbe DC, Tran TN, Triche TJ, Shimada J. Malignant rhabdoid tumor. A study with two established cell lines. Cancer 1993;71:2862–72.

123. Parham DM, Weeks DA, Beckwith JB. The clinicopathologic spectrum of putative extrarenal rhabdoid tumors. An analysis of 42 cases studied with immunohistochemistry or electron microscopy. Am J Surg Pathol 1994;18:1010–29.

123a.Rosson GB, Hazen-Martin DJ, Biegel JA, et al. Establishment and molecular characterization of five cell lines derived from renal and extrarenal malignant rhabdoid tumors. Mod Pathol 1998;11:1228–37.

124. Rosty C, Peter M, Zucman J, Validire P, Delattre O, Aurias A. Cytogenetic and molecular analysis of a t(1;22)(p36;q11.2) in a rhabdoid tumor with a putative homozygous deletion of chromosome 22. Genes Chromosomes Cancer 1998;21:82–9.

125. Schmidt D, Leuschner I, Harms D, Sprenger E, Schafer HJ. Malignant rhabdoid tumor. A morphological and flow cytometric study. Path Res Pract 1989;184:202–10.

126. Schofield DE, Beckwith JB, Sklar J. Loss of heterozygosity at chromosome regions 22q11-12 and 11p15.5 in renal rhabdoid tumors. Genes Chromosomes Cancer 1996;15:10–7.

127. Shashi V, Lovell MA, von Kap-herr C, Waldron P, Golden WL. Malignant rhabdoid tumor of the kidney: involvement of chromosome 22. Genes Chromosomes Cancer 1992;10:49–54.

128. Sotelo-Avila C, Gonzalez-Cruissi F, de Mello D, et al. Renal and extrarenal rhabdoid tumors in children: a clinicopathologic study of 14 patients. Semin Diagn Pathol 1986;3:151–63.

129. Weeks DA, Beckwith JB, Mierau GW, Luckey DW. Rhabdoid tumor of kidney. A report of 111 cases from the National Wilms' Tumor Study Pathology Center. Am J Surg Pathol 1989;13:439–58.

129a.White FV, Dehner LP, Belchis DA, et al. Congenital disseminated malignant rhabdoid tumor: a distinct clinicopathologic entity demonstrating abnormalities of chromosome 22q11. Am J Surg Pathol 1999;23:249–56.

130. Wick MR, Ritter JH, Dehner LP. Malignant rhabdoid tumors: a clinicopathologic review and conceptual discussion. Sem Diagn Pathol 1995;12:233–48.

Clear Cell Sarcoma

131. Bridge JA, Sreekantaiah C, Neff JR, Sandberg AA. Cytogenetic findings in clear cell sarcoma of tendons and aponeuroses. Malignant melanoma of soft parts. Cancer Genet Cytogenet 1991;52:101–106.

132. Chung EB, Enzinger FM. Malignant melanoma of soft parts. A reassessment of clear cell sarcoma. Am J Surg Pathol 1983;7:405–13.

133. Eckardt JJ, Pritchard DJ, Soule EH. Clear cell sarcoma. A clinicopathologic study of 27 cases. Cancer 1983;52:1482–8.

134. Enzinger FM. Clear cell sarcoma of tendons and aponeuroses: an analysis of 21 cases. Cancer 1965;18:1163–76.

135. Kindblom LG, Lodding P, Angervall L. Clear-cell sarcoma of tendons and aponeuroses. An immunohistochemical and electron microscopic analysis indicating neural crest origin. Virchows Arch [A] 1983;401:109–28.

136. Lucas DR, Nascimento AG, Sim FH. Clear cell sarcoma of soft tissues. Mayo Clinic experience with 35 cases. Am J Surg Pathol 1992;16:1197–204.

137. Montgomery EA, Meis JM, Ramos AG, et al. Clear cell sarcoma of tendons and aponeurosis: a clinicopathologic study of 58 cases with analysis of prognostic factors. Int J Surg Pathol 1993;1:59–62.

138. Mrozek K, Karakousis CP, Perez MC, Bloomfield CD. Translocation t(12;22)(q13;q12.2–12.3) in a clear cell sarcoma of tendons and aponeuroses. Genes Chromosomes Cancer 1993;6:249–52.

139. Reeves BR, Fletcher CD, Gusterson BA. Translocation t(12; 22)(q13; q13) is a nonrandom rearrangement in clear cell sarcoma. Cancer Genet Cytogenet 1992;64:101–3.

140. Stenman G, Kindblom LG, Angervall L. Reciprocal translocation t(12;22)(q13;q13) in clear-cell sarcoma of tendons and aponeuroses. Genes Chromosomes Cancer 1992;4:122–7.

141. Swanson PE, Wick MR. Clear cell sarcoma. An immunohistochemical analysis of six cases and comparison with other epithelioid neoplasms of soft tissue. Arch Pathol Lab Med 1989;113:55–60.

142. Travis JA, Bridge JA. Significance of both numerical and structural chromosomal abnormalities in clear cell sarcoma. Cancer Genet Cytogenet 1992;64:104–106.

143. Zucman J, Delattre O, Desmaze C, et al. EWS and ATF-1 gene fusion induced by t(12;22) translocation in malignant melanoma of soft parts. Nat Genet 1993;4:341–5.

Alveolar Soft Part Sarcoma

144. Auerbach HE, Brooks JJ. Alveolar soft part sarcoma. A clinicopathologic and immunohistochemical study. Cancer 1987;60:66–73.

145. Chetty R. Alveolar soft part sarcoma with psammoma bodies [Letter]. Histopathology 1990;17:188.

146. Christopherson WM, Foote FW Jr, Stewart FW. Alveolar soft-part sarcomas; structurally characteristic tumors of uncertain histogenesis. Cancer 1952;5:100–11.

147. Cullinane C, Thorner PS, Greenberg ML, Kwan Y, Kumar M, Squire J. Molecular genetic, cytogenetic, and immunohistochemical characterization of alveolar soft-part sarcoma. Implications for cell of origin. Cancer 1992;70:2444–50.

148. Enzinger FM, Weiss SW. Malignant soft tissue tumors of uncertain type: alveolar soft part sarcoma. In: Enzinger FM, Weiss SW, eds. Soft tissue tumors. 3rd ed. St. Louis: Mosby, 1995:1067.

149. Evans HL. Alveolar soft-part sarcoma. A study of 13 typical examples and one with a histologically atypical component. Cancer 1985;55:912–7.

150. Foschini MP, Eusebi V. Alveolar soft-part sarcoma: a new type of rhabdomyosarcoma? Semin Diagn Pathol 1994;11:58–68.

151. Heimann P, Devalck C, Debusscher C, Sariban E, Vamos E. Alveolar soft-part sarcoma: further evidence by FISH for the involvement of chromosome band 17q25. Genes Chromosomes Cancer 1998;23:194–7.

152. Hirose T, Kudo E, Hasegawa T, Abe J, Hizawa K. Cytoskeletal properties of alveolar soft part sarcoma. Hum Pathol 1990;21:204–11.

153. Lieberman PH, Brennan MF, Kimmel M, Erlandson RA, Garin CP, Flehinger BY. Alveolar soft-part sarcoma. A clinico-pathologic study of half a century. Cancer 1989;63:1–13.

154. Lillehei KO, Kleinschmidt DM, Mitchell DH, Spector E, Kruse CA. Alveolar soft part sarcoma: an unusually long interval between presentation and brain metastasis. Hum Pathol 1993;24:1030–4.

155. Marker P, Jensen ML, Siemssen SJ. Alveolar soft-part sarcoma of the oral cavity: report of a case and review of the literature. J Oral Maxillofac Surg 1995;53:1203–8.

156. Matsuno Y, Mukai K, Itabashi M, et al. Alveolar soft part sarcoma. A clinicopathologic and immunohistochemical study of 12 cases. Acta Pathol Jpn 1990;40:199–205.

157. Miettinen M, Ekfors T. Alveolar soft part sarcoma. Immunohistochemical evidence for muscle cell differentiation. Am J Clin Pathol 1990;93:32–8.

158. Mukai M, Torikata C, Iri H. Alveolar soft part sarcoma: an electron microscopic study especially of uncrystallized granules using a tannic acid-containing fixative. Ultrastruct Pathol 1990;14:41–50.

159. Nakashima Y, Kotoura Y, Kasakura K, Yamamuro T, Amitani R, Ohdera K. Alveolar soft-part sarcoma. A report of ten cases. Clin Orthop 1993;294:259–66.

160. Nielsen GP, Oliva E, Young RH, Rosenberg AE, Dickersin GR, Scully RE. Alveolar soft-part sarcoma of the female genital tract: a report of nine cases and review of the literature. Int J Gynecol Pathol 1995;14:283–92.

161. Ohno T, Park P, Higaki S, Miki H, Kamura S, Unno K. Smooth tubular aggregates associated with plasmalemmal invagination in alveolar soft part sarcoma. Ultrastruct Pathol 1994;18:383–8.

162. Ordonez NG, Ro JY, Mackay B. Alveolar soft part sarcoma. An ultrastructural and immunocytochemical investigation of its histogenesis. Cancer 1989;63:1721–36.

163. Pappo AS, Parham DM, Cain A, et al. Alveolar soft part sarcoma in children and adolescents: clinical features and outcome of 11 patients. Med Pediatr Oncol 1996;26:81–4.

164. Perel Y, Rivel J, Alos N, Pignol ML, Guillard JM. Alveolar soft part sarcoma. A rare tumor of unusual evolution in pediatrics. Am J Pediatr Hematol Oncol 1993;15:435–8.

165. Perry JR, Bilbao JM. Metastatic alveolar soft part sarcoma presenting as a dural-based cerebral mass. Neurosurgery 1994;34:168–70.

166. Rosai J, Dias P, Parham DM, Shapiro DN, Houghton P. MyoD1 protein expression in alveolar soft part sarcoma as confirmatory evidence of its skeletal muscle nature. Am J Surg Pathol 1991;15:974–81.

167. Sahin AA, Silva EG, Ordonez NG. Alveolar soft part sarcoma of the uterine cervix. Mod Pathol 1989;2:676–80.

168. Sciot R, Dal Cin P, De Vos R, et al. Alveolar soft-part sarcoma: evidence for its myogenic origin and for the involvement of 17q25. Histopathology 1993;23:439–44.

169. Sreekantaiah C, Li FP, Weidner N, Sandberg AA. Multiple and complex abnormalities in a case of alveolar soft-part sarcoma. Cancer Genet Cytogenet 1991;55:167–71.

170. Temple HT, Scully SP, O'Keefe RJ, Rosenthal DI, Mankin HJ. Clinical presentation of alveolar soft-part sarcoma. Clin Orthop 1994;300:213–8.

171. Tucker JA. Crystal-deficient alveolar soft part sarcoma. Ultrastruct Pathol 1993;17:279–86.

172. Wang NP, Bacchi CE, Jiang JJ, McNutt MA, Gown AM. Does alveolar soft-part sarcoma exhibit skeletal muscle differentiation? An immunocytochemical and biochemical study of myogenic regulatory protein expression. Mod Pathol 1996;9:496–506.

Synovial Sarcoma

173. Abenoza P, Manivel JC, Swanson PE, Wick MR. Synovial sarcoma: ultrastructural study and immunohistochemical analysis by a combined peroxidase-antiperoxidase/avidin-biotin-peroxidase complex procedure. Hum Pathol 1986;17:1107–15.

174. Brodsky JT, Burt ME, Hajdu SI, Casper ES, Brennan MR. Tenosynovial sarcoma. Clinicopathologic features, treatment, and prognosis. Cancer 1992;70:484–9.

175. Burke AP, Cowan D, Virmani R. Primary sarcomas of the heart. Cancer 1992;69:387–95.

176. Cagle LA, Mirra JM, Storm K, Roe DJ, Eilber FR. Histologic features relating to prognosis in synovial sarcoma. Cancer 1987;59:1810–14.

177. Carrillo R, Rodriguez-Peralto JL, Batsakis JG. Synovial sarcomas of the head and neck. Ann Otolaryngol Rhinol Laryngol 1992;101:367–70.

178. Choong PF, Pritchard DJ, Sim FH, Rock MG, Nascimento AG. Long-term survival in high-grade soft tissue sarcoma: prognostic factors in synovial sarcoma. Int J Oncol 1995;7:161–9.

179. Corson JM, Weiss LM, Banks-Schlegel SP, Pinkus GS. Keratin proteins and carcinoembryonic antigen in synovial sarcomas: an immunohistochemical study of 24 cases. Hum Pathol 1984;15:615–21.

180. Dal Cin P, Rao U, Jani-Sait S, Karakousis C, Sandberg AA. Chromosomes in the diagnosis of soft tissue tumors. I. Synovial sarcoma. Mod Pathol 1992;5:357–62.

181. Dardick I, Ramjohn S, Thomas MJ, Jeans D, Hammar SP. Synovial sarcoma. Inter-relationship of the biphasic and monophasic subtypes. Pathol Res Pract 1991;187:871–85.

182. Dei Tos AP, Wadden C, Calonje E, et al. Immunohistochemical demonstration of glycoprotein p30/32 MIC2 (CD99) in synovial sarcoma: a potential cause of diagnostic confusion. Appl Immunohistochem 1995;3:168–73.

183. Dickersin GR. Synovial sarcoma: a review and update, with emphasis on the ultrastructural characterization of the nonglandular component. Ultrastruct Pathol 1991;15:379–402.

184. El-Naggar AK, Ayala AG, Abdul-Karim FW, et al. Synovial sarcoma. A DNA flow cytometric study. Cancer 1990;65:2295–300.

185. Enzinger FM, Weiss SW. Soft tissue tumors, 3rd ed. St. Louis: Mosby, 1995:659–88.

186. Evans HL. Synovial sarcoma. A study of 23 biphasic and 17 probably monophasic examples. Pathol Annu 1980;15:309–31.

187. Farris KB, Reed RJ. Monophasic, glandular, synovial sarcomas and carcinomas of the soft tissues. Arch Pathol Lab Med 1982;106:129–32.

188. Fetsch JF, Meis JM. Synovial sarcoma of the abdominal wall. Cancer 1993;72:469–77.

189. Fisher C. Synovial sarcoma: ultrastructural and immunohistochemical features of epithelial differentiation in monophasic and biphasic tumors. Hum Pathol 1986;17:996–1008.

190. Fisher C, Schofield JB. S-100 protein positive synovial sarcoma. Histopathology 1991;19:375–7.

190a. Folpe AL, Schmidt RA, Chapman D, Gown AM. Poorly differentiated synovial sarcoma: immunohistochemical distinction from primitive neuroectodermal tumors and high-grade malignant peripheral nerve sheath tumors. Am J Surg Pathol 1998;22:673–82.

191. Gabbiani G, Kaye GI, Lattes R, Majno G. Synovial sarcoma. Electron microscopic study of a typical case. Cancer 1971;28:1031–9.

192. Gaertner E, Zeren H, Fleming MV, Colby TB, Travis WD. Biphasic synovial sarcomas arising in the pleural cavity. A clinicopathologic study of five cases. Am J Surg Pathol 1996;20:36–45.

193. Ghadially FN. Is synovial sarcoma a carcinosarcoma of connective tissue? Ultrastruct Pathol 1987;11:147–51.

194. Golouh R, Vuzevski V, Bracko M, Van Der Heul RO, Cervek J. Synovial sarcoma: a clinicopathological study of 36 cases. J Surg Oncol 1990;45:20–8.

195. Guillou L, Wadden C, Coindre JM, Krausz T, Fletcher CD. "Proximal-type" epithelioid sarcoma, a distinctive aggressive neoplasm showing rhabdoid features. Clinicopathologic, immunohistochemical, and ultrastructural study of a series. Am J Surg Pathol 1997;21:130–46

196. Guillou L, Wadden C, Kraus MD, Dei Tos AP, Fletcher CD. S-100 protein reactivity in synovial sarcomas—a potentially frequent diagnostic pitfall: immunohistochemical analysis of 100 cases. Appl Immunohistochem 1996;4:167–75.

197. Haagensen CD, Stout AP. Synovial sarcoma. Ann Surg 1944;120:826–42.

198. Karn CM, Socinski MA, Fletcher JA, Corson JM, Craighead JE. Cardiac synovial sarcoma with translocation (X;18) associated with asbestos exposure. Cancer 1994;73:74–8.

198a. Kawai A, Woodruff J, Healey JH, Brennan MF, Antonescu CR, Ladanyi M. SYT-SSX gene fusion as a determinant of morphology and prognosis in synovial sarcoma. N Engl J Med 1998;338:153–60.

199. Kindblom LG, Meis-Kindblom JM, Bertoni F, et al. Synovial sarcoma: identification of low and high risk groups [Abstract]. Mod Pathol 1996;9:8A.

200. Knight JC, Reeves BR, Smith S, et al. Cytogenetic and molecular analysis of synovial sarcoma. Int J Oncol 1992;1:747–52.

201. Krall RA, Kostianovsky M, Patchefsky AS. Synovial sarcoma. A clinical, pathological, and ultrastructural study of 26 cases supporting the recognition of a monophasic variant. Am J Surg Pathol 1981;5:137–51.

202. Ladenstein R, Treuner J, Koscielniak E, et al. Synovial sarcoma of childhood and adolescence. Report of the German CWS-81 study. Cancer 1993;71:3647–55.

203. Leader M, Patel J, Collins M, Kristin H. Synovial sarcomas. True carcinosarcomas? Cancer 1987;59:2096–8.

204. Limon J, Mrozek K, Mandahl N, et al. Cytogenetics of synovial sarcoma: presentation of ten new cases and review of the literature. Genes Chromosom Cancer 1991;3:338–45.

205. Lopes JM, Bjerkehagen B, Holm R, Bruland O, Sobrinho-Simoes M, Nesland JM. Immunohistochemical profile of synovial sarcoma with emphasis on the epithelial-type differentiation. A study of 49 primary tumours, recurrences, and metastases. Pathol Res Pract 1994;190:168–77.

206. Machen SK, Easley KA, Goldblum JR. Synovial sarcoma of the extremities. A clinicopathologic study of 34 cases including semi-quantitative analysis of spindled, epithelial and poorly differentiated areas Am J Surg Pathol 1999;23:268–75..

207. Mackenzie DH. Monophasic synovial sarcoma—a histological entity? Histopathology 1977;1:151–7.

208. Mackenzie DH. Synovial sarcoma. A review of 58 cases. Cancer 1966;19:169–80.

209. Mandahl N, Heim S, Arheden K, Rydholm A, Willen H, Mitelman F. Multiple karyotypical rearrangements, including t(X;18)(p11;q11), in a fibrosarcoma. Cancer Genet Cytogenet 1988;30:323–7.

210. Meis-Kindblom JM, Stenman G, Kindblom LG. Differential diagnosis of small round cell tumors. Sem Diagnostic Pathol 1996;13:213–41.

211. Mickelson MR, Brown GA, Maynard JA, Cooper RR, Bonfiglio M. Synovial sarcoma: an electron microscopic study of monophasic and biphasic forms. Cancer 1980;45:2109–18.

212. Miettinen M, Lehto VP, Virtanen I. Keratin in the epithelial-like cells of classical biphasic synovial sarcoma. Virchows Arch [Cell Pathol] 1982;40:157–61.

213. Miettinen M, Lehto VP, Virtanen I. Monophasic synovial sarcoma of spindle-cell type. Epithelial differentiation as revealed by ultrastructural features, content of prekeratin and binding of peanut agglutinin. Virchows Arch [Cell Pathol] 1983;44:187–99.

214. Miettinen M, Santavirta S, Slatis P. Intravascular synovial sarcoma. Hum Pathol 1987;18:1075–7.

215. Miettinen M, Virtanen I. Synovial sarcoma–a misnomer. Am J Surg Pathol 1984;117:18–25.

216. Milchgrub S, Ghandur-Mnaymneh L, Dorfman HD, Albores-Saavedra J. Synovial sarcoma with extensive osteoid and bone formation. Am J Surg Pathol 1993;17:357–63.

217. Mirra JM, Wang S, Bhuta S. Synovial sarcoma with squamous differentiation of its mesenchymal glandular elements. A case report with light-microscopic, ultramicroscopic, and immunologic correlation. Am J Surg Pathol 1984;8:791–6.

218. Nagao K, Ito H, Yoshida H. Chromosomal translocation t(X;18) in human synovial sarcomas analyzed by fluorescence in situ hybridization using paraffin-embedded tissue. Am J Pathol 1996;148:601–9.

218a. Nilsson G, Skytting B, Xie Y, et al. The SYT-SSX1 variant of synovial sarcoma is associated with a high rate of tumor cell proliferation and poor clinical outcome. Cancer Res 1999;59:3180–4.

219. Oda Y, Hashimoto H, Tsuneyoshi M, Takeshita S. Survival in synovial sarcoma. A multivariate study of prognostic factors with special emphasis on the comparison between early death and long-term survival. Am J Surg Pathol 1993;17:35–44.

220. Oda Y, Hashimoto H, Takeshita S, Tsuneyoshi M. The prognostic value of immunohistochemical staining for proliferating cell nuclear antigen in synovial sarcoma. Cancer 1993;72:478–85.

221. Ordonez NG, Mahfouz SM, Mackay B. Synovial sarcoma: an immunohistochemical and ultrastructural study. Hum Pathol 1990;21:733–49.

222. Pai S, Chinoy RF, Pradhan SA, D'Cruz AK, Kane SV, Yadav JN. Head and neck synovial sarcomas. J Surg Oncol 1993;54:82–6.

223. Pappa AS, Fontanesi J, Luo X, et al. Synovial sarcoma in children and adolescents: the St. Jude Children's Research Hospital experience. J Clin Oncol 1994;12:2360–6.

224. Poteat HJ, Corson JM, Fletcher JA. Detection of chromosome 18 rearrangement in synovial sarcoma by fluorescence in situ hybridization. Cancer Genet Cytogenet 1995;84:76–81.

225. Povysil C. Synovial sarcoma with squamous metaplasia. Ultrastruct Pathol 1984;7:207–13.

226. Ratnatunga N, Goodlad JR, Sankarakumaran N, Seimon R, Nagendran S, Fletcher CD. Primary biphasic synovial sarcoma of the orbit. J Clin Pathol 1992;45:265–7.

227. Rooser B, Willen H, Hugoson A, Rydholm A. Prognostic factors in synovial sarcoma. Cancer 1989;63:2182–5.

228. Roth JA, Enzinger FM, Tannenbaum M. Synovial sarcoma of the neck: a follow-up study of 24 cases. Cancer 1975;35:1243–53.

229. Salisbury JR, Isaacson PG. Synovial sarcoma: an immunohistochemical study. J Pathol 1985;147:49–57.

230. Schmidt D, Thum P, Harms D, Treuner J. Synovial sarcoma in children and adolescents. A report from the Kiel Pediatric Tumor Registry. Cancer 1991;67:1667–72.

231. Shaw GR, Lais CJ. Fatal intravascular synovial sarcoma in a 31 year old woman. Hum Pathol 1993;24:809–10.

232. Shmookler BM. Retroperitoneal synovial sarcoma. A report of 4 cases. Am J Clin Pathol 1982;77:686–91.

233. Shmookler BM, Enzinger FM, Brannon RB. Orofacial synovial sarcoma. A clinicopathologic study of 11 new cases and review of the literature. Cancer 1982;50:269–76.

234. Singer S, Baldini EH, Demetri GD, Fletcher JA, Corson JM. Synovial sarcoma: prognostic significance of tumor size, margin of resection, and mitotic activity for survival. J Clin Oncol 1996;14:1201–8.

235. Sumitomo M, Hirose T, Kudo E, Sano T, Shinomiya S, Hizawa K. Epithelial differentiation in synovial sarcoma. Correlation with histology and immunophenotypic expression. Acta Pathol Jpn 1989;39:381–7.

236. Turc-Carel C, Dal Cin P, Limon J, et al. Involvement of chromosome X in primary cytogenetic change in human neoplasia: nonrandom translocation in synovial sarcoma. Proc Natl Acad Sci USA 1987;84:1981–5.

237. Ueda T, Aozasa K, Tsujimoto M, et al. Prognostic significance of mast cells in soft tissue sarcoma. Cancer 1988;62:2416–9.

238. Van de Rijn M, Barr FG, Collins MH, Xiong QB, Fisher C. Absence of SYT-SSX fusion in products in soft tissue tumors other than synovial sarcoma. Am J Clin Pathol 1999;112:43–9.

238a. Van de Rijn M, Barr FG, Xiong Q, Hedges M, Shipley J, Fisher C. Poorly differentiated synovial sarcoma: an analysis of clinical, pathologic and molecular genetic features. Am J Surg Pathol, 1999;23:106–12.

239. Varela-Duran J, Enzinger FM. Calcifying synovial sarcoma. Cancer 1982;50:345–52.

240. Witkin GB, Miettinen M, Rosai J. A biphasic tumor of the mediastinum with features of synovial sarcoma. Am J Surg Pathol 1989;13:490–9.

241. Woodruff JM, Christensen WN. Glandular peripheral nerve sheath tumors. Cancer 1993;72:3618–28.

242. Wright PH, Sim FH, Soule EH, Taylor WF. Synovial sarcoma. J Bone Joint Surg (Am) 1982;64:112–22.

243. Yokoyama K, Shinohara N, Kondo M, Mashima T. Prognostic factors in synovial sarcoma: a clinicopathologic study of 18 cases. Jpn J Clin Oncol 1995;25:131–4.

244. Zeren H, Moran CA, Suster S, Fishback NF, Koss MN. Primary pulmonary sarcomas with features of monophasic synovial sarcoma. A clinicopathological, immunohistochemical and ultrastructural study of 25 cases. Hum Pathol 1995;26:474–80.

245. Zito RA. Synovial sarcoma: an Australian series of 48 cases. Pathology 1984;16:45–52.

Epithelioid Sarcoma

246. Arber DA, Kandalaft PL, Mehta P, Battifora H. Vimentin-negative epithelioid sarcoma. The value of an immunohistochemical panel that includes CD34. Am J Surg Pathol 1993;17:302–7.

247. Bliss BO, Reed RJ. Large cell sarcomas of tendon sheath. Malignant giant cell tumors of tendon sheath. Am J Clin Pathol 1968;49:776–81.

248. Bos GD, Pritchard DJ, Reiman HM, Dobyns JH, Ilstrup DM, Landon GC. Epithelioid sarcoma. An analysis of fifty-one cases. J Bone Joint Surg [Am] 1988;70:862–70.

249. Chase DR, Enzinger FM. Epithelioid sarcoma. Diagnosis, prognostic indicators, and treatment. Am J Surg Pathol 1985;9:241–63.

250. Daimaru Y, Hashimoto H, Tsuneyoshi M, Enjoji M. Epithelial profile of epithelioid sarcoma. An immunohistochemical analysis of eight cases. Cancer 1987;59:134–41.

251. el-Naggar AK, Garcia GM. Epithelioid sarcoma. Flow cytometric study of DNA content and regional DNA heterogeneity. Cancer 1992;69:1721–8.

252. Enzinger FM. Epithelioid sarcoma. A sarcoma simulating a granuloma or a carcinoma. Cancer 1970;26:1029–41.

253. Evans HL, Baer SC. Epithelioid sarcoma: a clinicopathologic and prognostic study of 26 cases. Semin Diagn Pathol 1993;10:286–91.

254. Fisher C. Epithelioid sarcoma: the spectrum of ultrastructural differentiation in seven immunohistochemically defined cases. Hum Pathol 1988;19:265–75.

255. Guillou L, Wadden C, Coindre JM, Krausz T, Fletcher CD. "Proximal-type" epithelioid sarcoma, a distinctive aggressive neoplasm showing rhabdoid features. Clinicopathologic, immunohistochemical, and ultrastructural study of a series. Am J Surg Pathol 1997;21:130–46.

256. Halling AC, Wollan PC, Pritchard DJ, Vlasak R, Nascimento AG. Epithelioid sarcoma: a clinicopathologic review of 55 cases. Mayo Clin Proc. 1996;71:636–42.

257. Huang DJ, Stanisic TH, Hansen KK. Epithelioid sarcoma of the penis. J Urol 1992;147:1370–2.

258. Ishida T, Oka T, Matsushita H, Machinami R. Epithelioid sarcoma: an electron-microscopic, immunohistochemical and DNA flow cytometric analysis. Virchows Arch [A] 1992;421:401–8.

259. Manivel JC, Wick MR, Dehner LP, Sibley RK. Epithelioid sarcoma. An immunohistochemical study. Am J Clin Pathol 1987;87:319–26.

260. Mills SE, Fechner RE, Bruns DE, Bruns ME, O'Hara MF. Intermediate filaments in eosinophilic cells of epithelioid sarcoma: a light-microscopic, ultrastructural, and electrophoretic study. Am J Surg Pathol 1981;5:195–202.

261. Mirra JM, Kessler S, Bhuta S, Eckardt J. The fibroma-like variant of epithelioid sarcoma. A fibrohistiocytic/myoid cell lesion often confused with benign and malignant spindle cell tumors. Cancer 1992;69:1382–95.

262. Pastel-Levy C, Bell DA, Rosenberg AE, Preffer F, Colvin RB, Flotte TJ. DNA flow cytometry of epithelioid sarcoma. Cancer 1992;70:2823–6.

263. Prat J, Woodruff JM, Marcove RC. Epithelioid sarcoma: an analysis of 22 cases indicating the prognostic significance of vascular invasion and regional lymph node metastasis. Cancer 1978;41:1472–87.

264. Quezado MM, Middleton LP, Bryant B, Lane K, Weiss SW, Merina MJ. Allelic loss on chromosome 22q in epithelioid sarcomas. Hum Pathol 1998;29:604–8.

265. Schmidt D, Harms D. Epithelioid sarcoma in children and adolescents. An immunohistochemical study. Virchows Arch [A] 1987;410:423–31.

266. Smith ME, Brown JI, Fisher C. Epithelioid sarcoma: presence of vascular-endothelial cadherin and lack of epithelial cadherin. Histopathology 1998;33:425–31.

267. Steinberg BD, Gelberman RH, Mankin HJ, Rosenberg AE. Epithelioid sarcoma in the upper extremity. J Bone Joint Surg [Am] 1992;74:28–35.

268. Ulbright TM, Brokaw SA, Stehman FB, Roth LM. Epithelioid sarcoma of the vulva. Evidence suggesting a more aggressive behavior than extra-genital epithelioid sarcoma. Cancer 1983;52:1462–9.

269. van de Rijn M. CD34: a review. Appl Immunohistochem 1994;2:71–80.

270. Weissmann D, Amenta PS, Kantor GR. Vulvar epithelioid sarcoma metastatic to the scalp. A case report and review of the literature. Am J Dermatopathol 1990;12:462–8.

271. Whitworth PW, Pollock RE, Mansfield PF, Couture J, Romsdahl MM. Extremity epithelioid sarcoma. Amputation vs local resection. Arch Surg 1991;126:1485–9.

272. Wick MR, Manivel JC. Epithelioid sarcoma and isolated necrobiotic granuloma: a comparative immunocytochemical study. J Cutan Pathol 1986;13:253–60.

✧✧✧

Index*

*Numbers in boldface indicate table and figure pages.

✧✧✧